T0325411

Common Contact Allergens

Common Contact Allergens

A Practical Guide to Detecting Contact Dermatitis

Edited by

John McFadden
Consultant Dermatologist
Department of Cutaneous Allergy
St John's Institute of Dermatology
King's College, Guy's Hospital
London, UK

Pailin Puangpet
Consultant Dermatologist
Occupational and Contact Dermatitis Clinic, Institute of Dermatology
Bangkok, Thailand

Korbkarn Pongpairoj
Consultant Dermatologist
Division of Dermatology, Department of Medicine, Faculty of Medicine
Chulalongkorn University and King Chulalongkorn Memorial Hospital
Thai Red Cross Society
Bangkok, Thailand

Supitchaya Thaiwat
Consultant Dermatologist
Contact Dermatitis clinic, Division of Dermatology, Department of Internal Medicine
Phramongkutklao Hospital
Bangkok, Thailand

Lee Shan Xian
Consultant Dermatologist
Department of Dermatology
Changi General Hospital
Singapore

WILEY Blackwell

This edition first published 2020 © 2020 by John Wiley & Sons Ltd

All rights reserved. No part of this publication may be reproduced, stored in a retrieval system, or transmitted, in any form or by any means, electronic, mechanical, photocopying, recording or otherwise, except as permitted by law. Advice on how to obtain permission to reuse material from this title is available at http://www.wiley.com/go/permissions.

The rights of John McFadden, Pailin Puangpet, Korbkarn Pongpairoj, Supitchaya Thaiwat, and Lee Shan Xian to be identified as the authors of editorial in this work has been asserted in accordance with law.

Registered Office(s)
John Wiley & Sons, Inc., 111 River Street, Hoboken, NJ 07030, USA
John Wiley & Sons Ltd, The Atrium, Southern Gate, Chichester, West Sussex, PO19 8SQ, UK

Editorial Office
9600 Garsington Road, Oxford, OX4 2DQ, UK

For details of our global editorial offices, customer services, and more information about Wiley products visit us at www.wiley.com.

Wiley also publishes its books in a variety of electronic formats and by print-on-demand. Some content that appears in standard print versions of this book may not be available in other formats.

Limit of Liability/Disclaimer of Warranty
The contents of this work are intended to further general scientific research, understanding, and discussion only and are not intended and should not be relied upon as recommending or promoting scientific method, diagnosis, or treatment by physicians for any particular patient. In view of ongoing research, equipment modifications, changes in governmental regulations, and the constant flow of information relating to the use of medicines, equipment, and devices, the reader is urged to review and evaluate the information provided in the package insert or instructions for each medicine, equipment, or device for, among other things, any changes in the instructions or indication of usage and for added warnings and precautions. While the publisher and authors have used their best efforts in preparing this work, they make no representations or warranties with respect to the accuracy or completeness of the contents of this work and specifically disclaim all warranties, including without limitation any implied warranties of merchantability or fitness for a particular purpose. No warranty may be created or extended by sales representatives, written sales materials or promotional statements for this work. The fact that an organization, website, or product is referred to in this work as a citation and/or potential source of further information does not mean that the publisher and authors endorse the information or services the organization, website, or product may provide or recommendations it may make. This work is sold with the understanding that the publisher is not engaged in rendering professional services. The advice and strategies contained herein may not be suitable for your situation. You should consult with a specialist where appropriate. Further, readers should be aware that websites listed in this work may have changed or disappeared between when this work was written and when it is read. Neither the publisher nor authors shall be liable for any loss of profit or any other commercial damages, including but not limited to special, incidental, consequential, or other damages.

Library of Congress Cataloging-in-Publication Data

Names: McFadden, John (Dermatologist), editor. | Puangpet, Pailin, editor. | Pongpairoj, Korbkarn, editor. | Thaiwat, Supitchaya, editor. | Lee, Shan Xian, editor.
Title: Common contact allergens : a practical guide to detecting contact dermatitis / edited by John McFadden, Pailin Puangpet, Korbkarn Pongpairoj, Supitchaya Thaiwat, Lee Shan Xian.
Description: Hoboken, NJ : Wiley-Blackwell, 2020. | Includes bibliographical references and index. |
Identifiers: LCCN 2019011947 (print) | LCCN 2019014062 (ebook) | ISBN 9781119405719 (Adobe PDF) | ISBN 9781119452812 (ePub) | ISBN 9781119405665 (hardback)
Subjects: | MESH: Dermatitis, Contact–diagnosis | Allergens–adverse effects | Patch Tests–methods
Classification: LCC RL244 (ebook) | LCC RL244 (print) | NLM WR 175 | DDC 616.97/3–dc23
LC record available at https://lccn.loc.gov/2019011947

Cover Design: Wiley
Cover Images: © AFPics/Shutterstock, © sdecoret/Shutterstock

Set in 9.5/12pt Minion by SPi Global, Pondicherry, India
Printed and bound in Singapore by Markono Print Media Pte Ltd

10 9 8 7 6 5 4 3 2 1

Dedications

John McFadden: To all my family, friends and colleagues. An especial dedication to Dr. Ian White who has been a teacher, mentor, colleague and friend at St John's for over 25 years.
Pailin Puangpet: For my family, teachers, friends and colleagues.
Korbkarn Pongpairoj: For all my beloved family, teachers, colleagues, and patients.
Supitchaya Thaiwat: I dedicate this book to my father, my other family members, my teachers, and my colleagues.
Lee Shan Xian: I would like to thank my family (especially my husband and son) for their unwavering support, my mentors, my friends/colleagues, and our patients for teaching me so much.

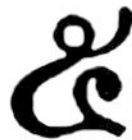

Contents

Others, 311

E-Supplements

List of Contributors

Dr. Mahbub M.U. Chowdhury
Consultant Dermatologist
The Welsh Institute of Dermatology
University Hospital Wales
Cardiff, Wales, UK
Setting up a Patch Test Practice

Dr. Elin Dafydd Owen
Cutaneous Allergy Fellow
The Welsh Institute of Dermatology
University Hospital Wales
Cardiff, Wales, UK
Setting up a Patch Test Practice

Bo Niklasson
CEO, President
Chemotechnique Diagnostics
Vellinge, Sweden
The Role of Providers of Patch Test Products

Associate Chapter Editors

Professor Klaus Ejner Andersen
Institute of Clinical Research
University of Southern Denmark
and
Department of Dermatology and Allergy Centre
Odense University Hospital
Odense, Denmark
Nickel

Dr. David Basketter
Toxicologist
DABMEB Consultancy Ltd.
Bedford, UK
Preservatives
para-Phenylenediamine
Immunology of Allergic Contact Dermatitis

Dr. Mike Beck
Emeritus Consultant Dermatologist
Contact Dermatitis Investigation Unit
Salford Royal NHS Foundation Trust
Manchester, UK
Patch Test Technique
History, Microhistory and Allergen Exposure

Dr. Johnny Bourke
Consultant Dermatologist
Department of Dermatology
South Infirmary Victoria University Hospital
Cork City, Ireland
Clioquinol
Neomycin

Professor Magnus Bruze
Professor of Occupational Dermatology
Department of Occupational and Environmental Dermatology
Lund University
Skåne University Hospital
Malmö, Sweden
Gold

Dr. Deirdre Buckley
Consultant Dermatologist
Department of Dermatology
Royal United Hospital
Bath, UK
Fragrances

Dr. John English
Consultant Dermatologist
Nottingham University Hospitals NHS Trust
Nottingham, UK
Colophonium
Epoxy Resin
PTBP Resin
Lanolin
Corticosteroids

Professor Chee Leok Goh
Clinical Professor
National Skin Centre
Singapore
Potassium Dichromate

Dr. Graham Johnston
Honorary Associate Professor
Department of Dermatology
University Hospitals of Leicester NHS Trust
Infirmary Square
Leicester, UK
Cobalt

Dr. Christopher Lovell
Consultant Dermatologist
Royal United Hospital
Combe Park
Bath, UK
Sesquiterpene Lactone and Compositae
Primin

Professor Howard Maibach
Department of Dermatology
University of California
San Francisco, CA, USA
Disperse Blue 106

Associate Professor Rosemary Nixon
Director, Occupational Dermatology Research and Education Centre
Skin and Cancer Foundation Inc.
Melbourne, VIC, Australia
Tosylamide Formaldehyde Resin

Dr. David Orton
Consultant Dermatologist
152 Harley Street Ltd
London, UK
Rubber Chemicals
Cetearyl Alcohol

Dr. Jason Williams
Consultant Dermatologist
Contact Dermatitis Investigation Unit
Salford Royal NHS Foundation Trust
Manchester, UK
Benzocaine

Preface

In many ways practising contact dermatitis resembles the work of a detective. They both require searching for clues in a systematic, detailed manner. They also both require a thorough grasp of relevant subject information and skills learnt from previous purposeful experience. This book aims to assist the physician in acquiring the skills necessary for optimal clinical practice in contact dermatitis.

The first section addresses methodology. Concepts such as microhistory and microexamination are introduced. We illustrate a detailed, systematic approach to contact dermatitis.

The second section gives a grounding in common non-allergic dermatitis/dermatoses. Approximately half of the patients seen in patch test clinics do not have allergic contact dermatitis, so recognising these other dermatitis/dermatoses is essential.

The third section involves common contact allergens that physicians are likely to encounter. Allergens are reported within their individual chapters. Key points followed by a synopsis of clinical disease are presented in a coherent, systematic way. Where appropriate, allergen profiling (potential sources of allergen exposure, routes of allergen exposure and clinical manifestations of contact allergy) is demonstrated. Bullet points have been color coded according to exposure sources. Throughout this section the emphasis is on helping the physician decide on the clinical relevance of the contact allergy identified by patch testing.

Electronic supplements for the allergen chapters give extra clinical, epidemiological, immunological and chemical material for an inquiring mind.

All but two of the chapters have been drafted by the five co-editors. This was a deliberate decision to keep the style and presentation consistent throughout the book. We have been fortunate to have, as associate chapter editors, some of the leading international experts in the chapters they have 'refereed', invariably improving the content.

We hope this book provides the methodology and background knowledge to assist the reader to practise contact dermatitis purposefully. Practising contact dermatitis can be fully rewarding and of great benefit to the physician's patient. We wish you every success.

John McFadden
Pailin Puangpet
Korbkarn Pongpairoj
Supitchaya Thaiwat
and
Lee Shan Xian

About the Companion Website

This book is accompanied by a companion website:

www.wiley.com/go/mcfadden/common_contact_allergens

Scan this QR code to visit the companion website:

The website includes E-Supplements

SECTION 1

Methodology

CHAPTER 1

Immunology of Allergic Contact Dermatitis

Allergic contact dermatitis is a T cell immune mediated inflammatory skin condition. It is characterized by the following immunological properties:

- *Immunological memory*: induction of sensitization. When a contact allergen penetrates and reacts covalently with protein in the skin, it is transported to the local lymph node by antigen presenting cells. There, it is presented to naive T cells through interactions between the haptenized antigen-peptide complex, Major Histocompatibility Complex (MHC) groove, and T cell receptor. On recognition of the antigen and in the presence of danger signals, a naive T cell will undergo clonal proliferation to produce memory and effector T cells.
- *Elicitation*: repeated exposure to the antigen will cause further clonal proliferation until a threshold is surpassed when the pool of cloned T cells recognizing the antigen is sufficiently large that when the antigen is encountered within the skin, the T cells will activate and initiate local dermal inflammation.
- The *Th1* and *Th17* immune pathways are predominantly involved with the production of pro-inflammatory cytokines such as IL-1, IL-2, tumor necrosis factor-α (TNF-α), α-interferon, IL-6, IL-8, IL-12, IL-17, and IL-23 [1].
- *Friedmann's principle*: the single most important factor in sensitization is allergen dose per unit area of skin (except for areas of skin less than 1 cm^2 when the aggregate dose is paramount). Therefore, someone who sprays perfume for 2 seconds on just a small area of the neck is more likely to become sensitized to the fragrance allergen(s) than someone who sprays the perfume for 2 seconds all over the torso [2].
- Contact allergens are *haptens*, which are protein reactive and bind chemically to proteins/peptides within the skin. Contact allergens/haptens are usually electrophilic and form covalent bonds with nucleophilic amino acids such as lysine, cysteine, and/or histidine [3]. Sometimes the contact allergen needs to be first oxidized (pre-hapten) or metabolized (pro-hapten) before becoming sufficiently electrophilic. The altered peptide/protein is then recognized by the immune system.
- *Danger signals* (Figure 1.1). Contact allergens/haptens also stimulate the innate immune system, which then alerts the adaptive immune system. It usually achieves innate immune activation through the generation of reactive oxygen species (ROS)/oxidative stress which then generates danger-associated molecular pattern (DAMP) molecules such as fibronectin and hyaluronan [4]. These DAMP molecules then activate pattern recognition receptors (PRRs) such as toll-like receptors (TLRs) 2 and 4, which leads to the stimulation of pro-inflammatory cytokines, the secretion of chemokines and recruitment of T cells to the skin, and an amplification of the immune response [1].
- Metal contact allergens appear to be unique in having the ability to directly stimulate TLRs, and hence the innate immune system, without generating DAMP molecules [5].
- *Immunological mechanisms* underpinning allergic contact dermatitis have similarities to the immune response to pathogenic bacteria and this explains why apparently evolutionarily wasteful responses (allergic contact dermatitis) have been preserved [1, 6].
- There is strong clinical evidence that the immune response to contact allergy consists of both a tolerizing and a sensitizing response, and that the tolerizing response decays with age at a faster rate than the sensitizing response. This explains why allergic contact dermatitis is more common in the elderly, when the T cell sensitizing response to experimental strong contact allergens such as dinitrochlorbenzene (DNCB) appears to decline [7].
- Exposure to contact allergens in the absence of danger signals should theoretically lead to tolerance. However, once clinical sensitization has occurred it has not so far been possible to reverse it [8].
- *Oral tolerance* to nickel through dental braces has probably occurred in many individuals; however, this effect will usually only happen if the individual has not had their ears pierced prior to dental braces being inserted such that they have significant prior skin exposure [9].
- In everyday life, most allergic contact dermatitis reactions are elicitation reactions and occur within 48 hours of exposure. A main exception to this is reaction to *p*-phenylenediamine in "henna beach tattoos", which is usually a primary sensitizing reaction occurring after 10–21 days, similar to an experimental DNCB sensitizing reaction.

Common Contact Allergens: A Practical Guide to Detecting Contact Dermatitis, First Edition. Edited by John McFadden, Pailin Puangpet, Korbkarn Pongpairoj, Supitchaya Thaiwat, and Lee Shan Xian.
© 2020 John Wiley & Sons Ltd. Published 2020 by John Wiley & Sons Ltd.
Companion website: www.wiley.com/go/mcfadden/common_contact_allergens

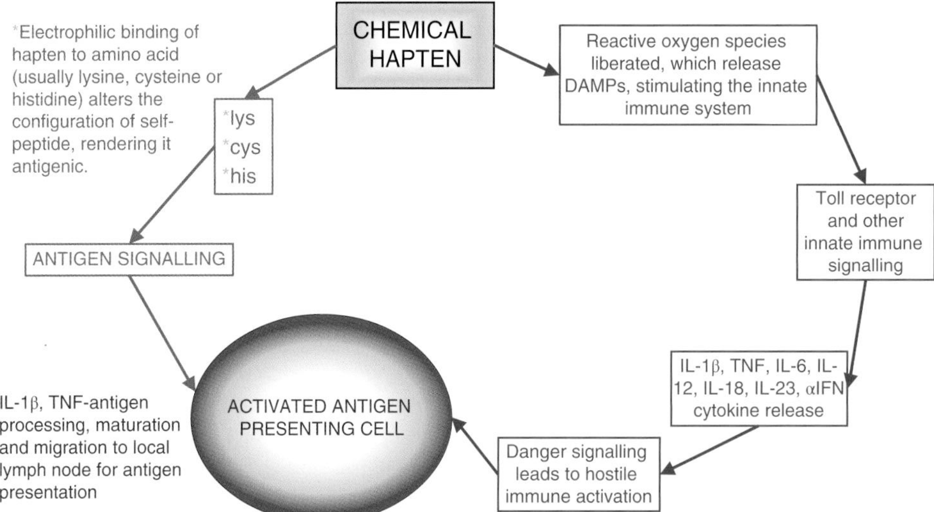

Figure 1.1 Dual signaling by haptens leading to contact sensitization. ⟶, antigen pathway; ⟶, danger pathway.

- By inference, sensitization to everyday agents such as cosmetic allergens are "quiet" events. Elicitation allergic contact dermatitis reactions occur when the threshold for response is surpassed, recognizing that the threshold will depend on the dose/concentration of the allergen factored with the extent/level of sensitization.
- The *level of sensitization* can increase through either repeated exposure to an allergen from a single source (e.g. *p*-phenylenediamine exposure from hair dye repeatedly applied every 1–2 months) or from exposure to an agent from multiple sources (e.g. methylisothiazolinone exposure from cosmetic creams, shampoos, and washing-up liquid).
- The immunological dose can increase through exposure to increased concentrations of an allergen (e.g. changing from blonde to black hair dye can increase the allergen exposure by a factor of 10 [10]), exposure to an allergen in the presence of an adjuvant (e.g. fragrance exposure in the presence of an aluminum salt in a deodorant, the aluminum salt acting as an adjuvant and increasing the danger signals generated), exposure to an allergen on skin which is already inflamed and where danger signals have already been generated (e.g. application of fragrance in an aftershave onto facial skin with seborrheic eczema), or increased time of exposure to an allergen (e.g. increased work hours in a construction unit leading to increased time of exposure to epoxy resin).
- Some contact allergens co-react from immunological cross-reaction due to chemical similarity, e.g. nickel and palladium, *p*-phenylenediamine and benzocaine. Some contact allergens co-react due to sensitization from same-source exposure, e.g. nickel and cobalt from exposure to low-carat gold jewelry.
- In patients with atopic dermatitis, contact sensitization occurs through the Th2 immune system and is therefore less efficient [11]. This may also explain how contact allergens and exposure to irritants can exacerbate atopic dermatitis (i.e. through Th2 stimulation) even without sensitization occurring (chemical atopy) [12].

References

1. McFadden, J.P., Puangpet, P., Basketter, D.A. et al. (2013). Why does allergic contact dermatitis exist? *British Journal of Dermatology* 168 (4): 692–699.
2. Rees, J.L., Friedmann, P.S., and Matthews, J.N. (1990). The influence of area of application on sensitization by dinitrochlorobenzene. *British Journal of Dermatology* 122 (1): 29–31.
3. Divkovic, M., Pease, C.K., Gerberick, G.F., and Basketter, D.A. (2005). Hapten-protein binding: from theory to practical application in the in vitro prediction of skin sensitization. *Contact Dermatitis* 53 (4): 189–200.
4. Galbiati, V., Papale, A., Galli, C.L. et al. (2014). Role of ROS and HMGB1 in contact allergen-induced IL-18 production in human keratinocytes. *Journal of Investigative Dermatology* 134 (11): 2719–2727.
5. Rachmawati, D., Bontkes, H.J., Verstege, M.I. et al. (2013). Transition metal sensing by Toll-like receptor-4: next to nickel, cobalt and palladium are potent human dendritic cell stimulators. *Contact Dermatitis* 68 (6): 331–338.
6. Martin, S.F. (2012). Allergic contact dermatitis: xenoinflammation of the skin. *Current Opinion in Immunology* 24 (6): 720–729.
7. McFadden, J.P., White, I.R., Basketter, D. et al. (2013). The cosmetic allergy conundrum: inference of an immunoregulatory response to cosmetic allergens. *Contact Dermatitis* 69 (3): 129–137.
8. van Hoogstraten, I.M., von Blomberg, B.M., Boden, D. et al. (1994). Non-sensitizing epicutaneous skin tests prevent subsequent induction of immune tolerance. *Journal of Investigative Dermatology* 102 (1): 80–83.
9. Van Hoogstraten, I.M., Andersen, K.E., Von Blomberg, B.M. et al. (1991). Reduced frequency of nickel allergy upon oral nickel contact at an early age. *Clinical and Experimental Immunology* 85 (3): 441–445.
10. Coenraads, P.J., Blomeke, B., Goebel, C., et al. (2016). Continuous usage of a hair dye product containing 2-methoxymethyl-para-phenylenediamine by hair-dye-allergic individual. *British Journal of Dermatology* 174(5): 1042–50.
11. Newell, L., Polak, M.E., Perera, J. et al. (2013). Sensitization via healthy skin programs Th2 responses in individuals with atopic dermatitis. *Journal of Investigative Dermatology* 133 (10): 2372–2380.
12. Puangpet, P., Lai-Cheong, J., and McFadden, J.P. (2013). Chemical atopy. *Contact Dermatitis* 68 (4): 208–213.

CHAPTER 2

Patch Test Technique

CHAPTER CONTENTS

Patch testing is an *in vivo* standard procedure to detect type IV hypersensitivity reactions to contact allergen(s) and determine the clinical relevance. The results from correct patch test techniques help in identifying and avoiding the true causative allergen(s). A positive patch test detects the immunological state of contact allergy. The diagnosis of allergic contact dermatitis depends on deducing clinical relevance. Patch testing within the context of the process of diagnosing allergic contact dermatitis is discussed in Chapter 3.

Patient expectations should be managed at the pre-patch test stage. In particular, a negative patch test and/or an inconclusive diagnosis at the post-patch test stage should be highlighted as possible outcomes.

Indications

- Where direct exposure allergic contact dermatitis (ACD) is suspected, e.g. to hair dye, perfume, gloves, jewelry.
- Acute or chronic dermatitis which is possibly related to occupational exposure.
- Recalcitrant chronic eczema.
- Hand eczema.
- Worsening of pre-existing eczema or exacerbation of endogenous eczema, such as atopic, seborrheic, or nummular eczema.
- When airborne ACD is suspected, e.g. perfumes, resins, preservatives and plants.
- Atypical, asymmetrical, or unpredictable flares of dermatitis to exclude by proxy ACD.
- Some delayed-type drug eruptions.
- Non-eczematous cutaneous reactions that may be manifestations of contact sensitization, such as lichenoid dermatitis and pseudolymphomatous reactions.
- To differentiate between angioedema and ACD mimicking angioedema.
- Discoid eczema.
- To exclude medicament allergy.
- Mucositis – conjunctivitis, stomatitis, vulvitis where ACD is suspected.
- Implants – loosening, rejection, association with localized or extensive rash [1, 2].

Cronin states "Ideally every patient with eczema should be patch tested and the importance of this investigation is now universally accepted"[3]. However, this statement should be seen as an ideal subject to practical constraint.

Patch test techniques

Patient information

- All patients should be informed about the purpose, procedure, benefits and potential side-effects of patch testing.
- The need to keep the back dry should be emphasized.
- Excessive exercise, wetting the testing areas, and sunlight should be avoided during the procedure. Excessive sunlight exposure in the 4 weeks prior to testing should also be avoided.

Common Contact Allergens: A Practical Guide to Detecting Contact Dermatitis, First Edition. Edited by John McFadden, Pailin Puangpet, Korbkarn Pongpairoj, Supitchaya Thaiwat, and Lee Shan Xian.
© 2020 John Wiley & Sons Ltd. Published 2020 by John Wiley & Sons Ltd.
Companion website: www.wiley.com/go/mcfadden/common_contact_allergens

Preparation of patch testing

1. Patch testing systems
   Patch testing is performed by applying chemical substances under occlusion on the patient's skin under standardized conditions. There is still no definite evidence to show which testing system is superior. Nowadays, there are many different systems available, including:
   - aluminum disks mounted on a non-occlusive hypoallergenic acrylic-based adhesive tape [4]
   - plastic chambers on hypoallergenic tape (Figure 2.1)
   - pre-packaged tests mounted on an acrylic-based adhesive tape.
2. Allergen selection
   - Standard/baseline series should be applied to all patients [5, 6].
   - The addition of a specific allergen, based on the history and clinical presentation of the dermatitis, may be needed [7, 8].
   - Extra series, when available, can be added to increase the sensitivity of the test if deemed clinically appropriate (e.g. hairstyling series in a beautician).
3. Vehicles
   The properties, solubility, and pH of an allergen determine the most suitable vehicle for use.
   - Petrolatum (pet.) can be mixed with most chemicals. First, petrolatum is stable. Second, it can prevent or decrease degradation, oxidization, and polymerization of the combined allergen [9, 10]. Third, it is inexpensive. Finally, it provides good occlusion. In general, water-insoluble agents are diluted in petrolatum. Acetone, methyl ethyl ketone, ethanol, and olive oil can be used as alternatives. Petroleum samples can be applied from a syringe to form a "snake" covering the maximum diameter of the chamber.
   - Aqueous solutions are more suitable vehicles for some substances, such as water for formaldehyde, methylchloroisothiazolinone, and methylisothiazolinone (MI). These are usually applied using a paper disc fixed onto the chamber with a small amount of pet. The application of too much petroleum may smother the upper layer of the disc on application of the patch to the back, thereby leading to a false-negative result.

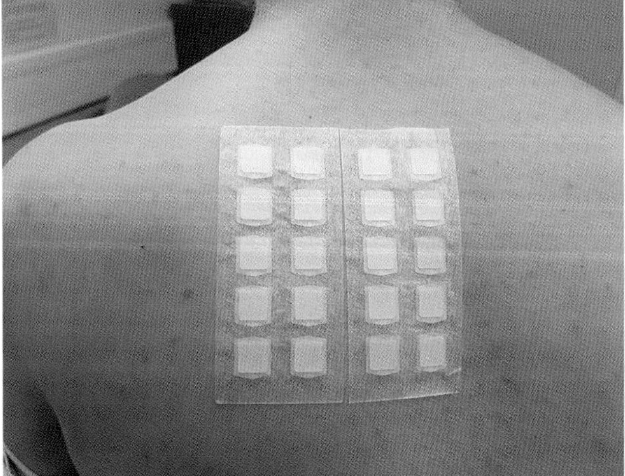

Figure 2.1 Patch test application using IQ® chamber system.

4. Concentrations
   - Commercial test substances are preferred.
   - A dilution series of allergens could be tested when investigating
     - a low number of highly suspected agents
     - new allergens.
   - Appropriate concentrations for patch testing of allergens in various preparations are shown in Table 2.1.

     Note: Testing patients' own products is only helpful when positive as there may be low sensitivity, e.g. a moisturizer may have MI at a concentration of 100 ppm, whereas the ideal concentration for MI for patch testing is 2000 ppm in aqueous solution.
   - Mixes of allergens
     Some allergens in the standard series, such as fragrances and rubber compounds are tested as mixtures. If practicable, subsequent additional testing to individual agents on the first reading should be performed if the patch test to the mix is positive.
   - Patch testing of a patient's own substance(s)
     - The important necessary information includes the patient's own sample(s), information leaflets, safety data sheets, and/or lists of ingredients, e.g. International Nomenclature of Cosmetic Ingredients (INCI) lists. This information may be found on the Internet or requested from the manufacturers.
     - Patch testing must not be done with unknown chemicals or extremely hazardous substances such as poisonous agents.
     - Strong acids or alkaline chemicals should be buffered in order to decrease the risk of cutaneous irritation and to allow allergen preparation in higher concentrations – in practice this will be outside the expertise of most centers.
     - Negative results may occur due to too low concentrations, whereas too high concentrations may lead to cutaneous irritation and active sensitization.
5. Storage
   In general, substances for patch testing should be kept at 2–8 °C and protected from light. A contact allergen with a particular property may need special storage conditions. For example, some diisothiocyanates should be stored at −18 °C. The expiry dates must be checked regularly [11, 12].

   Fragrances and acrylates are particularly volatile substances and should be stored in refrigerators in closed syringes. Preparation of these for patch testing should be performed immediately before application as prolonged exposure to air will lead to a theoretical lowering of allergen concentration.

Patch test application

1. Anatomical site
   - The upper back is the preferred site. Its flat surface is suitable for occlusion and a number of allergens can be tested due to an available large area.

Table 2.1 Different preparations of commonly used products and suitable concentrations for patch testing [20].

Preparation	Examples	Tested concentration	Notes
Leave-on products	Cosmetic preparations, protective creams, topical medicaments	"as is", i.e. undiluted	—
Rinse-off products	Liquid soap, shampoos, shower gels	1–10% in aq., depending on the formulation	—
Metal-working fluids	The most important allergens are biocides, rust preventives, emulsifiers, and tall oil derivatives	Test the metal-working fluid "as is" taken from the machine or a fresh dilution prepared from the concentrate	Testing only fluids may miss preservative and fragrance allergies
Water-based fresh metal-working fluids	The workplace concentration of water-based metal-working fluids is usually 4–8% in the circulatory system	5% concentration in aq. Adjusting the pH, the used water-based 4–8% metal-working fluids taken from the circulatory system can be tested if necessary	Other possible sources of impurities (e.g. oil) can be evaluated separately
Oil-based metal-working fluids		50% in olive oil (fresh and used)	—
Solid materials	Paper, textile, plastic, rubber, metal specimens of suitable shape, wood dust	"as is" Note: Samples can be fixed to the chambers with small amounts of pet.	Consider the use of large 12 mm diameter chambers —
Powdery materials, ground dust, scrapings or small cut pieces			Tested in chambers (first moistened with water or organic solvents)
Larger pieces	Glove material, textiles	"as is" Consider larger chambers	Test semi-open, cover with surgical test tape without a chamber
Plants		Concentrations of commercially available plant materials include sesquiterpene lactone mix 0.1% pet., primin 0.01% pet., tulipaline A 0.01% pet., and diallyl disulfide 1.0% pet. Fresh or dried plant material: use "as is" Plant materials (flower, leaf, or stem): patch test plant material "as is" with a drop of saline water or ethanol for each part of the plant because either water-soluble or alcohol-soluble allergens, or both, may be present	Consider the use of larger 12 mm chambers Some plants cause irritant reactions Active sensitization is a possible theoretical risk Plant material generally has more allergens during the summer compared to winter
Miscellaneous	Textiles, plastics, food, plants, perfumes, drugs, and grease	Thin-layer chromatograms, paper, "as is" [27]	Available only in a few centers in Europe
Unidentified material brought by patient			Do not test as may be caustic, noxious, or poisonous

- The outer surfaces of the upper arms or thighs can be used as alternatives.

2. Occlusion time

The latest International Contact Dermatitis Research Group (ICDRG) recommendation recommends an occlusion time of 2 days.

Patch test reading

1. Reading times

   Patch test reactions must be evaluated over at least two readings. Many options of reading times can be arranged with different levels of recommendation, as shown in Table 2.2.

2. Patch test reading

   The ICDRG reading criteria, which scores according to the morphology of patch test reactions, is used as a standard (Table 2.3 and Figure 2.2).

- Contact allergy is demonstrated with positive patch test reactions (reactions of at least 1+) at day 3 and/or later.
- Where necessary, a dose-response relationship between the strength of allergic reactions and a variety of concentrations differentiates a true positive result from an irritant reaction.
- Questionable reactions (?+) can sometimes be clinically relevant in an individual patient [6, 13] and may need further investigations such as repeated patch testing with different concentrations or a repeat open application test.
- False-positive reactions can give an appearance of skin which has been rubbed with "soap" (Figure 2.3). Pustular and follicular reactions may be either false or true positive reactions (Figures 2.4 and 2.5).

Table 2.2 Schedules of patch test reading and levels of recommendation [20].

Levels of recommendation	Days of patch test reading Day 2	Day 3	Day 4	Day 7	Notes
Optimum (ideal), but may be least practicable	✓	✓ (day 3 or day 4)		✓	A reading between day 5 and day 10 is necessary for some allergens, such as corticosteroids and aminoglycosides A reading around day 7 will pick up additionally 7–30% of contact allergies [28–30]
Fair alternative	X	✓ (day 3 or day 4)		✓	
Acceptable	✓	✓ (day 3 or day 4, prefer day 4)		X	False-negative results may occur
Possible but not generally recommended	X	X	✓	X	In order to increase detection of contact allergies, two readings on days 4 and 7 were required [28] A day 2 reading as the only single reading is not appropriate [31]

Table 2.3 The ICDRG patch test reading criteria [32].

Symbol	Morphology	Assessment
–	No reaction	Negative reaction
?+	Faint erythema only	Doubtful reaction
+	Erythema, infiltration, possibly papules	Weak positive reaction
++	Erythema, infiltration, papules, vesicles	Strong positive reaction
+++	Intense erythema, infiltrate, coalescing vesicles	Extreme positive reaction
IR	Various morphologies, e.g. soap effect, bulla, necrosis	Irritant reaction

- Positive reactions to corticosteroids can sometimes give an "edge" effect, with the periphery more raised and palpable than the center of the positive patch test reaction (Figure 2.6).
- A large blister reaction may indicate either a strong true "positive" reaction or a strong irritant "false" reaction to an inappropriately diluted agent.
- Rarely a non-eczematous true reaction may occur (e.g. an erythema multiforme-like reaction to *p*-phenylenediamine) which may be relevant to the morphology of the presenting dermatitis. At the first reading appointment equivocal patch test reactions, and surprisingly positive or surprisingly negative patch test reactions should be repeated.

Special considerations

False-negative and false-positive reactions

Although there is no definite contraindication for patch testing, physicians must be aware of the possibility of false-negative and/or false-positive reactions in some special situations. Patch testing, if necessary, could still be performed in these patients. Repeat patch testing may, however, give more information. The following may promote false-negative reactions:

- *Individual factors.* Immunosuppression [14–16], tanning, very active atopic dermatitis [17], active dermatitis
- *Environmental factors.* Ultraviolet (UV) light/sun exposure [18] – significant natural ultraviolet B (UVB) or therapeutic UV exposure to the back within the past 4 weeks or between the first and second readings.
- Medications:
  - systemic immunosuppressive drugs, e.g. corticosteroids more than 15 mg per day; azathioprine and cyclosporine – proceed with caution but if unsuspected negative test, consider re-testing when off immunosuppression [19].
  - Topical corticosteroids influence patch testing results only when they are applied to the patch test sites.
  - Antihistamines, disodium cromoglycate [19], and non-steroidal anti-inflammatory drugs (NSAIDs) usually have no effects on allergic patch test reactions [20].

Special groups

- Atopic dermatitis
  - Indications for patch testing are the same as for other patients.
  - Beware of false-positive/irritant reactions, especially to metals.
- Children
  - Indications for patch testing are the same as in adults [21].
  - A smaller selection of some contact allergens may be needed because of a smaller back.
  - Unless there is a history of exposure, exclude *p*-phenylenediamine and epoxy resin to reduce the possibility of active sensitization.
- Drug eruptions

  According to some types of drug eruptions, positive patch test results can confirm the culprit drug(s), whereas negative reactions cannot exclude the responsible medication. These include:

  1. delayed cutaneous adverse drug reactions (CADRs), including maculopapular exanthema, drug reaction with eosinophilia and systemic symptoms (DRESS),

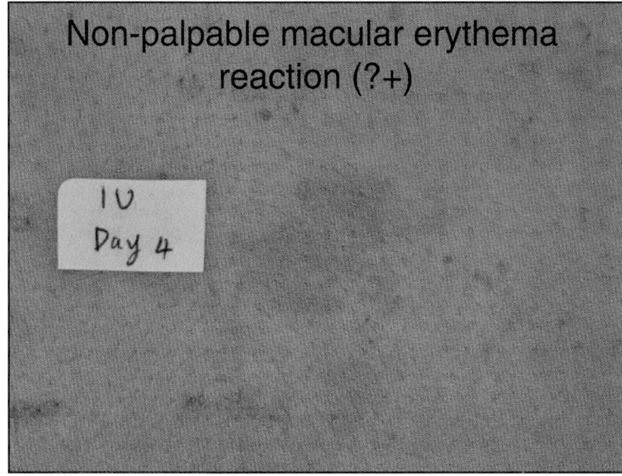

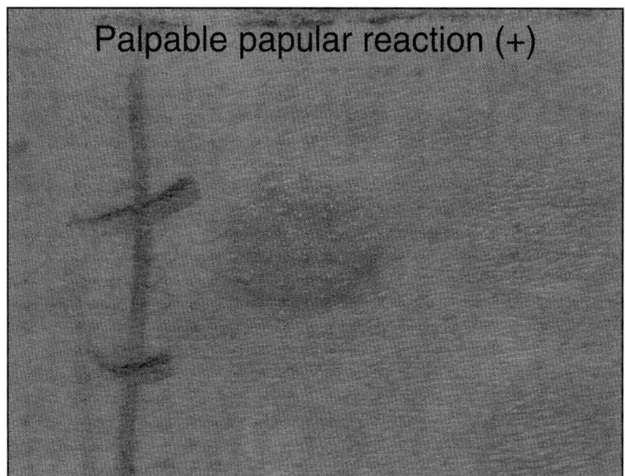

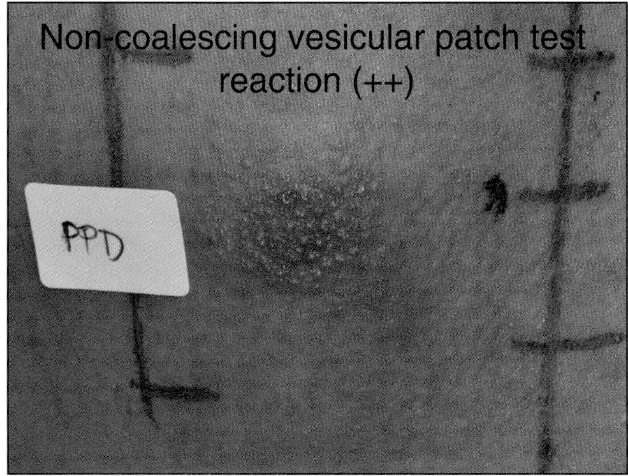

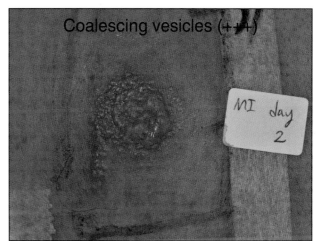

Figure 2.2 ICDRG criteria for scoring patch test reactions.

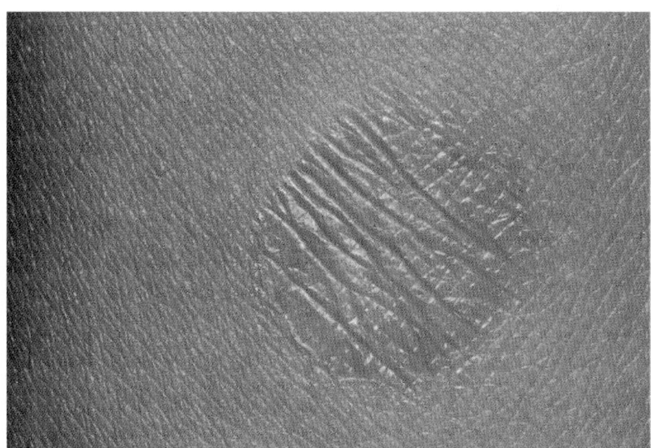

Figure 2.3 False-positive reactions with "soap" appearance.

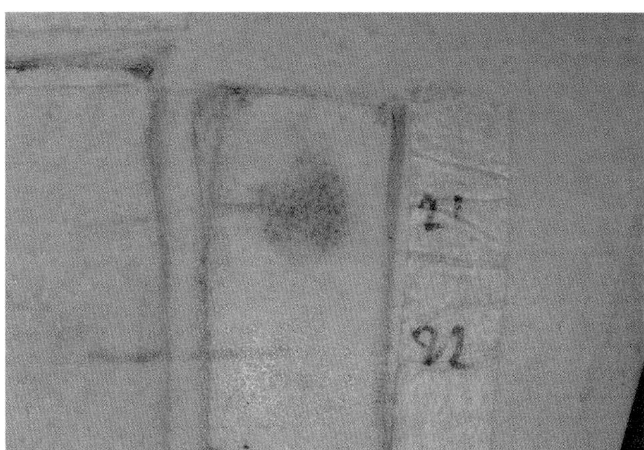

Figure 2.4 Irritant follicular patch test reaction to cobalt, most commonly seen in patients with atopic dermatitis.

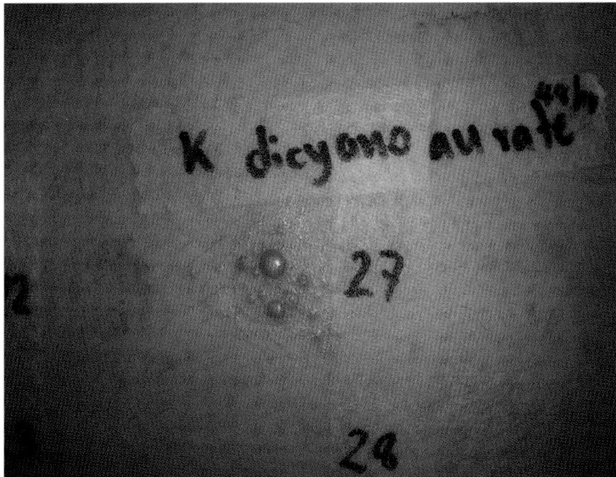

Figure 2.5 Pustular patch test reaction, most commonly seen with metals, which may be either true or false-positive reactions.

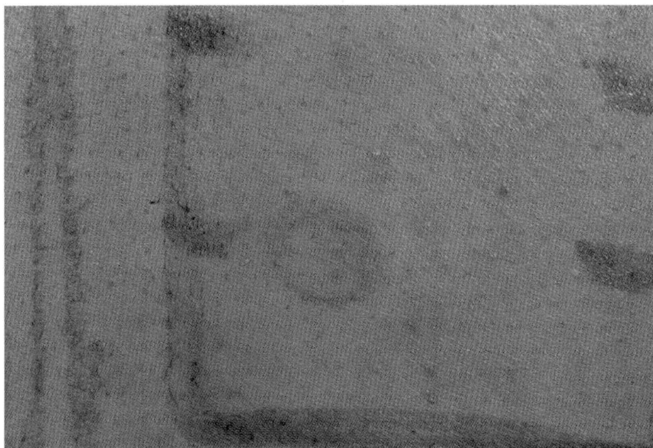

Figure 2.6 Edge effect, commonly seen in positive steroid patch test reactions.

Table 2.4 Allergen preparation in drug patch testing.

Allergen	Base	Control	Notes
Commercially available allergens such as antibiotics, anticonvulsants [33]	10% in pet.	Not required	—
Patient's own drug(s)	Mix with pet. until 10% wt/wt dilution[a]	Required [34]	The powder form (intravenous or capsules) is preferred over tablets
	Very low concentration: mix with 30% pet.[a]		

[a] Grind to a fine powder before mixing with pet.

acute generalized exanthematous pustulosis (AGEP), and Stevens–Johnson syndrome and toxic epidermal necrolysis (SJS/TEN) [22, 23]

2. ACD such as topical application or during manufacture/handling.

Some particular techniques are applied when performing patch testing for drug eruptions:

- Optimal time (seek specialist advice for DRESS and SJS/TEN)
  - At least 4–6 weeks after complete recovery from the CADRs.
  - A longer period may be required in DRESS [23].
- Allergen preparations are summarized in Table 2.4.
- Patch test reading
  - The morphology of reactions described in the ICDRG criteria, as well as other patterns resembling acute CADR(s), may be the presentation of positive patch test reactions [24].

Some special methods are applied only in fixed drug eruptions, including the following:

- Test sites: patch testing should be performed on two sites:
  - a resolved previous lesion (lesional patch test)
  - uninvolved skin, usually on the back (control)
- Duration: patch tests should be applied under occlusion for 6–24 hours.
- Reading time: at 24 and 48 hours (possibly at 6 hours).

Postponing patch testing

Patch tests, if possible, should be postponed in the following situations:

- severe and/or widespread active dermatitis
- systemic immunosuppressive drugs during tapering dosage: if on prednisolone of more than 15 mg per day postpone; if on other immunosuppressive proceed but note the immunosuppression the patient was on in the final summary of his/her patch test results
- recent topical corticosteroid application on the patch testing areas within the past 7 days [25]
- recent (4 weeks) natural sun with UVB or therapeutic ultraviolet exposure of the patch test sites
- active dermatitis at the test area
- pregnancy and lactation – patch testing during pregnancy and lactation is not known to be harmful but most dermatologists postpone during this time as a general precaution.

Interpretation

An assessment of contact allergy consists of two main steps. Step 1 is the interpretation of patch test reactions (Figure 2.7) and step 2 is the evaluation of clinical relevance (Table 2.5).

Adverse effects of patch testing

These adverse reactions can occur, even when the patch tests are performed correctly:

- pruritus
- irritant reactions
- transient localized hyper- or hypopigmentation
- occlusion folliculitis

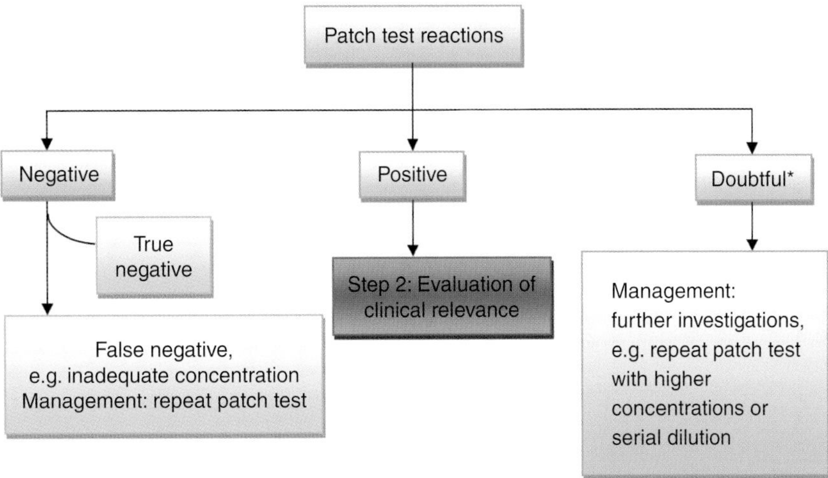

Figure 2.7 Interpretation of patch test reactions.

Table 2.5 The second step in the assessment of contact sensitization: evaluation of clinical relevance.

Clinical relevance	Interpretation
Present (current)	Gives the diagnosis of allergic contact dermatitis
Past	The patient has a past history of clinical contact dermatitis related to the positive patch test allergens
Unknown	Definite correlation cannot be confirmed due to inadequate information Management: re-evaluation of history, clinical examination, worksite visit Further investigations: use test, spot test, chemical analysis
Cross-reaction(s)	Sometimes (not always!) weaker patch test reaction than primary allergen Can occur without previous exposure or sensitization

exposure to allergen without reaction noted as 'exposed'

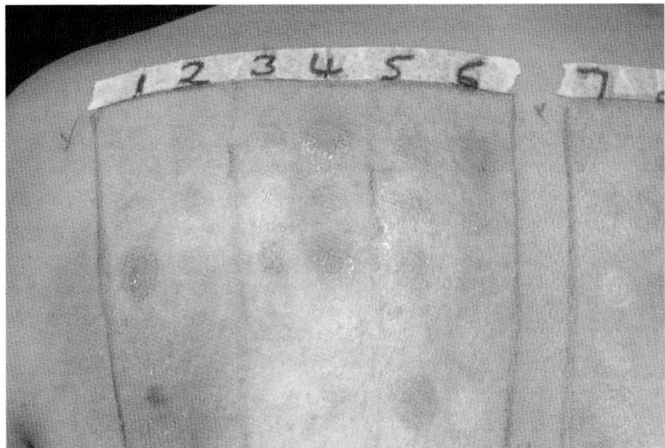

Figure 2.8 Angry back reaction. This is more likely to occur when the patient's dermatitis is extensive and active.

- scarring (very rare)
- flare-up of previous dermatitis

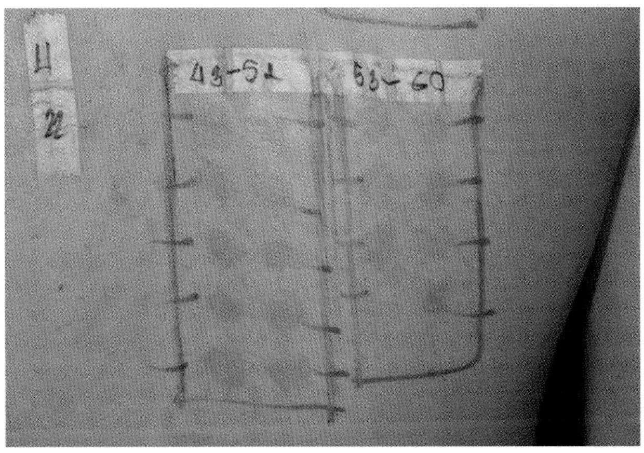

Figure 2.9 Uniform positive reactions in aluminum allergy (from aluminum in Finn Chambers®). Sometimes the reactions are annular in nature.

- persistence of patch test reactions which may last up to several weeks
- "angry back reaction": a non-specific inflammatory reaction with either sheeted inflammation or the appearance of multiple (false)-positive reactions (Figure 2.8). This is particularly likely to happen when the patient's dermatitis is active. Most chamber sites react, which may indicate contact allergy to the aluminum in Finn Chambers® (Figure 2.9).
- active sensitization
    - a positive patch test reaction after 2 weeks of an initially negative result at the same testing area indicates a late reaction which may be active sensitization or a late elicitation reaction.
    - diagnosis: no history of significant exposure and/or reaction. A quicker positive response at repeat patch testing may suggest the diagnosis of active sensitization [26].

Other *in vivo* tests

Other *in vivo* tests are shown in Table 2.6.

Table 2.6 Other *in vivo* tests.

Technique	Repeated open application test (ROAT) [35]	Semi-open test [36]	Open test [20]
Indication	A useful test for clarifying the clinical relevance of positive and doubtful patch test results	To test a patient's own product with suspected irritant properties, such as shampoos, detergents, and cooling fluids	Recommend as the first test for a poorly characterized substance
Techniques	Site: flexural area of the forearm below the antecubital fossa Frequency: 2 times/day Duration: until the patient develops a reaction or up to 2–4 weeks Size: 3 × 3 to 5 × 5 cm Amount: apply over the whole test area	Apply approximately 15 µl of a suspected allergen to an area of 1 × 1 cm using a cotton swab Wait until the substance is completely dry Look for wheals and flares (signs of contact urticaria) Cover with a permeable tape	Site: The volar forearm is usually tested, although the upper back and the upper arm are more reactive. Allergens: • "as is" or • dissolved in water or • some organic solvent (e.g. ethanol or acetone) Methods: 1. Drip a test substance onto the skin 2. Wait until the substance is dry. No occlusion
Reading	Positive reactions often start with follicular papules Erythema and vesicles can also be developed [37, 38]	Same as patch testing	First reading: evaluate at regular intervals during the first 30–60 minutes Second reading: at D3–D4 A negative open test may be due to inadequate penetration, therefore occlusive patch testing may be undertaken
Notes	Because it uses the principle of simulation of a real-life use situation, ROAT is sometimes the only demonstrable positive test in a patient with contact allergy	These two less standardized tests should be performed only by experienced clinicians who fully understand the hazards of the applied chemicals	

References

1 Schalock, P.C., Menne, T., Johansen, J.D. et al. (2012). Hypersensitivity reactions to metallic implants – diagnostic algorithm and suggested patch test series for clinical use. *Contact Dermatitis* 66 (1): 4–19.

2 Svedman, C., Ekqvist, S., Moller, H. et al. (2009). A correlation found between contact allergy to stent material and restenosis of the coronary arteries. *Contact Dermatitis* 60 (3): 158–164.

3 Cronin, E. (2001). *Foreword. Textbook of Contact Dermatitis*, 3e. Berlin: Springer.

4 Fischer, T. and Maibach, H. (1984). Finn chamber patch test technique. *Contact Dermatitis* 11 (3): 137–140.

5 Bruynzeel, D.P., Andersen, K.E., Camarasa, J.G. et al. (1995). The European standard series. European environmental and contact dermatitis research group (EECDRG). *Contact Dermatitis* 33 (3): 145–148.

6 Bruze, M., Conde-Salazar, L., Goossens, A. et al. (1999). Thoughts on sensitizers in a standard patch test series. The European Society of Contact Dermatitis. *Contact Dermatitis* 41 (5): 241–250.

7 Cronin, E. (1972). Clinical prediction of patch test results. *Transactions of the St John's Hospital Dermatological Society* 58 (2): 153–162.

8 Podmore, P., Burrows, D., and Bingham, E.A. (1984). Prediction of patch test results. *Contact Dermatitis* 11 (5): 283–284.

9 Bruze, M. and Fregert, S. (1983). Studies on purity and stability of photopatch test substances. *Contact Dermatitis* 9 (1): 33–39.

10 Isaksson, M., Gruvberger, B., Persson, L., and Bruze, M. (2000). Stability of corticosteroid patch test preparations. *Contact Dermatitis* 42 (3): 144–148.

11 Joy, N.M., Rice, K.R., and Atwater, A.R. (2013). Stability of patch test allergens. *Dermatitis* 24 (5): 227–236.

12 Siegel, P.D., Fowler, J.F., Law, B.F. et al. (2014). Concentrations and stability of methyl methacrylate, glutaraldehyde, formaldehyde and nickel sulfate in commercial patch test allergen preparations. *Contact Dermatitis* 70 (5): 309–315.

13 Andersen, K.E. and Andersen, F. (2008). The reaction index and positivity ratio revisited. *Contact Dermatitis* 58 (1): 28–31.

14 Johnson, M.W., Maibach, H.I., and Salmon, S.E. (1973). Brief communication: quantitative impairment of primary inflammatory response in patients with cancer. *Journal of the National Cancer Institute* 51 (3): 1075–1076.

15 van der Harst-Oostveen, C.J. and van Vloten, W.A. (1978). Delayed-type hypersensitivity in patients with mycosis fungoides. *Dermatologica* 157 (3): 129–135.

16 Grossman, J., Baum, J., Gluckman, J. et al. (1975). The effect of aging and acute illness on delayed hypersensitivity. *Journal of Allergy and Clinical Immunology* 55 (4): 268–275.

17 Thyssen, J.P., Linneberg, A., Ross-Hansen, K. et al. (2013). Filaggrin mutations are strongly associated with contact sensitization in individuals with dermatitis. *Contact Dermatitis* 68 (5): 273–276.

18 Seite, S., Zucchi, H., Moyal, D. et al. (2003). Alterations in human epidermal Langerhans cells by ultraviolet radiation: quantitative

and morphological study. *British Journal of Dermatology* 148 (2): 291–299.

19 Feuerman, E. and Levy, A. (1972). A study of the effect of prednisone and an antihistamine on patch test reactions. *British Journal of Dermatology* 86 (1): 68–71.

20 Johansen, J.D., Aalto-Korte, K., Agner, T. et al. (2015). European Society of Contact Dermatitis guideline for diagnostic patch testing – recommendations on best practice. *Contact Dermatitis* 73 (4): 195–221.

21 Moustafa, M., Holden, C.R., Athavale, P. et al. (2011). Patch testing is a useful investigation in children with eczema. *Contact Dermatitis* 65 (4): 208–212.

22 Santiago, F., Goncalo, M., Vieira, R. et al. (2010). Epicutaneous patch testing in drug hypersensitivity syndrome (DRESS). *Contact Dermatitis* 62 (1): 47–53.

23 Barbaud, A. (2014). Skin testing and patch testing in non-IgE-mediated drug allergy. *Current Allergy and Asthma Reports* 14 (6): 442.

24 Serra, D., Ramos, L., Brinca, A., and Goncalo, M. (2012). Acute generalized exanthematous pustulosis associated with acyclovir, confirmed by patch testing. *Dermatitis* 23 (2): 99–100.

25 Green, C. (1996). The effect of topically applied corticosteroid on irritant and allergic patch test reactions. *Contact Dermatitis* 35 (6): 331–333.

26 Bruze, M. (1984). Simultaneous patch test sensitization to 4 chemically unrelated compounds in a standard test series. *Contact Dermatitis* 11 (1): 48–49.

27 Bruze, M., Frick, M., and Persson, L. (2003). Patch testing with thin-layer chromatograms. *Contact Dermatitis* 48 (5): 278–279.

28 Macfarlane, A.W., Curley, R.K., Graham, R.M. et al. (1989). Delayed patch test reactions at days 7 and 9. *Contact Dermatitis* 20 (2): 127–132.

29 Jonker, M.J. and Bruynzeel, D.P. (2000). The outcome of an additional patch-test reading on days 6 or 7. *Contact Dermatitis* 42 (6): 330–335.

30 Isaksson, M., Andersen, K.E., Brandao, F.M. et al. (2000). Patch testing with corticosteroid mixes in Europe. A multicentre study of the EECDRG. *Contact Dermatitis* 42 (1): 27–35.

31 Uter, W.J., Geier, J., and Schnuch, A. (1996). Good clinical practice in patch testing: readings beyond day 2 are necessary: a confirmatory analysis. Members of the Information Network of Departments of Dermatology. *American Journal of Contact Dermatitis* 7 (4): 231–237.

32 Magnusson, B., Blohm, S.G., Fregert, S. et al. (1966). Routine patch testing. II. Proposed basic series of test substances for Scandinavian countries and general remarks on testing technique. *Acta Dermato-Venereologica* 46 (2): 153–158.

33 Barbaud, A., Trechot, P., Weber-Muller, F. et al. (2004). Drug skin tests in cutaneous adverse drug reactions to pristinamycin: 29 cases with a study of cross-reactions between synergistins. *Contact Dermatitis* 50 (1): 22–26.

34 Barbaud, A., Collet, E., Milpied, B. et al. (2013). A multicentre study to determine the value and safety of drug patch tests for the three main classes of severe cutaneous adverse drug reactions. *British Journal of Dermatology* 168 (3): 555–562.

35 Hannuksela, M. and Salo, H. (1986). The repeated open application test (ROAT). *Contact Dermatitis* 14 (4): 221–227.

36 Frosch, P.J., Geier, J., Uter, W., and Goossens, A. (2011). *Patch Testing with the Patients' Own Products* (eds. J. Johansen, P. Frosch and J.P. Lepoittevin) Contact Dermatitis. 5e. Berlin, Heidelberg: Springer.

37 Johansen, J.D., Bruze, M., Andersen, K.E. et al. (1998). The repeated open application test: suggestions for a scale of evaluation. *Contact Dermatitis* 39 (2): 95–96.

38 Johansen, J.D., Frosch, P.J., Svedman, C. et al. (2003). Hydroxyisohexyl 3-cyclohexene carboxaldehyde- known as Lyral: quantitative aspects and risk assessment of an important fragrance allergen. *Contact Dermatitis* 48 (6): 310–316.

CHAPTER 3

The Detective's Guide to Contact Dermatitis

CHAPTER CONTENTS

Key points

1. The four steps to diagnosing allergic contact dermatitis (ACD) are (i) *elimination* (or inclusion) of non-dermatitis dermatoses and non-allergic dermatitis, (ii) *perception* of a pre-patch test diagnosis, (iii) *detection* of contact allergy by patch testing, and (iv) *deduction* of a diagnosis of ACD by correlating the exposure to the allergen(s) in terms of dose, time, and contiguous aspects of the dermatitis.
2. The pre-patch test history should have a broad scope to check for exposure to a wide range of allergens.
3. In contrast, once a contact allergy(s) has been identified, the post-patch test history should have a narrow scope, focusing on exposure to the allergen in question and correlation with, in minute detail, the temporal aspects and distribution of the dermatitis (microhistory).
4. Contact allergy profiling is an important investigative tool in the diagnosis of ACD.

This is an abridged version of the paper "Diagnosing Allergic Contact Dermatitis through Elimination, Perception, Detection and Deduction" [1].

Introduction

The investigation of possible ACD is based on a systematic search for clues. A striking similarity between the skills of great fictional detectives such as Sherlock Holmes and those required to practice contact dermatitis has been noted by several authors. Goossens [2] comments on the detective skills involved in the assessment of contact dermatitis patients. Belsito (1999) [3] remarks on the need for diagnostic clues to solve puzzling clinical presentations. Here, we crystallize this concept further, reviewing how detection skills are utilized in diagnosing ACD.

The four steps involved are:

1. *elimination* (or inclusion) of non-allergic diagnoses
2. *perception* – reviewing the different scenarios of the pre-patch test diagnosis
3. *detection* – maximizing the sensitivity of the patch test investigation
4. *deduction* – achieving a diagnosis of ACD by associating the temporospatial nature of the allergen exposure to that of the dermatitis.

These four specific steps will be discussed within the context of differences between the pre- and post-patch test history and examination in the hands of the clinically experienced patch tester. The concept of contact allergy profiling as an investigative tool is also discussed.

Diagnosing ACD: a simple and obvious exercise?

The notion of ACD usually being not only from direct contact but also clinically obvious is a common but misplaced one.

Common Contact Allergens: A Practical Guide to Detecting Contact Dermatitis, First Edition. Edited by John McFadden, Pailin Puangpet, Korbkarn Pongpairoj, Supitchaya Thaiwat, and Lee Shan Xian.

© 2020 John Wiley & Sons Ltd. Published 2020 by John Wiley & Sons Ltd.

Companion website: www.wiley.com/go/mcfadden/common_contact_allergens

Table 3.1 Proposed ICDRG classification of the clinical presentations of contact allergy [4].

1. Direct exposure/contact dermatitis
2. Mimicking or exacerbation of pre-existing eczema
3. Multifactorial dermatitis, including ACD
4. By proxy
5. Mimicking angioedema
6. Airborne contact dermatitis
7. Photo-induced contact dermatitis
8. Systemic contact dermatitis
9. Non-eczematous contact dermatitis
10. Contact urticaria
11. Protein contact dermatitis
12. Respiratory/mucosal symptoms
13. Oral contact dermatitis
14. Erythroderma/exfoliative dermatitis
15. Minor forms of presentation
16. Extracutaneous manifestations

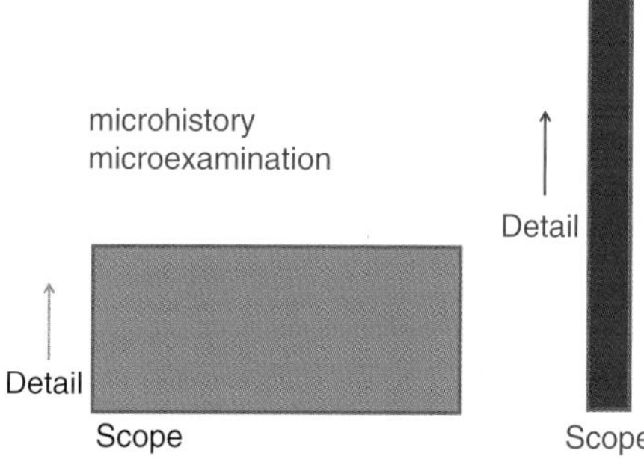

Figure 3.1 Pre-patch test scoping history and examination (blue) vs post-patch test history and examination (red). The pre-patch test history and examination should have a wide scope to screen for potential exposure to multiple allergens from different types of activities (see Table 3.2) and with different routes of exposure (see Table 3.3). In contrast, after patch testing, the scope narrows to focus on the potential allergen(s) identified through patch testing so that exposure to that allergen(s), and any potential associations with the dermatitis, can be assessed in minute detail (microhistory and microexamination).

The presentation of obvious axillary ACD to fragrance after deodorant use may be classical, but this is a relatively uncommon mode of presentation. For example, only 50% of patients presenting with ACD to hair dye will be aware of this possibility [4] and only 25% of patients found to be allergic to fragrance gave a pre-patch test history of reacting to fragrance/fragranced products (Thaiwat, unpublished observation). ACD to other allergens such as preservatives may be even less evident. ACD from direct contact is only one clinical presentation of contact allergy. A recent International Contact Dermatitis Research Group (ICDRG) classification documents 16 different clinical presentations of contact allergy (Table 3.1) [5].

Pre-patch test history and examination

Pre-patch test history: the need for a wide scope

There are two components to the pre-patch test history: first, regarding the nature of the dermatitis and, second, exposure to potential contact allergens. Questions regarding the location and temporal nature of the rash are essential, but ascertaining where the rash originated on the body is also important, as an underemphasized characteristic of ACD is its ability to spread [6].

The pre-patch test history of exposure to potential allergens should have a "wide scope" or extensive and wide anamnesis (Figure 3.1) [7] for the following reasons:

a. There are numerous contact allergens in the environment. Even the most basic baseline series contains at least nine groups of contact allergens, i.e. metals, fragrances, dyes, medicaments, plants, preservatives, rubber chemicals, resins, and vehicle excipients. In addition, there are also more specialized allergens represented in many different series (such as hairdressers, dental, medicaments, extra cosmetics, plastics/glues) which may need to be tested for, depending on the pre-patch test assessment.
b. There are at least 14 different specific aspects of everyday life where there is potential for contact allergen exposure (Table 3.2). In Section 3 we have arbitrarily grouped some of these together to give color coding for eight different sources of allergen exposure.
c. There are six different routes of exposure to contact allergens (Table 3.3). Whilst it is easy to remember direct contact and airborne contact, one can easily forget other routes, e.g. by proxy.
d. There are therefore many potential different permutations of how an individual can be exposed to contact allergens.

Table 3.2 Aspects of daily life with potential for contact allergen exposure.

1. The use of personal care products/cosmetics
2. Cosmetic procedures, e.g. hairstyling/dyeing, nail manicures, waxing
3. The home environment, including the use of household products, furnishings, and home decorating and cleaning
4. The work environment
5. Other environments, e.g. shops, friend's house
6. Leisure and sport activities
7. The wearing of clothes, shoes, gloves, and hats
8. The use of personal appliances such as spectacles, hearing aids, walking sticks, cutlery, scissors, pens, laptop computers, and mobile phones
9. The use of medications, herbal, and "alternative"agents
10. The wearing of jewelry and other ornamentation
11. Medical, dental, and surgical procedures
12. Travel, including car driving, cycling, and holiday environments
13. Dietary and mucosal exposure
14. Close physical intimacy
15. Other aspects of daily life

Table 3.3 Different routes of exposure to potential contact allergens.

Route of exposure	Examples
1. Direct exposure	Plaster applied to skin
2. Airborne exposure	Fragrance, epoxy, *parthenium*
3. Hand to face/body	Hand moisturizers, nail varnish
4. Systemic exposure	Certain fragrance chemicals
5. By proxy	Partner's aftershave
6. Mucosal exposure	Toothpaste, eye drops, dental amalgam

Pre-patch test examination: local and distal sites

Examination should include both local and distal site examination. Clues may be ascertained from both. For example, a patient presenting with a facial rash may show at the local site examination bilateral eyelid dermatitis consistent with an airborne exposure, but distally a patchy dermatitis on the neck and upper chest suggestive of nail varnish allergy from the hand to neck/body route of exposure and periungual/nail fold dermatitis from direct exposure to nail varnish. In addition, many patients will have pictures of acute exacerbations of their dermatitis stored on their mobile phones, adding a temporal aspect to the physical assessment (see Chapter 5).

The four steps in diagnosing ACD

Elimination (or inclusion) of non-allergic diagnoses

This step is equally as important as the others, as in most contact dermatitis clinics there is a positive patch test rate of only around 50–60% of patients tested and some patch test reactions are not of current relevance. There are three broad diagnostic groups to consider, the first being non-dermatitis dermatoses such as psoriasis and tinea. Tinea can easily be missed, especially if treatment/steroid modified. At St. John's, we see four patients with tinea manuum annually who have been referred for patch testing [8].

The second diagnosis to consider is endogenous or reactive dermatitis such as atopic and seborrheic dermatitis. ACD often co-exists with endogenous dermatitis, and indeed one clinical presentation of contact allergy is an apparent worsening of an endogenous dermatitis [5].

Finally, there is irritant contact dermatitis. Irritant exposure can occur within the home, work or leisure environment and can be additive. Both the intensity and duration of exposure to irritants are important. Irritant contact dermatitis may also be part of a multifactorial dermatitis, as it can co-exist with ACD and patients with a history of atopic dermatitis are also prone to developing irritant contact dermatitis [9].

Searching for diagnostic clues can help in this step. As an example, non-pustular psoriasis of the hands may be clinically evident with loosely bilateral areas which are well-defined and contain silvery scale, but sometimes this is not the case. However, there may be a family history, 30% of patients will have classical body plaques, and 85% will have plantar psoriasis. Manual workers with non-pustular palmar psoriasis are more likely to have involvement of the pressure areas of the hand (thenar and hypothenar eminences, palmar areas, volar aspects of the fingers, and margins of the palmar hand) [10].

Perception: pre-patch test diagnosis and the three scenarios principle

After an initial consultation and examination in a contact dermatitis clinic, it is common practice to formulate a working pre-patch test diagnosis. This is to ensure optimal testing with appropriate patch test series, amongst other considerations. A three scenarios approach can be a useful tool to reach such a working diagnosis.

Scenario 1: The diagnosis certain scenario. There is reasonable certainty of the diagnosis. For example, in a patient presenting with inflammation of the scalp 6 hours after hair dye application, a diagnosis of ACD may appear certain. However, irritant contact dermatitis can present in a similar manner: the hair dye process is alkaline, which can lead to delayed inflammation, and the presence of pre-existing scalp inflammation, e.g. seborrheic dermatitis, and exposure to hair dye for a prolonged time can both predispose to an irritant contact dermatitis. The principle is that one should attempt to form a differential diagnosis even when the diagnosis appears to be certain.

Scenario 2: The competing diagnoses scenario. If there is a differential diagnosis without there being a single strongly favored diagnosis, assess each competing diagnosis carefully for the one with the fewest irregularities. It is possible in this scenario that there may be coexisting diagnoses as well. Airborne ACD and facial seborrheic dermatitis may resemble each other but the absence of seborrheic eczema at other sites, especially the scalp, in the presence of significant facial involvement, together with a history of exposure to airborne allergens, e.g. methylisothiazolinone from wet paint, would favor a diagnosis of airborne ACD.

Scenario 3: The diagnosis unclear scenario. If at the end of pre-patch test consultation there is no working diagnosis, there should be a further search for clues in a systematic manner:

- Recheck the history. Sometimes, instead of taking a history chronologically from when the rash started to the present day, it may be worth taking the history in reverse chronology, i.e. from the present day and working back in time. When taken this way, some patients will remember or emphasize different details.
- Recheck the examination, ensuring that you examine as extensively as possible, i.e. examining areas away from the main rash as well as the main site of dermatosis, e.g. searching for psoriasis of the knees, elbows, scalp, and nails in a patient with facial dermatosis.
- Check for the possibility that topical/oral steroids or other immunosuppression could have made a dermatosis or infestation unrecognizable, i.e. "incognito."
- Check for the possibility of ACD by proxy, which usually presents in a bizarre way without clues in the history.

- Think of the mimicking diagnoses in dermatology: lupus, mycoses fungoides, syphilis, sarcoidosis, and ACD to the hair dye allergen *p*-phenylenediamine (PPD) can not only be great mimickers but also great disguisers. Exclude dermatitis artefacta.
- Perform extensive rather than limited patch test screening.
- Consider further investigations such as biopsy, microbiological tests, and chemical pathology screening.

The principle here is that if the diagnosis is unclear, one should keep searching for clues but in a systematic way.

Detection: optimizing the sensitivity of the patch test

Patch testing involves a controlled elicitation reaction to a contact allergen. It detects the immunological state of contact allergy [11]. ACD is the elicitation of an eczematous reaction to an allergen under clinical (normal life) conditions. The presence of contact allergy signifies the potential for a diagnosis of ACD, but this depends on the next phase of deduction. A negative patch test (assuming no error or false negative reaction occurred) excludes the possibility of ACD. One way of approaching patch testing is to simply order the baseline series for testing. However, one should be proactive to maximize the sensitivity of patch testing. There are several ways to enhance the sensitivity of patch testing:

a. Have a low threshold for adding extra series. As an example, the plant series should be added not only for gardeners or people who garden regularly, but also for patients who regularly use cosmetics with multiple plant material additives. Adding a fragrance series of the 26 individual fragrances listed in toiletries within the EU will increase the detection of fragrance allergy by more than 50% compared to testing with the standard series fragrance mixes alone [12].
b. When a specific allergy is suspected, add extra individual allergens to the baseline series to increase sensitivity. For example, if hair dye is suspected, adding in toluenediamine to the standard series, which normally relies only on the response to PPD, will increase the diagnosis of hair dye allergy by 15% [13]. A further example is adding amerchol and crude lanolin when lanolin allergy is suspected. Adding compositae mix in addition to the sesquiterpene lactone mix in the standard series will increase the detection of compositae allergy by over 20% [14].
c. Test with patients' own samples. These could include leave-on toiletries, clothing, woods, plastic materials (e.g. spectacle frames), and leaves of plants. Some agents (e.g. wash-off cosmetics, resins) need to be diluted and others (e.g. wood shavings) should be tested with a larger aluminum chamber. As an example, testing with shoe samples increases the sensitivity of detecting shoe contact allergy by up to 20% [15]. Patch testing with patients' own shoes should be performed using pieces of at least 1 cm^2 and less than 2 mm thick to minimize false negatives and irritant pressure reactions [16].
d. If medicament, fragrance, or metal allergy is suspected, deferring the last reading or adding in a further reading at 7 days will increase sensitivity [17–19].

Deduction: diagnosing ACD by associating the dermatitis with the allergen exposure

A sensitization induction reaction occurs at a minimum of 10–21 days after allergen exposure [20]. An elicitation reaction usually occurs within 48 hours of allergen exposure [20]. Most clinical cases of ACD reactions occur within 48 hours of exposure to the allergen and are therefore, by definition, elicitation reactions. It therefore follows that most cases of sensitization to contact allergens are quiet (sensitization to PPD from an extremely high dose in temporary beach tattoos being an exception). For an elicitation reaction to occur, this will depend on the extent of sensitization that has previously been induced as well as the immunological dose of the allergen. ACD reactions therefore occur when either of these increase to a certain threshold. Levels of sensitization will increase with repeated exposure to an allergen. Alternatively, the immunological dose may increase from alterations in the nature of exposure, e.g. increased frequency of application of a hair dye, longer exposure to hair dye or changing to a darker shade of hair dye (see the section on history, microhistory, and exposure sources).

Microhistory and microexamination

To diagnose ACD, the temporal and spatial exposure of the contact allergen identified as positive by patch testing needs to be causatively associated with the temporal and morphological aspects, as well as the localization of the dermatitis. Thus, the post-patch test history and examination differs from the pre-patch test history and examination, in some ways being its polar opposite. Instead of having a wide scope in order to explore the full possible range of exposure to potential allergens, the post-patch test history and examination now narrows the scope and focuses on exposure to the contact allergen(s) identified by patch testing and its relationship to the dermatitis in minute detail.

Likewise, a microexamination may reveal more clues. For example, fragrance ACD is characterized by axillary dermatitis involving the vault, and there may be local spread from the axilla to adjacent areas of the trunk, characteristic of fragrance ACD (Figure 3.2). A distal examination may reveal further clues; for example, dermatitis from ACD to airborne fragrance on the eyelids or from direct contact on the hands and neck.

Knowledge of contact dermatitis literature

Acquiring a working knowledge of contact dermatitis literature is a key requirement in optimizing practice. Journals such as the *American Journal of Clinical Dermatology*, *Contact Dermatitis*, *Dermatitis* and the *Journal of the American Academy of Dermatology* should be routinely reviewed to keep up to date

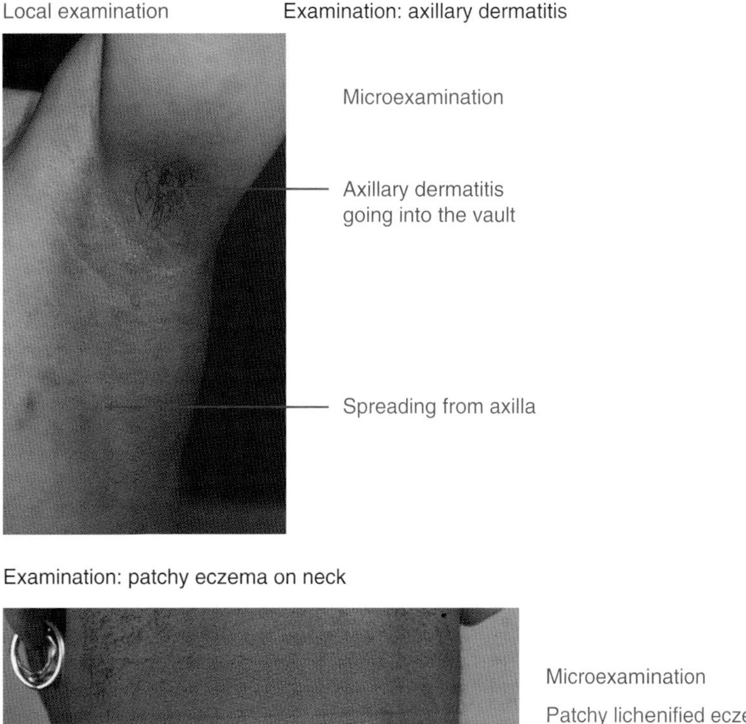

Figure 3.2 ACD to fragrance in a deodorant. Axillary dermatitis involving the axillary vault with apparent spread from the original site, which is characteristic of ACD.

with recent advances. The literature can be broadly divided into the following subheadings:

a. classical papers and reviews
b. patch test technique
c. epidemiological/incidence studies
d. case reports.

Just as lawyers need to know case law and precedents, knowledge of case literature is extremely important in the practice of contact dermatitis. Case reports could be related to new allergens, established allergens which are presenting in a novel way or reinforcing known presentations of established contact allergens.

Contact allergy profiling

Contact allergy profiling can be used as an important investigative tool in the diagnosis of ACD in the post-patch test analysis. For each standard contact allergen, the case literature and clinical experience can be used to compile a profile of the allergen with respect to:

a. the potential sources of exposure
b. the different routes of exposure
c. the various clinical manifestations of contact allergy to the specific agent.

For example, profiling fragrance reveals a very wide range of potential exposures from different aspects of daily life, routes of

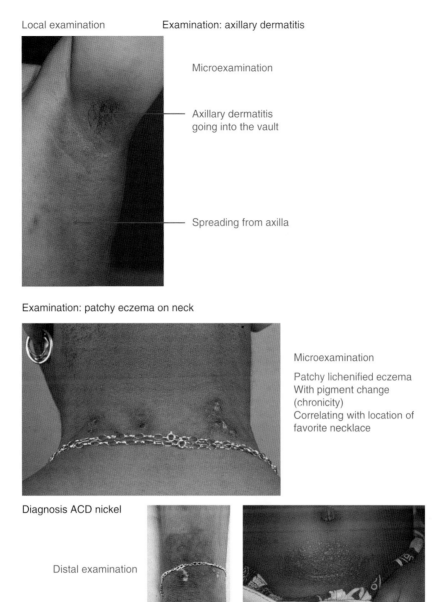

exposure, and multiple forms of clinical presentation. In contrast, the allergy profile of the hair dye chemical PPD shows a much more limited exposure profile from daily life and routes of exposure. However, known different clinical manifestations of contact allergy to PPD (n = 16) are even more numerous than that of contact allergy to fragrance. Examples of allergy profiling are given in Section 3.

Clinical experience

Stressing the importance of clinical experience may have become a cliché, but perhaps there is some evidence to support such a claim. Performance psychologists argue that most performers have practiced 1000 hours per year for 10 years before optimizing their sport, musical, or professional discipline (aggregate 10 000 hours) [21]. However, this practice needs to be purposeful (i.e. sustained, focused, and developmental). If this rule were applied to analytical medical skills and three patch test clinics were undertaken per week, then approximately 20 years would be needed to accumulate 10 000 hours of clinical experience to optimize skill set performance. Purposeful experience, however, requires interactions with colleagues and regular attendance at group meetings to discuss cases. Involvement with at least 200 cases per year has been recommended to maintain competence (www.bad.org.uk/shared/get-file.ashx?itemtype=document&id=1618). Membership of societies such as the American Contact Dermatitis Society and the European Society of Contact Dermatitis may also be beneficial.

Summary

Diagnosing ACD involves skills used in other fields of detection. The pre-patch test history and examination should include a wide scope to include questioning on the different aspects of daily life with potential for exposure to contact allergens. Examination should include both a local and distal aspect with respect to the anatomical location of the presenting rash. Step 1 involves the elimination/inclusion of non-allergic dermatological diagnoses. Step 2 involves perception: entertaining the different scenarios in a pre-patch test diagnosis. Step 3 involves the detection of contact allergy, utilizing the patch test process to increase its sensitivity. Step 4 involves deduction in order to diagnose ACD. The post-patch test microhistory and microexamination should focus in minute detail on the association of exposure to the allergen(s) identified by patch testing to the presenting dermatitis to be able to diagnose ACD. Clinical experience and knowledge of contact dermatitis case literature, in particular knowing the allergen's clinical profile, are essential tools in the practice of contact dermatitis.

References

1 Pongpairoj, K., Puangpet, P., Thaiwat, S., and McFadden, J.P. (2017). Diagnosing allergic contact dermatitis through elimination, perception, detection and deduction. *American Journal of Clinical Dermatology* 18 (5): 651–661.

2 Goossens, A. (2007). Art and science of patch testing. *Indian Journal of Dermatology, Venereology and Leprology* 73 (5): 289–291.

3 Belsito, D.V. (1999). A sherlockian approach to contact dermatitis. *Dermatologic Clinics* 17 (3): 705–713. x.

4 Ho, S.G., Basketter, D.A., Jefferies, D. et al. (2005). Analysis of para-phenylenediamine allergic patients in relation to strength of patch test reaction. *British Journal of Dermatology* 153 (2): 364–367.

5 Pongpairoj, K., Ale, I., Andersen, K.E. et al. (2016). Proposed ICDRG classification of the clinical presentation of contact allergy. *Dermatitis: Contact, Atopic, Occupational, Drug* 27 (5): 248–258.

6 Streit, M. and Braathen, L.R. (2001). Contact dermatitis: clinics and pathology. *Acta Odontologica Scandinavica* 59 (5): 309–314.

7 Goossens, A. (2001). Minimizing the risks of missing a contact allergy. *Dermatology* 202 (2): 186–189.

8 Smith, H.R., Holloway, D., Armstrong, D.K. et al. (2000). Association between tinea manuum and male manual workers. *Contact Dermatitis* 42 (1): 45.

9 Gittler, J.K., Krueger, J.G., and Guttman-Yassky, E. (2013). Atopic dermatitis results in intrinsic barrier and immune abnormalities: implications for contact dermatitis. *Journal of Allergy and Clinical Immunology* 131 (2): 300–313.

10 Kumar, B., Saraswat, A., and Kaur, I. (2002). Palmoplantar lesions in psoriasis: a study of 3065 patients. *Acta Dermato-Venereologica* 82 (3): 192–195.

11 Johansen, J.D., Aalto-Korte, K., Agner, T. et al. (2015). European Society of Contact Dermatitis guideline for diagnostic patch testing – recommendations on best practice. *Contact Dermatitis* 73 (4): 195–221.

12 Vejanurug, P., Tresukosol, P., Sajjachareonpong, P., and Puangpet, P. (2016). Fragrance allergy could be missed without patch testing with 26 individual fragrance allergens. *Contact Dermatitis* 74 (4): 230–235.

13 Basketter, D.A. and English, J. (2009). Cross-reactions among hair dye allergens. *Cutaneous and Ocular Toxicology* 28 (3): 104–106.

14 Bong, J.L., English, J.S., and Wilkinson, S.M. (2001). British contact dermatitis G. Diluted compositae mix versus sesquiterpene lactone mix as a screening agent for compositae dermatitis: a multicentre study. *Contact Dermatitis* 45 (1): 26–28.

15 Calnan, C.D. and Sarkany, I. (1959). Studies in contact dermatitis. IX. Shoe dermatitis. *Transactions of the St. John's Hospital Dermatological Society* 43: 8–26.

16 Matthys, E., Zahir, A., and Ehrlich, A. (2014). Shoe allergic contact dermatitis. *Dermatitis: Contact, Atopic, Occupational, Drug* 25 (4): 163–171.

17 Isaksson, M. and Bruze, M. (2003). Late patch-test reactions to budesonide need not be a sign of sensitization induced by the test procedure. *American Journal of Contact Dermatitis: Official Journal of the American Contact Dermatitis Society* 14 (3): 154–156.

18 Davis, M.D., Bhate, K., Rohlinger, A.L. et al. (2008). Delayed patch test reading after 5 days: the Mayo Clinic experience. *Journal of the American Academy of Dermatology* 59 (2): 225–233.
19 Higgins, E. and Collins, P. (2013). The relevance of 7-day patch test reading. *Dermatitis: Contact, Atopic, Occupational, Drug* 24 (5): 237–240.
20 Friedmann, P.S. (2007). The relationships between exposure dose and response in induction and elicitation of contact hypersensitivity in humans. *British Journal of Dermatology* 157 (6): 1093–1102.
21 Ericsson, K.A. and Lehmann, A.C. (1996). Expert and exceptional performance: evidence of maximal adaptation to task constraints. *Annual Review of Psychology* 47: 273–305.

CHAPTER 4

History, Microhistory, and Sources of Contact Allergen Exposure

CHAPTER CONTENTS

Key points

- The pre-patch test history consists of two parts:
  - The first part is asking about the nature of the rash. This includes ascertaining where the rash started and where it has spread to, when it started, symptomatology, a description of the rash, and whether the rash is intermittent or persistent. Information on the response to treatment, relationship to work, previous history of dermatitis, and general medical conditions and therapy should also be ascertained.
  - The second part involves screening for potential allergen exposures in different aspects of the patient's life, including personal care products, the domestic and occupational environment, travel and leisure pursuits, medicament agents and medical/dental procedures, use of personal appliances, clothing, jewellery and ornamentations, and other exposures. The pre-patch test history should have a wide scope to cover different aspects of daily life.
- In contrast, the post-patch test history (microhistory) should have a narrow scope to focus on exposures to the allergens to which the patient reacted positively on patch testing, to ascertain if exposures to the allergen(s) could be of current relevance to the dermatitis. In particular, to ascertain whether the dynamics of the exposure to the allergen(s) correlates with the development and progression of the dermatitis.
- Potential pitfalls in establishing relevance include when more than one allergy is identified, more than one source of allergen exposure is identified, the possibility of a missed allergen, indeterminate clinical relevance of the allergen exposure, and the presence of multifactorial dermatitis.
- A good working knowledge of potential allergen exposures in the different aspects of patients' daily activities is essential.

Introduction

Common misconceptions regarding allergic contact dermatitis (ACD) are that the history of the allergic reaction is self-evident and that allergen exposure is usually from a single source and due to direct contact. However, in practice, clues in the history (and examination) as to the source of ACD are often elusive. For example, only 25% of patients who have contact allergy to fragrance will give a positive history of reacting to fragrances or fragranced products on initial screening (Thaiwat, unpublished observation). One in three patients with allergy to hair dye chemicals will not give a history of reacting to hair dye [1]. Furthermore, direct contact is just one of six potential routes of allergen exposure.

In order to optimize the detection of clues, the contact dermatitis history has to (i) be systematic, (ii) have a wide scope regarding potential allergen exposure, and (iii) where relevant be of meticulous detail.

Fortunately, the history occurs in two stages.

1. *The pre-patch test (scoping) history*. This consists of a detailed history of the presenting dermatosis and then identifying potential allergen exposures. The history will cover several areas of daily life and therefore must have a "wide" scope.
2. *The post-patch test history (microhistory)*. When a contact allergen has been identified by a positive patch test, one

Common Contact Allergens: A Practical Guide to Detecting Contact Dermatitis, First Edition. Edited by John McFadden, Pailin Puangpet, Korbkarn Pongpairoj, Supitchaya Thaiwat, and Lee Shan Xian.

© 2020 John Wiley & Sons Ltd. Published 2020 by John Wiley & Sons Ltd.

Companion website: www.wiley.com/go/mcfadden/common_contact_allergens

should then go into minute detail regarding exposure to that allergen in relation to the development and progression of the dermatitis. The initial narrative and screening of potential allergen exposure from daily life is revisited in meticulous detail regarding exposure to the identified allergen to establish possible clinical relevance.

The immunological dose of allergen exposure

- Most cases of ACD present with *elicitation*, the sensitization phase being a silent phenomenon. For example, a patient may present a few weeks or a few months after using a new moisturizer before developing ACD to a preservative in the product, usually developing within 24–72 hours of the most recent exposure to it (as opposed to a sensitization reaction, which occurs 10–21 days after exposure). This may appear to be counter-intuitive as most experimental research on contact sensitization involves a first large single sensitizing dose of a potent allergen inducing an inflammatory reaction 10–21 days later [2]. However, most clinical cases of contact sensitization involve repeated low doses of exposure leading to clinically silent sensitization.
- Elicitation reactions can occur when the level of sensitization factored by the immunological dose (stimulus) of the contact allergen reaches a certain threshold. This could therefore occur through an increase in the level of sensitization from repeated exposure to the allergen. This is either from repeated exposure from a single source (e.g. monthly application of hair dye applied with the same brand, same shade of color, and for the same time) or from multiple sources (e.g. methylisothiazolinone [MI] in shampoo, liquid soap, dish-washing detergent, and from a recently painted wall). In this scenario, there may be no apparent change in exposure habits.[a]
- Alternatively, elicitation reactions can also occur when the immunological dose of allergen exposure increases. Examples of this in clinical practice include:
  a. *Increased concentration of allergen*, e.g. the patient changes his or her hair dye to a darker shade (darker dyes contain up to ten times higher concentrations of aromatic amine allergens compared to lighter shades), precipitating an acute ACD.
  b. *Increased exposure time* leading to increased cumulative exposure, e.g. a floor layer works overtime for a month, increasing his daily exposure to epoxy resin. Most contact allergens bind covalently to the skin and so may remain present for several days, in this case leading to increased levels of allergens within the skin.
  c. The immunological dose may also be affected by *how the allergen is delivered* to the skin. A fragrance chemical applied within a deodorant will have a bigger immunological dose than if delivered as part of fragranced water as the astringent in the deodorant will add to the danger signaling of the allergen.
  d. The immunological dose may be affected by *local skin factors*. For example, sweating will increase the amount of nickel released from jewelry or accelerator released from rubber in shoes. Occlusion from clothing or adhesive dressings will increase the penetration of fragrance sprayed onto the skin.

The dose of allergen required to cause sensitization or elicit an ACD reaction when applied to *skin which is already inflamed* will be lower than that applied to uninflamed skin, as the danger signaling and activation of the immune system is already in place, e.g. applying fragranced aftershave onto inflamed seborrheic eczema of the face.

The pre-patch test history

- *Ascertain when the dermatitis started.* This may be important for factors that the patient did not think of. For example, they may not have noticed that their facial dermatitis began a few weeks after their house was being decorated (with MI ACD from wall paint emission) (Figure 4.1).
- *Where did the rash start?* By the time the patient is seen, the condition would often have spread to other areas. It is therefore of vital importance to take the patient back to the time the condition *first* started and ascertain the primary site. By definition, the contact allergen must be in contact with this location to produce the dermatitis. It should be noted that both airborne and photocontact ACD will start on exposed areas (photocontact will tend to spare the submental and retroauricular areas).
- *Ascertain where the dermatitis has spread to.* ACD has the ability to spread, usually locally but occasionally distally as well, e.g. nickel ACD [4] on the earlobe spreading to the neck, ACD of the hand spreading up the arm, discoid dissemination of ACD from chromates in footwear. ACD to shoes can spread both locally and occasionally to the hands. Some forms of ACD, e.g. to nickel, have high susceptibility to undergo secondary spread [4]. Irritant contact dermatitis (ICD), in contrast, does not tend to spread.
- Ask the patient to *describe the rash.* The patient may complain of small or, more rarely, large blisters appearing. The dermatitis will often, in time, scale or have a drying effect.
- *What symptoms does the rash produce?* As with most other forms of dermatitis, pruritus is the main symptom but can vary in intensity from being barely present to burning/painful.
  - *Is the dermatitis a single event, intermittent or continuous?* Single-event ACD causes ACD after a single exposure. An example would be ACD to colophonium after exposure to adhesive tape. This is not strictly, in immunological terms, single exposure, as the patient would have required previous exposure to have immunological memory. They may have worn sticking plasters many years ago or could

[a] Levels of sensitization can also change through aging, which can alter sensitizing/regulatory immune functions favoring sensitization [3].

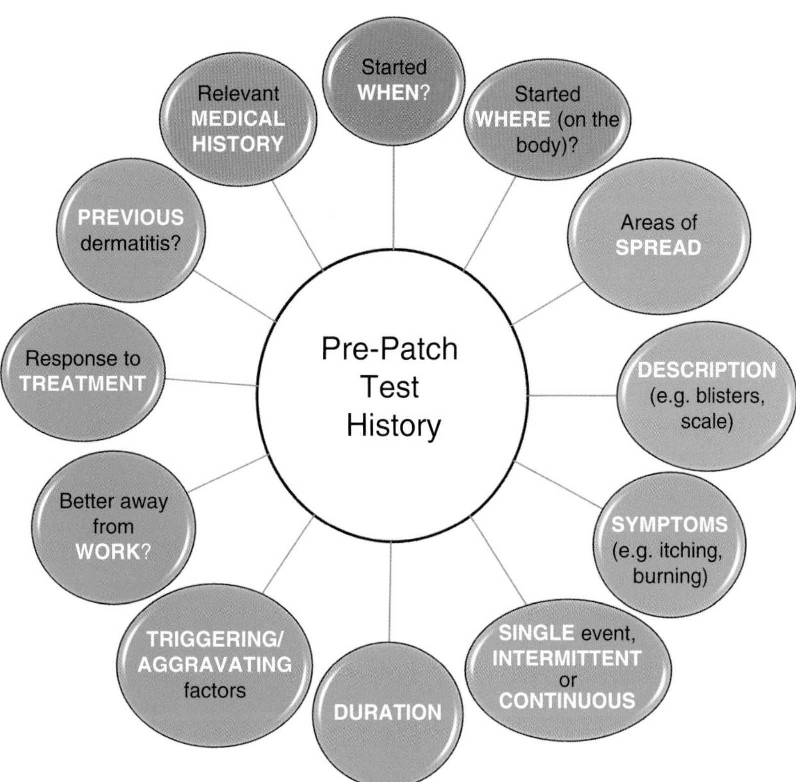

Figure 4.1 Pre-patch test history 1: characterization of the dermatitis/rash.

have been sensitized to colophonium from an alternative source. Intermittent ACD results from periodic exposure to the relevant allergen. Intermittent exposure can be defined as an exposure which does not occur on a daily basis. This can be subdivided into (i) regular intermittent exposure, e.g. dyeing hair every 4–6 weeks or riding a bike during the weekend, and (ii) irregular intermittent exposure, e.g. occasionally visiting a relative who has a primula plant, intermittent use of glues in fixing furniture around the house. Continuous ACD may be from daily exposure to cosmetic products, topical treatments, household goods, and agents in the domestic/work/leisure environment.

- *How long does the dermatitis last?* ACD tends to appear within 72 hours of exposure and lasts for days rather than hours or minutes.
- *Search further for triggering/aggravating factors.* These are more likely to be subtle than obvious.
- *Does the dermatitis get better away from work?* Ask about weekends and holidays. This will suggest an occupational element. However, the history may be misleading when there are multiple sources of exposure, e.g. airborne fragrance exposure both at work and at home.
- *What has been the response to treatment?* Eczema/dermatitis is usually responsive in some degree to topical/oral steroids. Medicament allergy can present as failure to respond to therapy/aggravation of dermatitis.
- *Previous dermatitis.* It is useful to establish a history of childhood atopic dermatitis, other previous dermatitis, and previous aggravating factors. Patients may present with idiopathic exacerbations of endogenous dermatitis such as seborrheic or atopic dermatitis. Occasionally, these exacerbations may be the clinical presentation of ACD. For example, MI ACD mimicking an exacerbation of seborrheic dermatitis. Patients with a long history of atopic dermatitis may be more at risk of developing ACD to topical medicaments.
- *General medical history and history of other non-dermatitic dermatological conditions.* Dermatitis may occur secondary to drugs or infections. ACD may complicate other dermatological diseases, e.g. psoriasis, leg ulceration.

The pre-patch test history: screening for potential allergen exposure

- The second part of the initial history consists of screening for potential allergen exposure, and any change in exposure, from different aspects of daily life (Figure 4.2). These include:
  a. use of personal care products (Table 4.1)
  b. agents in the domestic environment (excluding personal care products) (Table 4.2)
  c. agents in the work environment
  d. agents during travel and leisure pursuits (Table 4.3)
  e. medicament agents and medical/dental procedures
  f. use of personal appliances (Table 4.4)
  g. clothing, jewelry, and ornamentation (Table 4.5)
  h. agents in other environments.

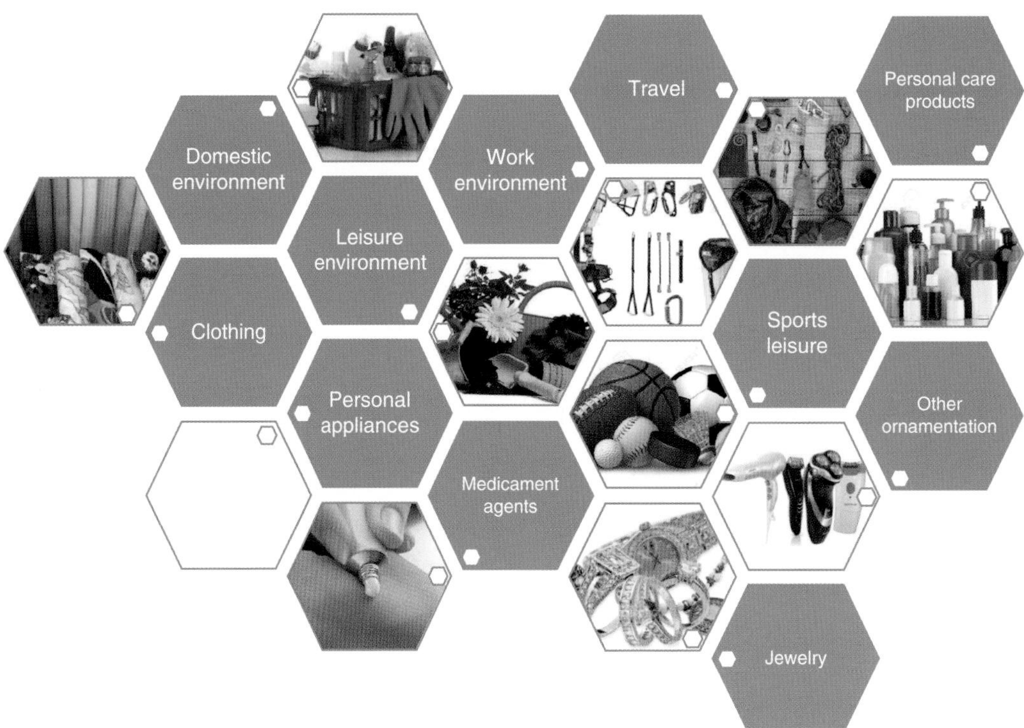

Figure 4.2 Pre-patch test history 2: screening for potential allergen exposure.

Personal care products

- Some examples of allergen exposure from personal care products, with reported clinical presentations, are given in Table 4.1.
- Although there is a multitude of chemicals in most cosmetics, the dominant allergens are preservatives, fragrances, and hair dye. It is also important to always ask about the wearing of nail varnish and the use of sculptured and stick-on nails.
- Different toiletries are usually used for specific parts of the body and can be leave-on or wash-off (including cleaning agents), and should be noted accordingly [5]. These include toiletries for the:
  a. scalp/hair
  b. eyes/periorbital region
  c. lips and mouth
  d. face (generally)
  e. hands
  f. nails
  g. feet
  h. genitals
  i. rest of the body, including the trunk and limbs.
- The environment in which the personal care product is applied may also influence exposure. For example, a woman, already silently sensitized to nail varnish resin, is applying nail varnish at leisure in her room. As she has plenty of time she is less likely to paint onto her nail fold and, therefore, is less likely to have an ACD reaction on the nail fold. However, prolonged exposure time to the resin fumes in a confined room makes her more likely to have an airborne periorbital ACD reaction. Conversely, the woman who hurriedly applies nail varnish on the train is more likely to smudge varnish onto the nail folds/periungual areas and, thus, is more likely to get an ACD involving the nail folds. However, the short application time in a relatively open area means that there is less airborne exposure to fumes and, therefore, a lower possibility of periorbital ACD reactions.
- Visits to the hairdresser/beautician/nail technician are an important source of personal care product exposure. The patient will usually not have immediate access to the product ingredients used.

Agents in the domestic environment

- This involves mainly housework and furnishings. Exposure to agents during childcare is mainly from personal care products, but there may also be some increased household product exposure. Cooking and gardening have, arbitrarily, been assigned to leisure (Table 4.3). Household decorating, household building, and furniture repair can lead to exposure to allergens and irritants akin to a building occupation. Car repair can also lead to allergen and irritant exposure akin to working as a mechanic.
- Questions such as “Is the housework performed regularly and how many times per week?” and “How many hours per week does the patient perform housework?” are of relevance. More hours worked over the course of a month will increase exposure to household goods and potentially increase the

Table 4.1 Some examples of reported allergens and clinical presentations of personal care product allergy.

Product	Reported allergens	Reported clinical manifestations
Shampoo	Fragrances MI MCI/MI Formaldehyde and the formaldehyde releasers; sodium lauryl ether sulfate [48] (probably a contained impurity) Cocamidopropyl betaine [49–51] Propylene glycol Vitamin E Parabens [52] Benzophenones Iodopropynylbutylcarbamate Methyldibromoglutaronitrile/phenoxyethanol Sodium *N*-methyl-*N*-(1-oxododecyl)-β-alaninate (anionic surfactant) [53] Zinc pyrithione [54] Ketoconazole [55] Selenium sulfide [56] Polidocanol (Laureth 9) [57] Triethanolamine polypeptide oleate [58] Disodium ricinoleamido MEA-sulfosuccinate [59] Captan Cocamide DEA (coconut DEA) Coco-betain Cocamidopropyl hydroxysultaine [60] Lauramide DEA Miranols [50] TEA-PEG-3 cocamide sulfate [61]	Dermatitis on the eyelids, face, forehead, neck, scalp [58], ears [60], postauricular area [59], upper trunk, and upper extremities [53, 62]; may extend to the abdomen [57] Facial edema and pruritus [55] Eyelid edema [52] Pustular psoriasis [54, 63]
Hair conditioner (the same allergens as shampoo but with these additional agents)	Panthenol [64]	Contact urticaria, facial swelling, erythema, and pruritus within a minute [64]
	Carvone/limonene [65]	Recurrent desquamative, red and itchy dermatitis on the preauricular cheeks [65]
	Protein hydrolysates [66, 67]	Contact urticaria [66, 67] (especially in atopic dermatitis) [66]
	Glutaraldehyde [68] (historical)	
Toothpaste	Cinnamyl alcohol [69] Benzyl alcohol [69] Cinnamal [69] Eugenol [69] L-carvone/limonene [69] Benzyl alcohol [69] Parabens [69] Fluoride [70] Cocamidopropyl betaine [71, 72] Triclosan [73] Peppermint oil [74] Aluminum hydroxide trihydrate [75][a] Aluminum hydroxide [75][a] Xantham gum [75][a] Menthol [75][a] Guar gum [75][a] Quinolone yellow [75][a] Benzalkonium chloride [75][a] Lemon balm [75][a] Anethole [76, 77] Azulene [77] Propolis [77] Isoeugenol [77] Spearmint oil [77] Vanillin [77]	Cheilitis: • upper and/or lower lip(s), angular area • constant or intermittent • 21% of ACD causing cheilitis reported to be due to toothpaste [69, 72, 74, 76] Blistering of buccal mucosa [73] Stomatitis [75] Glossitis [75] Perioral dermatitis [75] Immediate hypersensitivity [75] Dermatitis of the index finger [78]

(*Continued*)

Table 4.1 (Continued)

Product	Reported allergens	Reported clinical manifestations
Soap	MCI/MI [79, 80] Sodium cocoamphopropionate (a surfactant in disinfectant liquid soap) [81] Triclosan [82] Cocamidopropyl betaine and its impurities [83] Formaldehyde [84] Formaldehyde-releasing preservatives: • sodium hydroxymethylglycinate [85] • diazolidinylurea [86] 3-(dimethylamino) propylamine [87] Chloroxylenol (PCMX) [88] Methyldibromoglutaronitrile [89, 90] Sodium lauroyl sarcosinate [91] Undecylenamide diethanolamide [92] Fentichlor [93] (historical) Para-chloro-meta-xylenol [94] Monosulfiram (Tetmosol) [95] Irgasan [96] Lauryloxypropylamine [97] Metal salts: mercury (historical) [98] Halogenated salicylanilides [99] (historical) Lauryl ether sulfates [86] Cocamide DEA [86] Lauramide DEA [86] Chloroacetamide [86] Perfumes, musk ambrette [86] D&C Yellow No. 11(86) Lanolin [86] Colophonium [86] Parabens [100]	Sudden onset of follicular scaly pruritic papules, a few millimeters in size, on the periumbilical area, before spread to the back and arms [79] Hand eczema [101] Axillary dermatitis [92] Generalized dermatitis [86] Localized erythema multiforme-like lesions [102] Facial hyperpigmentation [86] Contact photoallergy [86, 93, 99] Immunological contact urticaria [82] Occupational contact dermatitis: • recurrent hand eczema [81, 83, 88, 89] • occasional sites of dermatitis include the scalp, flexures, forearms, wrist, face, and neck [83, 86, 91]
Deodorant/ antiperspirant	Benzethonium chloride [103] Usnic acid [104] Methenamine [105] Propanthine bromide Lanolin Paraben esters [106] Bisabolol (from German chamomile) [107] MI [108] Fragrances [109] HICC [110, 111] Alkyl glucosides [112] Aluminum [113] Hydrogenated castor oil [114, 115] Citronella oil [116] Farnesol [117] Zirconium [118, 119] Lichen acid mix [120] Zinc ricinoleate [121] Chloroacetamide [122] Propyl gallate [123] Cetearyl alcohol [124] Triclosan (Irgasan DP 300) [96, 103] Propellants: • trichloromonofluoromethane (Freon 11) [125] • dichlorofluoromethane (Freon 12) [125, 126] Stearamidoethyl diethylamine phosphate [127] Vitamin E [128]	Eczema on the contact areas, usually axilla and/or groin Usually bilateral axillary dermatitis, particularly of the vaults; if severe, may spread down the arms and trunk [129] Allergic granulomas (to metal salts) [118, 119] Urticaria-like lesions in the axilla and adjacent thorax [124] Scrotal and penile dermatitis from exposure by proxy to feminine hygiene spray (deodorant) Unilateral left forearm and upper arm ACD from by proxy exposure to fragrance from partner's deodorant Pigmented contact dermatitis [130] – very pronounced, reticulate, violet-brown pigmented macules surrounding a smooth, greyish, atrophic area in the axillae; patch test + to fragrance mix 1 May cause a pre-existing endogenous axillary dermatitis to flare [129] Acute dermatitis of the foot where deodorant/antiperspirant was applied [105] Pruritus may be an early sign of developing ACD Irritant dermatitis is common Deodorants may be the most common source of sensitization and ACD to fragrance [109]

Table 4.1 (Continued)

Product	Reported allergens	Reported clinical manifestations
Perfume [131]	*Myroxylon pereirae* Fragrance mix I (geraniol, cinnamal, cinnamyl alcohol, isoeugenol, eugenol, hydroxycitronellal, amyl cinnamal, oak moss, sorbitan sesquioleate) Fragrance mix II (HICC, citral, farnesol, coumarin, citronellol, hexyl cinnamal), essential oils (tea tree oil, peppermint oil, lavender oil, ylang-ylang oil, jasmine absolute), sandalwood oil, *evernia prunastri*, bergamot oil Propolis "Emerging" fragrance allergens: hydroperoxides of linalool, oxidized limonene Sources of fragrance-related airborne ACD: plants, citrus fruits, essential oils Occupational: • healthcare workers: *Myroxylon pereirae* in soaps, antiseptic cleansers, emollient creams • dentists: eugenol in mouthwashes, dressings, impression materials and periodontal packings • food handlers: cinnamal, cinnamic alcohol, *Myroxylon pereirae* in spices and essential oils • beauticians • hairdressers Hobbies: soapmaking (airborne ACD)	Distribution: • any part of the body can be affected • "atomizer sign": axilla, face, hands, neck • well-circumscribed areas: wrist, behind the ear, neck • widespread: nummular pattern to erythroderma, airborne ACD • Men and individuals with a history of atopic dermatitis are more likely to have scattered and generalized lesions Presentations: • most common presentation is patchy dermatitis with eczematous papules • vesicles • chronic forms: lichenified pruritic plaques • itch • contact urticaria • delayed hypersensitivity • ICD • photo-allergic dermatitis • pustular lesions [132] • pigmented contact dermatitis, Berloque dermatitis • by proxy: unilateral, bizarre or irregular distribution; no obvious pattern to flare of eczema • systemic contact dermatitis • respiratory tract irritation • asthma exacerbation
Eye makeup remover	Sodium cocoamphoacetate [133] Cocamidopropyl betaine [134] Derivatives of cocamidopropyl betaine [135] Can also contain benzyl alcohol, propylene glycol, colorants, botanical agents, preservatives, fragrance	Facial dermatitis [133] Eyelid dermatitis [134, 135]
Mascara	Carba mix Rosin (colophonium) [106, 136] PPD in tinting mascara [137] Shellac [138–140] Quaternium-22 [141] Prime yellow carnauba wax [142] Coathylene [142] Black iron oxide [143] Yellow iron oxide [144] Can also contain propylene glycol, carnauba wax, isopropyl myristate, fragrance, preservatives including MI	Eyelid dermatitis [138, 144] with [143]/without periorbital dermatitis Upper and lower eyelid but predominant upper eyelid involvement is sometimes possible [140] Eyelids and periorbital involvement/spread [144] Periorbital edema [129] Loss of eyelashes [137] Associated conjunctivitis Irritant dermatitis can occur [129]
Eyeliner	1,3-butylene glycol and shellac [145] Nickel [146] Can also contain fragrance, coloring agents, carnauba wax	Recurrent severe itchy swelling of the eyelids, followed by erythema and scaling Irritant dermatitis can occur [129] Eyelid dermatitis
Eyeshadow	Colophonium [129, 136] Nickel [147] (controversial) Lanolin [129] Can also contain tocopherol acetate, sorbitan sesquioleate, coloring agents, fragrance	Eyelid dermatitis and edema; can occasionally spread to involve the whole face [129]
Eyelash curler	Nickel [148] Rubber accelerators Black rubber [149]	Bilateral upper eyelid dermatitis Not suspected by the patient Can spread from eyelids to other areas of the face [149]
Eye cream (see also face creams/ moisturisers)	Vitamin K1 [150] Chloroacetamide sodium benzoate Can also contain fragrances, preservatives, botanical agents	Bilateral eyelid dermatitis

(*Continued*)

Table 4.1 (Continued)

Product	Reported allergens	Reported clinical manifestations
Lip balm/lipstick	Lip balm: • carnauba wax [151, 152] • propolis [152] Lipstick: • candelilla wax [153] • benzophenone [154] • glyceryl monoisostearate monomyristate [155] • gallate: propyl gallate [156–158], dodecyl gallate [159], octyl gallate [160] • lanolin alcohols [161] • balsams [161] • dithiodimorpholine [161] • microcrystalline wax [161] • D&C Red No. 7 [162] • pentaerythritol rosinate [163] • ester gum [164] • ricinoleic acid [164] • 2-hexyldecanoic acid (isopalmitate) [165] • glyceryl ricinoleate [121] • ditrimethylolpropane triethylhexanoate [166] • bisabolol [167] • polyvinylpyrrolidone/hexadecene copolymer [167] • propylene glycol ricinoleate [168] • di-isostearyl malate [169] • macademia nut oil [169] • isopalmityl diglyceryl sebacate [170] • oleyl alcohol [171]	Cheilitis [29, 151, 153–156, 158, 162–164, 166] Perioral dermatitis [161] Pseudoangioedema: edema of the periorbital areas, lips, nose and face [161] Contact leukoderma [157, 172] Allergic contact stomatitis [159]
Nail varnish	Tosylamide formaldehyde resin (TSFR) [173, 174] Phthalic anhydride/trimellitic anhydride/glycols copolymer [175, 176] Nitrocellulose [177] Benzophenone-2 (nail varnish remover) [178] Acrylates Colophonium Metal in glitter Adipic acid	Dermatitis of the eyelids [179], chin, cheeks, lower half of the face, anterior/lateral sides of the neck [177], upper chest [180], periungual and perianal areas [174] Cheilitis [181] Eyelid dermatitis with periorbital discoid lupus erythematosus [182] Seborrheic dermatitis-like eruption [180] Note: because nail varnish is usually used as a barrier coat on nickel-containing metals [183], it is a potential allergen in patients with nickel allergy [184].
Wet wipes	MI [185–188] (historical) MCI/MI [189, 190] (historical) Polyhexamethylene biguanide [191] Polyaminopropyl biguanide [192] Panthenol [193] Quaternium-15(188) Sodium hydroxymethylglycinate [85] Methyldibromoglutaronitrile [194] Iodopropynyl butylcarbamate [195] Disinfectant; *N*-benzyl-*N*,*N*-dihydroxyethyl-*N*-cocosalkyl-ammonium chloride [196] Note: 2-bromo-2-nitropropane-1,3-diol is a potential allergen and is a common ingredient but contact allergy from wet wipes has not been reported	Eczema at the sites of contact, e.g. face [185, 193], hands [186, 195, 197], vulvar [198], and perianal areas [195, 199–201] Forehead, cheeks and periorbital areas Dyshidrotic eczema of the hands [201] Contact urticaria syndrome [192] Lymphomatoid contact dermatitis [188]

DEA, diethanolamide; HICC, hydroxyisohexyl 3-cyclohexene carboxaldehyde; MCI, methylchloroisothiazolinone; MI, methylisothiazolinone; PCMX, *p*-chloro-*m*-xylenol; TSFR, tosylamide formaldehyde resin.

[a] Reported as contained in the product rather than as a case report, false eyelash glue – cyanoacrylate, eyelash and eyebrow tints – same as for hair dye allergens.

dose of allergen (and irritant) exposure. Specific tasks need to be probed, together with identifying which agents are used – dish washing, floor surface cleaning, dusting, hoovering, waxing, polishing, and window cleaning.

- Wearing of gloves and the type of gloves should be recorded.
- Temporal aspects can be important, e.g. relatives or friends coming to visit and stay may be preceded by an increase in housework. Some patients undertake periodic thorough house cleaning or "spring cleaning."
- Poorly ventilated rooms can lead to an increase in airborne exposure to household agents such as bleach and fragrance in air fresheners.

Table 4.2 Some examples of reported sensitizers in the domestic environment.

Domestic environment	Reported allergens[a]	Reported clinical manifestations
Washing-up liquid	Geraniol [202] Coconut DEA [203] MI [204] Limonene MCI/MI 2-bromo-2-nitropropane-1,3-diol Cocamidopropyl betaine Linalool Hexyl cinnamal Butylphenylmethylpropional [205][b]	Hand dermatitis [202, 203] with [203]/without forearm involvement
Scented products, air freshener, scented candles	Volatile organic compounds: fragrances [206–208] such as limonene [209–211], linalool [212], chamomile [213] Biocides: BIT (reported in occupational contact allergy) [214]	ACD [207] Photoallergic reaction [207] Airborne contact dermatitis [207] Occupational contact dermatitis can cause eczema on the face, hands, forearms, and feet [214]. Others (may be non-allergic): acute rhinitis [213], respiratory tract irritation, asthma [215], headache, vomiting [206] Scented products can trigger the symptoms of patients with unexplained multimorbidity with sensitivities (but not usually allergic) [216].
Wall paints/ decorations	Isothiazolinones [217]: • MI [218–220] • benzisothiazolinone [221] • octylisothiazolinone [222] MCI/MI [223] Aliphatic polyisocyanates based on HDI [224] Triglycidyl isocyanurate [225] Trimethylolpropane triacrylate (UV-cured paint) [226] Acrylates (lacquers for wood surface coating) [227] HDI [228] iodopropynyl butylcarbamate [229] Chloroacetamide [230]	Airborne ACD [218, 220] Acute severe facial dermatitis and airway difficulty [219] Hypersensitivity pneumonitis [225] Occupational airborne contact allergy: • occupational conjunctivitis [226] • occupational asthma [225] • acute life-threatening extrinsic allergic alveolitis [228]
Sofa	Dimethylfumarate [231] Chromate PTBP-FR MI (contained in leather care product) [232]	Generalized eczematous lesions with lichenification on both the arms and trunk, but most prominently on the buttocks, the posterior sides of both thighs, and the dorsolateral aspects of the lower legs [232] Severe, pruritic, papulovesicular, eczematous dermatitis affecting sites of contact with the sofa (back, arms, and thighs) [231] Blistering and lichenoid eruptions were also observed A few patients presented with contact urticaria, worsening of pre-existing asthma, wheezing and sneezing, especially when on or around the chair or sofa Patients complained of itching and stinging shortly after sitting on the chair or sofa or when entering the room with the furniture, and even thick covers may not prevent the rash from flaring [233] Widespread leukoderma affecting the back, lasting 2 years after withdrawal of the sofa [234] Resistant to treatment [235]
Toilet seat	Pine [236] Teak [237] Plastic [238] Varnish/rosin [239] Polyurethane foam/isocyanates [240]	Buttock and thigh dermatitis, usually sharply defined and arciform in a toilet seat distribution [236] Variants: pseudolymphomatoid morphology [237] Psoriasiform dermatitis [238] Can be caused by irritant dermatitis from harsh cleansers [241]
Wax polish	Dipentene [242] Colophonium	Highly pruritic erythematous scaly lesions with hyperkeratotic fissures on the digital pulps, periungual, and hypothenar areas of the right hand (one case report: the patient had worked as a car mechanic and painter) [242]

(Continued)

Table 4.2 (Continued)

Domestic environment	Reported allergens[a]	Reported clinical manifestations
Cleaning products	Fragrances: oxidized D-limonene [209, 243], geraniol, linalool, hexyl cinnamal, butylphenyl methylpropional [205], pinene [244], hydroxycitronellal [245] Eugenol [244] Disinfectants: aldehydes (glutaraldehyde, ortho-phthaldehyde) [244] Preservatives: formaldehyde [246], sodium hydroxymethylglycinate [85], isothiazolinones [244], MCI/MI, 2-bromo-2-nitropropane-1,3-diol [205], 1,2-benzisothiazolin-3-one [205] Solvents: propylene glycol and glycol ethers [247, 248] Water softeners: EDTA (uncertain mechanism but irritant is unlikely) [249] Quaternary ammonium compounds: benzalkonium chloride [244] Amine compounds: monoethanolamine [244] Chloramines T [244] Chlorine-irritant [250] Acryl polymers, polyethylene (in waxes in film formers and polishes to provide surface care) [244] Microbial enzymes [251] (type 1 allergy) Surfactants: cocamidopropyl betaine [205]	Most cleaning agents irritate the mucous membranes and skin, and occasionally cause sensitization [244]. ACD, eczema [248] Respiratory symptoms: occupational asthma and rhinitis (can be either irritant or allergic reactions) [244, 249, 252–256]
Washing powder	Tinopal CH 3566 (an optical whitener) [257] Chromate (alkaline sourcing agents) note controversial [258] Proteolytic enzymes (improve the cleaning efficacy of washing powders) [259–264]	Textile dermatitis [257] Pigmented contact dermatitis [265] Perioral dermatitis [266] Asthma and rhinitis; occupational (healthcare) [259] and consumer [263]

BIT, 1,2-benzisothiazolin-3-one; EDTA, ethylenediamine tetraacetic acid; HDI, hexamethylene di-isocyanate; MCI, methylchloroisothiazolinone; MI, methylisothiazolinone; PTBP-FR, *p*-tert-butyl-phenol formaldehyde resin.

[a] Limonene is a potential allergen and is widely used as a fragrance in many leave-on cosmetic and household products such as machine-cleaning detergents, surface cleaners, dishwashing liquids, and hand cleansers [209–211].

[b] Reported as contained in the products rather than actual case report.

- Exposure to household agents may contribute to multiple sources of allergen exposure, e.g. fragrance exposure from personal care products (shampoo, perfume spray), household products (cleaning agents, air fresheners), and in the work environment (e.g. liquid soap).
- ACD from furnishings will usually not be apparent to the patient. Household maintenance, known in some countries as 'do-it-yourself', can lead to exposure to potential allergens, e.g. in glues and paint.

Occupational exposure

- The occupational relevance for each standard allergen is covered in Section 3, chapters 10–36. Detailed descriptions of occupational dermatitis can be found in specialized texts. Some principles and specific examples are given here.
- A specific part of the history refers to occupation. "Is the dermatitis better away from work?" However, this can cover different time periods such as:
  a. the weekend
  b. several days off between shifts
  c. a holiday of one to several weeks
  d. prolonged absence from work (often health-related).

  Short periods such as the weekend or a few days may not be long enough for an improvement in ACD to be noticed.
- Irritant dermatitis tends to fade and return more slowly than allergic dermatitis.
- As a very rough generalization, irritant dermatitis may tend to affect more work personnel than ACD.
- A substitute for a workplace visit is for the patients to bring in photographs on their mobile phone (though some workplaces forbid the use of photography).
- During history taking, the patient may use terms which are specific or even unique to his workplace and not familiar to the doctor. Time may be needed for clarification.
- A detailed description of washing facilities and agents should be garnered. Inadequate hygiene may lead to hazardous levels of exposure to work-related allergens and irritants. In contrast, over-washing and excessive exposure to liquid soaps and cleaning agents may also lead to ICD.
- A detailed history of protective clothing should be taken. Inadequate protective clothing can predispose to contact dermatitis. For example, gaps between a glove and sleeve cover may leave the skin unprotected against irritants and allergens.

Table 4.3 Some examples of allergens in leisure pursuits, their sources and clinical features in previous reports.

Leisure activity	Source	Reported allergens	Reported clinical manifestations
Swimming[a]	Swimming pool water (disinfectant)	Chlorinated water: Di-Halo®, sodium hypochlorite, lithium hypochlorite [267] Bromine-based disinfectant (spa pool water): Halobrome® [268] Both chlorine and bromine: BCDMH [269]	Recurrent generalized eczema with pruritic papules and vesicles within 6–24 hours after swimming
	Flocculant	Aluminum chloride [270]	Severe itching over the entire body and rash
	An oxidizing agent used to "shock" hot tubs and swimming pools	Potassium peroxymonosulfate [271]	Itchy erythematous macules, papules, and patches on the trunk and extremities within 12 hours
	Swim fins	DPPD [272]	Recurrent eczema on the dorsal aspects of both feet and thighs
	Swimming cap	MBT [273]	
	Swimming goggles	Black foam rubber padding [274] Phenol-formaldehyde resin, benzoyl peroxide [275] Thiourea derivatives [276] IPPD, CPPD, DPPD [277]	Severe itching, erythema, swelling of the eyelids and periorbital skin, minimal conjunctivitis [274, 275]
Diving[a]/snorkeling[a]	Diving suit, wet suit	Thiourea derivatives: diethylthiourea [278, 279], dibutylthiourea [280], diphenylthiourea [281] PTBP-FR [17, 282] Zinc diethyldithiocarbamate [282] Nickel [283] (controversial) Tego 103G disinfectant [284]	Dermatitis on the whole body, especially the axillary folds and groin but sparing the face, hands and feet [278] Generalized itchy erythematous vesicular eruption [282] Itchy, scaly erythematous rash on the contact sites with a clear cut-off at non-exposure areas [284]
	Diving mask	BT-DEC, thiuram mix, TMTM [285] IPPD [286]	Pruritic, erythematous and scaly facial dermatitis at the contact areas [285] Recurrent facial itching and redness within 10 minutes [286]
	Diver's footgear	Dibutylthiourea [287]	
Running[a]/jogging[a]/ walking[a]	Shoes	Ethylbutylthiourea [288] MBT Dibenzothiazole disulfide [289]	
	Creams	Eucalyptus [290] Arnica Palmitoyl hydrolysed milk Palmitoyl collagen amino acids Lipacide-cas [291]	
	Athletic tape and adhesive	PTBP-FR [292]	
Cycling[a]	Bicycle handgrips	*N*-isopropyl-*N*-phenyl-4-phenylenediamine (main sensitizer in black rubber) [293]	Severe pruritic erythematous vesicles on the palms and flexural aspects of the fingers, recurrent dyshidrosiform eruption [293]
	Anti-chafing cream	MI [204]	Groin dermatitis [204]
Gardening[a]	Plants	Published examples include: *Fabaceae* family, runner bean (allergen = diallyl disulfide) [294]	Contact urticaria, swelling of the face, anterior neck, dorsal aspects of hands, and arms [294]
		Acanthaceae family, *Pachystachys lutea* (golden shrimp plant, lollipop plant) [295]	Dermatitis on the dorsal aspects of the fingers and hands with spread to the forearms, face, chest, and thighs [295]
		Anacardiaceae family, *Toxicodendron succedaneum* (rhus tree) [296]	Facial dermatitis (in younger patients) Dermatitis on the upper limbs (in older patients)
		Araceae family, *Zantedeschia aethiopica* [297]	Pruritus, erythema, and edema of both hands [297]
		Araliaceae family, *Hedera helix* [298–301]	Acute linear edematous and vesiculobullous lesions on both arms and legs [298], hand dermatitis, extensive dermatitis

(Continued)

Table 4.3 (Continued)

Leisure activity	Source	Reported allergens	Reported clinical manifestations
		Compositae (*Asteraceae*) family [302, 303], e.g. asters, sunflowers, daisies	Edematous dermatitis on both hands and distal forearms [303] ACD
	Gloves	Thiuram and other rubber accelerators Potassium dichromate [302]	Severe chronic vesicular hand eczema [302]
	Fertilizer (plant growth regulator)	Cyanamide (Dormex) [304]	Intensely pruritic, severe vesicles and bullae on the left hand, right wrist, chin, and right ear
Cooking	Examples include: • pizza • olives [306]	Diallyl disulfide Ammonium persulfate [305]	Hand eczema [305]
			Contact urticaria [306] Recurrent eczema of the hands, ventral forearms, and elbows [307]
	Garlic	Diallyl disulfide	Hand dermatitis [308–312] Systemic contact dermatitis [313] Airborne ACD [314]
	Fish [315], wheat flour [316], asparagus [317], coriander [318], fresh foods [319]	Protein	Protein contact dermatitis [315–318] Contact urticaria ACD
	Churros (fritter) making [320]	Nickel	Itching, scaling, redness and vesicles on the right forearm and fingers of the left hand
	Bakery	Sodium metabisulfite [321] Dodecyl gallate [321] Emulsifying agent [322]	Dermatitis of both hands with [322]/ without [321] forearm involvement
	Cakes	Sodium carboxymethyl cellulose (sodium cellulose glycolate) [323]	Recurrent hand dermatitis
Musical instruments	Brass, flute	Exotic woods Flavonoids in exotic rose wood Brass Metals Nickel [324]	Eczema on the contact sites: mouth, face, and hands
	Trumpet, cornet	Thiuram [325] Nickel [326]	Recurrent lip swelling [325], cheilitis [326]
	Violin, viola	Chin rest: exotic woods, varnishes (propolis) [327], nickel [328, 329], PPD [330] Violin bow: rubber [331] Strings: rosin (colophonium) [332, 333], metals [333] Fingerboards: ebony wood [327, 334] Others: turpentine [334], as part of polysensitization, [335] chromium, PPD [336]	Fiddler's neck [330, 334]: supraclavicular neck dermatitis, a lichenified plaque below the left angle of the mandible [328] Fiddler's finger [329] Hand dermatitis [331]
	Guitar	Nickel (guitar strings) [337, 338] Chromium PPD [336]	Eczema on the fingertips of the left hand
	Tuba	Nickel (possible: palladium, cobalt) [339]	Cheilitis
	Saxophone, clarinet	Wood reed [340] Cane reed, *arundo donax* [341, 342]	Cheilitis [340, 341]
	Cello	Nickel Chromate Colophonium Propolis PPD [336, 343]	Finger dermatitis (right thumb, index, and middle finger) [343]
	Recorder	African blackwood [344]	Cheilitis
	Violin and cello	Rosin (colophony) [345]	Dry, fissured hand dermatitis
	Others	Woodwind instruments: nickel, exotic woods, cane reeds Brass instruments: nickel, chromium [336]	

Table 4.3 (Continued)

Leisure activity	Source	Reported allergens	Reported clinical manifestations
Contact Sport	Shin guards[b][346]	Thiourea Carbamix Mercaptomix Black rubber mix *n*-(cyclohexylthio)phtalimide Urea-formaldehyde resin Azo dyes	Bilateral eruption involving the anterior shins coinciding with the areas of contact Can be extremely pruritic, vesicular Can spread to other areas of the lower legs

BCDMH, 1-bromo-3-chloro-5,5-dimethyl hydantoin; BT-DEC, 2-benzothiazolyl-*N*,*N*-diethylthiocarbamylsulfide; CPPD, *N*-cyclohexyl-*N*-phenyl-1,4-phenylenediamine; DPPD, *N*,*N*-diphenyl-1,4-paraphenylenediamine; IPPD, *N*-isopropyl-*N*-phenylparaphenylenediamine; MBT, mercaptobenzothiazole; MI, methylisothiazolinone; PTBP-FR, *p*-tert-butylphenol formaldehyde resin; PPD, *p*-phenylenediamine; TMTM, tetramethylthiuram monosulfide.

[a] Contact allergy to sunscreen is possible for all outdoor hobbies.

[b] Can be irritant in etiology [347, 348].

Table 4.4 Some examples of causative agents and clinical presentations of ACD to personal appliances.

Personal appliance	Reported allergens	Reported clinical manifestations
Spectacle frames	Nickel [349] Palladium [350] Plasticisers: • triethylene glycol *bis*-(2-ethylhexanoate) [351] • triphenyl phosphate [352] • tricresyl phosphate [353] • solvent Orange 60 dye [354] Ultraviolet inhibitors: • phenylsalicylate [355, 356] • resorcinol monobenzoate [356] Agents for polishing spectacle frames: • colophonium [357] • turpentine [358] *p*-tert-butyl phenol [359] Aliphatic isocyanate (wax) [360] Abietic acid Diethyl phthalate Anthraquinone Brown-black dye Butyl acrylate Epoxy resin Ethylene glycol monomethyl ether acetate Methylethylketone (solvents) [353] Disperse azo dyes [361] Cellulose acetate (plastic) [353] Tea tree oil (passively transferred by spectacles to cause eyelid dermatitis) [362] MI [363]	Retroauricular dermatitis: [354] • the most common form of presentation • can be chronic and persistent • can spread (in one case to the dorsal aspects of the hands and chest) [351] • can be severe, exudative [354] • important complications: ear cellulitis and facial erysipelas [351] Dermatitis on both sides of the nose bridge [355] Dermatitis involving the medial eyebrows, lower forehead and cheeks [353] Persistent bilateral temporal region eczema [351] Leukoderma of the temporal and retroauricular areas [359] Repeated facial edema [364] Repeated facial erysipelas [365] Eyelid dermatitis [362] Tip: Test scrapings from the spectacle frame in pet. with a large (12 mm) chamber
Contact lenses	Merthiolate [366] Thimerosal [367] 2-hydroxyethyl-acrylate [368] Triethylene glycol diacrylate [369] Phenyl mercuric nitrate Ammoniated mercury Benzethonium chloride Disodium cocoamphodipropionate [370] Antimicrobial agents [371]	Allergic contact conjunctivitis without dermatitis [366] Itching and burning of the eyes Watery discharge from the eyes Eyelid dermatitis [370] Localized dyshidrosiform vesicles limited to a palm and index fingertip without eye or eyelid involvement [367] Recurrent localized hand dermatitis [368] Systemic allergic dermatitis of the lips
Hearing aids	Acrylics [372, 373]: polyethylene glycol dimethacrylate [372], 2-hydroxyethyl methacrylate [372], methylmethacrylate monomer [374, 375], triethyleneglycol dimethacrylate [376], urethane dimethacrylate [376] Finish coat [372] PTBP-FR [377] Gold [378] Benzyl alcohol [379] Epoxy resin [380] Plastic mold [378] Cochlear implantation: silicone [381] polyethylene terephthalate mesh [382]	Localized dermatitis on the auricular and preauricular areas [375, 378] and/or otitis externa (can be acute or chronic) [372, 375, 376, 383] Dermatitis over the skin flap (cochlear implantation) [382]

(Continued)

Table 4.4 (Continued)

Personal appliance	Reported allergens	Reported clinical manifestations
Earplugs	Mercaptobenzothiazole, tetramethylthiuram disulfide (rubber earplugs) [384] Azodicarbonamide [385]	Localized eczema [384] Recurrent bilateral otitis externa [385]
Bindi	PVC PTBP-FR Epoxy resins Disperse Blue 124 Disperse Blue 106 Nickel [386] Thimerosal and gallate mix [387, 388] Sandalwood ("chandan" bindi) [389]	Erythema [390] Eczema [387, 390, 391] Contact leukoderma [387, 390] Hyperpigmentation [390]: slate gray pigmentation with erythema, infiltration and papulation; circumscribed pigmented macular lesion [389] Foreign body granuloma [390]
Mobile phones	Nickel [392–397] Chromium [392, 398] Cobalt [394] Cell phone cover: plastics and glues [399]	Dermatitis on the contact sites: unilateral ear, lateral cheek, preauricular [400], and/or unilateral facial dermatitis [399, 401], anterolateral aspects of both thighs Bilateral symmetrical facial and outer thigh dermatitis has been reported in a patient using two mobile phones [402]. Dermatitis on the legs (related to carrying a mobile phone in pockets) [403] Intermittent pruritic scaly papules below the umbilicus and between both breasts [404] Breast eczema (where mobile phone carried) [405]
Computer accessories	Plastic components of the computer mouse: • diethyl phthalate [406] • dimethyl phthalate • resorcinol monobenzoate (a UV absorber) [407] Mouse pad/mat [408]: neoprene rubber – diphenyl thiourea Keyboard wrist rest pad [409–411]: • neoprene rubber • mercaptans • thiurams • dialkyl thiourea	Pruritic, scaly, erythematous, vesicular patches and plaques on the palmar side of the hand(s) directly in contact with the allergens (may be unilateral or bilateral) [412]

MI, methylisothiazolinone; PTBP-FR, *p*-tert-butylphenol formaldehyde resin; PVC, polyvinylchloride.

- Conversely, protective equipment can also cause ACD. This includes masks (resins, thioureas, rubber accelerators, methylhydroxystearate, silicone rubber, contamination with disinfectant, promotion of ACD through an occlusive effect) [6–13], protective clothing (dyes, resins, biocides) [14–18], shoes/boots [19], and gloves. [20]
- Gloves are not always effective barriers to contact allergens. For example, latex gloves are a poor barrier to MI permeation when compared to nitrile gloves [21]. Vinyl and latex gloves gave poor prevention against the penetration of *p*-phenylenediamine (PPD) over 60 minutes when compared to nitrile gloves [22].
- Sparing of an area of the face that is covered (e.g. by masks) may lead to a suspicion of airborne contact dermatitis.
- A past history of atopic dermatitis predisposes to work-related ICD. Skin atopy has been estimated to at least double the skin effects of occupational irritants [23]. Whether there is also a predisposition to ACD in some circumstances is a more controversial issue [24].
- Conversely, occupational irritant and ACD can, in some circumstances, reactivate atopic dermatitis [25, 26].

Travel and leisure pursuits

- *Hobbies*: These are numerous but most do involve some exposure to contact allergens and irritants (see Table 4.3).
- *Cars*: Examples of ACD related to cars are given below.
  a. A woman developed generalized truncal eczema from ACD to uncured epoxy resin in her car seat [27]. Leather and plastic chemicals may also be present.
  b. A man with intractable palm eczema had ACD from the plastic chemical resorcinol monobenzoate in his car steering wheel [28]. He was also patch test positive to *Myroxylon pereirae*, which contains resorcinol monobenzoate.
  c. A 53-year-old woman developed dermatitis on her left shoulder where her skin was in contact with a blue car safety belt. She was patch test positive to Disperse Blue 106 and Disperse Dye 153 [29].
  d. Car windscreen repair kits commonly contain acrylates as contact allergens. ACD often presents as widespread fingertip dryness, vesicles, and desquamation. Sometimes, only the thumb and adjacent finger of the dominant hand

Table 4.5 Some examples of reported allergens and clinical features of ACD related to clothing and personal ornamentation.

Clothing/ ornamentation	Reported allergen	Common sources	Reported clinical manifestations
Textiles [45, 413]	Disperse dyes [414]	Non-cellulosic fibers (acetate polyester, nylon, cellulose acetate triacetate fibers)	Most common: extremities (upper > lower) especially the hands, followed by the trunk, face, genitals, buttocks, and folds Often atypical and polymorphic presentations: • persistent or transient erythematous wheals • generalized pruritus with excoriations [47] • prurigo-like eczema • diffuse itching • erythema multiforme-like eruptions • purpuric dermatitis • pigmented contact dermatitis [47] • nummular dermatitis • erythroderma • pseudolymphoma Some Disperse Orange dyes are primary active sensitizers presenting with late patch test reactions at 10 or more days
		Textile necklace [415]	Dermatitis around the neck Recall dermatitis on the neck after patch testing has been reported in a patient with orange/yellow textile necklace allergy The patch test showed +++ positive reactions to PPD, Disperse Orange 1 and Disperse Yellow 3 as well as a ++ positive reaction to Disperse Yellow 9 [415].
	Reactive dyes	Natural fibers (wool, silk, 100% cotton and linen), rayon, polyamides	Acute and explosive dermatitis [44], chronic subacute dermatitis [47] Common sites [45]: areas with frequent perspiration and friction: • bed linens, furniture: upper back, posterior thighs • apparel: antecubital folds, popliteal folds, medial thighs, anterior and posterior axillary lines, waistbands, posterior neck and upper back
	Sodium metabisulfite (used in bleaching and dyeing jeans)	Jeans	
	Rubber chemicals: carbamates, thiurams, mercaptobenzothiazole	Elastic (these allergens are generally not found in Spandex, except for mercaptobenzothiazole in Elastane®)	
	Chromates (trivalent and hexavalent chromium)	Tanned leather	
	Cobalt	Metallic dyes	
	Corticosteroids, propylene glycol, lanolin, bacitracin, neomycin, and other components of topical medicaments	Mesh of bras, knitted parts of socks, and rarely washed garments like jackets	
	Formaldehyde resins [44]	Cellulosic fibers (wool, cotton, rayon)	Subacute and chronic dermatitis Typical sites: confined only to the areas where the clothes fit snugly: • dermatitis of the anterior and posterior axillary folds, sparing the vault • atypical presentation: papular and follicular lesions [47]
Watch straps	PTBP-FR [416]	Leather adhesive	Band-like vesicular dermatitis on the wrist Non-eczematous interface/lichenoid dermatitis confined to the area of the watch strap (from PTBP-FR) [416]
	Formaldehyde [417]	Leather watch strap in small amounts	
	Nickel, cobalt	Buckle	
	Others: • Chromate • PPD mix • DPPD and CPPD [418] • IPPD [419] • Dyes		

(Continued)

Table 4.5 (Continued)

Clothing/ ornamentation	Reported allergen	Common sources	Reported clinical manifestations
Hats	Chromate PTBP resin Dyes		Dermatitis on hat band area
Wedding/ engagement rings	Nickel Cobalt Gold Palladium Iridium [420] Platinum, mercury [421]		Dermatitis under ring area Irritant (e.g. liquid soap, washing-up liquid may get under the ring, causing ICD; other allergens can also get occluded under the ring, causing dermatitis (e.g. fragrance) [422] Umbilical rings can also cause ACD with spread to the adjacent areas of the abdomen [423] When ring dermatitis occurs, patients will often change their rings to another finger, where ACD also develops [421].
Earrings [424, 425]	Nickel Cobalt Gold Silver Platinum Palladium		Earlobe adjacent to pierced area May react to post worn after intial piercing, and/or to earrings Secondary spread to periauricular areas One case showed dermatitis sparing the earlobe but affecting the neck inferior and slightly posterior to the ear; here, the hoop of the earring was nickel positive but the post part, fitting inside the pierced earlobe, was negative for nickel [426] A report of persisting granulomatous lesions [427] Can be irritant dermatitis (shampoo infiltrates pierced area) ACD to metal earrings can become secondarily infected/impetiginized [424] The risk of metal allergy increases statistically with the number of piercings [428]
Bracelets	Metal: cobalt, nickel Rubber Disperse Black 1 IPPD Black rubber [429] Woods, e.g. rosewood [430], cocobolo [431], *Dalbergia nigra* [432]		Band-like dermatitis under the area of contact With loose fitting metals, bracelet dermatitis can cover large areas of the forearm, wrist and base of hand
Shoes [433]	Thiuram mix (1% pet.) MBT (2.0% pet.) Mercapto mix (1.0% pet.) Thiourea (0.1% pet.) Carbamates Dialkyl thioureas Black rubber mix	Accelerators	ACD to the upper part of the shoe gives the characteristic clinical picture of a rash limited to the dorsa of the toes and adjacent surface of the foot Often the big toe is the principal site of involvement, especially its medial and dorsal aspects, while the interdigital spaces and plantar surfaces are usually unaffected [434] Allergy to the sole of the shoe causes dermatitis on weight-bearing areas with sparing of the instep region, proximal palmar aspects of the toes and interdigital areas [435]. Rash corresponds exactly to the webbing or straps of the causative shoe Variants include sides of the feet, the heel area, and the anterior part of the sole [436] Complicating factors include dyshidrosis, stasis dermatitis, and bacterial and fungal infections Local spread and spread to the hands can occur [436]
	4-tert-butylphenol formaldehyde resin (1.0% pet.) Colophonium Dodecylmercaptan Epoxy resins (only rarely reported) Benzoyl peroxide (glue catalyst) Dibutyl phthalate (plasticizer)	Adhesives	
	Chromate Vegetable tannins (rare allergens) Formaldehyde (uncommon tanning agent) Glutaraldehyde (uncommon tanning agent)	Tanning agents	
	Dimethylfumarate	Anti-mold	
	PPD Disperse Orange 3 Acid Yellow 36 Disperse Red 1 Disperse Blue 106/124 mix	Dyes	
	Nickel (buckle) Cobalt	Metal	

Table 4.5 (Continued)

Clothing/ ornamentation	Reported allergen	Common sources	Reported clinical manifestations

Gloves [437]	Accelerators
	• Mercaptobenzothiazole
	• *N*-Cyclohexyl–2-benzothiazylsulfenamide
	• Morpholinylmercaptobenzothiazole
	• Dibenzothiazyldisulfide
	• Zinc diethyldithiocarbamate
	• Zinc dibutyldithiocarbamate
	• Zinc dimethyldithiocarbamate
	• 1,3-diphenylguanidine
	• Tetraethylthiuram disulfide
	• Tetramethylthiuram monosulfide
	• Tetramethythiuram disulfide
	• Dipentamethylenethiuram disulfide
	• Dibutyl thiourea
	• Diphenyl thiourea
	• Diethyl thiourea
	
	Antioxidants
	• Bisphenol A
	• Methylcyclohexyldimethylphenol
	• 4,4′-thio-*bis*-(6-*tert*-butyl-*meta*-cresol)
	• BHA
	• 2-tertiary-butyl-4-methylphenol
	• 4,4′-dihydroxydiphenyl ether
	• *N*-isopropyl-*N*′-phenyl-paraphenylenediamine
	• *N*-cyclohexyl-*N*′-phenyl-paraphenylenediamine
	
	Antimicrobials
	• Cetylpyridinium chloride
	
	Latex[b]
		Rubber/synthetic (neoprene and nitrile) gloves	Hand dermatitis, which may have some of the following features:
			• abrupt cut-off adjacent to the wrist
			• diffuse or patchy eczema on the dorsal aspects of the hands and fingers [438]
			• Thenar and hypothenar eminence involvement may also occur [439]
			• Variants:
			  ◦ may extend onto the forearm
			  ◦ may only involve finger pulps
			
			Study clinical patterns:
			The highest frequency of rubber ACD was found in the following patterns of involvement in hand dermatitis: dorsa hands +/– dorsa aspect fingers 6/40 (15%), fingers only 5/51 (9%), all hands involved 9/57 (9%), palms +/– palmar aspect fingers 7/115 (6%) [440]
			
			Contact urticaria can be caused by latex, starch, casein, accelerators, and di (2-ethylhexyl)phthalate

	Plasticisers • Poly(adipic acid-*co*-1,2-propylene glycol) • Adipic polyester • Di-(*n*-octyl) tin-*bis*-(2-ethylhexylmaleate) (stabilizer) • Tricresyl phosphate • Triphenyl phosphate • Methyldichlorobenzenesulfonate • Epoxy resin[a] Antioxidants • Bisphenol A Antimicrobials/preservatives • 1,2 benzisothiazolinone • Formaldehyde[a] Coloring agents • Pigment Orange 34 (single case) • Di-(2-ethylhexyl)phthalate	Plastic gloves	
	Chromate	Leather gloves	
	Single case reacted to several dyes: Disperse Orange 3, Acid Red 118, Direct Orange 34, Disperse Red 17, Disperse Blue 35, Disperse Orange and 4-aminoazobenzene	Textile gloves	

BHA, butylated hydroxyanisole; CPPD, *N*-cyclohexyl-*N*′-phenyl-1,4-phenylenediamine; DPPD, *N,N*′-diphenyl-1,4-paraphenylenediamine; IPPD, *N*-isopropyl-*N*-phenylparaphenylenediamine; PTBP-FR, *p*-tert-butylphenol formaldehyde resin; PPD, *p*-phenylenediamine.

[a] Not confirmed.

[b] Latex causing contact dermatitis – controversial and disputed.

are affected. Other times, there can be spread to the palm, dorsal fingers, and perionychium. Gloves can be contaminated as well [30, 31].

e) ACD to rubber tires from isopropyl-*p*-phenylenediamine (IPPD)/black rubber, mercapto chemicals, resorcinol, and chromium from the metal part of the wheel have all been reported, though this is usually observed in an occupational setting [32–35].

- *Cycling*:
  - See Table 4.3, e.g. black rubber from bike handles, MI in anti-chafing cream.
  - Lycra (spandex) contains polyurethane, and azo dyes can also be present.
- *Holidays*:
  - Holidays often involve leisure pursuits (see Table 4.3).
  - They also involve living in a hotel or other domestic environment (see Table 4.2) and the use of hotel/different personal care products (see Table 4.1).
  - Sunscreens are commonly used on sunny holidays. Sunscreen agents can cause both contact and photocontact dermatitis. Preservatives, fragrances, and bases contained within the sunscreen creams can also cause ACD. Photodermatoses such as polymorphic light eruption and actinic dermatitis can present on holiday, as can photo-aggravated endogenous dermatitis.
  - In assessing dermatitis presenting during a seaside holiday, a working knowledge of aquatic dermatoses is helpful.

Medicament agents and medical/dental procedures

- Several contact allergens are contained within topical medicated agents and emollients, including the active pharmacological agents (including antibiotics and corticosteroids), preservatives (such as parabens), and vehicles (such as lanolin).
- Herbal and over-the-counter medicated agents are another potential source of contact allergen exposure, e.g. arnica and chamomile are both potential *Compositae* contact allergens.
- A very careful history of anything else applied with the intention of helping the rash must be taken. This includes the use of their own or friends' medicaments and topical agents found in the cupboard at home or elsewhere!
- There are standardized "dental series" to be tested alongside the baseline series for both dental patients and staff where contact dermatitis is suspected. Allergens include metals, rubber, acrylates, preservatives, and flavors.
- A recent review of ACD in dermatologic surgery [36] identified many examples of potential contact allergens in the medical setting, including:
  a. antiseptics
  b. permanent markers
  c. local anesthetic agents
  d. rubber gloves
  e. metals in instruments
  f. suture materials (rare)
  g. acrylates in electrosurgical plates, prosthetic procedures, adhesives, surgical strips for wound closure, and from the use of 2-octylcyanoacrylate in surgical wound glues
  h. common allergens in wound dressings
  i. topical antibiotics, particularly when applied to surgical wounds
  j. topical corticosteroids used to treat post-operative dermatitis
  k. other agents in topical medicated preparations, such as fragrance [37].
- ACD to ultrasonic gel has been reported with propylene glycol, imidazolidinyl urea, methyldibromoglutaronitrile, and parabens being implicated as causative agents [38–40].
- Similarly, ACD to propylene glycol in electrocardiographic gel has been described [41]. ACD to para-tertiary butyl phenol (PTBP) resin in electrocardiographic adhesives has also been described [42].

Personal appliances

- Examples are summarized in Table 4.4.
- As with other aspects, a history of when the appliance was first used is important.
- Sweat or sweating can release allergens. For example, if headphones are worn whilst exercising in the gym, potential allergen chemicals are more likely to be released than whilst the individual is sedentary.
- Nickel is more readily released from agents such as spectacle frames the older they are and the longer they have been used [43].

Clothing items and ornamentation

- Examples are summarized in Table 4.5.
- Sweat helps to release allergens. For example, in temperate climates there may be a seasonal element to ACD caused by gloves or shoes as individuals sweat more during the summer.
- Pressure, friction, warmth, and perspiration are potentiating factors [44].
- Primary sensitization can be due to chemicals cross-reacting with allergens in textiles rather than due to the textiles themselves. These causative agents include hair dye (PPD, aminophenol, and diaminotoluene sulfate) in hairdressers and, rarely, formaldehyde in healthcare workers, embalmers, cabinet makers, and machinists. Primary sensitization is sometimes caused by PPD in temporary black henna tattoos [45].
- The allergens in medicament ointments are difficult to wash by laundry detergent and water and can be retained in clothing [46].
- Unusual manifestations including atopic dermatitis-like textile contact dermatitis and lichen amyloidosis-like lesions have been reported [47].

The post-patch test history: microhistory

- The *microhistory* consists of detailed probing of the identified allergen from patch testing in respect of the history and exposure in daily life.

- *Clinical relevance*: diagnosing ACD involves the correlation of:
  1. the temporal, anatomical, and morphological aspects of the dermatitis with
  2. the temporal, anatomical, qualitative, and quantitative exposure to the contact allergens in question.
- *Onset of dermatitis*. Was the patient significantly exposed to the allergen at the time of onset of the dermatitis?
- *Location of origin of dermatitis*. Could the allergen exposure explain the location of onset of the dermatitis?
- *Progression of dermatitis*. Does the allergen exposure conform to the progression of the dermatitis, whether single event, intermittent or continuous?
- *Detailed analysis of allergen exposure*. During the initial history, it is adequate to record if an agent such as a perfume spray is used. However, if a potentially relevant allergen has been identified, it may then be necessary to question this in much greater detail as there is tremendous variety in how people use different agents. As an illustration, Loretz et al. reported on the variation in the usage of six common cosmetics, such as perfume spray, by 800 adult individuals [5]. They found very large interindividual variation in terms of the amount of cosmetic used. When comparing individuals on the 10th and 90th centiles regarding the amount of daily cosmetic used, i.e. not the extremes of amounts used, there could still be as much as 40 times difference for some cosmetics. However, when comparing the amount of cosmetic used per application, the difference could go above five times and even over 40 times for one agent. In addition, there were differences as to where the perfume spray was applied, with the neck being the most common area, followed by the arms, torso, and legs. Just recording the use of perfume spray may not effectively characterize the full nature of allergen exposure.
- *Sources of allergen exposure*. One should closely analyze exposure to the particular allergen identified in respect of different daily activities. For example, in an individual with hand and face dermatitis, ACD to fragrance may be most easily explained through personal care product use (fragrance spray, shampoo), but other potential sources of exposure such as domestic (washing-up liquid), work (diffuser), leisure (use of gym shampoo), medical/dental procedures (exposure to eugenol), and travel (use of hotel toiletries) may also be relevant.
- *Routes of allergen exposure*. To use fragrance allergy as an example again, the relevant route of contact may be through direct contact (fragrance sprayed directly onto the skin) but other potential routes should also be considered, such as airborne (sprays, scented candles), hands to face/neck, by proxy (from partner), mucosal (flavor in toothpaste) or systemic (foods containing *Myroxylon pereirae* agents).

Potential pitfalls

- *More than one allergen identified*. Each allergen should be assessed separately regarding potential relevance of exposure with regards to the history of the dermatitis as well as potential sources and routes of exposure. It is not unusual to have more than one clinically relevant contact allergy identified.
- *More than one source of allergen exposure identified*. Each source should be assessed individually. It is not unusual for some allergens, e.g. fragrance, to have more than one clinically relevant source of exposure and in a few, e.g. ACD to MI, the majority of cases will have more than one source of clinically relevant exposure.
- *Missed allergen*. This diagnosis should be entertained when there is a highly suspicious history and negative patch testing. This could either be due to the known incompleteness of screening agents (e.g. screening for fragrance allergy with the fragrance mixes alone, plant allergy screening with commercial preparations alone) or difficulty in documenting all potential sources of allergen exposure (e.g. in an occupational setting where there is no full documentation of potential allergen exposure).
- *Indeterminate clinical relevance of allergen*. One needs to clearly delineate to the patient the diversity of potential exposure for a particular allergen. With plant allergens, pictorial illustrations can be helpful.
- *Multifactorial dermatitis*. It is not uncommon for allergic, irritant contact, and endogenous dermatitis to all contribute to the dermatitis (e.g. hairdresser's hand dermatitis), and they can adversely interact with each other and worsen the prognosis. The contribution of the contact allergy will not be fully confirmed until after complete avoidance for at least 1–2 months.

Summary

A history in relation to ACD consists of two parts. There is an initial history taken of the dermatitis together with screening for potential allergen exposure. Post-patch testing the history becomes focused to meticulous detail on the allergen identified by patch testing, in particular the source, route, and nature of exposure in relation to the nature and characteristics of the dermatitis. Diagnosis of ACD depends on rational correlation of the allergen exposure with the dermatitis. An understanding and knowledge of both the basic immunological principles involved and contact dermatitis literature in respect of the contact allergen's profile (sources of exposure, routes of exposure, and types of clinical presentation) are required.

References

1 Ho, S.G., Basketter, D.A., Jefferies, D. et al. (2005). Analysis of para-phenylenediamine allergic patients in relation to strength of patch test reaction. *British Journal of Dermatology* 153 (2): 364–367.

2 Kanerva, L., Tarvainen, K., Pinola, A. et al. (1994). A single accidental exposure may result in a chemical burn, primary sensitization and allergic contact dermatitis. *Contact Dermatitis* 31 (4): 229–235.

3 McFadden, J.P., White, I.R., Basketter, D. et al. (2013). The cosmetic allergy conundrum: inference of an immunoregulatory response to cosmetic allergens. *Contact Dermatitis* 69 (3): 129–137.

4 Calnan, C.D. (1956). Nickel dermatitis. *British Journal of Dermatology* 68 (7): 229–236.

5 Loretz, L., Api, A.M., Barraj, L. et al. (2006). Exposure data for personal care products: hairspray, spray perfume, liquid foundation, shampoo, body wash, and solid antiperspirant. Food and chemical toxicology: an international journal published for the British industrial. *Biological Research Association* 44 (12): 2008–2018.

6 Wenk, K.S. and Ehrlich, A. (2010). Allergic contact dermatitis from epoxy resin in solder mask coating in an individual working with printed circuit boards. *Dermatitis: Contact, Atopic, Occupational, Drug* 21 (5): 288–290.

7 Iwata, M., Tanizaki, H., Fujii, H. et al. (2015). Contact urticaria due to a face mask coated with disinfectant liquid spray. *Acta Dermato-Venereologica* 95 (5): 628–629.

8 Munoz, C.A., Gaspari, A., and Goldner, R. (2008). Contact dermatitis from a prosthesis. *Dermatitis: Contact, Atopic, Occupational, Drug* 19 (2): 109–111.

9 Donovan, J. and Skotnicki-Grant, S. (2007). Allergic contact dermatitis from formaldehyde textile resins in surgical uniforms and nonwoven textile masks. *Dermatitis: Contact, Atopic, Occupational, Drug* 18 (1): 40–44.

10 Elmer, K.B. and George, R.M. (1999). Contact urticaria to the MCU-2A/P gas mask. *Military Medicine* 164 (5): 377–378.

11 Wigger-Alberti, W., Hofmann, M., and Elsner, P. (1997). Contact dermatitis caused by triglycidyl isocyanurate. *American Journal of Contact Dermatitis: Official Journal of the American Contact Dermatitis Society* 8 (2): 106–107.

12 Bruze, M. and Kestrup, L. (1994). Occupational allergic contact dermatitis from diphenylguanidine in a gas mask. *Contact Dermatitis* 31 (2): 125–126.

13 Benton, E.C., White, I.R., and McFadden, J.P. (2012). Allergic contact dermatitis to methyl hydroxystearate in a rubber respirator. *Contact Dermatitis* 67 (4): 238–239.

14 Scheman, A.J. (1998). Allergic contact dermatitis from basic red 46 in flame-retardant work clothing. *Contact Dermatitis* 38 (6): 340.

15 Foti, C., Zambonin, C.G., Cassano, N. et al. (2009). Occupational allergic contact dermatitis associated with dimethyl fumarate in clothing. *Contact Dermatitis* 61 (2): 122–124.

16 Laing, M.E., Hackett, C.B., and Murphy, G.M. (2005). Unusual allergen in nurse uniform trousers. *Contact Dermatitis* 52 (5): 293.

17 Nagashima, C., Tomitaka-Yagami, A., and Matsunaga, K. (2003). Contact dermatitis due to para-tertiary-butylphenol-formaldehyde resin in a wetsuit. *Contact Dermatitis* 49 (5): 267–268.

18 Tarvainen, K., Jolanki, R., Henriks Eckerman, M.L., and Estlander, T. (1998). Occupational allergic contact dermatitis from isophoronediamine (IPDA) in operative-clothing manufacture. *Contact Dermatitis* 39 (1): 46–47.

19 Romaguera, C., Grimalt, F., and Vilaplana, J. (1989). Eczematous and purpuric allergic contact dermatitis from boots. *Contact Dermatitis* 21 (4): 269.

20 Heese, A., van Hintzenstern, J., Peters, K.P. et al. (1991). Allergic and irritant reactions to rubber gloves in medical health services. Spectrum, diagnostic approach, and therapy. *Journal of the American Academy of Dermatology* 25 (5 Pt 1): 831–839.

21 Espasandin-Arias, M. and Goossens, A. (2014). Natural rubber gloves might not protect against skin penetration of methylisothiazolinone. *Contact Dermatitis* 70 (4): 249–251.

22 Antelmi, A., Young, E., Svedman, C. et al. (2015). Are gloves sufficiently protective when hairdressers are exposed to permanent hair dyes? An in vivo study. *Contact Dermatitis* 72 (4): 229–236.

23 Coenraads, P.J. and Diepgen, T.L. (1998). Risk for hand eczema in employees with past or present atopic dermatitis. *International Archives of Occupational and Environmental Health* 71 (1): 7–13.

24 Sutthipisal, N., McFadden, J.P., and Cronin, E. (1993). Sensitization in atopic and non-atopic hairdressers with hand eczema. *Contact Dermatitis* 29 (4): 206–209.

25 Williams, J., Cahill, J., and Nixon, R. (2007). Occupational autoeczematization or atopic eczema precipitated by occupational contact dermatitis? *Contact Dermatitis* 56 (1): 21–26.

26 Puangpet, P., Lai-Cheong, J., and McFadden, J.P. (2013). Chemical atopy. *Contact Dermatitis* 68 (4): 208–213.

27 Wurpts, G. and Merk, H.F. (2010). Allergy to car seat. *Der Hautarzt; Zeitschrift fur Dermatologie, Venerologie, und Verwandte Gebiete* 61 (11): 933–934.

28 Jordan, W.P. Jr. (1973). Resorcinol monobenzoate, steering wheels, Peruvian balsam. *Archives of Dermatology* 108 (2): 278.

29 Guin, J.D. (2001). Seat-belt dermatitis from Disperse Blue dyes. *Contact Dermatitis* 44 (4): 263.

30 Fremlin, G. and Sansom, J. (2014). Acrylate-induced allergic contact dermatitis in a car windscreen repairer. *Occupational Medicine* 64 (7): 557–558.

31 Le Coz, C.J. (2003). Occupational allergic contact dermatitis from polyurethane/methacrylates in windscreen repair chemical. *Contact Dermatitis* 48 (5): 275–276.

32 Abbate, C., Polito, I., Puglisi, A. et al. (1989). Dermatosis from resorcinal in tyre makers. *British Journal of Industrial Medicine* 46 (3): 212–214.

33 Zina, A.M., Bedello, P.G., Cane, D. et al. (1987). Dermatitis in a rubber tyre factory. *Contact Dermatitis* 17 (1): 17–20.

34 Burrows, D. (1981). Chromium dermatitis in a tyre fitter. *Contact Dermatitis* 7 (1): 55–56.

35 Foussereau, J. and Cavelier, C. (1977). Has N-isopropyl-N'-phenyl-paraphenylenediamine a place among standard allergens? Importance of this allergen in rubber intolerance. *Dermatologica* 155 (3): 164–167.

36 Butler, L. and Mowad, C. (2013). Allergic contact dermatitis in dermatologic surgery: review of common allergens. *Dermatitis: Contact, Atopic, Occupational, Drug* 24 (5): 215–221.

37 Buckley, D.A., Rycroft, R.J., White, I.R., and McFadden, J.P. (2002). Fragrance as an occupational allergen. *Occupational Medicine* 52 (1): 13–16.

38 Eguino, P., Sanchez, A., Agesta, N. et al. (2003). Allergic contact dermatitis due to propylene glycol and parabens in an ultrasonic gel. *Contact Dermatitis* 48 (5): 290.

39 Erdmann, S.M., Sachs, B., and Merk, H.F. (2001). Allergic contact dermatitis due to methyldibromo glutaronitrile in Euxyl K 400 in an ultrasonic gel. *Contact Dermatitis* 44 (1): 39–40.

40 Ando, M., Ansotegui, J., Munoz, D., and Fernandez de Corres, L. (2000). Allergic contact dermatitis from imidazolidinyl urea in an ultrasonic gel. *Contact Dermatitis* 42 (2): 109–110.

41 Uter, W. and Schwanitz, H.J. (1996). Contact dermatitis from propylene glycol in ECG electrode gel. *Contact Dermatitis* 34 (3): 230–231.

42 Avenel-Audran, M., Goossens, A., Zimerson, E., and Bruze, M. (2003). Contact dermatitis from electrocardiograph-monitoring electrodes: role of *p*-tert-butylphenol-formaldehyde resin. *Contact Dermatitis* 48 (2): 108–111.

43 Walsh, G. and Mitchell, J.W. (1998). The leaching of nickel from new and used metal spectacle frames. *Ophthalmic & Physiological Optics: Journal of the British College of Ophthalmic Opticians* 18 (4): 372–377.
44 Reich, H.C. and Warshaw, E.M. (2010). Allergic contact dermatitis from formaldehyde textile resins. *Dermatitis: Contact, Atopic, Occupational, Drug* 21 (2): 65–76.
45 Mobolaji-Lawal, M. and Nedorost, S. (2015). The role of textiles in dermatitis: an update. *Current Allergy and Asthma Reports* 15 (4): 17.
46 Nedorost, S., Kessler, M., and McCormick, T. (2007). Allergens retained in clothing. *Dermatitis: Contact, Atopic, Occupational, Drug* 18 (4): 212–214.
47 Lazarov, A., Cordoba, M., Plosk, N., and Abraham, D. (2003). Atypical and unusual clinical manifestations of contact dermatitis to clothing (textile contact dermatitis): case presentation and review of the literature. *Dermatology Online Journal* 9 (3): 1.
48 Van Haute, N. and Dooms-Goossens, A. (1983). Shampoo dermatitis due to cocobetaine and sodium lauryl ether sulphate. *Contact Dermatitis* 9 (2): 169.
49 Welling, J.D., Mauger, T.F., Schoenfield, L.R., and Hendershot, A.J. (2014). Chronic eyelid dermatitis secondary to cocamidopropyl betaine allergy in a patient using baby shampoo eyelid scrubs. *JAMA Ophthalmology* 132 (3): 357–359.
50 Brand, R. and Delaney, T.A. (1998). Allergic contact dermatitis to cocamidopropylbetaine in hair shampoo. *Australasian Journal of Dermatology* 39 (2): 121–122.
51 Korting, H.C., Parsch, E.M., Enders, F., and Przybilla, B. (1992). Allergic contact dermatitis to cocamidopropyl betaine in shampoo. *Journal of the American Academy of Dermatology* 27 (6 Pt 1): 1013–1015.
52 Cooper, S.M. and Shaw, S. (1998). Allergic contact dermatitis from parabens in a tar shampoo. *Contact Dermatitis* 39 (3): 140.
53 Kato, K., Igawa, K., Nishizawa, A. et al. (2016). Allergic contact dermatitis induced by the anionic surfactant, sodium N-methyl-N-(1-oxododecyl)-beta-alaninate, contained in a daily-use shampoo. *Journal of the European Academy of Dermatology and Venereology* 30(11): e123–e124.
54 Jo, J.H., Jang, H.S., Ko, H.C. et al. (2005). Pustular psoriasis and the Kobner phenomenon caused by allergic contact dermatitis from zinc pyrithione-containing shampoo. *Contact Dermatitis* 52 (3): 142–144.
55 Liu, J. and Warshaw, E.M. (2014). Allergic contact dermatitis from ketoconazole. *Cutis* 94 (3): 112–114.
56 Eisenberg, B.C. (1955). Contact dermatitis from selenium sulfide shampoo. *AMA Archives of Dermatology* 72 (1): 71–72.
57 Grills, C.E. and Cooper, S.M. (2007). Polidocanol: a potential contact allergen in shampoo. *Contact Dermatitis* 56 (3): 178.
58 Sasseville, D. and Moreau, L. (2005). Allergic contact dermatitis from triethanolamine polypeptide oleate condensate in eardrops and shampoo. *Contact Dermatitis* 52 (4): 233.
59 Tan, B.B., Lear, J.T., and English, J.S. (1996). Allergic contact dermatitis from disodium ricinoleamido MEA-sulfosuccinate in shampoo. *Contact Dermatitis* 35 (5): 307.
60 Guin, J.D. (2000). Reaction to cocamidopropyl hydroxysultaine, an amphoteric surfactant and conditioner. *Contact Dermatitis* 42 (5): 284.
61 Andersen, K.E., Roed-Petersen, J., and Kamp, P. (1984). Contact allergy related to TEA-PEG-3 cocamide sulfate and cocamidopropyl betaine in a shampoo. *Contact Dermatitis* 11 (3): 192–193.
62 Zirwas, M. and Moennich, J. (2009). Shampoos. *Dermatitis: Contact, Atopic, Occupational, Drug* 20 (2): 106–110.
63 Nielsen, N.H. and Menne, T. (1997). Allergic contact dermatitis caused by zinc pyrithione associated with pustular psoriasis. *American Journal of Contact Dermatitis: Official Journal of the American Contact Dermatitis Society* 8 (3): 170–171.
64 Schalock, P.C., Storrs, F.J., and Morrison, L. (2000). Contact urticaria from panthenol in hair conditioner. *Contact Dermatitis* 43 (4): 223.
65 Quertermous, J. and Fowler, J.F. Jr. (2010). Allergic contact dermatitis from carvone in hair conditioners. *Dermatitis: Contact, Atopic, Occupational, Drug* 21 (2): 116–117.
66 Niinimaki, A., Niinimaki, M., Makinen-Kiljunen, S., and Hannuksela, M. (1998). Contact urticaria from protein hydrolysates in hair conditioners. *Allergy* 53 (11): 1078–1082.
67 Freeman, S. and Lee, M.S. (1996). Contact urticaria to hair conditioner. *Contact Dermatitis* 35 (3): 195–196.
68 Jaworsky, C., Taylor, J.S., Evey, P., and Handel, D. (1987). Allergic contact dermatitis to glutaraldehyde in a hair conditioner. *Cleveland Clinic Journal of Medicine* 54 (5): 443–444.
69 Lavy, Y., Slodownik, D., Trattner, A., and Ingber, A. (2009). Toothpaste allergy as a cause of cheilitis in Israeli patients. *Dermatitis: Contact, Atopic, Occupational, Drug* 20 (2): 95–98.
70 Foti, C., Romita, P., Ficco, D. et al. (2014). Allergic contact cheilitis to amine fluoride in a toothpaste. *Dermatitis: Contact, Atopic, Occupational, Drug* 25 (4): 209.
71 Jacob, S.E. and Amini, S. (2008). Cocamidopropyl betaine. *Dermatitis: Contact, Atopic, Occupational, Drug* 19 (3): 157–160.
72 Agar, N. and Freeman, S. (2005). Cheilitis caused by contact allergy to cocamidopropyl betaine in '2-in-1 toothpaste and mouthwash'. *Australasian Journal of Dermatology* 46 (1): 15–17.
73 Robertshaw, H. and Leppard, B. (2007). Contact dermatitis to triclosan in toothpaste. *Contact Dermatitis* 57 (6): 383–384.
74 Lim, S.W. and Goh, C.L. (2000). Epidemiology of eczematous cheilitis at a tertiary dermatological referral centre in Singapore. *Contact Dermatitis* 43 (6): 322–326.
75 Sainio, E.L. and Kanerva, L. (1995). Contact allergens in toothpastes and a review of their hypersensitivity. *Contact Dermatitis* 33 (2): 100–105.
76 Poon, T.S. and Freeman, S. (2006). Cheilitis caused by contact allergy to anethole in spearmint flavoured toothpaste. *Australasian Journal of Dermatology* 47 (4): 300–301.
77 Francalanci, S., Sertoli, A., Giorgini, S. et al. (2000). Multicentre study of allergic contact cheilitis from toothpastes. *Contact Dermatitis* 43 (4): 216–222.
78 Ghosh, S.K. and Bandyopadhyay, D. (2011). Concurrent allergic contact dermatitis of the index fingers and lips from toothpaste: report of three cases. *Journal of Cutaneous Medicine and Surgery* 15 (6): 356–357.
79 Concha-Garzon, M.J., Solano-Lopez, G., Montes, A. et al. (2015). Follicular allergic contact dermatitis due to methylchloroisothiazolinone/methylisothiazolinone (MCI/MI) in a rinse-off soap product. *Clinical and Experimental Dermatology* 40 (6): 690–691.
80 Schlichte, M.J. and Katta, R. (2014). Methylisothiazolinone: an emergent allergen in common pediatric skin care products. *Dermatology Research and Practice* 2014: 132564.
81 Hagvall, L., Brared-Christensson, J., and Inerot, A. (2014). Occupational contact dermatitis caused by sodium cocoamphopropionate in a liquid soap used in fast-food restaurants. *Contact Dermatitis* 71 (2): 122–124.

82 Ozkaya, E. and Kavlak Bozkurt, P. (2013). An unusual case of triclosan-induced immunological contact urticaria. *Contact Dermatitis* 68 (2): 121–123.
83 Suuronen, K., Pesonen, M., and Aalto-Korte, K. (2012). Occupational contact allergy to cocamidopropyl betaine and its impurities. *Contact Dermatitis* 66 (5): 286–292.
84 Zemtsov, A., Taylor, J.S., Evey, P., and Dijkstra, J. (1990). Allergic contact dermatitis from formaldehyde in a liquid soap. *Cleveland Clinic Journal of Medicine* 57 (3): 301–303.
85 Russell, K. and Jacob, S.E. (2010). Sodium hydroxymethylglycinate. *Dermatitis* 21 (2): 109–110.
86 Dooms-Goossens, A. and Blockeel, I. (1996). Allergic contact dermatitis and photoallergic contact dermatitis due to soaps and detergents. *Clinics in Dermatology* 14 (1): 67–76.
87 Knopp, E. and Watsky, K. (2008). Eyelid dermatitis: contact allergy to 3-(dimethylamino)propylamine. *Dermatitis: Contact, Atopic, Occupational, Drug* 19 (6): 328–333.
88 Berthelot, C. and Zirwas, M.J. (2006). Allergic contact dermatitis to chloroxylenol. *Dermatitis: Contact, Atopic, Occupational, Drug* 17 (3): 156–159.
89 Bruze, M., Gruvberger, B., and Zimerson, E. (2006). A clinically relevant contact allergy to methyldibromo glutaronitrile at 1% (0.32 mg/cm) detected by a patch test. *Contact Dermatitis* 54 (1): 14–17.
90 Diba, V.C., Chowdhury, M.M., Adisesh, A., and Statham, B.N. (2003). Occupational allergic contact dermatitis in hospital workers caused by methyldibromo glutaronitrile in a work soap. *Contact Dermatitis* 48 (2): 118–119.
91 Zemtsov, A. and Fett, D. (2005). Occupational allergic contact dermatitis to sodium lauroyl sarcosinate in the liquid soap. *Contact Dermatitis* 52 (3): 166–167.
92 Christersson, S. and Wrangsjo, K. (1992). Contact allergy to undecylenamide diethanolamide in a liquid soap. *Contact Dermatitis* 27 (3): 191–192.
93 Jeanmougin, M., Manciet, J.R., and Dubertret, L. (1992). Contact fentichlor photoallergy from soap for handwashing. *Annales de Dermatologie et de Venereologie* 119 (12): 983–985.
94 Libow, L.F., Ruszkowski, A.M., and DeLeo, V.A. (1989). Allergic contact dermatitis from para-chloro-meta-xylenol in Lurosep soap. *Contact Dermatitis* 20 (1): 67–68.
95 Dick, D.C. and Adams, R.H. (1979). Allergic contact dermatitis from monosulfiram (Tetmosol)soap. *Contact Dermatitis* 5 (3): 199.
96 Roed-Petersen, J., Auken, G., and Hjorth, N. (1975). Contact sensitivity to Irgasan DP 300. *Contact Dermatitis* 1 (5): 293–294.
97 Lachapelle, J.M. and Tennstedt, D. (1975). Occupational soap dermatitis: contact allergic reaction to lauryloxypropylamine. *Contact Dermatitis* 1 (4): 260.
98 Blank, I.H. (1956). Allergic hypersensitivity to an antiseptic soap. *Journal of the American Medical Association* 160 (14): 1225–1226.
99 Molloy, J.F. (1966). Photosensitizers in soaps. *Journal of the American Medical Association* 195 (10): 878.
100 Verhaeghe, I. and Dooms-Goossens, A. (1997). Multiple sources of allergic contact dermatitis from parabens. *Contact Dermatitis* 36 (5): 269–270.
101 Timm-Knudson, V.L., Johnson, J.S., Ortiz, K.J., and Yiannias, J.A. (2006). Allergic contact dermatitis to preservatives. *Dermatology Nursing/Dermatology Nurses' Association* 18 (2): 130–136.
102 Ajith, C., Dogra, S., and Handa, S. (2005). Localized erythema multiforme-like contact dermatitis from laundry bar soap. *Contact Dermatitis* 52 (2): 112–113.
103 Fisher, A.A. (1973). Allergic reaction to feminine hygiene sprays. *Archives of Dermatology* 108 (6): 801–802.
104 Heine, A. and Tarnick, M. (1987). Allergic contact eczema caused by usnic acid in deoderant sprays. *Dermatologische Monatschrift* 173 (4): 221–225.
105 Gonzalez-Perez, R., Gonzalez-Hermosa, R., Aseginolaza, B. et al. (2003). Allergic contact dermatitis from methenamine in an antiperspirant spray. *Contact Dermatitis* 49 (5): 266.
106 Skog, E. (1980). Incidence of cosmetic dermatitis. *Contact Dermatitis* 6 (7): 449–451.
107 Russell, K. and Jacob, S.E. (2010). Bisabolol. *Dermatitis: Contact, Atopic, Occupational, Drug* 21 (1): 57–58.
108 Amaro, C., Santos, R., and Cardoso, J. (2011). Contact allergy to methylisothiazolinone in a deodorant. *Contact Dermatitis* 64 (5): 298–299.
109 Heisterberg, M.V., Menne, T., Andersen, K.E. et al. (2011). Deodorants are the leading cause of allergic contact dermatitis to fragrance ingredients. *Contact Dermatitis* 64 (5): 258–264.
110 Jacob, S.E. (2008). Allergic contact dermatitis from lyral in an aerosol deodorant. *Dermatitis: Contact, Atopic, Occupational, Drug* 19 (4): 216–217.
111 Hendriks, S.A., Bousema, M.T., and van Ginkel, C.J. (1999). Allergic contact dermatitis from the fragrance ingredient Lyral in underarm deodorant. *Contact Dermatitis* 41 (2): 119.
112 Gijbels, D., Timmermans, A., Serrano, P. et al. (2014). Allergic contact dermatitis caused by alkyl glucosides. *Contact Dermatitis* 70 (3): 175–182.
113 Garg, S., Loghdey, S., and Gawkrodger, D.J. (2010). Allergic contact dermatitis from aluminium in deodorants. *Contact Dermatitis* 62 (1): 57–58.
114 Shaw, D.W. (2009). Allergic contact dermatitis from 12-hydroxystearic acid and hydrogenated castor oil. *Dermatitis: Contact, Atopic, Occupational, Drug* 20 (6): E16–E20.
115 Taghipour, K., Tatnall, F., and Orton, D. (2008). Allergic axillary dermatitis due to hydrogenated castor oil in a deodorant. *Contact Dermatitis* 58 (3): 168–169.
116 Davids, M.G., Hodgson, G.A., and Evans, E. (1978). Contact dermatitis from an ostomy deodorant. *Contact Dermatitis* 4 (1): 11–13.
117 Goossens, A. and Merckx, L. (1997). Allergic contact dermatitis from farnesol in a deodorant. *Contact Dermatitis* 37 (4): 179–180.
118 Hurley, H.J. Jr. and Shelley, W.B. (1958). The zirconium deodorant granuloma: an allergic disorder. *Henry Ford Hospital Medical Bulletin* 6 (3): 279–290.
119 Shelley, W.B. and Hurley, H.J. (1958). The allergic origin of zirconium deodorant granulomas. *British Journal of Dermatology* 70 (3): 75–101.
120 Sheu, M., Simpson, E.L., Law, S.V., and Storrs, F.J. (2006). Allergic contact dermatitis from a natural deodorant: a report of 4 cases associated with lichen acid mix allergy. *Journal of the American Academy of Dermatology* 55 (2): 332–337.
121 Magerl, A., Heiss, R., and Frosch, P.J. (2001). Allergic contact dermatitis from zinc ricinoleate in a deodorant and glyceryl ricinoleate in a lipstick. *Contact Dermatitis* 44 (2): 119–121.
122 Taran, J.M. and Delaney, T.A. (1997). Contact allergy to chloroacetamide. *Australasian Journal of Dermatology* 38 (2): 95–96.

123 Kraus, A.L., Stotts, J., Altringer, L.A., and Allgood, G.S. (1990). Allergic contact dermatitis from propyl gallate: dose response comparison using various application methods. *Contact Dermatitis* 22 (3): 132–136.

124 Corazza, M., Lombardi, A.R., and Virgili, A. (1997). Non-eczematous urticarioid allergic contact dermatitis due to Eumulgin L in a deodorant. *Contact Dermatitis* 36 (3): 159–160.

125 van Ketel, W.G. (1976). Allergic contact dermatitis from propellants in deodorant sprays in combination with allergy to ethyl chloride. *Contact Dermatitis* 2 (2): 115–119.

126 Valdivieso, R., Pola, J., Zapata, C. et al. (1987). Contact allergic dermatitis caused by freon 12 in deodorants. *Contact Dermatitis* 17 (4): 243–245.

127 Taylor, J.S., Jordan, W.P., and Maibach, H.I. (1984). Allergic contact dermatitis from stearamidoethyl diethylamine phosphate: a cosmetic emulsifier. *Contact Dermatitis* 10 (2): 74–76.

128 Aeling, J.L., Panagotacos, P.J., and Andreozzi, R.J. (1973). Letter: Allergic contact dermatitis to vitamin E aerosol deodorant. *Archives of Dermatology* 108 (4): 579–580.

129 Cronin, E. Chapter 4. In: (1980). *Cosmetic Dermatitis*, 96–171. Edinburgh: Churchill Livingstone.

130 Pincelli, C., Magni, R., and Motolese, A. (1993). Pigmented contact dermatitis from deodorant. *Contact Dermatitis* 28 (5): 305–306.

131 Cheng, J. and Zug, K.A. (2014). Fragrance allergic contact dermatitis. *Dermatitis* 25 (5): 232–245.

132 Verma, A., Tancharoen, C., Tam, M.M., and Nixon, R. (2015). Pustular allergic contact dermatitis caused by fragrances. *Contact Dermatitis* 72 (4): 245–248.

133 Goossens, A., Bruze, M., Gruvberger, B. et al. (2006). Contact allergy to sodium cocoamphoacetate present in an eye make-up remover. *Contact Dermatitis* 55 (5): 302–304.

134 Ross, J.S. and White, I.R. (1991). Eyelid dermatitis due to cocamidopropyl betaine in an eye make-up remover. *Contact Dermatitis* 25 (1): 64.

135 Du-Thanh, A., Siret-Alatrista, A., Guillot, B., and Raison-Peyron, N. (2011). Eyelid contact dermatitis due to an unsuspected eye make-up remover. *Journal of the European Academy of Dermatology and Venereology* 25 (1): 112–113.

136 Fisher, A.A. (1988). Allergic contact dermatitis due to rosin (colophony) in eyeshadow and mascara. *Cutis* 42 (6): 507–508.

137 Wachsmuth, R. and Wilkinson, M. (2006). Loss of eyelashes after use of a tinting mascara containing PPD. *Contact Dermatitis* 54 (3): 169–170.

138 Shaw, T., Oostman, H., Rainey, D., and Storrs, F. (2009). A rare eyelid dermatitis allergen: shellac in a popular mascara. *Dermatitis: Contact, Atopic, Occupational, Drug* 20 (6): 341–345.

139 Le Coz, C.J., Leclere, J.M., Arnoult, E. et al. (2002). Allergic contact dermatitis from shellac in mascara. *Contact Dermatitis* 46 (3): 149–152.

140 Gallo, R., Marro, I., and Pavesi, A. (2005). Allergic contact dermatitis from shellac in mascara. *Contact Dermatitis* 53 (4): 238.

141 Scheman, A.J. (1998). Contact allergy to quaternium-22 and shellac in mascara. *Contact Dermatitis* 38 (6): 342–343.

142 Chowdhury, M.M. (2002). Allergic contact dermatitis from prime yellow carnauba wax and coathylene in mascara. *Contact Dermatitis* 46 (4): 244.

143 Saxena, M., Warshaw, E., and Ahmed, D.D. (2001). Eyelid allergic contact dermatitis to black iron oxide. *American Journal of Contact Dermatitis: Official Journal of the American Contact Dermatitis Society* 12 (1): 38–39.

144 Zugerman, C. (1985). Contact dermatitis to yellow iron oxide. *Contact Dermatitis* 13 (2): 107–109.

145 Magerl, A., Pirker, C., and Frosch, P.J. (2003). Allergic contact eczema from shellac and 1,3-butylene glycol in an eyeliner. *Journal der Deutschen Dermatologischen Gesellschaft: Journal of the German Society of Dermatology* 1 (4): 300–302.

146 Travassos, A.R., Bruze, M., Dahlin, J., and Goossens, A. (2011). Allergic contact dermatitis caused by nickel in a green eye pencil. *Contact Dermatitis* 65 (5): 307–308.

147 Goh, C.L., Ng, S.K., and Kwok, S.F. (1989). Allergic contact dermatitis from nickel in eyeshadow. *Contact Dermatitis* 20 (5): 380–381.

148 Henke, U. and Boehncke, W.H. (2005). Eyelid dermatitis caused by an eyelash former. *Contact Dermatitis* 53 (4): 237.

149 McKenna, K.E. and McMillan, C. (1992). Facial contact dermatitis due to black rubber. *Contact Dermatitis* 26 (4): 270–271.

150 Lopez-Lerma, I. and Vilaplana, J. (2013). Contact dermatitis to vitamin K1 in an eye cream. *Annals of Allergy, Asthma & Immunology: Official Publication of the American College of Allergy, Asthma, & Immunology* 111 (3): 227–228.

151 Alrowaishdi, F., Colomb, S., Guillot, B., and Raison-Peyron, N. (2013). Allergic contact cheilitis caused by carnauba wax in a lip balm. *Contact Dermatitis* 69 (5): 318–319.

152 Jacob, S.E., Chimento, S., and Castanedo-Tardan, M.P. (2008). Allergic contact dermatitis to propolis and carnauba wax from lip balm and chewable vitamins in a child. *Contact Dermatitis* 58 (4): 242–243.

153 Barrientos, N., Abajo, P., Moreno de Vega, M., and Dominguez, J. (2013). Contact cheilitis caused by candelilla wax contained in lipstick. *Contact Dermatitis* 69 (2): 126–127.

154 Aguirre, A., Izu, R., Gardeazabal, J. et al. (1992). Allergic contact cheilitis from a lipstick containing oxybenzone. *Contact Dermatitis* 27 (4): 267–268.

155 Asai, M., Kawada, A., Aragane, Y., and Tezuka, T. (2001). Allergic contact cheilitis due to glyceryl monoisostearate monomyristate in a lipstick. *Contact Dermatitis* 45 (3): 173.

156 Athavale, N.V. and Srinivas, C.R. (1994). Contact cheilitis from propyl gallate in lipstick. *Contact Dermatitis* 30 (5): 307.

157 Pandhi, D., Vij, A., and Singal, A. (2011). Contact depigmentation induced by propyl gallate. *Clinical and Experimental Dermatology* 36 (4): 366–368.

158 Ozkaya, E., Topkarci, Z., and Ozarmagan, G. (2007). Allergic contact cheilitis from a lipstick misdiagnosed as herpes labialis: subsequent worsening due to Zovirax contact allergy. *Australasian Journal of Dermatology* 48 (3): 190–192.

159 Gamboni, S.E., Palmer, A.M., and Nixon, R.L. (2013). Allergic contact stomatitis to dodecyl gallate? A review of the relevance of positive patch test results to gallates. *Australasian Journal of Dermatology* 54 (3): 213–217.

160 Giordano-Labadie, F., Schwarze, H.P., and Bazex, J. (2000). Allergic contact dermatitis from octyl gallate in lipstick. *Contact Dermatitis* 42 (1): 51.

161 de Darko, E. and Osmundsen, P.E. (1984). Allergic contact dermatitis to Lipcare lipstick. *Contact Dermatitis* 11 (1): 46.

162 Ha, J.H., Kim, H.O., Lee, J.Y., and Kim, C.W. (2003). Allergic contact cheilitis from D & C red no 7 in lipstick. *Contact Dermatitis* 48 (4): 231.

163 Ichihashi, K., Soga, F., Katoh, N., and Kishimoto, S. (2003). Allergic contact cheilitis from pentaerythritol rosinate in a lipstick. *Contact Dermatitis* 49 (4): 213.

164 Inoue, A., Shoji, A., and Aso, S. (1998). Allergic lipstick cheilitis due to ester gum and ricinoleic acid. *Contact Dermatitis* 39 (1): 39.
165 Kimura, M. and Kawada, A. (1999). Contact dermatitis due to 2-hexyldecanoic acid (isopalmitate) in a lipstick. *Contact Dermatitis* 41 (2): 99–100.
166 Miura, M., Isami, M., Yagami, A., and Matsunaga, K. (2011). Allergic contact cheilitis caused by ditrimethylolpropane triethylhexanoate in a lipstick. *Contact Dermatitis* 64 (5): 301–302.
167 Pastor, N., Silvestre, J.F., Mataix, J. et al. (2008). Contact cheilitis from bisabolol and polyvinylpyrrolidone/hexadecene copolymer in lipstick. *Contact Dermatitis* 58 (3): 178–179.
168 Sowa, J., Suzuki, K., Tsuruta, K. et al. (2003). Allergic contact dermatitis from propylene glycol ricinoleate in a lipstick. *Contact Dermatitis* 48 (4): 228–229.
169 Sugiura, K. and Sugiura, M. (2009). Di-isostearyl malate and macademia nut oil in lipstick caused cheilitis. *Journal of the European Academy of Dermatology and Venereology* 23 (5): 606–607.
170 Suzuki, K., Matsunaga, K., and Suzuki, M. (1999). Allergic contact dermatitis due to isopalmityl diglyceryl sebacate in a lipstick. *Contact Dermatitis* 41 (2): 110.
171 Tan, B.B., Noble, A.L., Roberts, M.E. et al. (1997). Allergic contact dermatitis from oleyl alcohol in lipstick cross-reacting with ricinoleic acid in castor oil and lanolin. *Contact Dermatitis* 37 (1): 41–42.
172 Ghosh, S. and Mukhopadhyay, S. (2009). Chemical leukoderma: a clinico-aetiological study of 864 cases in the perspective of a developing country. *British Journal of Dermatology* 160 (1): 40–47.
173 Ozkaya, E. and Mirzoyeva, L. (2009). Tosylamide/formaldehyde resin allergy in a young boy: exposure from bitter nail varnish used against nail biting. *Contact Dermatitis* 60 (3): 171–172.
174 Lazzarini, R., Duarte, I., de Farias, D.C. et al. (2008). Frequency and main sites of allergic contact dermatitis caused by nail varnish. *Dermatitis: Contact, Atopic, Occupational, Drug* 19 (6): 319–322.
175 Gach, J.E., Stone, N.M., and Finch, T.M. (2005). A series of four cases of allergic contact dermatitis to phthalic anhydride/trimellitic anhydride/glycols copolymer in nail varnish. *Contact Dermatitis* 53 (1): 63–64.
176 Moffitt, D.L. and Sansom, J.E. (2002). Allergic contact dermatitis from phthalic anhydride/trimellitic anhydride/glycols copolymer in nail varnish. *Contact Dermatitis* 46 (4): 236.
177 Castelain, M., Veyrat, S., Laine, G., and Montastier, C. (1997). Contact dermatitis from nitrocellulose in a nail varnish. *Contact Dermatitis* 36 (5): 266–267.
178 Boehncke, W.H., Schmitt, M., Zollner, T.M., and Hensel, O. (1997). Nail polish allergy. An important differential diagnosis in contact dermatitis. *Deutsche Medizinische Wochenschrift* 122 (27): 849–852.
179 Guin, J.D. (2004). Eyelid dermatitis: a report of 215 patients. *Contact Dermatitis* 50 (2): 87–90.
180 Liden, C., Berg, M., Farm, G., and Wrangsjo, K. (1993). Nail varnish allergy with far-reaching consequences. *British Journal of Dermatology* 128 (1): 57–62.
181 Freeman, S. and Stephens, R. (1999). Cheilitis: analysis of 75 cases referred to a contact dermatitis clinic. *American Journal of Contact Dermatitis: Official Journal of the American Contact Dermatitis Society* 10 (4): 198–200.
182 Trindade, M.A., Alchorne, A.O., da Costa, E.B., and Enokihara, M.M. (2004). Eyelid discoid lupus erythematosus and contact dermatitis: a case report. *Journal of the European Academy of Dermatology and Venereology* 18 (5): 577–579.
183 Ozkaya, E. and Ekinci, A. (2010). Metal contact sites: a hidden localization for nail varnish allergy? *Clinical and Experimental Dermatology* 35 (4): e137–e140.
184 Shergill, B. and Goldsmith, P. (2004). Nail varnish is a potential allergen in nickel allergic subjects. *Clinical and Experimental Dermatology* 29 (5): 545–546.
185 Isaksson, M. and Persson, L. (2015). 'Mislabelled' make-up remover wet wipes as a cause of severe, recalcitrant facial eczema. *Contact Dermatitis* 73 (1): 56–59.
186 Schwensen, J.F., Menne, T., Friis, U.F., and Johansen, J.D. (2015). Undisclosed methylisothiazolinone in wet wipes for occupational use causing occupational allergic contact dermatitis in a nurse. *Contact Dermatitis* 73 (3): 182–184.
187 Chang, M.W. and Nakrani, R. (2014). Six children with allergic contact dermatitis to methylisothiazolinone in wet wipes (baby wipes). *Pediatrics* 133 (2): e434–e438.
188 Mendese, G., Beckford, A., and Demierre, M.F. (2010). Lymphomatoid contact dermatitis to baby wipes. *Archives of Dermatology* 146 (8): 934–935.
189 Kazandjieva, J., Gergovska, M., and Darlenski, R. (2014). Contact dermatitis in a child from methlychloroisothiazolinone and methylisothiazolinone in moist wipes. *Pediatric Dermatology* 31 (2): 225–227.
190 Gardner, K.H., Davis, M.D., Richardson, D.M., and Pittelkow, M.R. (2010). The hazards of moist toilet paper: allergy to the preservative methylchloroisothiazolinone/methylisothiazolinone. *Archives of Dermatology* 146 (8): 886–890.
191 Leysen, J., Goossens, A., Lambert, J., and Aerts, O. (2014). Polyhexamethylene biguanide is a relevant sensitizer in wet wipes. *Contact Dermatitis* 70 (5): 323–325.
192 Creytens, K., Goossens, A., Faber, M. et al. (2014). Contact urticaria syndrome caused by polyaminopropyl biguanide in wipes for intimate hygiene. *Contact Dermatitis* 71 (5): 307–309.
193 Chin, M.F., Hughes, T.M., and Stone, N.M. (2013). Allergic contact dermatitis caused by panthenol in a child. *Contact Dermatitis* 69 (5): 321–322.
194 Sanchez-Perez, J., Del Rio, M.J., Jimenez, Y.D., and Garcia-Diez, A. (2005). Allergic contact dermatitis due to methyldibromo glutaronitrile in make-up removal wipes. *Contact Dermatitis* 53 (6): 357–358.
195 Schollnast, R., Kranke, B., and Aberer, W. (2003). Anal and palmar contact dermatitis caused by iodopropynyl butylcarbamate in moist sanitary wipes. *Der Hautarzt; Zeitschrift fur Dermatologie, Venerologie, und Verwandte Gebiete* 54 (10): 970–974.
196 Placucci, F., Benini, A., Guerra, L., and Tosti, A. (1996). Occupational allergic contact dermatitis from disinfectant wipes used in dentistry. *Contact Dermatitis* 35 (5): 306.
197 Boyapati, A., Tam, M., Tate, B. et al. (2013). Allergic contact dermatitis to methylisothiazolinone: exposure from baby wipes causing hand dermatitis. *Australasian Journal of Dermatology* 54 (4): 264–267.
198 Foote, C.A., Brady, S.P., Brady, K.L. et al. (2014). Vulvar dermatitis from allergy to moist flushable wipes. *Journal of Lower Genital Tract Disease* 18 (1): E16–E18.
199 Gonzalez-Perez, R., Sanchez-Martinez, L., and Piqueres Zubiaurrre, T. (2014). Urtaran Ibarzabal a, Soloeta Arechavala R. Patch testing in patients with perianal eczema. *Actas Dermo-Sifiliograficas* 105 (7): 694–698.

200 Admani, S., Matiz, C., and Jacob, S.E. (2014). Methylisothiazolinone: a case of perianal dermatitis caused by wet wipes and review of an emerging pediatric allergen. *Pediatric Dermatology* 31 (3): 350–352.

201 de Groot, A.C., van Ulsen, J., and Weyland, J.W. (1991). Peri-anal allergic contact eczema with dyshidrotic eczema of the hands due to the use of Kathon CG moist toilet wipes. *Nederlands Tijdschrift voor Geneeskunde* 135 (23): 1048–1049.

202 Murphy, L.A. and White, I.R. (2003). Contact dermatitis from geraniol in washing-up liquid. *Contact Dermatitis* 49 (1): 52.

203 Pinola, A., Estlander, T., Jolanki, R. et al. (1993). Occupational allergic contact dermatitis due to coconut diethanolamide (cocamide DEA). *Contact Dermatitis* 29 (5): 262–265.

204 McFadden, J.P., Mann, J., White, J.M. et al. (2013). Outbreak of methylisothiazolinone allergy targeting those aged >/=40 years. *Contact Dermatitis* 69 (1): 53–55.

205 Magnano, M., Silvani, S., Vincenzi, C. et al. (2009). Contact allergens and irritants in household washing and cleaning products. *Contact Dermatitis* 61 (6): 337–341.

206 Kim, S., Hong, S.H., Bong, C.K., and Cho, M.H. (2015). Characterization of air freshener emission: the potential health effects. *Journal of Toxicological Sciences* 40 (5): 535–550.

207 Bridges, B. (2002). Fragrance: emerging health and environmental concerns. *Flavour and Fragrance Journal* 17 (5): 361–371.

208 Johansen, J.D., Andersen, T.F., Thomsen, L.K. et al. (2000). Rash related to use of scented products. A questionnaire study in the Danish population. Is the problem increasing? *Contact Dermatitis* 42 (4): 222–226.

209 Pesonen, M., Suomela, S., Kuuliala, O. et al. (2014). Occupational contact dermatitis caused by D-limonene. *Contact Dermatitis* 71 (5): 273–279.

210 Matura, M., Skold, M., Borje, A. et al. (2006). Not only oxidized R-(+)- but also S-(−)-limonene is a common cause of contact allergy in dermatitis patients in Europe. *Contact Dermatitis* 55 (5): 274–279.

211 Matura, M., Goossens, A., Bordalo, O. et al. (2002). Oxidized citrus oil (R-limonene): a frequent skin sensitizer in Europe. *Journal of the American Academy of Dermatology* 47 (5): 709–714.

212 Skold, M., Borje, A., Harambasic, E., and Karlberg, A.T. (2004). Contact allergens formed on air exposure of linalool. Identification and quantification of primary and secondary oxidation products and the effect on skin sensitization. *Chemical Research in Toxicology* 17 (12): 1697–1705.

213 Scala, G. (2006). Acute, short-lasting rhinitis due to camomile-scented toilet paper in patients allergic to compositae. *International Archives of Allergy and Immunology* 139 (4): 330–331.

214 Dias, M., Lamarao, P., and Vale, T. (1992). Occupational contact allergy to 1, 2-benzisothiazolin-3-one in the manufacture of air fresheners. *Contact Dermatitis* 27 (3): 205–207.

215 Anonymous (2002). Hazardous pleasant odors. Scented substances cause asthma in asthma patients. *MMW Fortschritte der Medizin* 144 (44): 14.

216 Genuis, S.J. and Tymchak, M.G. (2014). Approach to patients with unexplained multimorbidity with sensitivities. *Canadian Family Physician Medecin de Famille Canadien* 60 (6): 533–538.

217 Lundov, M.D., Kolarik, B., Bossi, R. et al. (2014). Emission of isothiazolinones from water-based paints. *Environmental Science & Technology* 48 (12): 6989–6994.

218 Wright, A.M. and Cahill, J.L. (2015). Airborne exposure to methylisothiazolinone in paint causing allergic contact dermatitis: an Australian perspective. *Australasian Journal of Dermatology*.

219 Alwan, W., White, I.R., and Banerjee, P. (2014). Presumed airborne contact allergy to methylisothiazolinone causing acute severe facial dermatitis and respiratory difficulty. *Contact Dermatitis* 70 (5): 320–321.

220 Madsen, J.T. and Andersen, K.E. (2014). Airborne allergic contact dermatitis caused by methylisothiazolinone in a child sensitized from wet wipes. *Contact Dermatitis* 70 (3): 183–184.

221 Schwensen, J.F., Lundov, M.D., Bossi, R. et al. (2015). Methylisothiazolinone and benzisothiazolinone are widely used in paint: a multicentre study of paints from five European countries. *Contact Dermatitis* 72 (3): 127–138.

222 Mose, A.P., Frost, S., Ohlund, U., and Andersen, K.E. (2013). Allergic contact dermatitis from octylisothiazolinone. *Contact Dermatitis* 69 (1): 49–52.

223 Kristensen, D., Hein, H.O., and Weismann, K. (2002). Airborne contact allergy provoked by kathon in water-based plastic paint. *Ugeskrift for Laeger* 164 (18): 2411–2413.

224 Aalto-Korte, K., Pesonen, M., Kuuliala, O. et al. (2010). Contact allergy to aliphatic polyisocyanates based on hexamethylene-1,6-diisocyanate (HDI). *Contact Dermatitis* 63 (6): 357–363.

225 Sastre, J., Carnes, J., Garcia del Potro, M. et al. (2011). Occupational asthma caused by triglycidyl isocyanurate. *International Archives of Occupational and Environmental Health* 84 (5): 547–549.

226 Mancuso, G. and Berdondini, R.M. (2008). Occupational conjunctivitis as the sole manifestation of airborne contact allergy to trimethylolpropane triacrylate contained in a UV-cured paint. *Contact Dermatitis* 59 (6): 372–373.

227 Saval, P., Kristiansen, E., Cramers, M., and Lander, F. (2007). Occupational allergic contact dermatitis caused by aerosols of acrylate monomers. *Contact Dermatitis* 57 (4): 276.

228 Bieler, G., Thorn, D., Huynh, C.K. et al. (2011). Acute life-threatening extrinsic allergic alveolitis in a paint controller. *Occupational Medicine* 61 (6): 440–442.

229 Jensen, C.D., Thormann, J., and Andersen, K.E. (2003). Airborne allergic contact dermatitis from 3-iodo-2-propynyl-butylcarbamate at a paint factory. *Contact Dermatitis* 48 (3): 155–157.

230 Bogenrieder, T., Landthaler, M., and Stolz, W. (2001). Airborne contact dermatitis due to chloroacetamide in wall paint. *Contact Dermatitis* 45 (1): 55.

231 Doumit, J., Gavigan, G., and Pratt, M. (2012). Allergic contact dermatitis from dimethyl fumarate after contact with a Chinese sofa. *Journal of Cutaneous Medicine and Surgery* 16 (5): 353–356.

232 Vandevenne, A., Vanden Broecke, K., and Goossens, A. (2014). Sofa dermatitis caused by methylisothiazolinone in a leather-care product. *Contact Dermatitis* 71 (2): 111–113.

233 Susitaival, P., Winhoven, S.M., Williams, J. et al. (2010). An outbreak of furniture related dermatitis ('sofa dermatitis') in Finland and the UK: history and clinical cases. *Journal of the European Academy of Dermatology and Venereology* 24 (4): 486–489.

234 Vives, R., Ana, V., Hervella, M., and Yanguas, J. (2011). Leukoderma after Chinese sofa dermatitis. *Contact Dermatitis* 64 (1): 58–59.

235 Lynch, M. and Collins, P. (2010). Sofa dermatitis presenting as a chronic treatment resistant dermatitis. *Irish Medical Journal* 103 (4): 119–120.

236 Holme, S.A., Stone, N.M., and Mills, C.M. (2005). Toilet seat contact dermatitis. *Pediatric Dermatology* 22 (4): 344–345.
237 Ezzedine, K., Rafii, N., and Heenen, M. (2007). Lymphomatoid contact dermatitis to an exotic wood: a very harmful toilet seat. *Contact Dermatitis* 57 (2): 128–130.
238 Heilig, S., Adams, D.R., and Zaenglein, A.L. (2011). Persistent allergic contact dermatitis to plastic toilet seats. *Pediatric Dermatology* 28 (5): 587–590.
239 Raison-Peyron, N., Nilsson, U., Du-Thanh, A., and Karlberg, A.T. (2013). Contact dermatitis from unexpected exposure to rosin from a toilet seat. *Dermatitis: Contact, Atopic, Occupational, Drug* 24 (3): 149–150.
240 Turan, H., Saricaoglu, H., Turan, A., and Tunali, S. (2011). Polyurethane toilet seat contact dermatitis. *Pediatric Dermatology* 28 (6): 731–732.
241 Litvinov, I.V., Sugathan, P., and Cohen, B.A. (2010). Recognizing and treating toilet-seat contact dermatitis in children. *Pediatrics* 125 (2): e419–e422.
242 Martins, C., Goncalo, M., and Goncalo, S. (1995). Allergic contact dermatitis from dipentene in wax polish. *Contact Dermatitis* 33 (2): 126–127.
243 Karlberg, A.T. and Dooms-Goossens, A. (1997). Contact allergy to oxidized d-limonene among dermatitis patients. *Contact Dermatitis* 36 (4): 201–206.
244 Quirce, S. and Barranco, P. (2010). Cleaning agents and asthma. *Journal of Investigational Allergology & Clinical Immunology* 20 (7): 542–550.
245 Heydorn, S., Andersen, K.E., Johansen, J.D., and Menne, T. (2003). A stronger patch test elicitation reaction to the allergen hydroxycitronellal plus the irritant sodium lauryl sulfate. *Contact Dermatitis* 49 (3): 133–139.
246 Bauer, A. (2013). Contact dermatitis in the cleaning industry. *Current Opinion in Allergy and Clinical Immunology* 13 (5): 521–524.
247 Choi, H., Schmidbauer, N., Spengler, J., and Bornehag, C.G. (2010). Sources of propylene glycol and glycol ethers in air at home. *International Journal of Environmental Research and Public Health* 7 (12): 4213–4237.
248 Choi, H., Schmidbauer, N., Sundell, J. et al. (2010). Common household chemicals and the allergy risks in pre-school age children. *PLoS One* 5 (10): e13423.
249 Laborde-Casterot, H., Villa, A.F., Rosenberg, N. et al. (2012). Occupational rhinitis and asthma due to EDTA-containing detergents or disinfectants. *American Journal of Industrial Medicine* 55 (8): 677–682.
250 Bernard, A. (2007). Chlorination products: emerging links with allergic diseases. *Current Medicinal Chemistry* 14 (16): 1771–1782.
251 Sarlo, K., Kirchner, D.B., Troyano, E. et al. (2010). Assessing the risk of type 1 allergy to enzymes present in laundry and cleaning products: evidence from the clinical data. *Toxicology* 271 (3): 87–93.
252 Siracusa, A., De Blay, F., Folletti, I. et al. (2013). Asthma and exposure to cleaning products – a European academy of allergy and clinical immunology task force consensus statement. *Allergy* 68 (12): 1532–1545.
253 Dumas, O., Siroux, V., Luu, F. et al. (2014). Cleaning and asthma characteristics in women. *American Journal of Industrial Medicine* 57 (3): 303–311.
254 Zock, J.P., Kogevinas, M., Sunyer, J. et al. (2002). Asthma characteristics in cleaning workers, workers in other risk jobs and office workers. *European Respiratory Journal* 20 (3): 679–685.
255 Walters, G.I., Moore, V.C., McGrath, E.E. et al. (2013). Agents and trends in health care workers' occupational asthma. *Occupational Medicine* 63 (7): 513–516.
256 Folletti, I., Zock, J.P., Moscato, G., and Siracusa, A. (2014). Asthma and rhinitis in cleaning workers: a systematic review of epidemiological studies. *Journal of Asthma: Official Journal of the Association for the Care of Asthma* 51 (1): 18–28.
257 Osmundsen, P.E. and Alani, M.D. (1971). Contact allergy to an optical whitener, "CPY", in washing powders. *British Journal of Dermatology* 85 (1): 61–66.
258 Weiler, K.J. and Russel, H.A. (1986). Chromate eczema in food, domestic and cleaning occupations. *Dermatosen in Beruf und Umwelt Occupation and Environment* 34 (5): 135–139.
259 Adisesh, A., Murphy, E., Barber, C.M., and Ayres, J.G. (2011). Occupational asthma and rhinitis due to detergent enzymes in healthcare. *Occupational Medicine* 61 (5): 364–369.
260 Schweigert, M.K., Mackenzie, D.P., and Sarlo, K. (2000). Occupational asthma and allergy associated with the use of enzymes in the detergent industry – a review of the epidemiology, toxicology and methods of prevention. *Clinical and Experimental Allergy: Journal of the British Society for Allergy and Clinical Immunology* 30 (11): 1511–1518.
261 Hole, A.M., Draper, A., Jolliffe, G. et al. (2000). Occupational asthma caused by bacillary amylase used in the detergent industry. *Occupational and Environmental Medicine* 57 (12): 840–842.
262 Gottmann-Luckerath, I. and Steigleder, G.K. (1972). Hypersensitivity to enzyme containing washing powders and detergent enzymes. *Archiv fur dermatologische Forschung* 245 (1): 63–68.
263 Belin, L., Hoborn, J., Falsen, E., and Andre, J. (1970). Enzyme sensitisation in consumers of enzyme-containing washing powder. *Lancet* 2 (7684): 1153–1157.
264 Newhouse, M.L., Tagg, B., Pocock, S.J., and McEwan, A.C. (1970). An epidemiological study of workers producing enzyme washing powders. *Lancet* 1 (7649): 689–693.
265 Trattner, A., Hodak, E., and David, M. (1999). Screening patch tests for pigmented contact dermatitis in Israel. *Contact Dermatitis* 40 (3): 155–157.
266 Arutjunow, V. (1978). Perioral dermatitis – an allergic disease? *Der Hautarzt; Zeitschrift fur Dermatologie, Venerologie, und verwandte Gebiete* 29 (2): 89–91.
267 Sasseville, D., Geoffrion, G., and Lowry, R.N. (1999). Allergic contact dermatitis from chlorinated swimming pool water. *Contact Dermatitis* 41 (6): 347–348.
268 Fitzgerald, D.A., Wilkinson, S.M., Bhaggoe, R. et al. (1995). Spa pool dermatitis. *Contact Dermatitis* 33 (1): 53.
269 Dalmau, G., Martinez-Escala, M.E., Gazquez, V. et al. (2012). Swimming pool contact dermatitis caused by 1-bromo-3-chloro-5,5-dimethyl hydantoin. *Contact Dermatitis* 66 (6): 335–339.
270 Stenveld, H. (2012). Allergic to pool water. *Safety and Health at Work* 3 (2): 101–103.
271 Salvaggio, H.L., Scheman, A.J., and Chamlin, S.L. (2013). Shock treatment: swimming pool contact dermatitis. *Pediatric Dermatology* 30 (4): 494–495.

272 Seyfarth, F., Krautheim, A., Schliemann, S., and Elsner, P. (2009). Sensitization to para-amino compounds in swim fins in a 10-year-old boy. *Journal der Deutschen Dermatologischen Gesellschaft: Journal of the German Society of Dermatology* 7 (9): 770–772.

273 Cronin, E. Chapter 14. In: (1980). *Contact Dermatitis*, 714–770. New York: Churchill Livingstone.

274 Vaswani, S.K., Collins, D.D., and Pass, C.J. (2003). Severe allergic contact eyelid dermatitis caused by swimming goggles. *Annals of Allergy, Asthma & Immunology: Official Publication of the American College of Allergy, Asthma, & Immunology* 90 (6): 672–673.

275 Azurdia, R.M. and King, C.M. (1998). Allergic contact dermatitis due to phenol-formaldehyde resin and benzoyl peroxide in swimming goggles. *Contact Dermatitis* 38 (4): 234–235.

276 Alomar, A. and Vilaltella, I. (1985). Contact dermatitis to dibutylthiourea in swimming goggles. *Contact Dermatitis* 13 (5): 348–349.

277 Romaguera, C., Grimalt, F., and Vilaplana, J. (1988). Contact dermatitis from swimming goggles. *Contact Dermatitis* 18 (3): 178–179.

278 Kroft, E.B. and van der Valk, P.G. (2007). Allergic contact dermatitis as a result of diethylthiourea. *Contact Dermatitis* 57 (3): 194–195.

279 Adams, R.M. (1982). Contact allergic dermatitis due to diethylthiourea in a wetsuit. *Contact Dermatitis* 8 (4): 277–278.

280 Gudi, V.S., White, M.I., and Ormerod, A.D. (2004). Allergic contact dermatitis from dibutylthiourea in a wet suit. *Dermatitis: Contact, Atopic, Occupational, Drug* 15 (1): 55–56.

281 Boehncke, W.H., Wessmann, D., Zollner, T.M., and Hensel, O. (1997). Allergic contact dermatitis from diphenylthiourea in a wet suit. *Contact Dermatitis* 36 (5): 271.

282 Martellotta, D., Di Costanzo, L., Cafiero, M. et al. (2008). Contact allergy to p-tert-butylphenol formaldehyde resin and zinc diethyldithiocarbamate in a wet suit. *Dermatitis: Contact, Atopic, Occupational, Drug* 19 (2): E3–E4.

283 Corazza, M. and Virgili, A. (1998). Allergic contact dermatitis due to nickel in a neoprene wetsuit. *Contact Dermatitis* 39 (5): 257.

284 Munro, C.S., Shields, T.G., and Lawrence, C.M. (1989). Contact allergy to Tego 103G disinfectant in a deep-sea diver. *Contact Dermatitis* 21 (4): 278–279.

285 Bergendorff, O. and Hansson, C. (2007). Contact dermatitis to a rubber allergen with both dithiocarbamate and benzothiazole structure. *Contact Dermatitis* 56 (5): 278–280.

286 Tuyp, E. and Mitchell, J.C. (1983). Scuba diver facial dermatitis. *Contact Dermatitis* 9 (4): 334–335.

287 Foussereau, J., Herve-Bazin, B., Cavelier, C., and Certin, J.F. (1982). A case of allergy to dibutylthiourea caused by diver's footgear (author's transl.). *Dermatosen in Beruf und Umwelt Occupation and Environment* 30 (2): 58–59.

288 Fisher, A.A. (1993). Allergic contact dermatitis: practical solutions for sports-related rashes. *Physician and Sportsmedicine* 21: 65–72.

289 Jung, J.H., McLaughlin, J.L., Stannard, J., and Guin, J.D. (1988). Isolation, via activity-directed fractionation, of mercaptobenzothiazole and dibenzothiazyl disulfide as 2 allergens responsible for tennis shoe dermatitis. *Contact Dermatitis* 19 (4): 254–259.

290 Vilaplana, J. and Romaguera, C. (2000). Allergic contact dermatitis due to eucalyptol in an anti-inflammatory cream. *Contact Dermatitis* 43 (2): 118.

291 de Leeuw, J. and den Hollander, P. (1987). A patient with a contact allergy to jogging cream. *Contact Dermatitis* 17 (4): 260–261.

292 Shono, M., Ezoe, K., Kaniwa, M.A. et al. (1991). Allergic contact dermatitis from para-tertiary-butylphenol-formaldehyde resin (PTBP-FR) in athletic tape and leather adhesive. *Contact Dermatitis* 24 (4): 281–288.

293 Ozkaya, E. and Elinc-Aslan, M.S. (2011). Black rubber sensitization by bicycle handgrips in a child with palmar hyperhidrosis. *Dermatitis: Contact, Atopic, Occupational, Drug* 22 (4): E10–E12.

294 Narayan, S. and Sansom, J.E. (2002). Contact urticaria from runner bean (*Phaseolus coccineus*). *Contact Dermatitis* 47 (4): 243.

295 Paulsen, E., Andersen, S.L., and Andersen, K.E. (2009). Occupational contact dermatitis from golden shrimp plant (*Pachystachys lutea*). *Contact Dermatitis* 60 (5): 293–294.

296 Rademaker, M. and Duffill, M.B. (1995). Allergic contact dermatitis to *Toxicodendron succedaneum* (rhus tree): an autumn epidemic. *New Zealand Medical Journal* 108 (997): 121–123.

297 Minciullo, P.L., Fazio, E., Patafi, M., and Gangemi, S. (2007). *Allergic contact dermatitis due to Zantedeschia aethiopica. Contact Dermatitis* 56 (1): 46–47.

298 Lurquin, E., Swinnen, I., and Goossens, A. (2012). Allergic contact dermatitis caused by *Hedera helix arborescens* and not by *Hedera helix* L. *Contact Dermatitis* 66 (6): 352–353.

299 Garcia, M., Fernandez, E., Navarro, J.A. et al. (1995). Allergic contact dermatitis from *Hedera helix* L. *Contact Dermatitis* 33 (2): 133–134.

300 Jones, J.M., White, I.R., White, J.M., and McFadden, J.P. (2009). Allergic contact dermatitis to English ivy (*Hedera helix*) – a case series. *Contact Dermatitis* 60 (3): 179–180.

301 Ozdemir, C., Schneider, L.A., Hinrichs, R. et al. (2003). Allergic contact dermatitis to common ivy (*Hedera helix* L.). *Der Hautarzt; Zeitschrift fur Dermatologie, Venerologie, und verwandte Gebiete* 54 (10): 966–969.

302 English, J. (2011). Case study 1 – a 54-year-old male gardener with chronic hand eczema. *Clinical and Experimental Dermatology* 36 (Suppl): 3–4.

303 Corazza, M., Miscioscia, R., Lauriola, M.M. et al. (2008). Allergic contact dermatitis due to cineraria hybrid in an amateur gardener housewife. *Contact Dermatitis* 59 (2): 128–129.

304 Foti, C., Bonamonte, D., Conserva, A. et al. (2008). Allergic contact dermatitis with a fertilizer containing hydrogen cyanamide (Dormex). *Cutaneous and Ocular Toxicology* 27 (1): 1–3.

305 Lembo, S., Lembo, C., Patruno, C. et al. (2014). Pizza makers' contact dermatitis. *Dermatitis: Contact, Atopic, Occupational, Drug* 25 (4): 191–194.

306 Williams, J., Roberts, H., and Tate, B. (2007). Contact urticaria to olives. *Contact Dermatitis* 56 (1): 52–53.

307 Wong, G.A. and King, C.M. (2004). Occupational allergic contact dermatitis from olive oil in pizza making. *Contact Dermatitis* 50 (2): 102–103.

308 Bleumink, E., Doeglas, H.M., Klokke, A.H., and Nater, J.P. (1972). Allergic contact dermatitis to garlic. *British Journal of Dermatology* 87 (1): 6–9.

309 Lembo, G., Balato, N., Patruno, C. et al. (1991). Allergic contact dermatitis due to garlic (*Allium sativum*). *Contact Dermatitis* 25 (5): 330–331.

310 Papageorgiou, C., Corbet, J.P., Menezes-Brandao, F. et al. (1983). Allergic contact dermatitis to garlic (*Allium sativum* L.). Identification of the allergens: the role of mono-, di-, and trisulfides present in garlic. A comparative study in man and animal (Guinea-pig). *Archives of Dermatological Research* 275 (4): 229–234.

311 McFadden, J.P., White, I.R., and Rycroft, R.J. (1992). Allergic contact dermatitis from garlic. *Contact Dermatitis* 27 (5): 333–334.
312 Kanerva, L., Estlander, T., and Jolanki, R. (1996). Occupational allergic contact dermatitis from spices. *Contact Dermatitis* 35 (3): 157–162.
313 Burden, A.D., Wilkinson, S.M., Beck, M.H., and Chalmers, R.J. (1994). Garlic-induced systemic contact dermatitis. *Contact Dermatitis* 30 (5): 299–300.
314 Bassioukas, K., Orton, D., and Cerio, R. (2004). Occupational airborne allergic contact dermatitis from garlic with concurrent type I allergy. *Contact Dermatitis* 50 (1): 39–41.
315 Kaae, J., Menne, T., and Thyssen, J.P. (2013). Severe occupational protein contact dermatitis caused by fish in 2 patients with filaggrin mutations. *Contact Dermatitis* 68 (5): 319–320.
316 Foti, C., Mistrello, G., Cassano, N. et al. (2012). Occupational protein contact dermatitis from wheat flour with IgE reactivity against alpha-amylase inhibitor. *Contact Dermatitis* 67 (5): 316–318.
317 Rieker, J., Ruzicka, T., Neumann, N.J., and Homey, B. (2004). Protein contact dermatitis to asparagus. *Journal of Allergy and Clinical Immunology* 113 (2): 354–355.
318 Kanerva, L. and Soini, M. (2001). Occupational protein contact dermatitis from coriander. *Contact Dermatitis* 45 (6): 354–355.
319 Vester, L., Thyssen, J.P., Menne, T., and Johansen, J.D. (2012). Occupational food-related hand dermatoses seen over a 10-year period. *Contact Dermatitis* 66 (5): 264–270.
320 Sanz-Sanchez, T., Sanchez-Perez, J., Cordoba, S., and Garcia-Diez, A. (2001). Occupational nickel dermatitis in fritter making. *Contact Dermatitis* 45 (1): 46.
321 Lee, A. and Nixon, R. (2001). Contact dermatitis from sodium metabisulfite in a baker. *Contact Dermatitis* 44 (2): 127–128.
322 Vincenzi, C., Stinchi, C., Ricci, C., and Tosti, A. (1995). Contact dermatitis due to an emulsifying agent in a baker. *Contact Dermatitis* 32 (1): 57.
323 Hamada, T. and Horiguchi, S. (1978). Allergic contact dermatitis due to sodium carboxymethyl cellulose. *Contact Dermatitis* 4 (4): 244.
324 Gasenzer, E.R. and Neugebauer, E.A. (2012). Contact allergies in musicians. *Deutsche Medizinische Wochenschrift* 137 (51–52): 2715–2721.
325 Hallai, N., Meirion Hughes, T., and Stone, N. (2004). Contact allergy to thiuram in a musician. *Contact Dermatitis* 51 (3): 154.
326 Thomas, P., Rueff, F., and Przybilla, B. (2000). Cheilitis due to nickel contact allergy in a trumpet player. *Contact Dermatitis* 42 (6): 351–352.
327 Lieberman, H.D., Fogelman, J.P., Ramsay, D.L., and Cohen, D.E. (2002). Allergic contact dermatitis to propolis in a violin maker. *Journal of the American Academy of Dermatology* 46 (2 Suppl Case Reports): S30–S31.
328 Caero, J.E. and Cohen, P.R. (2012). Fiddler's neck: Chin rest-associated irritant contact dermatitis and allergic contact dermatitis in a violin player. *Dermatology Online Journal* 18 (9): 10.
329 Alvarez, M.S. and Brancaccio, R.R. (2003). Multiple contact allergens in a violinist. *Contact Dermatitis* 49 (1): 43–44.
330 Bork, K. (1993). Allergic contact dermatitis on a violinist's neck from para-phenylenediamine in a chin rest stain. *Contact Dermatitis* 28 (4): 250–251.
331 Herro, E.M., Friedlander, S.F., and Jacob, S.E. (2011). Violin bow-associated rubber allergy in a child. *Dermatitis: Contact, Atopic, Occupational, Drug* 22 (4): 223–224.
332 Fisher, A.A. (1981). Allergic contact dermatitis in a violinist. The role of abietic acid – a sensitizer in rosin (colophony) – as the causative agent. *Cutis* 27 (5): 466, 8, 73.
333 Buckley, D.A. and Rogers, S. (1995). Fiddler's fingers': violin-string dermatitis. *Contact Dermatitis* 32 (1): 46–47.
334 Kuner, N. and Jappe, U. (2004). Allergic contact dermatitis from colophonium, turpentine and ebony in a violinist presenting as fiddler's neck. *Contact Dermatitis* 50 (4): 258–259.
335 Murphy, J., Clark, C., Kenicer, K., and Green, C. (1999). Allergic contact dermatitis from colophony and Compositae in a violinist. *Contact Dermatitis* 40 (6): 334.
336 Gambichler, T., Boms, S., and Freitag, M. (2004). Contact dermatitis and other skin conditions in instrumental musicians. *BMC Dermatology* 4: 3.
337 Friis, U.F., Menne, T., Jellesen, M.S. et al. (2012). Allergic nickel dermatitis caused by playing the guitar: case report and assessment of nickel release from guitar strings. *Contact Dermatitis* 67 (2): 101–103.
338 Smith, V.H., Charles-Holmes, R., and Bedlow, A. (2006). Contact dermatitis in guitar players. *Clinical and Experimental Dermatology* 31 (1): 143–145.
339 Vine, K. and DeLeo, V. (2011). Dermatologic manifestations of musicians: a case report and review of skin conditions in musicians. *Cutis* 87 (3): 117–121.
340 Mariano, M., Patruno, C., Lembo, S., and Balato, N. (2010). Contact cheilitis in a saxophonist. *Dermatitis: Contact, Atopic, Occupational, Drug* 21 (2): 119–120.
341 Inoue, A., Shoji, A., and Yashiro, K. (1998). Saxophonist's cane reed cheilitis. *Contact Dermatitis* 39 (1): 37.
342 McFadden, J.P., Ingram, M.J., and Rycroft, R.J. (1992). Contact allergy to cane reed in a clarinetist. *Contact Dermatitis* 27 (2): 117.
343 O'Hagan, A.H. and Bingham, E.A. (2001). Cellist's finger dermatitis. *Contact Dermatitis* 45 (5): 319.
344 Pfohler, C., Hamsch, C., and Tilgen, W. (2008). Allergic contact dermatitis of the lips in a recorder player caused by African blackwood. *Contact Dermatitis* 59 (3): 180–181.
345 Angelini, G. and Vena, G.A. (1986). Allergic contact dermatitis to colophony in a violoncellist. *Contact Dermatitis* 15 (2): 108.
346 Sommer, S., Wilkinson, S.M., and Dodman, B. (1999). Contact dermatitis due to urea-formaldehyde resin in shin-pads. *Contact Dermatitis* 40 (3): 159–160.
347 Weston, W.L. and Morelli, J.G. (2006). Dermatitis under soccer shin guards: allergy or contact irritant reaction? *Pediatric Dermatology* 23 (1): 19–20.
348 Powell, D. and Ahmed, S. (2010). Soccer shin guard reactions: allergic and irritant reactions. *Dermatitis: Contact, Atopic, Occupational, Drug* 21 (3): 162–166.
349 Sun, C.C. (1987). Allergic contact dermatitis of the face from contact with nickel and ammoniated mercury in spectacle frames and skin-lightening creams. *Contact Dermatitis* 17 (5): 306–309.
350 Suhonen, R. and Kanerva, L. (2001). Allergic contact dermatitis caused by palladium on titanium spectacle frames. *Contact Dermatitis* 44 (4): 257–258.
351 Andersen, K.E., Vestergaard, M.E., and Christensen, L.P. (2014). Triethylene glycol bis (2-ethylhexanoate) – a new contact allergen identified in a spectacle frame. *Contact Dermatitis* 70 (2): 112–116.
352 Carlsen, L., Andersen, K.E., and Egsgaard, H. (1986). Triphenyl phosphate allergy from spectacle frames. *Contact Dermatitis* 15 (5): 274–277.

353 Nakada, T. and Maibach, H.I. (1998). Eyeglass allergic contact dermatitis. *Contact Dermatitis* 39 (1): 1–3.

354 Yeo, L., Kuuliala, O., White, I.R., and Alto-Korte, K. (2011). Allergic contact dermatitis caused by solvent Orange 60 dye. *Contact Dermatitis* 64 (6): 354–356.

355 Sonnex, T.S. and Rycroft, R.J. (1986). Dermatitis from phenyl salicylate in safety spectacle frames. *Contact Dermatitis* 14 (5): 268–270.

356 Nakagawa, M., Kawai, K., and Kawai, K. (1992). Cross-sensitivity between resorcinol, resorcinol monobenzoate and phenyl salicylate. *Contact Dermatitis* 27 (3): 199–200.

357 Thorneby-Andersson, K. and Hansson, C. (1994). Allergic contact dermatitis from colophony in waxes for polishing spectacle frames. *Contact Dermatitis* 31 (2): 126–127.

358 Jordan, W.P. (1972). Turpentine in eyeglasses. *Contact Dermatitis Newsletter* 309.

359 Crepy, M.N., Bensefa-Colas, L., Krief, P. et al. (2011). Facial leukoderma following eczema: a new case induced by spectacle frames. *Contact Dermatitis* 65 (4): 243–245.

360 Vilaplana, J., Romaguera, C., and Grimalt, F. (1987). Allergic contact dermatitis from aliphatic isocyanate on spectacle frames. *Contact Dermatitis* 16 (2): 113.

361 Batchelor, R.J. and Wilkinson, S.M. (2006). Contact allergy to disperse dyes in plastic spectacle frames. *Contact Dermatitis* 54 (1): 66–67.

362 Williams, J.D., Nixon, R.L., and Lee, A. (2007). Recurrent allergic contact dermatitis due to allergen transfer by sunglasses. *Contact Dermatitis* 57 (2): 120–121.

363 El-Houri, R.B., Christensen, L.P., Persson, C. et al. (2016). Methylisothiazolinone in a designer spectacle frame – a surprising finding. *Contact Dermatitis* 75 (5): 310–312.

364 Ebeling, F. (1999). Repeated facial edemas. *Duodecim; Laaketieteellinen Aikakauskirja* 115 (13): 1417–1419.

365 Hecksteden, K., Stuck, B.A., Klimek, L., and Laszig, R. (2005). Relapsing facial erysipelas caused by nickel allergy. Significance of allergy diagnostics in ENT practice. *HNO* 53 (6): 557–559.

366 Pedersen, N.B. (1978). Allergic contact conjunctivitis from merthiolate in soft contact lenses. *Contact Dermatitis* 4 (3): 165.

367 Sertoli, A., Di Fonzo, E., Spallanzani, P., and Panconesi, E. (1980). Allergic contact dermatitis from thimerosol in a soft contact lens wearer. *Contact Dermatitis* 6 (4): 292–293.

368 Peters, K. and Andersen, K.E. (1986). Allergic hand dermatitis from 2-hydroxyethyl-acrylate in contact lenses. *Contact Dermatitis* 15 (3): 188–189.

369 Podmore, P. and Storrs, F.J. (1989). Contact lens intolerance; allergic conjunctivitis? *Contact Dermatitis* 20 (2): 98–103.

370 Donshik, P.C. and Ehlers, W.H. (1991). The contact lens patient and ocular allergies. *International Ophthalmology Clinics* 31 (2): 133–145.

371 Cressey, B.D. and Scheinman, P.L. (2012). Systemic allergic dermatitis of the lips resulting from allergy to an antimicrobial agent in a contact lens disinfecting solution. *Contact Dermatitis* 67 (4): 239–240.

372 Sood, A. and Taylor, J.S. (2004). Allergic contact dermatitis from hearing aid materials. *Dermatitis: Contact, Atopic, Occupational, Drug* 15 (1): 48–50.

373 Koefoed-Nielsen, B. and Pedersen, B. (1993). Allergy caused by light-cured ear-moulds. *Scandinavian Audiology* 22 (3): 193–194.

374 Di Berardino, F., Pigatto, P.D., Ambrosetti, U., and Cesarani, A. (2009). Allergic contact dermatitis to hearing aids: literature and case reports. *Contact Dermatitis* 60 (5): 291–293.

375 Marshall, M., Guill, A., and Odom, R.B. (1978). Hearing aid dermatitis. *Archives of Dermatology* 114 (7): 1050–1051.

376 Meding, B. and Ringdahl, A. (1992). Allergic contact dermatitis from the earmolds of hearing aids. *Ear and Hearing* 13 (2): 122–124.

377 Matrolonardo, M., Loconsole, F., Conte, A., and Rantuccio, F. (1993). Allergic contact dermatitis due to para-tertiary-butylphenol-formaldehyde resin in a hearing aid. *Contact Dermatitis* 28 (3): 197.

378 O'Donoghue, N.B., Rustin, M.H., and McFadden, J.P. (2004). Allergic contact dermatitis from gold on a hearing-aid mould. *Contact Dermatitis* 51 (1): 36–37.

379 Shaw, D.W. (1999). Allergic contact dermatitis to benzyl alcohol in a hearing aid impression material. *American Journal of Contact Dermatitis: Official Journal of the American Contact Dermatitis Society* 10 (4): 228–232.

380 Word, A.P., Nezafati, K.A., and Cruz, P.D. Jr. (2011). Ear dermatitis + epoxy reactivity = hearing aid allergy? *Dermatitis: Contact, Atopic, Occupational, Drug* 22 (6): 350–354.

381 Puri, S., Dornhoffer, J.L., and North, P.E. (2005). Contact dermatitis to silicone after cochlear implantation. *The Laryngoscope* 115 (10): 1760–1762.

382 Lung, H.L., Huang, L.H., Lin, H.C., and Shyur, S.D. (2009). Allergic contact dermatitis to polyethylene terephthalate mesh. *Journal of Investigational Allergology & Clinical Immunology* 19 (2): 161–162.

383 Onder, M., Onder, T., Ozunlu, A. et al. (1994). An investigation of contact dermatitis in patients with chronic otitis externa. *Contact Dermatitis* 31 (2): 116–117.

384 Deguchi, M. and Tagami, H. (1996). Contact dermatitis of the ear due to a rubber earplug. *Dermatology* 193 (3): 251–252.

385 Yates, V.M. and Dixon, J.E. (1988). Contact dermatitis from azodicarbonamide in earplugs. *Contact Dermatitis* 19 (2): 155–156.

386 Baxter, K.F. and Wilkinson, S.M. (2002). Contact dermatitis from a nickel-containing bindi. *Contact Dermatitis* 47 (1): 55.

387 Gupta, D. and Thappa, D.M. (2015). Dermatoses due to Indian cultural practices. *Indian Journal of Dermatology* 60 (1): 3–12.

388 Laxmisha, C., Nath, A.K., and Thappa, D.M. (2006). Bindi dermatitis due to thimerosal and gallate mix. *Journal of the European Academy of Dermatology and Venereology* 20 (10): 1370–1372.

389 Tewary, M. and Ahmed, I. (2006). Bindi dermatitis to 'chandan' bindi. *Contact Dermatitis* 55 (6): 372–374.

390 Lilly, E. and Kundu, R.V. (2012). Dermatoses secondary to Asian cultural practices. *International Journal of Dermatology* 51 (4): 372–379; quiz 9-82.

391 Dwyer, C.M. and Forsyth, A. (1994). Allergic contact dermatitis from bindi. *Contact Dermatitis* 30 (3): 174.

392 Richardson, C., Hamann, C.R., Hamann, D., and Thyssen, J.P. (2014). Mobile phone dermatitis in children and adults: a review of the literature. *Pediatric Allergy, Immunology, and Pulmonology* 27 (2): 60–69.

393 Jacob, S.E., Goldenberg, A., Pelletier, J.L. et al. (2015). Nickel allergy and our children's health: a review of indexed cases and a view of future prevention. *Pediatric Dermatology* 32 (6): 779–785.

394 Aquino, M., Mucci, T., Chong, M. et al. (2013). Mobile phones: potential sources of nickel and cobalt exposure for metal allergic patients. *Pediatric Allergy, Immunology, and Pulmonology* 26 (4): 181–186.

395 Jensen, P., Johansen, U.B., Johansen, J.D., and Thyssen, J.P. (2013). Nickel may be released from iPhone([R]) 5. *Contact Dermatitis* 68 (4): 255–256.

396 Jensen, P., Johansen, J.D., Zachariae, C. et al. (2011). Excessive nickel release from mobile phones – a persistent cause of nickel allergy and dermatitis. *Contact Dermatitis* 65 (6): 354–358.

397 Berk, D.R. and Bayliss, S.J. (2011). Cellular phone and cellular phone accessory dermatitis due to nickel allergy: report of five cases. *Pediatric Dermatology* 28 (3): 327–331.

398 Tan, S. and Nixon, R. (2011). Allergic contact dermatitis caused by chromium in a mobile phone. *Contact Dermatitis* 65 (4): 246–247.

399 Williams, P.J., King, C., and Arslanian, V. (2012). Allergic contact dermatitis caused by a cell phone cover. *Australasian Journal of Dermatology* 53 (1): 76–77.

400 Lee, D.Y. and Yang, J.M. (2010). Preauricular eczema: a sign of cellular phone dermatitis. *Clinical and Experimental Dermatology* 35 (2): 201–202.

401 Livideanu, C., Giordano-Labadie, F., and Paul, C. (2007). Cellular phone addiction and allergic contact dermatitis to nickel. *Contact Dermatitis* 57 (2): 130–131.

402 Ozkaya, E. (2011). Bilateral symmetrical contact dermatitis on the face and outer thighs from the simultaneous use of two mobile phones. *Dermatitis: Contact, Atopic, Occupational, Drug* 22 (2): 116–118.

403 Guarneri, F., Guarneri, C., and Cannavo, S.P. (2010). An unusual case of cell phone dermatitis. *Contact Dermatitis* 62 (2): 117.

404 Suarez, A., Chimento, S., and Tosti, A. (2011). Unusual localization of cell phone dermatitis. *Dermatitis: Contact, Atopic, Occupational, Drug* 22 (5): 277–278.

405 Dannepond, C. and Armingaud, P. (2012). Breast eczema: mobile phones must not be overlooked. *Annales de Dermatologie et de Venereologie* 139 (2): 142–143.

406 Capon, F., Cambie, M.P., Clinard, F. et al. (1996). Occupational contact dermatitis caused by computer mice. *Contact Dermatitis* 35 (1): 57–58.

407 Goossens, A., Blondeel, S., and Zimerson, E. (2002). Resorcinol monobenzoate: a potential sensitizer in a computer mouse. *Contact Dermatitis* 47 (4): 235–235.

408 Garcia-Morales, I., Garcia Bravo, B., and Camacho Martinez, F. (2003). Occupational contact dermatitis caused by a personal-computer mouse mat. *Contact Dermatitis* 49 (3): 172.

409 Johnson, R.C. and Elston, D.M. (1997). Wrist dermatitis: contact allergy to neoprene in a keyboard wrist rest. *American Journal of Contact Dermatitis: Official Journal of the American Contact Dermatitis Society* 8 (3): 172–174.

410 Bassiri, S. and Cohen, D.E. (2002). Bilateral palmar dermatitis. *American Journal of Contact Dermatitis: Official Journal of the American Contact Dermatitis Society* 13 (2): 75–76.

411 Yokota, M., Fox, L.P., and Maibach, H.I. (2007). Bilateral palmar dermatitis possible caused by computer wrist rest. *Contact Dermatitis* 57 (3): 192–193.

412 Ghasri, P. and Feldman, S.R. (2010). Frictional lichenified dermatosis from prolonged use of a computer mouse: case report and review of the literature of computer-related dermatoses. *Dermatology Online Journal* 16 (12): 3.

413 Coman, G., Blattner, C.M., Blickenstaff, N.R. et al. (2014). Textile allergic contact dermatitis: current status. *Reviews on Environmental Health* 29 (3): 163–168.

414 Malinauskiene, L., Bruze, M., Ryberg, K. et al. (2012). Contact allergy from disperse dyes in textiles: a review. *Contact Dermatitis* 68 (2): 65–75.

415 Nygaard, U., Kralund, H.H., and Sommerlund, M. (2013). Allergic contact dermatitis induced by textile necklace. *Case Reports in Dermatology* 5 (3): 336–339.

416 Ozkaya-Bayazit, E. and Buyukbabani, N. (2001). Non-eczematous pigmented interface dermatitis from para-tertiary-butylphenol-formaldehyde resin in a watchstrap adhesive. *Contact Dermatitis* 44 (1): 45–46.

417 Kanerva, L., Jolanki, R., and Estlander, T. (1996). Allergic contact dermatitis from leather strap of wrist watch. *International Journal of Dermatology* 35 (9): 680–681.

418 Romaguera, C., Aguirre, A., Diaz Perez, J.L., and Grimalt, F. (1986). Watch strap dermatitis. *Contact Dermatitis* 14 (4): 260–261.

419 Foussereau, J., Cavelier, C., and Protois, J.C. (1988). A case of allergic isopropyl-p-phenylenediamine (IPPD) dermatitis from a watch strap. *Contact Dermatitis* 18 (4): 253.

420 Gamboni, S.E., Simmons, I., Palmer, A., and Nixon, R.L. (2013). Allergic contact dermatitis to indium in jewellery: diagnosis made possible through the use of the contact allergen Bank Australia. *Australasian Journal of Dermatology* 54 (2): 139–140.

421 Kawai, K., Zhang, X.M., Nakagawa, M. et al. (1994). Allergic contact dermatitis due to mercury in a wedding ring and a cosmetic. *Contact Dermatitis* 31 (5): 330–331.

422 Cordoba, S., Sanchez-Perez, J., and Garcia-Diez, A. (2000). Ring dermatitis as a clinical presentation of fragrance sensitization. *Contact Dermatitis* 42 (4): 242.

423 Pazzaglia, M., Vincenzi, C., Montanari, A., and Tosti, A. (1998). Sensitization to nickel from an umbilical ring. *Contact Dermatitis* 38 (6): 345.

424 Gaul, J.E. (1967). Development of allergic nickel dermatitis from earrings. *Journal of the American Medical Association* 200 (2): 176–178.

425 Nakada, T., Iijima, M., Nakayama, H., and Maibach, H.I. (1997). Role of ear piercing in metal allergic contact dermatitis. *Contact Dermatitis* 36 (5): 233–236.

426 Shore, R.N. and Berger, B.J. (1974). Letter: earring dermatitis sparing the ears. *Archives of Dermatology* 109 (1): 95.

427 Goossens, A., De Swerdt, A., De Coninck, K. et al. (2006). Allergic contact granuloma due to palladium following ear piercing. *Contact Dermatitis* 55 (6): 338–341.

428 Ehrlich, A., Kucenic, M., and Belsito, D.V. (2001). Role of body piercing in the induction of metal allergies. *American Journal of Contact Dermatitis: Official Journal of the American Contact Dermatitis Society* 12 (3): 151–155.

429 Lodi, A., Chiarelli, G., Mancini, L.L. et al. (1996). Allergic contact dermatitis from a rubber bracelet. *Contact Dermatitis* 34 (2): 146.

430 Hausen, B.M. (1982). Rosewood allergy due to an arm bracelet and a recorder. *Dermatosen in Beruf und Umwelt Occupation and Environment* 30 (6): 189–192.

431 Moratinos, M.M., Tevar, E., and Conde-Salazar, L. (2005). Contact allergy to a cocobolo bracelet. *Dermatitis: Contact, Atopic, Occupational, Drug* 16 (3): 139–141.

432 Dias, M. and Vale, T. (1992). Contact dermatitis from a Dalbergia nigra bracelet. *Contact Dermatitis* 26 (1): 61–62.

433 Matthys, E., Zahir, A., and Ehrlich, A. (2014). Shoe allergic contact dermatitis. *Dermatitis: Contact, Atopic, Occupational, Drug* 25 (4): 163–171.

434 Epstein, E. (1969). Shoe contact dermatitis. *Journal of the American Medical Association* 209 (10): 1487–1492.

435 Cronin E. Chapter 4. In:*Clothing and Textiles*. Edinburgh: Churchill Livingstone; 1980 36–93.
436 Calnan, C.D. and Sarkany, I. (1959). Studies in contact dermatitis. IX. Shoe dermatitis. *Transactions of the St John's Hospital Dermatological Society* 43: 8–26.
437 Rose, R.F., Lyons, P., Horne, H., and Mark Wilkinson, S. (2009). A review of the materials and allergens in protective gloves. *Contact Dermatitis* 61 (3): 129–137.
438 Fisher, A.A. (1992). Allergic contact reactions in health personnel. *Journal of Allergy and Clinical Immunology* 90 (5): 729–738.
439 Nedorost, S. (2009). Clinical patterns of hand and foot dermatitis: emphasis on rubber and chromate allergens. *Dermatologic Clinics* 27 (3): 281–287, vi.
440 Cronin, E. (1985). Clinical patterns of hand eczema in women. *Contact Dermatitis* 13 (3): 153–161.

CHAPTER 5

Microexamination

CHAPTER CONTENTS

Introduction

- In order to detect diagnostic clues in contact dermatitis, careful examination of the patient is required. “Microexamination” is a meticulous and systematic contact dermatitis examination.
- Examination can be divided into:
  1. *Local*: involving the anatomical area of presenting dermatitis
  2. *Distal* anatomical sites: For example, if a patient with eyelid dermatitis is found to be allergic to nail varnish resin, particular distal sites of interest would include the lower area of the face, the neck, the “V area” of the front of the chest, the lips and the nail folds, all potential areas of contact dermatitis to nail varnish resin in addition to the periorbital area. This can also be helpful in diagnosing endogenous or non-dermatitis dermatoses. The local/distal elements to examination are illustrated in Tables 5.5–5.8 of this chapter.
  3. *Temporal*: Patients often have photographic records of acute exacerbations or unusual elements to their dermatitis. This can now be used as a third dimension to the objective examination/assessment of the dermatitis.

Microexamination

- To illustrate this concept of microexamination further, two essential anatomical areas for examination, the hands and the head and neck, are reviewed. Even when not part of the local examination, these two regions are mandatory areas for distal site examination (see Figures 5.1 and 5.2).

Microexamination of the hands

General principles

- *Often heterogeneous and multifactorial*: Hand dermatitis is generally accepted to consist of a heterogeneous group of dermatitis of differing etiologies including endogenous, irritant, and allergic, with often multiple causative factors. Patterns of dermatitis may therefore vary.
- *Acute, chronic, and “acute on chronic”*: Morphological assessment can determine acute features of dermatitis (e.g. vesiculation, marked erythema, exudation), chronic dermatitis (e.g. scaling, fissuring, lichenification), or a combination of both.
- *Local spread of allergic contact dermatitis (ACD) may hide a distinctive pattern of ACD*: Although several distinctive

Common Contact Allergens: A Practical Guide to Detecting Contact Dermatitis, First Edition. Edited by John McFadden, Pailin Puangpet, Korbkarn Pongpairoj, Supitchaya Thaiwat, and Lee Shan Xian.

© 2020 John Wiley & Sons Ltd. Published 2020 by John Wiley & Sons Ltd.

Companion website: www.wiley.com/go/mcfadden/common_contact_allergens

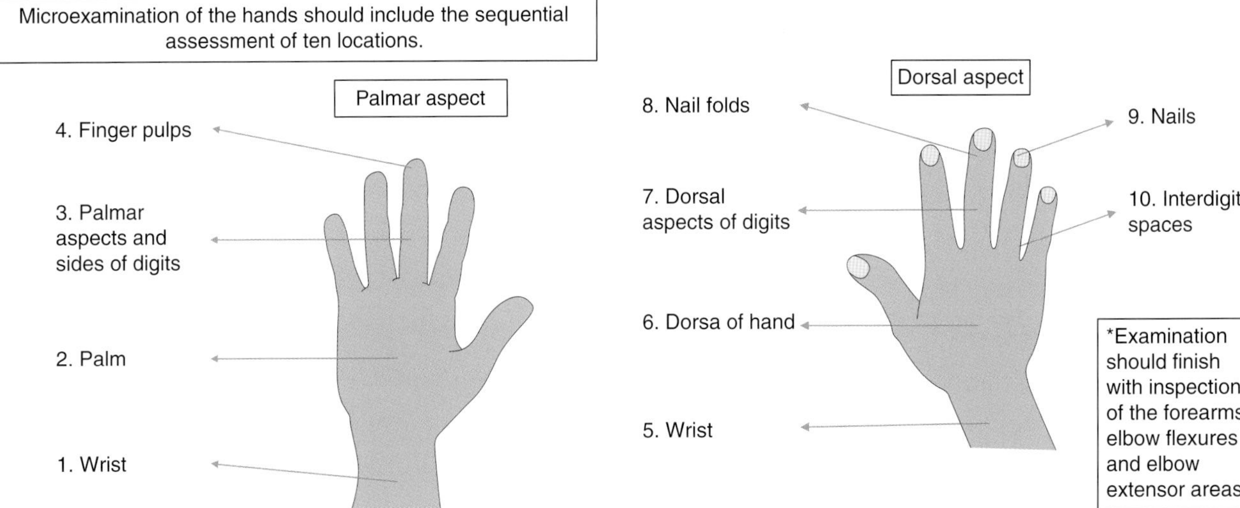

Figure 5.1 Microexamination of the hands.

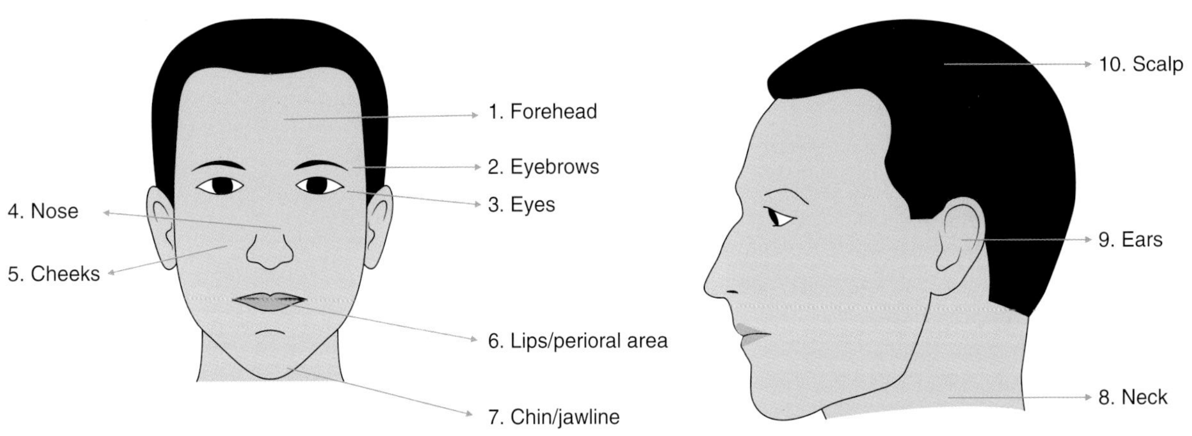

Figure 5.2 Microexamination of the head and neck.

patterns of ACD have been described, e.g. glove dermatitis, these may be concealed by local secondary spread of ACD, particularly in chronic ACD.

- *Classification of hand eczema by morphological type*: The Danish Contact Dermatitis Group has proposed a classification of hand eczema based on morphological subtypes after testing the concept on 710 patients [128]: vesicular, rare eruptions (5.9% of total group), vesicular, repeated eruptions (31.8%), dry fissured (31.8%), hyperkeratotic palmar (7.4%), nummular (7.9%), pulpitis (1.1%), and non-classifiable (8.8%).
- *ACD is more common in vesicular type dermatitis*: The Danish Contact Dermatitis Group found that irritant contact dermatitis (ICD) was most frequent in the dry fissured (44%), pulpitis (42%), and nummular (41%) subtypes, whereas ACD was the more common diagnosis in vesicular, rare eruptions (24%), and vesicular, repeated eruptions (35%). Another group also found an association between vesicular hand dermatitis and contact allergy [129], the most frequent sensitizers being metals, fragrances, and preservatives.
- *Patients with hand dermatitis should always be patch tested*: Cronin (1985) studied the patterns of hand eczema in 263 sequentially patch tested patients and concluded that one could not predict the presence of ACD based on pattern alone (although ICD affected the palmar area to a lesser degree) [130]. In another study by Cronin (1972), 25 women were diagnosed with rubber glove dermatitis but in none was the diagnosis made before patch testing, and in some they had suffered several years before rubber ACD was diagnosed by patch testing [131].
- *The "apron pattern" of hand dermatitis is almost always endogenous*: A localized eczema of the central palm spreading

proximally from the interdigital areas toward the base of the hand ("apron pattern") is probably always endogenous [131]. However, as with other endogenous dermatitis, it may coexist with allergic and/or ICD.

- *Atopic hand dermatitis is often complicated by ICD*: This is particularly noted in an occupational setting [132]. The association of atopic dermatitis with barrier (filaggrin) defects may be one major factor.
- *Psoriasis and tinea are important diagnoses to eliminate*: See Chapter 8.
- *It is useful to get patients to demonstrate how they hold objects*: This is because there is a great degree of variation, which would affect the clinical pattern of ACD (e.g. pens, mobile phones).

10-point local examination of the hands

- Examination of the hands should include the sequential assessment of ten locations (Figure 5.1):

Palmar aspect

1. Wrists
2. Palms
3. Palmar aspects and sides of digits
4. Finger pulps

Dorsal aspect

5. Wrists
6. Dorsa of hand
7. Dorsal aspects of digits
8. Nail folds
9. Nails
10. Dorsal interdigital areas

Examination should finish with inspection of the forearms, and elbow flexures and extensors.

The sections below provide further elaboration in conjunction with Tables 5.1 and 5.2.

Table 5.1 Some examples of ACD affecting the hands.

	Direct contact (allergens in brackets)	Others (by proxy, systemic)
Wrists/lower forearm (examination points 1 and 5)	Bracelet/bangle/wristband (metal, rubber, plastic, wood) Wearable health devices (nickel, acrylates) Watch (metal, chromate, *p*-tertiary butyl-phenol formaldehyde (PTBP) resin, rubber) Clothing dyes Rubber gloves Perfume Sunscreen chemicals affecting the dorsal aspects, causing ACD and/or photoallergic contact dermatitis Topical medicaments Orthopedic wrist splint (neoprene) Keyboard wrist rest (neoprene)	By proxy: nickel (partner's watch from holding hands)
Palms, palmar aspects and sides of digits (examination points 2 and 3)	Occupational exposures (multiple agents) Coins Rubber gloves Gripped objects[a] Affected in vesicular hand eczema, which has the strongest association with contact allergy (metals, fragrance, isothiazolinones) Hyperkeratotic hand eczema often affects palmar aspects Squash ball (black rubber) Escalator rail (black rubber) Medicament allergy from applying medicated creams onto others	By proxy: primin and other plant chemicals left on door knobs, furniture Systemic: can involve the palms especially, with vesiculation (nickel, sesquiterpene lactone)
Finger pulps (examination point 4)	Plants Resins (epoxy resins, acrylates) Metals Rubber gloves Can be affected in vesicular hand eczema Medicament allergy from applying medicated creams onto others	
Dorsal aspects of hands and digits (examination points 6 and 7)	Ring dermatitis can be due to metal ACD Rubber gloves Sunscreen chemicals causing ACD and/or photoallergic contact dermatitis	
Nail folds and nail plate (examination points 8 and 9)	Nail varnish (resins) Sculptured and ultraviolet (UV)-cured nails (acrylates) Nail extensions (ethyl cyanoacrylate) Nail folds can be affected in vesicular hand eczema	
Dorsal interdigital spaces (examination point 10)	Billiard cue (resin) Spread from ring dermatitis	

Medicament allergy can complicate all dermatitis conditions of the hand. Dry fissured eczema can affect all areas of the hands.
[a] Pattern of dermatitis dependent on individual's method of gripping object (e.g. bag, racket, utensil).

Table 5.2 Some examples of non-allergic dermatoses affecting the hands, which may be part of a differential diagnosis for ACD.

	Irritant contact dermatitis	Endogenous/other eczemas	Non-dermatitis dermatoses, others
Wrists/lower forearm (examination points 1 and 5)	Bracelets can cause ICD	Atopic dermatitis (flexural aspects)	Lichen planus (flexural aspects) Wristwatch tinea
Palms, palmar aspects and sides of digits (examination points 2 and 3)	Common site of involvement (acute, cumulative, or mechanical ICD), though less frequent than dorsal aspect Handling of plants	"Apron pattern" of palmar dermatitis supports endogenous eczema	Pustular/palmoplantar psoriasis Lichen planus Erythema multiforme Infections, e.g. tinea manuum, secondary syphilis, coxsackie virus Keratodermas Keratolysis exfoliativa Bazex's syndrome
Finger pulps (examination point 4)	Can occur with alstroemeria and bulbous plants such as narcissus/hyacinth/onion/garlic	Atopic dermatitis	Psoriasis Vasculitic infarcts
Dorsal aspects of hands and digits (examination points 6 and 7)	Common site of involvement (acute or cumulative ICD) Ring dermatitis can be due to ICD	Atopic dermatitis Nummular eczema Chronic actinic dermatitis (CAD)	Connective tissue disorders, e.g. dermatomyositis, scleroderma Acanthosis nigricans Ochronosis Actinic change Photodermatoses, e.g. porphyria, actinic prurigo, drug photosensitivity, pellagra Granuloma annulare Erythema multiforme Infections, e.g. orf Phytophotodermatitis
Nail folds and nail plate (examination points 8 and 9)	Chronic exposure to irritant substances (e.g. detergents, bulbs, and spices) can cause nail changes and paronychia Solvents used to remove enamel or cuticles can cause paronychia Formaldehyde-containing nail hardeners are irritant and can cause painful onycholysis	Atopic dermatitis can affect the nail folds and cause secondary nail dystrophy	Psoriasis Lichen planus Connective tissue disorders Darier's disease Bazex's syndrome Infections, e.g. onychomycosis, bacterial/candidal paronychia Metabolic conditions, e.g. thyroid disease Drug-induced nail disorders, e.g. tetracycline-induced onycholysis
Dorsal interdigital spaces (examination point 10)	Common site of involvement, especially cumulative ICD Frequent use of liquid soaps/detergents	Atopic dermatitis	Interdigital pilonidal sinus/foreign body granuloma Infections, e.g. scabies, candida Drug phototoxicity, e.g. doxycycline Phytophotodermatitis

Examination points 1 and 5: wrists/lower forearm

- *Bracelets* can be made of metal, rubber, plastic or wood and all can give ACD reactions. One case of ACD to Indian rosewood, a quinone-containing hardwood, showed acute changes with erythema, edema, and blistering [133]. Another three patients had ACD to "silver-oak" wooden bracelets [134]. All reacted on patch testing to the wood shavings. ACD to a hospital identification bracelet developed 2 hours post-operatively with erythema and edema on the wrist extending to the digits [135]. Identification bracelets can occasionally cause severe ACD – plastic chemicals such as dibutyl phthalate, resorcinol monobenzoate, and benzoyl peroxide have been implicated. ACD to loose-fitting metal bangles can give a wide band of dermatitis due to the bangles moving over a wider area of the wrist/forearm.
- *Wrist watch* ACD can be due to the metal component (nickel), chromate or PTBP resin from a leather strap. However, of 21 watches bought in Bangkok in 2015, only one and three were positive to nickel and cobalt spot tests, respectively [136]. The eczema may be bilateral if the watch is transferred to the other wrist due to the eczema.
- *Clothing*: The wrist area (flexor and extensor aspects) is one of the target areas for azo clothing dye ACD.
- The classic "*rubber glove*" dermatitis shows a sharply delineated band of eczema on the wrist/upper forearm corresponding

to the upper border of the glove, associated with eczema on the dorsa of the hands and flexor and extensor aspects of the wrists and not extending beyond the covered areas of the glove. However, this classic distribution was seen in very few patients in Cronin's series (1980), with the majority having a non-specific pattern of eczema. She remarks that in most patients, rubber glove allergy could not have been made without patch testing [137].

- The flexural aspect of the lower forearm/wrist is the second most common site for perfume spray to be applied [87].
- Occupational: Inadequate cover from gloves and/or protective clothing can lead to ACD or ICD from noxious chemicals in an occupational environment. Occupational ACD can lead to flares of atopic dermatitis, with the wrist being one target area [138].
- Uncommon/rare presentations in the literature:
  - *Medicaments* (see also Figure 5.3): A 34-year-old man presented with a combination of leukoderma and pigmented contact dermatitis on the flexural aspects of his wrist and lower forearm from a topical herbal preparation for chronic wrist pain [139].
  - A 47-year-old man developed ACD on the wrist area to neoprene from an orthopedic *wrist splint* [140].
  - *ACD to keyboard wrist rests*: Neoprene ACD with dermatitis on the flexural aspects of both wrists with secondary spread to the extremities and face [141].
  - *Photoallergic contact dermatitis*: An outbreak involving the wrists from wearing brosimum wood bracelets was described [142].
  - *Keyboard wrist pads*: Two Japanese workers spending 6 hours or more daily on a computer for several years developed sclerotic thickened wrist pads on the ulnar side of the flexor aspect of the wrist from persistent application of that area to their desks (pressure/mechanical irritant effect) [143].
  - ICD from a *tight elasticated bracelet* giving a linear erythematous vesicular dermatitis on the wrist has been reported [144]. Rubber wrist bands are usually more likely to cause ACD than ICD.
- Wrist flexural eczema is commonly observed in atopic dermatitis.
- Itchy violaceous polygonal papules of the flexural aspects of the wrists are observed in lichen planus.
- Wrist watch tinea (*Trichophyton rubrum*, candida) can mimic nickel ACD but often begins as a small circumscribed scaly area which grows [145].

Examination points 2 and 3: palms, palmar aspects, and sides of digits

- A few examples of distinctive patterns of palmar and digital ACD are given:
  - There are multiple causes of occupational ACD affecting the palmar area of the hand, e.g. cutting oils, essential oils, and hairdressing chemicals.
  - Coin dermatitis can affect the palmar holding area and palmar digits and pulps [146].
  - Squash ball dermatitis from ACD to black rubber affects the central palmar area of the non-dominant hand [147].
  - ACD to black rubber affecting the palmar aspects of the fingers of the right hand, from intermittently holding an escalator rail [148].
  - ACD to acrylates presenting with left palmar involvement alone in a nurse through kneading whilst holding dental cement in the left hand (rubber gloves providing inadequate protection from acrylate permeation) [149].
  - ACD to primula is often characterized by linear erythematous lesions with vesicles or blisters, but can occasionally present with lichenoid papules on the thumbs and wrists [150].
- *Holding and gripping objects*: Ask the patient to demonstrate as there is much inter-individual variation. The pressure areas of the hands have been described as the thenar and hypothenar eminences, and the margins of the palmar areas of the digits [151]. These areas are twice as likely to be involved in manual workers with palmar psoriasis compared to non-manual workers. The grip areas for bag handles often involve the palmar digits and adjacent palmar areas. A walking stick may be gripped like a bag or held with the palmar area and first three digits. Reading a book will often involve the palmar digits and thenar areas of both hands, whilst holding a mobile phone may involve the palmar digits/pulps and the thenar eminence or mid palm, depending on the size of the phone and the size of the hand. It can be helpful to ask the patient to demonstrate their holding technique. Whilst some ACD from rods, sticks, and handles (e.g. bicycles, pushchairs, rackets, steering wheels, and handbags) may give a pattern reflecting contact, this may not necessarily be evident if secondary spread has occurred.
- *Vesicular hand eczema* (Figure 5.4) is characterized by vesicular eczema on the palms and palmar aspects and sides of digits (and occasionally the dorsal digital skin adjacent to the nail folds). This type of hand eczema has the strongest association with contact allergy [128, 129]. Nickel, cobalt, fragrance, and the isothiazolinones are the most commonly associated allergens [129]. Although direct contact is the most common mode of exposure, other modes should be considered, e.g. by proxy, vesicular hand dermatitis in sesquiterpene lactone sensitive patients from oral ingestion of compositae. Associations with atopy and ingested metal are postulated but remain controversial [152]. Patients with tinea pedis are significantly at risk of developing outbreaks of vesicular hand eczema [153].
- *Hyperkeratotic hand eczema* is defined as well-demarcated hyperkeratosis on the palms, possibly extending to the palmar aspects of the fingers [154]. It is distinguished from psoriasis by (i) being less inflamed, (ii) absence of silvery scale, and (iii) lack of evidence of psoriasis on distal examination. It does not evolve into psoriasis. Interestingly, there is an inverse association with smoking, whereas pustular psoriasis occurs almost exclusively amongst smokers/ex-smokers [155]. The most common contact allergies detected in this group were nickel (13%), the

(a)

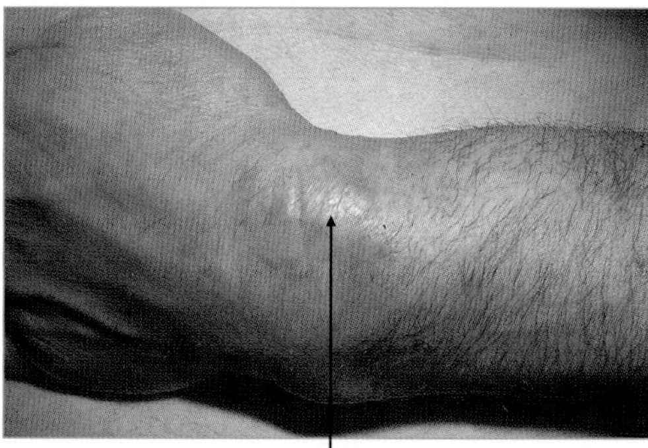

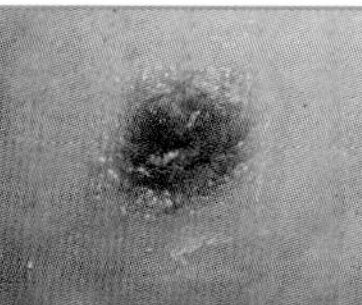

This patient developed localized erythema and edema at the site of application of topical diphenhydramine cream to relieve itch after an insect bite. He demonstrated a +++ patch test reaction to the cream. Apart from prescription topical medications, over-the-counter topicals and herbal preparations should be enquired about as well.

(b)

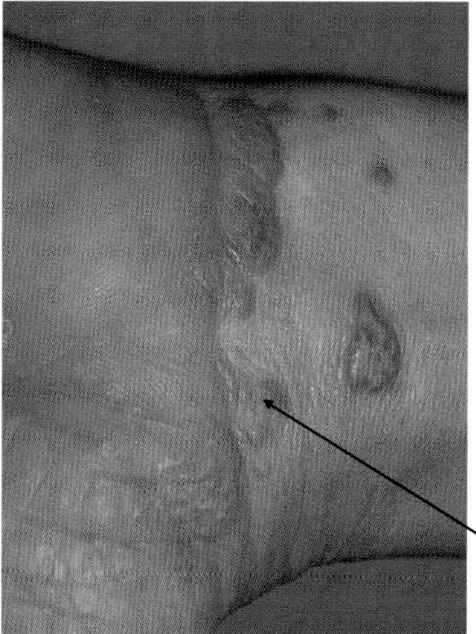

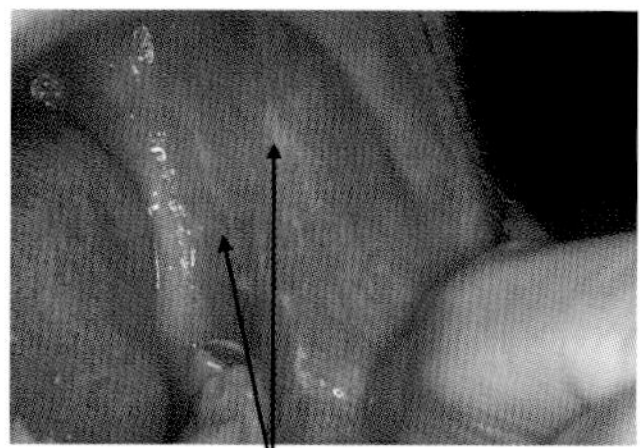

Check the buccal mucosa for Wickham's striae. The scalp, nails and genitals can be involved as well.
Violaceous polygonal shiny flat-topped papules and plaques with overlying Wickham's striae. Lichen planus classically affects the flexural aspects of the wrists.

(c)

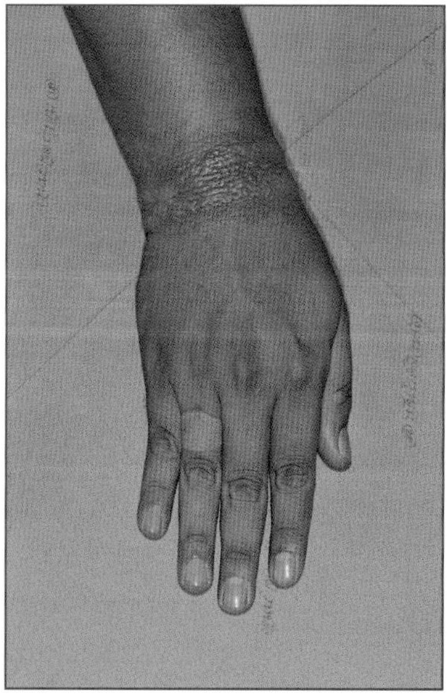

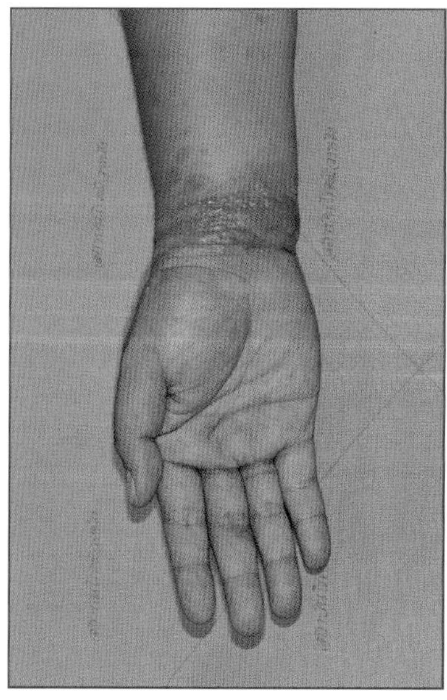

Figure 5.3 Examples of dermatoses affecting the wrist. (a) Contact dermatitis to topical diphenhydramine cream. (b) Lichen planus affecting the wrist. (c) ACD from wooden bangle coated with lacquer tree resin.

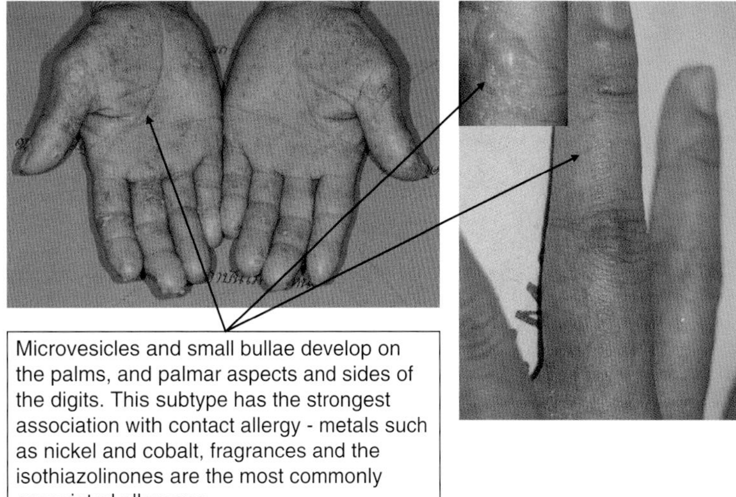

Vesicular hand eczema/pompholyx
Microvesicles and small bullae develop on the palms, and palmar aspects and sides of the digits. This subtype has the strongest association with contact allergy - metals such as nickel and cobalt, fragrances and the isothiazolinones are the most commonly associated allergens.

Figure 5.4 Vesicular hand eczema.

isothiazolinones (6.7%), methyldibromoglutaronitrile (5.9%), and potassium dichromate (5%) (NB: clinical relevance is not commented upon) [129].

- *Chronic fissured eczema* is defined as dry eczema, usually with scaling and possibly hyperkeratotic areas and fissures, with a limited number of vesicles, on the sides and palmar aspects of the palm or palmar aspects of the fingers [154]. All areas of the hands can be affected. This morphology is typically seen in chronic hand eczema [154]. The most common allergens detected in this group were nickel (16.5%), methylchloroisothiazolinone/methylisothiazolinone (MCI/MI) (10.4%), cobalt (6.3%) and fragrances (fragrance mix 1 6.1%, fragrance mix 2 5.9%). Rubber accelerator allergy is twice as common in this group compared to the vesicular subtype and three times more common compared to the hyperkeratotic subtype [129].
- In a group mainly consisting of homemakers, irritant exposure was considered relevant in over 50% with palmar hand dermatitis [130].
- *Mechanical* trauma from occupational-related pressure, vibration or repeated handling of objects such as paper, cardboard, and fabric can cause ICD, sometimes presenting as a hyperkeratotic variant.
- *Endogenous dermatitis* can give an "apron pattern" of palmar dermatitis.
- *Filaggrin null-mutations* may manifest with hyperlinear palms.
- *Tinea manuum* can be characterized by fine scaling within the palmar creases.

Examination point 4: finger pulps

- ACD to plants, resins (e.g. epoxy resin, acrylates), and metals can all present as pulpitis.
- Allergic and irritant occupational contact dermatitis to alstroemeria in two florists was described as a pruriginous dry pulpitis with hyperkeratosis and fissuring localized to the first three digits of both hands, extending to the palmar aspect of the right hand in one patient. Occasional episodes of pruriginous vesiculation of the fingers had also been experienced [156].
- *Tulip fingers*: In ACD in tulip pickers, the pulps of the thumb and index finger are most frequently involved but it can occasionally spread to other parts of the body [157].
- *Bulb dermatitis*: Handling other bulbous plants such as narcissus, hyacinth, garlic, and onion can give rise to both ACD and ICD [158]. "Garlic fingers" involves the thumb, as well as the second and third finger pulps of the non-dominant hand which hold the garlic whilst it is being cut. Garlic juice may run to affect the adjacent areas of these digits.
- Patients with pulpitis were more likely to be allergic to methacrylates compared to patients with hand dermatitis without pulpitis [129]. In a dental worker with ACD to methacrylate, dermatitis started on the right index finger pulp before spreading [159].
- The finger pulps may be involved as part of vesicular or chronic fissured hand eczema.
- Rare cases of ACD from the literature:
  - Pulpitis of all digits was a manifestation of occupational ACD to benzisothiazolinone in a shoe glue [160].
  - Photoallergic contact dermatitis affecting the right thumb and adjacent two digits in carers administering chlorpromazine drops [161].
- ICD can also present as pulpitis – in one large study 41% of hand eczema patients with pulpitis were diagnosed with ICD [128].
- Digital pulpitis has been proposed as a singular manifestation of atopic dermatitis [162] and can also be a manifestation of *psoriasis*.

Examination points 6 and 7: dorsal aspects of the hands and digits

- In Cronin's survey of 263 consecutive women with hand eczema (1985), only 18 (7%) had eczema confined to the dorsal aspects of the hands and digits. However, this group had the highest incidence of contact with irritants (75%) [130]. In contrast, a study of 164 patients with occupational hand dermatitis found that dorsal hand, finger, and nail fold involvement was associated with ACD [163].
- A large study of 714 consecutive patients with hand dermatitis found that patients with a history of atopy were more likely to have dorsal hand involvement [164].
- *Ring dermatitis* (dorsal and palmar digits) may be either irritant (especially if loose-fitting rings) or ACD to metal.
- Of 65 cement workers with hand dermatitis, the majority suffering from ICD, hyperkeratosis of the dorsa of the hand around the metacarpophalangeal joints was noted to be a common finding [165].
- *Hyperkeratosis* of the knuckles and dorsal aspects of the hands and feet has been described as an occupational dermatosis amongst carpet-fitters [166].
- *Nummular eczema* is one of the six clinical subtypes of hand eczema as defined by the Danish Contact Dermatitis Group [154]. The well-circumscribed lesions are characterized by erythema, keratosis, and vesicles, and are often located on the dorsal aspects of the hands and fingers. The lesions are frequently colonized/infected with *Staphylococcus aureus* [154]. Nummular eczema is often associated with involvement of the feet/lower legs. Although associations with ICD [128] and metal contact allergy [167] have been reported, it is considered to be primarily an endogenous dermatitis.
- *Photodermatoses* such as actinic dermatitis, porphyria, actinic prurigo (24% of cases) [168], photoaggravated dermatoses, photoallergic contact dermatitis, and drug photosensitivity frequently affect the dorsa of the hands.
- *Non-dermatitis dermatoses* involving the dorsa of the hand include scleroderma, dermatomyositis (Gottron's papules), subtypes of acanthosis nigricans and lesions associated with solar damage, e.g. solar keratoses.

Examination points 8 and 9: nail folds and nail plate

- The frequency of nail fold involvement in patients with ACD to tosylamide formaldehyde nail varnish varies between reports; whilst most state it is a minority, one report found, on close inspection, some form of nail involvement in 11/18 patients [169].
- Acrylate ACD (Figure 5.5) from sculptured and UV-cured nails more commonly affects the nail unit when compared to tosylamide formaldehyde nail varnish ACD, although facial and eyelid involvement can also be seen [170]. Onychodystrophy, paronychia, onycholysis, (rarely) permanent loss of nails, and eczematous reactions of the surrounding skin can occur [170].
- ACD to ethyl cyanoacrylate from nail extensions also predominantly presents with nail unit dermatitis; onychodystrophy, onycholysis, paronychia, and nail bed hyperkeratosis can occur, as can eyelid involvement [170]. Other resins used in nail cosmetics can occasionally cause ACD affecting the nail unit.

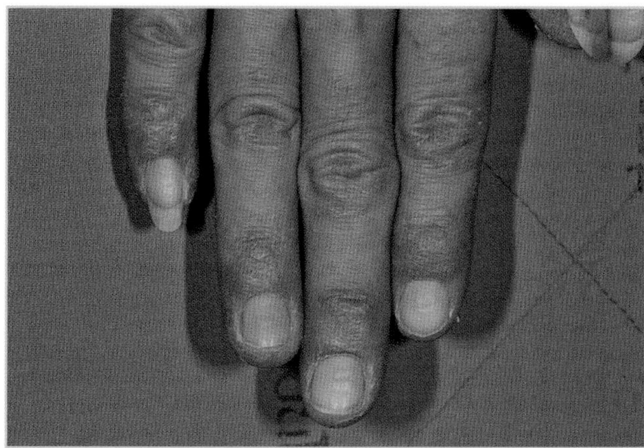

Figure 5.5 Allergic contact dermatitis to acrylates in nail gel affecting the nail fold.

- Chronic exposure to irritant substances (e.g. detergents, bulbs, and spices), if able to penetrate the nail unit barrier, can cause onycholysis, longitudinal ridging, and paronychia [170].
- Solvents used to remove enamel or cuticles can also cause irritant paronychial dermatitis [171].
- Formaldehyde-containing nail hardeners are irritant and can result in painful onycholysis [172].
- A prospective study of 39 patients with connective tissue disorders found nail changes in 27 (69%). The most common abnormalities observed were longitudinal nail ridging ($n = 11$), periungual erythema ($n = 10$), periungual telangiectasia ($n = 11$), and ragged cuticles ($n = 10$) [173].
- Non-dermatitis dermatoses, infections (e.g. bacterial paronychia, candida, tinea), general dermatoses involving the nails (e.g. lichen planus, psoriasis, Darier's), drug-induced nail disease, and primary nail disorders should all be considered in the differential diagnosis. Photo-onycholysis can be drug-induced (e.g. tetracyclines, griseofulvin) or spontaneous [174].

Examination point 10: dorsal interdigital spaces

- Unusual dermatoses can occur, e.g. fissured eczema affecting the first interdigital space associated with hyperkeratotic hand eczema from ACD to resin in a billiard cue was observed [175].
- Interdigital dermatitis is often associated with low-grade irritant dermatitis from over-use of liquid soaps/detergents, as this location has the lowest thickness of skin. 2275 hairdressing apprentices were examined a median of 6 weeks after the start of their training [176]. Skin changes were noted in 821 (36%). The interdigital sites were most commonly affected (664, 81% of those affected). Interdigital eczema can be regarded as a potential precursor of more severe hand dermatitis in hairdressers, and probably of irritant hand dermatitis in wet work occupations in general.

- 51 out of 79 ball-bearing workers with major exposure to the irritant kerosene were found to have erythema and desquamation in the interdigital spaces [177].
- Interdigital pilonidal sinuses/foreign body granulomas from hair can occur in hairdressers and sheep shearers [178].
- Scabies and candida infections can target the interdigital spaces.
- Three adolescent patients developed bilateral phototoxic dermatitis on the dorsal thenar spaces while taking doxycycline. Identification of this "heart sign" (dorsal thenar spaces are affected so that when apposing both thumbs and second digits a 'heart' is formed) should alert clinicians to the possibility of drug phototoxicity [179].

Microexamination of the head and neck

General principles

- ACD of the head and neck can occur from all six potential routes of exposure to contact allergens (direct contact, airborne, hand to face, by proxy, systemic, and mucosal).
- Airborne ACD tends to affect the eyelids, but can also affect the head and neck (except for the scalp).
- Photodermatoses including photoallergic ACD can spare the upper eyelids, retroauricular regions, and the area under the chin.
- *Facial psoriasis* can involve different areas of the face; in a large series, the following areas were involved (in decreasing order of frequency) [180]: upper forehead (76%), lower forehead (52%), periauricular (48%), ears (39%), cheeks (39%), nasolabial folds (19%), perioral (12%), and eyelids (5.5%).

  Facial psoriasis is associated with scalp involvement in 94% of cases. There are three types: centrofacial, peripheral facial, and mixed type. The centrofacial type is associated with extensive disease affecting the whole body, whilst the peripheral type is associated with extensive scalp disease.

  Facial psoriasis is a marker for severe psoriasis – it is associated with prolonged disease, early onset, pruritus, nail and joint involvement, a positive family history, and positive Koebner's response.
- Rosacea tends to affect the midface including the forehead, nose, cheeks, and chin. There is often characteristic sparing of the periocular skin (even with ocular involvement).
- Be wary of unusual non-allergic presentations, e.g. bilateral lichenified lower eyelid dermatitis as a manifestation of lichen simplex chronicus [181], cheilitis as a phototoxic reaction to sweet oranges, [182] or factitious disease presenting as severe crusted cheiltis [183].

10-point local examination of the head and neck

- Examination of the head and neck should include the sequential assessment of ten locations (Figure 5.2):
  1. forehead (central, lateral)
  2. eyebrows (including glabella)
  3. eyes (upper and lower eyelids, periocular)
  4. nose (root, bridge, apex, alae nasi, alae nasi sulci, nasolabial folds, septum)
  5. cheeks (medial, malar area, zygomatic arch, hollows)
  6. lips (upper lip, lower lip, angles of mouth, vermilion border, perioral area, philtrum)
  7. chin (chin, mentolabial sulcus, jawline)
  8. neck (anterior, sides, dorsa, submental area)
  9. ears (pre-auricular, retroauricular, pinna, lobes)
  10. scalp (frontal, temporal, parietal, occipital, including scalp margins)

The following sections provide further elaboration in conjunction with Tables 5.3 and 5.4.

Examination point 1: forehead

- Scalp dermatoses can spread to involve the forehead.
- ACD to hair dye and other hair products can affect the forehead, particularly the scalp margin.
- ACD to hats, caps, or helmets. ACD to hat bands manifests as a band-like eruption on the forehead and contact areas of the scalp, which is often vesicular. Putative allergens include chromate and PTBP resin [184].
- *Bindi dermatoses* affecting the kumkum mark on the central area of the forehead can be due to ACD, hyperpigmentation, leukoderma or foreign body granulomas [185, 186]. ACD to tefillin can also affect the forehead.
- *Pigmented erythema* on the forehead and zygoma cheek area can be a manifestation of contact dermatitis or chronic irritancy, or be due to the effects of UV light [187]. Pigmented or actinic *lichen planus* is often a differential.
- *Seborrheic eczema* tends to particularly target the median forehead and areas adjacent to the scalp and eyebrows, whereas *airborne ACD*, *CAD* and *atopic dermatitis* tend to give a more even involvement.
- Unusual case reports include:
  - a case of acute psoriasiform ACD of the forehead and scalp related to the use of a cap [188]
  - a case of hyperpigmentation on the forehead following baptism due to a phototoxic reaction to chrism [189]
  - Hailey-Hailey disease secondary to koebnerization from a crash helmet [190]
  - a "prayer nodule" on the mid-forehead [191].

Examination point 2: eyebrows/glabella

- Tinting of the eyebrows and/or eyelashes is currently a relatively common procedure in Europe and America and can lead to ACD to hair dye [192].
- The glabella and eyebrows are key areas of involvement in facial seborrheic dermatitis.
- There are multiple reports of granulomatous reactions to eyebrow tattooing [193].
- Granulomatous diseases (e.g. sarcoidosis, leprosy) can affect the eyebrows.
- Opportunistic infections (e.g. mycobacterium, microsporum) have been reported to occur with eyebrow tattooing and threading [194, 195].

Table 5.3 Some examples of ACD affecting the head and neck.

Part affected	Direct contact (allergens in brackets)	Airborne	Others (by proxy, hand to face/neck, mucosal, systemic[a])
1. Forehead	Hair dye/other haircare products Hats/caps/helmets/headbands Bindi Tefillin Topical medicaments/medicated balms Sunscreen chemicals[b]	As per periocular region	Hand to face: nail products/varnish[c]
2. Eyebrows/glabella	Tinting of eyebrows *p*-phenylenediamine (PPD) Waxing of eyebrows (colophonium) Glabella: sunscreen chemicals[b]		Hand to face: nail products/varnish[c]
3. Periocular region	Hair dye/other haircare products, e.g. shampoo, conditioner Cosmetics, e.g. eye liner, eye shadow, mascara, face/eye creams, eye makeup remover (can contain metals like nickel and gold) Eyelash curlers (nickel, black rubber) False eyelash glue (cyanoacrylate) Eyelash dye Topical medicaments/eyedrops Sunscreen chemicals[b] Wet wipes Swimming/work goggles Spectacle frames Contact lenses	Fragrance Preservatives Resins, e.g. nail varnish Plants Woods Drug inhalers Pharmaceuticals in an occupational setting	Hand to face: nail products/varnish[c], rubber, plants, e.g. ivy Secondary spread of nickel ACD from distal sites
4. Nose	Spectacle frames Eyeglass pads Masks Sunscreen chemicals[b] Medicaments, e.g. steroid nasal sprays	Relative sparing of the nose	Hand to face: nail products/varnish[c] (affecting the nasolabial sulci)
5. Cheeks	Cosmetics, e.g. blushers, rouge, moisturizers, creams Cosmetic cleansers, wet wipes Perfume Sunscreen chemicals[b] Mobile phones Masks Spectacle frames Hair-bearing areas: • shaving creams/gels/foam • electric razors (nickel) • aftershaves/fragranced lotions	As per periocular region	By proxy: fragrance from various sources, affecting the cheeks and adjacent areas Hand to face: nail products/varnish[c], rubber, plants
6. Lips/perioral area (see also Table 5.6)	Cosmetics, e.g. lipsticks Sunscreen chemicals contained in lip products[b] Topical medicaments Non-steroidal anti-inflammatory drugs (NSAIDs) Dyeing/waxing of mustache area Toothpastes Toothbrush material Mouthwashes Dental material (rubber, colophonium) Adhesives for orthodontic braces Masks Nasal cannula Musical instruments Chewing on pens/rubber items/other utensils Diallyl disulfide causing ACD and photoallergic contact dermatitis, foods	Can be involved in advanced cases	Hand to face: nail products/varnish[c] Mucosal: toothpaste, mouthwash, dental material, metal braces, flavorings in food

Table 5.3 (Continued)

Part affected	Direct contact (allergens in brackets)	Airborne	Others (by proxy, hand to face/neck, mucosal, systemic[a])
7. Chin/ jawline	Cosmetics, e.g. blushers, rouge, moisturizers, creams Cosmetic cleansers, wet wipes Perfume Mobile phones Masks Helmet straps Sunscreen chemicals[b] Hair-bearing areas: • shaving creams/gels/foam • electric razors (nickel) • aftershaves/fragranced lotions	Can be involved in advanced cases	Hand to face: nail products/varnish[c]
8. Neck	Hair-cleaning agents Hair dye Necklace (metal, wood, fabric dyes) Lanyard Stethoscope Fiddler's neck Perfume Sunscreen chemicals[b] Clothing dye Clothing labels/tags Hoop, drop, and chandelier earrings	Can be involved in advanced cases	Hand to neck: nail products/varnish[c], rubber, plants
9. Ears (see also Table 5.8)	Hair dye Sunscreen chemicals[b] Hearing aids Earplugs Instruments to pick at the ear (metal, wood) Topical medicaments Earrings Mobile phones Spectacle frames Headwear, head sets	Can be involved in advanced cases	Hand to face: nail products/varnish[c], rubber, plants
10. Scalp	Hair pin/clasp (metal) Headwear, e.g. headbands, elasticated hair nets, bathing caps Hair-cleaning agents Hair gel Hair dye Bleaches and other hair chemicals Wig adhesives, prosthetic hair pieces Medicaments, e.g. minoxidil scalp lotion, diphencyprone		

Medicament ACD can affect any part of the head and neck (usually direct contact but can be airborne, e.g. inhalers).

[a] Systemic contact dermatitis can affect all areas of the head and neck.

[b] Can cause both ACD and photoallergic contact dermatitis.

[c] Possible routes of transfer: airborne, by proxy, hand to face/neck.

Examination point 3: periocular region

- Periocular dermatitis is often a result of multiple factors (e.g. ACD superimposed on a primary endogenous eczema such as atopic dermatitis) [1, 32]. However, most studies have found ACD to be the most common cause, ranging from 30% to 77%, followed by atopic dermatitis and ICD [1] (Table 5.5).

Examination point 4: nose

- ACD to spectacle frames can involve the bridge of the nose. ACD to eyeglass pads typically presents as small annular lesions or spreads to cause more diffuse dermatitis.
- Nasal involvement as part of ACD to a facemask [196].
- ACD/photoallergic contact dermatitis to sunscreen products can involve the nose (e.g. amongst outdoor sportsmen/ women).
- Medicament ACD from nasal spray (budesonide): A 9-year-old boy presented with erythema, edema and scaling around the nose and complaints of severe pruritus. The lesions persisted for 2 years and had started 3 weeks after beginning treatment with a budesonide nasal spray [197].
- Sparing of the nasal skin has been reported as a common finding in airborne ACD (the "beak sign") [198].

Table 5.4 Some examples of non-allergic dermatoses affecting the head and neck, which may be part of a differential diagnosis for ACD.

Part affected	Irritant contact dermatitis	Endogenous/other eczemas	Non-dermatitis dermatoses, others
1. Forehead	Pigmented erythema can be a manifestation of chronic irritancy	Atopic dermatitis Seborrheic dermatitis CAD	Psoriasis Lichen planus Rosacea Occlusion acne from hair gel Melasma/ochronosis Herpes zoster
2. Eyebrows/glabella		Seborrheic dermatitis	Granulomatous tissue reaction to eyebrow tattooing Sarcoidosis Infections, e.g. mycobacterium with eyebrow tattooing/threading, leprosy
3. Periocular region	Direct contact, e.g. cleansing agents, mascara/other cosmetics Airborne, e.g. chemical fumes	Atopic dermatitis Seborrheic dermatitis Lichen simplex chronicus preferentially affecting the lower eyelids [181]	Psoriasis Connective tissue disorders, e.g. dermatomyositis, lupus erythematosus (LE) Rosacea (Morbihan's disease) Angioedema Infections, e.g. tinea faciei, cellulitis
4. Nose		Seborrheic dermatitis CAD	Psoriasis Connective tissue disorders, e.g. Wegener's granulomatosis, LE Rosacea Sarcoidosis Granuloma faciale Infections, e.g. tuberculosis (TB), leprosy, leishmaniasis
5. Cheeks		Seborrheic dermatitis Eczematous photodermatoses	Psoriasis Lichen planus LE Non-eczematous photodermatoses Acne vulgaris/rosacea Melasma/ochronosis Sarcoidosis Granuloma faciale Infections, e.g. tinea faciei, cellulitis/erysipelas, slapped cheek syndrome
6. Lips/perioral area (see also table 5.6)	Lip licking, angular cheilitis from saliva Lipsticks Medication Mechanical ICD from wind instruments Sweet oranges (irritant + phototoxic) [182]	Atopic cheilitis, often affecting the philtrum as well Seborrheic dermatitis	Actinic cheilitis Angular cheilitis (infective and/or nutritional) Exfoliative cheilitis Plasma cell cheilitis Cheilitis granulomatosa Psoriasis Lichen planus Discoid lupus erythematosus (DLE) Lupus miliaris disseminatus faciei Actinic prurigo Rosacea Melasma/ochronosis Sarcoidosis Periorofacial dermatitis (including the granulomatous variant) Herpes simplex virus infection Erythema multiforme/Stevens–Johnson syndrome Factitious [183]
7. Chin/jawline	Shaving rash (irritant +/− allergic)		Acne vulgaris/rosacea Pseudofolliculitis barbae

Table 5.4 (Continued)

Part affected	Irritant contact dermatitis	Endogenous/other eczemas	Non-dermatitis dermatoses, others
8. Neck (see also Table 5.7)	Clothing labels/tags Shampoo Moisturizers/bath oil containing benzalkonium chloride Local herbal preparations Fiddler's neck	Atopic dermatitis Seborrheic dermatitis Lichen simplex chronicus	Psoriasis Acanthosis nigricans Acne keloidalis nuchae Ochronosis
9. Ears (see also Table 5.8)	Shampoos can infiltrate ear-piercing sites	Atopic dermatitis Seborrheic dermatitis	Psoriasis Juvenile spring eruption Inflammatory disorders, e.g. chondrodermatitis nodularis helicis, relapsing polychondritis, red ear syndrome, DLE Infections, e.g. otitis externa, pseudomonas, leprosy, cutaneous TB, Lyme borreliosis Paraneoplastic, e.g. Bazex's syndrome
10. Scalp	Hair dye (alkaline process) "Hot combing" Hair straighteners/relaxers Minoxidil scalp lotion	Seborrheic dermatitis	Psoriasis Lichen planus LE Erosive pustular dermatoses Infections, e.g. tinea capitis, cellulitis, folliculitis, herpes zoster

- Unusual case reports of ACD:
  - ACD to snuff tobacco presenting as nasal dermatitis has been reported [199].
  - Erythema and scaling of the tip of the nose after an injection of acrylate fillers [200].
- Seborrheic dermatitis typically affects the alae nasi folds.
- Nasal skin involvement is common in CAD but uncommon in atopic dermatitis (H. Fassihi, personal communication).
- Rosacea, sarcoidosis, connective tissue disorders (Wegener's granulomatosis, LE) and TB can all commonly involve the nasal skin.

Examination points 5 and 7: cheeks and chin/jawline

- A common site of involvement for direct contact ACD to cosmetics and cosmetic cleansers/wipes, as well as airborne ACD (together with the eyelids and forehead). ACD to wet wipes in young children commonly affects the cheeks and perioral area [201].
- The malar and zygoma areas are commonly involved in ACD to cosmetic blushers or rouge [202].
- ACD to face moisturizers/creams often extends to the lateral area of the cheeks but stops short of the scalp margin by 0.5–1 cm as the topicals are typically applied with a small gap from the scalp (the "moisturizer sign") (Figure 5.6).
- The cheek (and forehead) area has been associated with fragrance contact allergy. This may be due to both airborne and direct contact exposures [203].
- ACD to mobile phones can affect the lateral area of the cheek(s).
- ACD to surgical and face masks can affect the cheek area.
- ACD to spectacle frames can affect the midcheek area.
- ACD affecting the hairbearing areas of the face can occur due to shaving creams/gels, aftershaves/fragranced lotions and nickel in electric razors [204].
- The cheeks can be involved in photoallergic contact dermatitis.
- Seborrheic dermatitis commonly affects the central areas of the cheeks.
- The rash in LE is often termed a "malar" rash because of cheek involvement.
- Involvement as part of photodermatoses.
- Both erythematotelangiectatic and papulopustular rosacea tend to affect the central/malar areas of the cheeks [205].
- Of 80 cases of tinea faciei, 52.5% affected the cheeks and 15% involved the mandible area [206].

Examination point 6: lips and perioral area

- ACD of the lips can often spread to the perioral area (Figure 5.7).
- ACD to cosmetics is a common cause of ACD in the perioral area.
- Mustache dye can cause ACD, whilst waxing of this area can cause both ACD and ICD.
- Dental agents can also cause ACD in the perioral area, e.g. rubber [207].
- ACD to an oxygen facemask showed marked perioral involvement [196].
- The philtrum is a key target area for atopic dermatitis.
- Non-allergic causes of dermatitis affecting the perioral area include atopic dermatitis, periorofacial dermatitis (including the granulomatous variant), lupus miliaris disseminatus faciei, rosacea, and sarcoidosis (Table 5.6).

Examination point 8: neck

- Common contact allergens include hair-cleaning products, hair dye, fragrance, clothing dye, and nail varnish (Table 5.7).

Table 5.5 Local and distal site findings in examples of disorders causing periocular lesions.

Local findings	Distal findings
Allergic contact dermatitis: periocular region	
• **Direct contact allergic contact dermatitis or secondary spread from local/distal sites** [1–6]	
– Pruritus > burning sensation – Erythema, edema, oozing, coalescing papules – Marked periorbital edema in severe cases – Vesiculation on the eyelids is uncommon	– Evidence of ACD distally (e.g. neck, wrists, and hands with ACD to fragrance) – Periocular area can be site of secondary spread of ACD from elsewhere (e.g. nickel) [7]
Notes: – *Important sources/allergens: • topical ophthalmic medications, antibiotics, phenylephrine hydrochloride, thimerosal, drop bottle bulb used to administer eyedrops (mercaptobenzothiazole) [8], metals in glitter/cosmetic products (nickel), face cream, hair dye, eyelash tint, false eyelash glue/cyanoacrylate (which can cause severe edema), eyelash curlers (nickel, black rubber), fragrances, preservatives • shampoos, hair conditioners, eye makeup remover, mascaras, eye liner, eye shadow, eye cream, and wet wipes: see Table 4.1 • swimming and other sports: see Table 4.3 • spectacle frames: see Table 4.4	
➢ **Illustrative example: Hair and eyelash dye**	
– Periocular dermatitis and severe facial edema may be presenting complaint, and may be mistaken for angioedema (pseudoangioedema) [9]	– Other potential areas of involvement: scalp, forehead, periauricular region and neck – Distant site involvement can be present in ACD to PPD (e.g. the knuckles, elbows, knees, penis, and scrotum have been involved in mustache dye allergy) [10]
Notes: – *Important allergens: PPD [11], resorcinol [11], *m*-aminophenol [11], *p*-aminophenol [11], 2-amino-4-hydroxyethylaminoanisole sulfate [12], *p*-toluenediamine [13], *p*-toluenediamine sulfate [14], toluene-2,5-diamine [15], 2-hydroxyethylamino-5-nitroanisole, 3-nitro-*p*-hydroxyethyl-aminophenol [16], 4-amino-3-nitrophenol [17]. Occasionally, tertiary non-dye chemicals are the putative allergens in hair dye preparations, e.g. Laureth-12 [18], benzyl alcohol [19].	
➢ **Illustrative example: Eyedrops** [20, 21]	
– Eyelid edema – Conjunctivitis – Pruritic erythematous and edematous lesions on both cheeks	
Notes: – *Reported sources/allergens [22, 23]: ○ anti-glaucoma eyedrops (dorzolamide [20], timolol [21]), β-adrenergic blockers [24], α-2 adrenergic agonists (apraclonidine, brimonidine), carbonic anhydrase inhibitors (dorzolamide), mydriatics, phenylephrine (can cause systemic ACD and persistent patch test reactions) [25], β-interferon [26], antibiotics (gentamicin [27], chloramphenicol, vancomycin, sodium colistimethate), antiviral drugs, antihistamines (pheniramine maleate), anesthetics (tetracaine), enzymatic cleaners, preservatives (thimerosal, parabens), antioxidants (pirenoxine, sodium bisulfate), prostaglandins (latanoprost), NSAIDs (trometamol), mucolytics (*N*-acetylcysteine), bismuth oxide [23] ○ for contact lenses: see Table 4.4.	
• **Airborne allergic contact dermatitis** [1]	
– Classical presentation: dermatitis on exposed areas including the face, "V area" of neck and chest – The upper eyelids are particularly susceptible – In contrast to photoallergic contact dermatitis, the areas behind the ears ("Wilkinson's triangle"), under the chin, eyelids, and nasolabial folds are also involved – In patients wearing glasses, dermatitis can be present at the edge of the nose due to occlusion – Acute and/or chronic eczema signs – Severe cases can have swelling as the predominant sign (pseudoangioedema), especially MI from wet paint	– Dermatitis on the exposed forearms and hands can occur – Sweat can cause allergen trapping, leading to cutaneous reactions on covered sites – Fragrances: can involve multiple sites; hands (43%), face/neck (36%), generalized involvement (17%), both hands and face (5%), legs (4%), anogenital area (3%) and axillae (1%) [28] – Epoxy resin: possible associated hand involvement, especially the digit pulps; involvement of the face (56%), hands (50%), and arms (37%) [29]; knee and elbow involvement in floor layers – Nail varnish: annular lesions on the lower forehead, auricular/retroauricular areas, lips, neck, and chest; possible involvement of the face and neck (72%), associated nail folds (9%), palms (4.5%), periungual toenails (3%), and uncommonly the scalp, perianal/genital region, lower limbs, and soles [30] – Plants: *Compositae* ACD affects the hands only in 36%, hands and face in 24%, generalized involvement in 20%, and the face only in 11% [31]

Notes:

- *Important sources/allergens [1, 32]:
  - fragrances, resins, nail varnish, preservatives, drugs and plants, particularly the *Asteraceae (Compositae)* family
  - air fresheners, scented candles and wall paints: see Table 4.2
  - other causes include wood, plastics, rubber, glues, industrial and pharmaceutical chemicals, metals, pesticides, animal feed additives, agricultural dusts, potassium dichromate/cement, cigarette smoke, UV-cured ink, multifunctional acrylic monomers, tripropylene glycol diacrylate (occupational) [33], and chlorpromazine (from crushed tablets).

➢ **Illustrative example: Colophonium resin from soldering flux** [34]	
– Eyelid dermatitis	– Other potential areas of involvement: rest of face, ears, neck, arms, and hands
Notes: – Airborne ACD to colophonium can also occur from exposure to wood dust. – Soldering flux can also cause ICD. – Patch test to scrapings of flux residue.	
• **Hand to face transfer**	
Manual transfer of some allergens noted, e.g. rubber [35]	
• **Photoallergic contact dermatitis** [1]	
– Eczematous eruption	– Rashes on exposed areas – Some patients may have clinical signs of coexisting photodermatoses such as CAD and polymorphic light eruption (PLE) (over 50% of photoallergic patients had an underlying photodermatosis, mainly CAD and PLE, in one study [36])

Notes:

- *Reported photoallergens [37–39]:
  - the most common photoallergens are sunscreens (organic UV absorbers)
  - other reported photocontact/photoaggravating allergens include MI, fragrances, antimicrobial agents (bithionol, chlorhexidine diacetate, dichlorophen, fentichlor, hexachlorophene, sulfanilamide), antiseptics (triclosan, trichlorocarbanilide, tribromosalicylanilide), topical NSAIDs, topical antihistamines (promethazine), and thioureas/thiocarbamide.
- Photopatch testing is essential for diagnosis (responsible action spectrum: wavelengths 320–400 nm).

Irritant contact dermatitis [6, 32]	
• **Direct contact irritant contact dermatitis**	
– May be difficult to distinguish from ACD but usually no vesicles or secondary spread	– ICD from wet wipes may also involve the forehead and cheeks
• **Airborne irritant contact dermatitis**	
– The upper eyelids are particularly susceptible	

Notes:

- *Important causative agents:
  - Direct contact: hair dye, shampoo, eye makeup remover, mascara, wet wipes
  - airborne irritants can be from the work (industrial solvents) or home environment (cleaning agents).
- Clinical symptoms:
  - burning and stinging sensations > pruritus
  - these sensations can occur within minutes; cutaneous lesions may be minimal.

(Continued)

Table 5.5 (Continued)

Local findings	Distal findings
Examples of endogenous dermatitis	
• **Atopic dermatitis** [1, 6]	
– Particularly affects upper eyelids – Lichenification, brown discoloration – Dennie-Morgan (infraorbital) folds – Can get loss of eyelashes – Mucoid discharge – Periocular milia – Complications: ∘ Secondary infection, which may be extensive: *Staphylococcal* infection (golden crusting) or herpes (clustered vesicles) ∘ Ocular complications: blepharitis, punctate keratitis, keratoconjunctivitis, keratoconus, uveitis, anterior subcapsular cataracts, retinal detachment, herpes infection	– Flexural eczema – Scalp, hand, and foot involvement – Hyperlinear palms – Pityriasis alba – Keratosis pilaris
Notes: – Pruritus is a major feature and is often aggravated by heat, sweat, and wool. – Associated asthma, hay fever. – Raised serum IgE.	
• **Seborrheic dermatitis** [6]	
– Pruritus is variable – Eyelids (including anterior ciliary area), glabella, eyebrows, and lower forehead – Greasy, adherent scaling debris and patchy erythema – In severe cases, small ulcers and pinpoint bleeding can be seen after removal of the debris – Can get loss or displacement of eyelashes – Keratoconjunctivitis sicca occurs in one-third of patients – Complications: ∘ Recurrent *Staphylococcal* infection is common ∘ Ocular complications: meibomianitis, recurrent hordeola, conjunctivitis, keratitis	– Other potential areas of involvement: scalp (particularly along anterior hairline), external ears/retroauricular areas, nasolabial folds, sternal area, axillae, and groin flexures – Patchy, subtle-to-intense erythema with fine white or adherent yellow greasy scales
Notes: – Male > female. – May be seen in association with untreated acquired immunodeficiency syndrome (AIDS) and neurological diseases such as Parkinson's disease, epilepsy, and multiple sclerosis.	
Examples of non-dermatitis dermatoses	
• **Psoriasis** [1, 40]	
– Psoriasiform blepharitis – Non-specific conjunctivitis is the most common form of conjunctivitis with psoriasis, and can occur with or without eyelid margin rashes – Coexists with seborrheic dermatitis in sebopsoriasis (uncommon to have periocular psoriasis in the absence of seborrheic dermatitis)	– Scalp, elbows, knees, hands, feet, and nails for evidence of psoriasis – Scalp, sternal area, and flexures for evidence of sebopsoriasis

• **Dermatomyositis** [41]	
– Heliotrope rash: ○ Upper eyelids, usually symmetrical ○ Periorbital erythema, often associated with edema – Facial erythema	– Alopecia – Gottron's sign, Gottron's papules – Inverse Gottron's sign/papules: ○ erythema or papules on palmar aspects of hand joints ○ associated with acute/subacute interstitial lung disease – Mechanic's hands: most characteristic cutaneous marker of anti-synthetase syndrome – Periungual changes: erythema, dilated capillary loops, cuticular hyperplasia/hemorrhages – V-sign – Shawl sign – Other cutaneous manifestations: flagellate erythema, vesiculo-bullous lesions, calcinosis cutis, panniculitis, cutaneous ulcers
Notes: – Cutaneous lesions may present with or without muscle symptoms (amyopathic dermatomyositis). – Can be a manifestation of internal malignancy such as cancer of the nasopharynx/ovary/gallbladder [42] and hemophagocytic lymphohistiocytosis [43].	
• **Lupus erythematosus** [44]	
– Discoid rash – Heliotrope rash [45] – Periorbital mucinosis [46] – Neonatal lupus [47, 48] ○ Periorbital involvement is very common ○ Characteristic: 'owl eyes' or 'raccoon eyes' (confluent, scaly periorbital erythema), non-scarring subacute cutaneous lupus (annular, erythematous, and polycyclic lesions)	– Alopecia – Malar rash – Photosensitive rash – Generalized maculopapular rash; may subsequently develop toxic epidermolytic necrosis (TEN) or TEN-like eruption – Subacute cutaneous lupus (psoriasiform, annular polycyclic) – DLE (can be lichenoid) – Lupus profundus – Chilblain lupus – Non-specific skin lesions: vasculitis, bullous lesions, Raynaud's phenomenon, erythema multiforme, leg ulcers, urticaria, panniculitis, periungual telangiectasia, nail fold infarction, pyoderma gangrenosum
Notes: – Skin lesions are the initial manifestation in 25% of cases. – Careful history taking, physical examination, and investigations (including serology tests) to rule out systemic involvement are mandatory.	
• **Tinea faciei** [49]	
– Usually: unilateral confluent erythematous plaques, some eyelash ± eyebrow loss, upper eyelid swelling – Minority: vesiculation, annular/'ring' appearance – Scaling: varies from nil to hyperkeratotic	– Usually no abnormalities
Notes: – Host: usually in children. – Source: exposure to animals. – Duration: usually more than 1 month. – *Easily missed diagnosis: initially misdiagnosed as eczema, impetigo, or herpes.	

* signifies importance

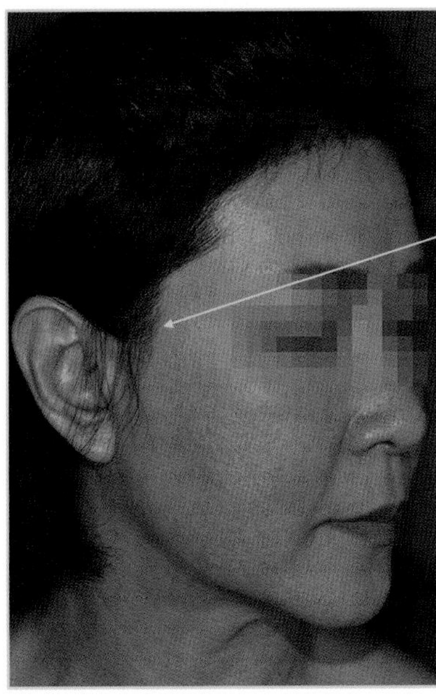

The "moisturizer sign"
Allergic contact dermatitis to face moisturizers/face creams. Note the sparing of the hairline and periorbital area. Face creams are not usually applied up to the scalp to avoid contaminating the hair (the "moisturizer sign").

Figure 5.6 The "moisturizer sign".

Cheilitis secondary to allergic contact dermatitis to fragrance in lipsticks. Lip products often contain sunscreen chemicals, which can cause both allergic contact dermatitis and photoallergic contact dermatitis.

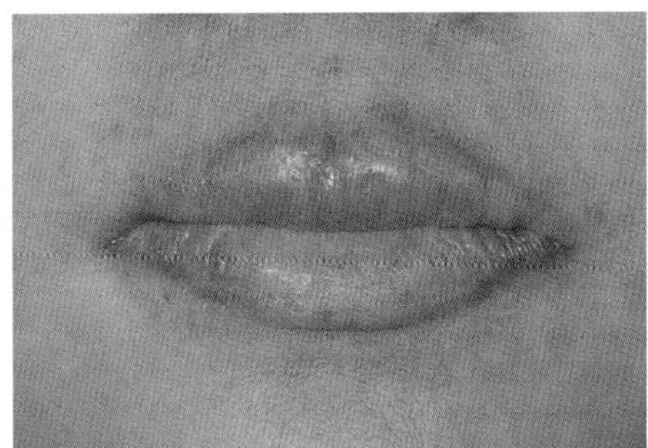

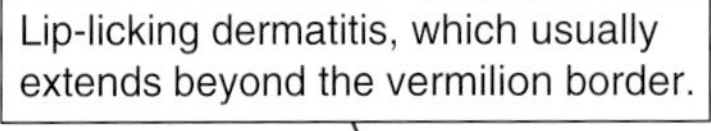

Lip-licking dermatitis, which usually extends beyond the vermilion border.

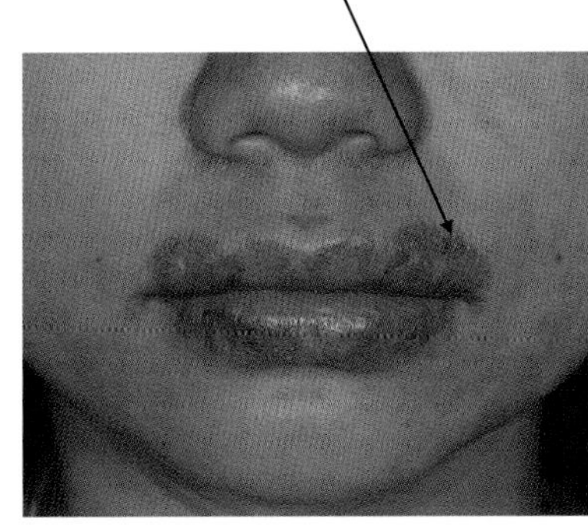

Figure 5.7 Examples of dermatitis affecting the lips/perioral area.

Examination point 9: ears

- The "ear lobe sign" can be observed in patients with ACD to substances applied to the face. The ear lobe is spared on the ipsilateral side of the face of the applying hand, whilst the ear lobe is involved on the contralateral side [208] (Table 5.8).

Examination point 10: scalp

- The patch tests of 1320 patients with scalp dermatitis were analyzed. The majority of relevant reactions were to agents in hair-cleaning/washing products, hair dye and bleaches, and medicaments [209]. ACD to hair-cleaning products (e.g. shampoos) can spread to the rest of the head and neck, and even involve the trunk. ACD to hair dye is more pronounced on the scalp margins (including the ear and neck) than within the scalp itself. It can affect the periocular area or cause widespread rashes involving the head and neck.
- Another study found that metals from hair pins and clasps were another source of ACD. They also found that scalp pruritus, rather than erythema, was a common dominant manifestation of scalp ACD. In their series, pre-existing scalp conditions were commonly observed, being present in over 80% of patients with scalp ACD [210].
- ACD to nickel in a headband involved the retroauricular areas and frontal area of the scalp, with spread to the face [211].
- ACD to hair gel can give varied manifestations, e.g. erythema and oozing of the forehead and anterior part of the scalp, erythema and edema of the upper eyelids, erythema and lichenification of the neck, scalp margin, and helix, and papular erythema of the forehead and sides of the neck [212].

Table 5.6 Local and distal site findings in examples of disorders affecting the lips.

Local findings	Distal findings
Allergic contact dermatitis: cheilitis [50]	
– Symptoms variable but characteristically presents with pain or burning sensations of the tongue or buccal mucosa, and painful swelling or blistering of the lips – Cheilitis or circumoral dermatitis with or without stomatitis – Lipstick/lip salve dermatitis may: ○ involve only the vermilion, or extend to the perioral areas with/without involvement of the angles of the mouth ○ present with persistent irritation and scaling, or as an acute reaction with edema and vesicles	– Other potential areas of involvement: ○ Fragrances: eyelids, axillae, hands, generalized (face/trunk) ○ Nail varnish: eyelids, lower face, neck, "V area" of chest ○ Lanolin: face, hands, legs
Notes: – * mportant exposure sources are lip products/cosmetics, topical medicaments, toothpastes, mouthwashes, dental material, and musical appliances. – * mportant allergens include [51, 52]: fragrances (cinnamal, evernia prunastri, isoeugenol, limonene, *Myroxylon pereirae*), nail varnish, shellac, colophonium, preservatives, lanolin, dodecyl gallate, octyl gallate, benzoic acid, sunscreen agents, nickel, acrylates in adhesives for orthodontic braces [53], *Arundo donax* in musical reeds [54], toothbrush material [55], nasal cannulae [56], occasionally diallyl disulfide [57], olive oil [58], betel [59], honey [60], rosemary [61], castor oil [62] in foods. – Contact urticaria of the lips can occasionally occur from food exposure. Patients give a history of itching, stinging, tingling and/or edema of the lips shortly after contact with the offending foods (orange, artichoke, mango, apple, potato, carrot, tomato, kiwi).	
• **Photoallergic contact dermatitis**	
– Usually lower lip cheilitis, but cases affecting both the upper and lower lip have been reported	– Photoallergic contact dermatitis at other sites – Photodermatoses at other sites: photoallergic contact dermatitis frequently occurs in patients with other photodermatoses
Notes: – Sunscreen chemicals are often contained in lip products such as lipsticks and lip moisturizers. – Photoallergic cheilitis has been reported with NSAIDs and garlic/diallyl disulfide [63, 64].	
Irritant contact dermatitis [65]	
– Eczematous/exfoliative cheilitis at the sites of contact	– Usually no abnormalities
Notes: – The most common causes include lip licking, lipsticks, and medications. – Lip licking dermatitis often involves the lips and perioral area with a sharp cut-off. It is more common in younger age groups [66]. Predisposing factors include a history of atopic dermatitis and the use of flavored lip salves. – Isolated case of mechanical ICD from playing the trumpet [67].	
Examples of endogenous dermatitis	
• **Atopic cheilitis**	
– Can be a sole manifestation of atopic dermatitis [68], one of the minor criteria of Hanifin and Rajka [69] – The philtrum is usually also involved	– See Table 5.5

(*Continued*)

Table 5.6 (Continued)

Local findings	Distal findings
Examples of non-dermatitis dermatoses	
• **Actinic cheilitis** [70]	
– Most frequently affects a portion of or the entire vermilion border of the lower lip due to more sunlight exposure – Atrophy: the earliest sign – Poorly defined atrophic, erosive, or keratotic plaques	– May demonstrate photodamaged skin (search for evidence of distal actinic changes)
Notes: – UVB-induced intra-epithelial neoplasm. – Premalignant: invasive, metastasizing squamous cell carcinoma can develop in pre-existing actinic cheilitis.	
• **Angular cheilitis**	
– Can vary from small rhagades limited to the corner of the mouth with slight involvement of adjacent skin (Type 1) to more extensive involvement (Type II) to several rhagades radiating into adjacent skin (Type III) to no rhagades but erythema of adjacent skin (Type IV) – Types I and II most common [71]	– Evidence of anemia (erythema affecting the digital palms, conjunctival pallor, koilonychia) – Signs associated with systemic causes of angular cheilitis (see Notes)
Notes: – Predisposing factors: dentures, atopic background [71]. – Associated with mixed growth of organisms: *Staphylococcus aureus* 82.5% of cases, candida 48%, streptococci 14% [71]. – Associated nutritional deficiencies including iron, vitamins $B_2/B_6/B_{12}$, folic acid, niacin, and zinc [72]. – Systemic causes of angular cheilitis include diabetes, Down's syndrome, xerostomia, eating disorders, Sjögren's syndrome, systemic lupus erythematosus (SLE), inflammatory bowel disease, glucagonoma, Plummer–Vinson disease and secondary syphilis [72].	
• **Exfoliative cheilitis**	
– Upper and lower lips, vermilion border	– Usually no abnormalities
Notes: – Stress and some psychiatric conditions are associated with the onset of the disease [73]. Some cases have been speculated to be factitious [74]. – Exfoliative cheilitis has been reported in association with metal dental implants and mercury amalgam. Patch tests showed positive results for palladium, gold, nickel, copper, and thimerosal *(Note: controversial.)* [75].	
• **Cheilitis granulomatosa** [76, 77]	
– The first presentation is acute diffuse swelling of the upper lip (and, less often, the lower lip). The first episode of edema usually subsides completely in hours to days. – Recurrent painless swelling of one or both lips: swelling increases in duration and gradually becomes firmer, then persists.	– Associated signs may be found in patients with: ∘ orofacial granulomatosis: more diffuse facial swelling ∘ Melkersson–Rosenthal syndrome: facial palsy, fissured tongue (others: swelling of the gingival/buccal/palatal mucosa, sublingual areas, tongue, pharynx, and larynx; regional lymph node enlargement).
Notes: – Idiopathic, or may be an early manifestation of Crohn's disease, sarcoidosis, or infectious disorders such as TB. Can be associated with allergens such as benzoates and cinnamates. – Patients with Melkersson–Rosenthal syndrome may have a genetic predisposition (autosomal dominant with variable expression).	

• **Lichen planus** [78]	
– Can be asymptomatic, but pain, burning sensations, and xerostomia have all been reported – Lower > upper lip, inner border of the lower vermilion – Erosions, mild keratosis, atrophy, reticular pattern, plaques – Look for Wickham's striae on buccal mucosa	– Cutaneous lesions may be present (predilection sites: wrists, lower back, legs)
Notes: – Epidemiology: mean age 72 years old, male > female. – Injuries superimposed on lip lesions increase the risk of malignant transformation.	
• **Discoid lupus erythematosus** [79]	
– External edge of lower lip – Erythema, thickening, or atrophic macules with peripheral extension (similar to cutaneous lesions)	
• **Actinic prurigo** [80]	
– Lower lip involved, upper lip also affected in 10% – Scaling, fissures, erythema, edema, ulceration, adjacent hyperpigmentation – Some cases: extensive exudates with yellow crusting	– Symmetrical involvement of the sun-exposed areas of the skin, particularly the face, with polymorphic erythematous macules, papules, and plaques in varying stages of evolution (present in less than half of actinic prurigo cheilitis patients)
• **Herpes simplex virus infection** [81]	
– Primary infection: o Oral and/or perioral lesions often appear within 1–2 days after the onset of prodromal symptoms o Vesicles and/or ulcers may appear on any mucosal surfaces, but rarely affect the gingiva – Recurrent infection: o Recurrent herpes labialis affecting the mucocutaneous junction of the lip is the most common presentation	– Systemic symptoms ("prodrome") in primary infection: fever, malaise, headache, gastrointestinal symptoms, lymphadenopathy – Erythema multiforme – Immunocompromised hosts may have atypical presentations and can have disseminated infection
Notes: – Recurrent infection can be reactivated by cold, sunlight, stress, trauma, or immunosuppression.	

* signifies importance

Table 5.7 Local and distal site findings in examples of disorders affecting the neck.

Local findings	Distal findings
Allergic contact dermatitis: neck	
Notes: – *Important sources/allergens: fragrances, hair dye, nickel and other metals, resins, textile dyes, preservatives. – *Less common allergens include 2-monomethylol phenol in clothing/footwear labels/tags [82, 83], turpentine, and ebony [84]. ACD to potassium monopersulfate (MPS) used in spa and pool "shock" treatments affects the neck and below [85]. – Both direct contact and airborne ACD, as well as photoallergic contact dermatitis, can affect the neck.	
➢ **Illustrative example: Necklace**	
– Sides of neck, back of neck (if ACD to clasp of necklace), upper anterior chest	– Other sites of contact: earlobes, wrist, fingers, periumbilical region
➢ **Illustrative example: Fragrance**	
– Sides of neck – Prominent plaque over Adam's apple area ("atomizer sign") [86]	– Other areas of application: wrist, trunk – Other exposed sites (airborne)
Notes: – The neck is the most frequent area of perfume fine spray application [87].	
➢ **Illustrative example: Clothing/textile dyes**	
– Sides and back of neck with accentuation at the neck fold (if from shirt) – Generalized (if from scarf)	– Other potential areas of involvement: axillae, wrist, and groin
➢ **Illustrative example: Nail varnish**	
– Sides of neck – Annular patches	– Other potential areas of involvement: eyelids, lower face, anterior chest, and periungual areas; less commonly the ears, lips, and perianal region
Irritant contact dermatitis	
• **Clothing labels/tags**	
– Label dermatitis/clothing tag pruritus [83]: pruritus and excoriated dermatitis affecting areas where clothing label/tag has been in contact with neck	– Similar lesions at sites of clothing labels/tags elsewhere, e.g. lumbar area
Notes: – Associated with atopic background. – Clothing labels/tags can cause both ACD and ICD (see above).	
• **Surfactants**	
– Neck dermatitis from surfactant in shampoos [88]. – Severe inflammation and desquamation of neck from benzalkonium chloride in bath oil [89]. – Benzalkonium chloride in moisturizers has been reported to cause flexural ICD involving the neck.	– Forehead can be involved (surfactant in shampoos) [88]. – Other body flexures can be involved (benzalkonium chloride).
Others	
– Inflammation and soreness at nape of neck from hair relaxer [90] – Local herbal preparations, e.g. garlic necklace to aid cold symptoms: dermatitis especially on and adjacent to neck flexures (anterior/lateral neck) [91] – Fiddler's neck: can be ICD and/or ACD	
Examples of endogenous dermatitis	
• **Atopic dermatitis** [92]	
– Anterior neck folds (minor feature according to Hanifin and Rajka criteria) – Flexural eczema, lichenification	– See Table 5.5

• **Seborrheic dermatitis**	
– Annular patches and/or eczema on neck	– Other potential areas of involvement: scalp/scalp margin, face, sternal area/upper chest, upper back, body flexures
• **Lichen simplex chronicus and prurigo nodularis** [93]	
– Lichen simplex chronicus: ○ Usually located on the dorsal aspect of the neck ○ Primary excessive scratching leads to lichenification ○ Thickened and often hyperpigmented, centrally lichenified plaque – Prurigo nodularis: ○ Intensely pruritic chronic circumscribed papules and nodules with lichenification ○ Picker's nodules: hard nodules with a warty, excoriated, pigmented dark-red surface with central crusting and an irregular hyperpigmented ring	
Examples of non-dermatitis dermatoses	
• **Psoriasis**	
– Dorsa of neck, scalp margin	– Other potential areas of involvement: scalp, plaques at elbows and knees, nail changes
• **Acanthosis nigricans**	
– Gray, brown, or black velvety plaques	
Notes: – May be associated with obesity (with or without endocrine disorders), insulin resistance (subclinical or clinical), and malignancy.	– Other potential areas of involvement: face, axillae, groin, flexural aspects of extremities – Tripe palms in malignancy-associated acanthosis nigricans
• **Acne keloidalis nuchae** [94]	
– Chronic scarring folliculitis, perifolliculitis, and follicular papules that coalesce into firm plaques and nodules on the posterior neck and occiput	– Usually no abnormalities
Notes: – A multifactorial disease of young black men, beginning after adolescence.	

Table 5.8 Local and distal site findings in examples of disorders affecting the ears.

Local findings	Distal findings
	Allergic contact dermatitis: ears
• **Direct contact allergic contact dermatitis**	
➢ **Illustrative example: Hair dye**	
– Particularly upper ear	– Other potential areas of involvement: forehead, periorbital region, neck
➢ **Illustrative example: Hearing aids**	
– Localized dermatitis on the auricular and pre-auricular areas [95, 96] and/or otitis externa (can be acute or chronic) [95, 97–99] – Dermatitis over the skin flap for cochlear implants [100]	– Usually no abnormalities
Notes: – *Important sources/allergens: see Table 4.4.	
➢ **Illustrative example: Earplugs**	
– Localized dermatitis [101] – Recurrent bilateral otitis externa [102]	– Usually no abnormalities
Notes: – *Important allergens: mercaptobenzothiazole, tetramethylthiuram disulfide in rubber earplugs, [101] azodicarbonamide [102].	
➢ **Illustrative example: Topical medicaments**	
Localized dermatitis +/– secondary spread	
Notes: – *Important allergens: local anesthetic agents, antibiotics (neomycin, gentamicin), tixocortol pivalate, NSAIDs, methyl salicylate, additives (crotamiton, diisopropanolamine, L-menthol, parabens, modified resins), herbal medicaments/plants. (*Note: Benzalkonium chloride ICD more frequent than ACD.*) – *Important photoallergens: ketoprofen, benzophenone 3. – Becoming more common with advancing age [103].	
➢ **Illustrative example: Earrings** [104, 105]	
– May react to 'post' worn after initial piercing and/or to earrings – Dermatitis on the earlobe adjacent to pierced area, can have secondary spread to periauricular areas – There has been a report of persisting granulomatous lesions [106] – Can become secondarily infected/impetiginized [104]	– Usually no abnormalities – One case showed dermatitis sparing the earlobe but affecting the neck inferior and slightly posterior to the ear; here, the hoop of the earring was nickel positive but the post portion, fitting inside the pierced earlobe, was negative for nickel [107]
Notes: – *Important allergens: nickel, cobalt, gold, silver, platinum, palladium. – Metal allergy statistically increases with the number of piercings [108].	
➢ **Illustrative example: Mobile phones** [109]	
– Pre-auricular skin and a small sharply demarcated area on the anti-tragus of the ear	
➢ **Illustrative example: Spectacle frames**	
– Retroauricular dermatitis is the most common presentation [110] – Leukoderma of the retroauricular and temporal areas has been reported [111]	– Dermatitis can spread to the adjacent areas
Notes: – Important rare complication: cellulitis [112].	

• **Photoallergic contact dermatitis**	
– Eczematous inflammation of the sun-exposed areas of the ears	– Other sun-exposed areas
Notes: – *Important allergens: sunscreen chemicals, topical medicaments.	
Irritant contact dermatitis	
– Shampoos can infiltrate ear piercings	
Examples of endogenous dermatitis	
• **Atopic dermatitis**	
– Ear lobe flexure often involved – Recurrent pseudocysts of the auricle in a patient with active facial and ear atopic dermatitis has been reported [113]	– See Table 5.5
• **Seborrheic dermatitis**	
– Symmetrical erythema and scaling on the ears and retroauricular areas [114]	– See Table 5.5
Examples of non-dermatitis dermatoses	
• **Juvenile spring eruption** [115]	
– Inflammation of the outer helices	– Usually no abnormalities
Notes: – Usually in boys and young men in April, thought to be a benign local variant of juvenile spring eruption.	
• **Inflammatory disorders**	
➢**Chondrodermatitis nodularis helicis** [116]	
– Superior pole of helix at the transition from the vertical to the horizontal course of the ear margin (much less frequent: antihelix, scapha, concha) – Bilateral or multiple lesions on one ear – Painful, firm, lentil to cherry-sized solid or cystic nodule – Keratosis, ulceration, or central crusting may occur	– Usually no abnormalities
Notes: – Average age: 58–72 years old (childhood: exceptional cases). – Characteristic pain is an important diagnostic clue. – An association with autoimmune diseases such as dermatomyositis and scleroderma has been discussed.	
➢**Relapsing polychondritis** [117]	
– Sudden onset – Intermittent inflammation of the ear leading to structural deformities	– Other skin signs: oral aphthosis, nodules on limbs, purpura, papules, sterile pustules, superficial phlebitis, livedo reticularis, limb ulcerations and distal necrosis, erythema multiforme – Joint pain (the second most common clinical feature) – Nasal chondritis (found in 24% at the time of diagnosis) and laryngotracheal involvement – Cardiopulmonary and neurological involvement (vasculitis)
Notes: – A rare multisystemic disease. – 30% associated with autoimmune diseases: anti-neutrophil cytoplasmic antibody (ANCA)-associated vasculitides, mouth and genital ulcers with inflamed cartilage (MAGIC) syndrome.	
➢**Red ear syndrome** [118]	
– Recurrent unilateral (> bilateral) erythema and edema	– Face may be involved

(Continued)

Table 5.8 (Continued)

Local findings	Distal findings
Notes: – Red ear syndrome is divided into: ∘ primary: isolated or in association with primary headache ∘ secondary: underlying organic disease such as disorders of the ear, mandibular joint or cervical spine. – Attacks occur spontaneously or are triggered by factors such as mechanical trauma, heat, or cold stimuli. – Usually accompanied by dysaesthesia and cephalalgia.	
➢ **Discoid lupus erythematosus** [119]	
– Well-demarcated, scaly, erythematous macules or papules which gradually develop into an indurated discoid plaque with adherent scale which is painful to remove – Squamous cell carcinoma can arise in long-standing lesions [120] – Follicular plugging	– 5–10% of DLE patients develop SLE
• **Infections**	
➢ **Otitis externa** [121]	
– Acute otitis externa: ∘ Cause: usually an infectious condition ∘ Predisposing factors: impacted ear wax, chronic dermatologic conditions such as psoriasis and atopic dermatitis ∘ Hallmark: pain is worse with traction on the pinna or palpation of the tragus – Chronic otitis externa (3–5%): ∘ duration: lasting >/= 3 months ∘ causes: non-infectious dermatitic, allergic, and autoimmune causes>chronic infection such as fungi or bacteria ∘ findings: maculopapular rash with excoriations, eczema, hyperkeratosis, lichenification	– Regional lymphadenitis
Notes: – Otitis externa is an inflammatory condition of the external ear canal, with or without infection.	
➢ **Leprosy** [122, 123]	
– Ear lobe thickening	– Skin lesions: numerous, symmetric, poorly defined, mildly hypopigmented/erythematous/flesh-colored papules and nodules, minimal anesthesia, leonine facies, loss of eyelashes and eyebrows (madarosis), erythema nodosum leprosum
➢ **Cutaneous tuberculosis** [124, 125]	
– Lupus vulgaris (LV) may exclusively involve the ear lobe and pinna – Squamous cell carcinoma may develop in long-standing LV – Primary cutaneous TB (from primary inoculation from ear piercing): an ulcerative lesion	– Other predilection sites for LV: head (particularly cheeks and nose), neck, buttocks, extremities – Regional lymphadenitis
Notes: – LV: ∘ post-primary, paucibacillary form of TB caused by hematogenous, lymphatic, or contiguous spread from elsewhere in the body ∘ 10–20% have active pulmonary TB or TB of the bones and joints.	

➢**Lyme borreliosis** [126]	
– Erythema migrans and lymphocytomas, when located on the ear (or breast), are characteristic – Erythema migrans: o acute stage o expanding round-to-oval, sharply demarcated, red to bluish-red lesion, target-like appearance ("bull's eye") – Borrelial lymphocytoma: o subacute stage o B-cell pseudolymphoma o typically found on earlobe (children), areola (adults), scrotum, or anterior axillary fold o soft, non-tender bluish-red nodule or sharply demarcated plaque, often with slightly atrcphic surface	– Extracutaneous manifestations possible in acute stage: fatigue, malaise, arthralgia, myalgia, headache, regional lymphadenopathy, fever
• **Paraneoplastic**	
➢**Acrokeratosis paraneoplastica (Bazex's syndrome)** [127]	
– Psoriasiform lesions	– Psoriasiform eruptions on the nose and cheeks – Acral lesions: initial stage – palmoplantar hyperkeratosis, later stage – psoriasiform – Symmetrical onychodystrophy
Notes: – Associated with squamous cell carcinoma of the upper aerodigestive tract, lung cancer.	

* signifies importance

- ACD to wig adhesives and metal in hair clasps usually manifests as local dermatitis. This is in contrast with ACD to hair dye, hair gel, and hair-cleaning agents, which often affects the scalp margins [213, 214].
- Both ACD and ICD can occur to minoxidil scalp lotion. Reported clinical manifestations of minoxidil ACD include erythema and edema of the scalp and face, a vesicular rash of the retroauricular areas and photoaggravated dermatitis of the scalp, forehead, and periocular area [215]. Scalp ACD can occasionally cause hair loss [216].
- Psoriasis and seborrheic dermatitis can affect both the scalp and scalp margins. Non-dermatitis dermatoses in the differential diagnosis of inflammatory scalp disease include tinea, lupus, and lichen planus.

References

1 Wolf, R., Orion, E., and Tüzün, Y. (2014). Periorbital (eyelid) dermatides. *Clinics in Dermatology* 32 (1): 131–140.

2 Landeck, L., John, S.M., and Geier, J. (2014). Periorbital dermatitis in 4779 patients – patch test results during a 10-year period. *Contact Dermatitis* 70 (4): 205–212.

3 Guin, J.D. (2004). Eyelid dermatitis: a report of 215 patients. *Contact Dermatitis* 50 (2): 87–90.

4 Feser, A., Plaza, T., Vogelgsang, L., and Mahler, V. (2008). Periorbital dermatitis-a recalcitrant disease: causes and differential diagnoses. *British Journal of Dermatology* 159 (4): 858–863.

5 Landeck, L., Schalock, P.C., Baden, L.A., and Gonzalez, E. (2010). Periorbital contact sensitization. *American Journal of Ophthalmology* 150 (3): 366–70.e2.

6 Zug, K.A., Palay, D.A., and Rock, B. (1996). Dermatologic diagnosis and treatment of itchy red eyelids. *Survey of Ophthalmology* 40 (4): 293–306.

7 Calnan, C.D. (1956). Nickel dermatitis. *British Journal of Dermatology* 68 (7): 229–236.

8 Calnan, C.D. and Cronin, E. (1981). False positive reaction to mercaptobenzthiazole from rubber in eyedrop bottle. *Contact Dermatitis* 7 (5): 283–284.

9 Tukenmez Demirci, G., Kivanc Altunay, I., Atis, G., and Kucukunal, A. (2012). Allergic contact dermatitis mimicking angioedema due to paraphenylendiamine hypersensitivity: a case report. *Cutaneous and Ocular Toxicology* 31 (3): 250–252.

10 Chan, H.P. and Maibach, H.I. (2008). Moustache p-phenylenediamine dye allergic contact dermatitis with distant site involvement – an atypical presentation. *Contact Dermatitis* 58 (3): 179–180.

11 Kim, H. and Kim, K. (2015). Prevalence of potent skin sensitizers in oxidative hair dye products in Korea. *Cutaneous and Ocular Toxicology* 1–4.

12 Madsen, J.T. and Andersen, K.E. (2016). 2-Amino-4-hydroxyethylaminoanisole sulfate – a coupler causing contact allergy from use in hair dyes. *Contact Dermatitis* 74 (2): 102–104.

13 Krasteva, M., Bons, B., Ryan, C., and Gerberick, G.F. (2009). Consumer allergy to oxidative hair coloring products: epidemiologic data in the literature. *Dermatitis: Contact, Atopic, Occupational, Drug* 20 (3): 123–141.

14 Yazar, K., Boman, A., and Liden, C. (2012). P-Phenylenediamine and other hair dye sensitizers in Spain. *Contact Dermatitis* 66 (1): 27–32.

15 Sosted, H., Rustemeyer, T., Goncalo, M. et al. (2013). Contact allergy to common ingredients in hair dyes. *Contact Dermatitis* 69 (1): 32–39.

16 Dejobert, Y., Piette, F., and Thomas, P. (2006). Contact dermatitis to 2-hydroxyethylamino-5-nitroanisole and 3-nitro-p-hydroxyethyl aminophenol in a hair dye. *Contact Dermatitis* 54 (4): 217–218.

17 Blanco, R., de la Hoz, B., Sanchez-Fernandez, C., and Sanchez-Cano, M. (1998). Allergy to 4-amino-3-nitrophenol in a hair dye. *Contact Dermatitis* 39 (3): 136.

18 Field, S., Hazelwood, E., Bourke, B., and Bourke, J.F. (2007). Allergic contact dermatitis from tertiary-butylhydroquinone and Laureth 12 in a hair dye. *Contact Dermatitis* 56 (2): 116.

19 Carrascosa, J.M., Domingo, H., Soria, X., and Ferrandiz, C. (2006). Allergic contact dermatitis due to benzyl alcohol in a hair dye. *Contact Dermatitis* 55 (2): 124–125.

20 Lee, S.J. and Kim, M. (2015). Allergic contact dermatitis caused by dorzolamide eyedrops. *Clinical Ophthalmology* 9: 575–577.

21 Otero-Rivas, M.M., Ruiz-Gonzalez, I., Valladares-Narganes, L.M. et al. (2015). A case of contact dermatitis caused by timolol in anti-glaucoma eyedrops. *Contact Dermatitis* 73 (4): 256–257.

22 Tabar, A.I., Garcia, B.E., Rodriguez, A. et al. (1993). Etiologic agents in allergic contact dermatitis caused by eyedrops. *Contact Dermatitis* 29 (1): 50–51.

23 Chaudhari, P.R. and Maibach, H.I. (2007). Allergic contact dermatitis from ophthalmics: 2007. *Contact Dermatitis* 57 (1): 11–13.

24 Nino, M., Napolitano, M., and Scalvenzi, M. (2010). Allergic contact dermatitis due to the beta-blocker betaxolol in eyedrops, with cross-sensitivity to timolol. *Contact Dermatitis* 62 (5): 319–320.

25 Erdmann, S.M., Sachs, B., and Merk, H.F. (2002). Allergic contact dermatitis from phenylephrine in eyedrops. *American Journal of Contact Dermatitis* 13 (1): 37–38.

26 Pigatto, P.D., Bigardi, A., Legori, A. et al. (1991). Allergic contact dermatitis from beta-interferon in eyedrops. *Contact Dermatitis* 25 (3): 199–200.

27 Sanchez-Perez, J., Lopez, M.P., De Vega Haro, J.M., and Garcia-Diez, A. (2001). Allergic contact dermatitis from gentamicin in eyedrops, with cross-reactivity to kanamycin but not neomycin. *Contact Dermatitis* 44 (1): 54.

28 Buckley, D.A., Rycroft, R.J., White, I.R., and McFadden, J.P. (2000). Contact allergy to individual fragrance mix constituents in relation to primary site of dermatitis. *Contact Dermatitis* 43 (5): 304–305.

29 Rademaker, M. (2000). Occupational epoxy resin allergic contact dermatitis. *Australasian Journal of Dermatology* 41 (4): 222–224.

30 Lazzarini, R., Duarte, I., de Farias, D.C. et al. (2008). Frequency and main sites of allergic contact dermatitis caused by nail varnish. *Dermatitis: Contact, Atopic, Occupational, Drug* 19 (6): 319–322.

31 Ross, J.S., du Peloux Menage, H., Hawk, J.L., and White, I.R. (1993). Sesquiterpene lactone contact sensitivity: clinical patterns of Compositae dermatitis and relationship to chronic actinic dermatitis. *Contact Dermatitis* 29 (2): 84–87.

32 Besra, L., Jaisankar, T.J., Thappa, D.M. et al. (2013). Spectrum of periorbital dermatoses in South Indian population. *Indian Journal of Dermatology, Venereology and Leprology* 79 (3): 399–407.

33 Whitfeld, M. and Freeman, S. (1991). Allergic contact dermatitis to ultra violet cured inks. *Australasian Journal of Dermatology* 32 (2): 65–68.

34 Mathias, C.G. and Adams, R.M. (1984). Allergic contact dermatitis from rosin used as soldering flux. *Journal of the American Academy of Dermatology* 10 (3): 454–456.

35 Calnan, C.D. (1975). Rubber sensitivity presenting as eyelid oedema. *Contact Dermatitis* 1 (2): 124–125.
36 Darvay, A., White, I.R., Rycroft, R.J. et al. (2001). Photoallergic contact dermatitis is uncommon. *British Journal of Dermatology* 145 (4): 597–601.
37 de Groot, A.C. and Roberts, D.W. (2014). Contact and photocontact allergy to octocrylene: a review. *Contact Dermatitis* 70 (4): 193–204.
38 Goncalo, M., Ferguson, J., Bonevalle, A. et al. (2013). Photopatch testing: recommendations for a European photopatch test baseline series. *Contact Dermatitis* 68 (4): 239–243.
39 Victor, F.C., Cohen, D.E., and Soter, N.A. (2010). A 20-year analysis of previous and emerging allergens that elicit photoallergic contact dermatitis. *Journal of the American Academy of Dermatology* 62 (4): 605–610.
40 Young Park, J., Hyun Rim, J., Beom Choe, Y., and Il Youn, J. (2004). Facial psoriasis: comparison of patients with and without facial involvement. *Journal of the American Academy of Dermatology* 50 (4): 582–584.
41 Muro, Y., Sugiura, K., and Akiyama, M. (2015). Cutaneous manifestations in dermatomyositis: key clinical and serological features-a comprehensive review. *Clinical Reviews in Allergy & Immunology*.
42 Jurcic, P. (2015). Dermatomyositis as the first manifestation of gallbladder adenocarcinoma: case report and literature overview. *World Journal of Surgical Oncology* 13: 127.
43 Thomas, A., Appiah, J., Langsam, J. et al. (2013). Hemophagocytic lymphohistiocytosis associated with dermatomyositis: a case report. *Connecticut Medicine* 77 (8): 481–485.
44 Kole, A.K. and Ghosh, A. (2009). Cutaneous manifestations of systemic lupus erythematosus in a tertiary referral center. *Indian Journal of Dermatology* 54 (2): 132–136.
45 Erras, S., Benjilali, L., and Essaadouni, L. (2012). Periorbital edema as initial manifestation of chronic cutaneous lupus erythematosus. *Pan African Medical Journal* 12: 57.
46 Morales-Burgos, A., Sanchez, J.L., Gonzalez-Chavez, J. et al. (2010). Periorbital mucinosis: a variant of cutaneous lupus erythematosus? *Journal of the American Academy of Dermatology* 62 (4): 667–671.
47 Lee, L.A. (2004). Neonatal lupus: clinical features and management. *Paediatric Drugs* 6 (2): 71–78.
48 Inzinger, M., Salmhofer, W., and Binder, B. (2012). Neonatal lupus erythematosus and its clinical variability. *Journal of the German Society of Dermatology* 10 (6): 407–411.
49 Basak, S.A., Berk, D.R., Lueder, G.T., and Bayliss, S.J. (2011). Common features of periocular tinea. *Archives of Ophthalmology* 129 (3): 306–309.
50 Ophaswongse, S. and Maibach, H.I. (1995). Allergic contact cheilitis. *Contact Dermatitis* 33 (6): 365–370.
51 Strauss, R.M. and Orton, D.I. (2003). Allergic contact cheilitis in the United Kingdom: a retrospective study. *American Journal of Contact Dermatitis* 14 (2): 75–77.
52 O'Gorman, S.M. and Torgerson, R.R. (2015). Contact allergy in cheilitis. *International Journal of Dermatology*.
53 Tabor, D., Smith, V.M., and Wilkinson, S.M. (2015). Chronic cheilitis caused by acrylates used as an adhesive for an orthodontic brace. *Contact Dermatitis* 72 (2): 115–116.
54 Inoue, A., Shoji, A., and Yashiro, K. (1998). Saxophonist's cane reed cheilitis. *Contact Dermatitis* 39 (1): 37.
55 Forward, E., Harris, V., and Smith, S.D. (2018). A novel case of a brush with discomfort: allergic contact dermatitis caused by mercaptobenzothiazole in rubber components of a toothbrush. *Contact Dermatitis* 78 (6): 424–425.
56 Wright, R.C. and Fregert, S. (1983). Allergic contact dermatitis from epoxy resin in nasal canulae. *Contact Dermatitis* 9 (5): 387–389.
57 Ekeowa-Anderson, A.L., Shergill, B., and Goldsmith, P. (2007). Allergic contact cheilitis to garlic. *Contact Dermatitis* 56 (3): 174–175.
58 Beukers, S.M., Rustemeyer, T., and Bruynzeel, D.P. (2008). Cheilitis due to olive oil. *Contact Dermatitis* 59 (4): 253–255.
59 Chiu, C.S. and Tsai, Y.L. (2008). Cheilitis granulomatosa associated with allergic contact dermatitis to betel quid. *Contact Dermatitis* 58 (4): 246–247.
60 Pasolini, G., Semenza, D., Capezzera, R. et al. (2004). Allergic contact cheilitis induced by repeated contact with propolis-enriched honey. *Contact Dermatitis* 50 (5): 322–323.
61 Guin, J.D. (2001). Rosemary cheilitis: one to remember. *Contact Dermatitis* 45 (1): 63.
62 le Coz, C.J. and Ball, C. (2000). Recurrent allergic contact dermatitis and cheilitis due to castor oil. *Contact Dermatitis* 42 (2): 114–115.
63 Canelas, M.M., Cardoso, J.C., Goncalo, M., and Figueiredo, A. (2010). Photoallergic contact dermatitis from benzydamine presenting mainly as lip dermatitis. *Contact Dermatitis* 63 (2): 85–88.
64 Scheman, A. and Gupta, S. (2001). Photoallergic contact dermatitis from diallyl disulfide. *Contact Dermatitis* 45 (3): 179.
65 Lim, S.W. and Goh, C.L. (2000). Epidemiology of eczematous cheilitis at a tertiary dermatological referral Centre in Singapore. *Contact Dermatitis* 43 (6): 322–326.
66 Hisa, T., Hamada, T., Hirachi, Y. et al. (1995). Senile lip licking. *Dermatology* 191 (4): 339–340.
67 Raza, N. and Dar, N.R. (2008). Trumpet cheilitis in a novice musician. *Archives of Dermatology* 144 (5): 690–691.
68 Pugliarello, S., Cozzi, A., Gisondi, P., and Girolomoni, G. (2011). Phenotypes of atopic dermatitis. *Journal of the German Society of Dermatology* 9 (1): 12–20.
69 Wahab, M.A., Rahman, M.H., Khondker, L. et al. (2011). Minor criteria for atopic dermatitis in children. *Mymensingh Medical Journal* 20 (3): 419–424.
70 Wood, N.H., Khammissa, R., Meyerov, R. et al. (2011). Actinic cheilitis: a case report and a review of the literature. *European Journal of Dentistry* 5 (1): 101–106.
71 Oza, N. and Doshi, J.J. (2017). Angular cheilitis: a clinical and microbial study. *Indian Journal of Dental Research* 28 (6): 661–665.
72 Park, K.K., Brodell, R.T., and Helms, S.E. (2011). Angular cheilitis, Part 2: Nutritional, systemic, and drug-related causes and treatment. *Cutis* 88 (1): 27–32.
73 Mani, S.A. and Shareef, B.T. (2007). Exfoliative cheilitis: report of a case. *Journal* 73 (7): 629–632.
74 Taniguchi, S. and Kono, T. (1998). Exfoliative cheilitis: a case report and review of the literature. *Dermatology* 196 (2): 253–255.
75 Pigatto, P.D., Berti, E., Spadari, F. et al. (2011). Photoletter to the editor: Exfoliative cheilitis associated with titanium dental implants and mercury amalgam. *Journal of Dermatological Case Reports* 5 (4): 89–90.
76 Critchlow, W.A. and Chang, D. (2014). Cheilitis granulomatosa: a review. *Head and Neck Pathology* 8 (2): 209–213.
77 van der Waal, R.I., Schulten, E.A., van de Scheur, M.R. et al. (2001). Cheilitis granulomatosa. *Journal of the European Academy of Dermatology and Venereology* 15 (6): 519–523.

78 Nuzzolo, P., Celentano, A., Bucci, P. et al. (2016). Lichen planus of the lips: an intermediate disease between the skin and mucosa? Retrospective clinical study and review of the literature. *International Journal of Dermatology*.

79 Guillet, G., Constant, D., Cales, D., and Helenon, R. (1985). Cheilitis and labial lesions of lupus in the French Indies. *International Journal of Dermatology* 24 (1): 66–67.

80 Plaza, J.A., Toussaint, S., Prieto, V.G. et al. (2016). Actinic prurigo cheilitis: a clinicopathologic review of 75 cases. *American Journal of Dermatopathology* 38 (6): 418–422.

81 Stoopler, E.T. and Sollecito, T.P. (2014). Oral mucosal diseases: evaluation and management. *The Medical Clinics of North America* 98 (6): 1323–1352.

82 Ziaj, S., Zaheri, S., and Wakelin, S. (2014). Contact dermatitis caused by a footwear label with a positive patch test reaction to 2-monomethylol phenol. *Contact Dermatitis* 71 (4): 253–254.

83 Veien, N.K. (2003). Label dermatitis. *American Journal of Contact Dermatitis* 14 (2): 104.

84 Kuner, N. and Jappe, U. (2004). Allergic contact dermatitis from colophonium, turpentine and ebony in a violinist presenting as fiddler's neck. *Contact Dermatitis* 50 (4): 258–259.

85 Yankura, J.A., Marks, J.G. Jr., Anderson, B.E., and Adams, D.R. (2008). Spa contact dermatitis. *Dermatitis: Contact, Atopic, Occupational, Drug* 19 (2): 100–101.

86 Jacob, S.E. and Castanedo-Tardan, M.P. (2008). A diagnostic pearl in allergic contact dermatitis to fragrances: the atomizer sign. *Cutis* 82 (5): 317–318.

87 Loretz, L., Api, A.M., Barraj, L. et al. (2006). Exposure data for personal care products: hairspray, spray perfume, liquid foundation, shampoo, body wash, and solid antiperspirant. *Food and Chemical Toxicology* 44 (12): 2008–2018.

88 Oiso, N., Fukai, K., and Ishii, M. (2005). Irritant contact dermatitis from benzalkonium chloride in shampoo. *Contact Dermatitis* 52 (1): 54.

89 Storer, E., Koh, K.J., and Warren, L. (2004). Severe contact dermatitis as a result of an antiseptic bath oil. *Australasian Journal of Dermatology* 45 (1): 73–75.

90 Kaur, B.J., Singh, H., and Lin-Greenberg, A. (2002). Irritant contact dermatitis complicated by deep-seated staphylococcal infection caused by a hair relaxer. *Journal of the National Medical Association* 94 (2): 121–123.

91 Esfahani, A. and Chamlin, S.L. (2017). Garlic dermatitis on the neck of an infant treated for nasal congestion. *Pediatric Dermatology* 34 (4): e212–e213.

92 Jacob, S.E., Goldenberg, A., Nedorost, S. et al. (2015). Flexural eczema versus atopic dermatitis. *Dermatitis: Contact, Atopic, Occupational, Drug* 26 (3): 109–115.

93 Lotti, T., Buggiani, G., and Prignano, F. (2008). Prurigo nodularis and lichen simplex chronicus. *Dermatologic Therapy* 21 (1): 42–46.

94 Ogunbiyi, A. and George, A. (2005). Acne keloidalis in females: case report and review of literature. *Journal of the National Medical Association* 97 (5): 736–738.

95 Marshall, M., Guill, A., and Odom, R.B. (1978). Hearing aid dermatitis. *Archives of Dermatology* 114 (7): 1050–1051.

96 O'Donoghue, N.B., Rustin, M.H., and McFadden, J.P. (2004). Allergic contact dermatitis from gold on a hearing-aid mould. *Contact Dermatitis* 51 (1): 36–37.

97 Onder, M., Onder, T., Ozunlu, A. et al. (1994). An investigation of contact dermatitis in patients with chronic otitis externa. *Contact Dermatitis* 31 (2): 116–117.

98 Sood, A. and Taylor, J.S. (2004). Allergic contact dermatitis from hearing aid materials. *Dermatitis: Contact, Atopic, Occupational, Drug* 15 (1): 48–50.

99 Meding, B. and Ringdahl, A. (1992). Allergic contact dermatitis from the earmolds of hearing aids. *Ear and Hearing* 13 (2): 122–124.

100 Lung, H.L., Huang, L.H., Lin, H.C., and Shyur, S.D. (2009). Allergic contact dermatitis to polyethylene terephthalate mesh. *Journal of Investigational Allergology & Clinical Immunology* 19 (2): 161–162.

101 Deguchi, M. and Tagami, H. (1996). Contact dermatitis of the ear due to a rubber earplug. *Dermatology* 193 (3): 251–252.

102 Yates, V.M. and Dixon, J.E. (1988). Contact dermatitis from azodicarbonamide in earplugs. *Contact Dermatitis* 19 (2): 155–156.

103 Green, C.M., Holden, C.R., and Gawkrodger, D.J. (2007). Contact allergy to topical medicaments becomes more common with advancing age: an age-stratified study. *Contact Dermatitis* 56 (4): 229–231.

104 Gaul, J.E. (1967). Development of allergic nickel dermatitis from earrings. *Journal of the American Medical Association* 200 (2): 176–178.

105 Nakada, T., Iijima, M., Nakayama, H., and Maibach, H.I. (1997). Role of ear piercing in metal allergic contact dermatitis. *Contact Dermatitis* 36 (5): 233–236.

106 Goossens, A., De Swerdt, A., De Coninck, K. et al. (2006). Allergic contact granuloma due to palladium following ear piercing. *Contact Dermatitis* 55 (6): 338–341.

107 Shore, R.N. and Letter, B.B.J. (1974). Earring dermatitis sparing the ears. *Archives of Dermatology* 109 (1): 95.

108 Ehrlich, A., Kucenic, M., and Belsito, D.V. (2001). Role of body piercing in the induction of metal allergies. *American Journal of Contact Dermatitis* 12 (3): 151–155.

109 Wohrl, S., Jandl, T., Stingl, G., and Kinaciyan, T. (2007). Mobile telephone as new source for nickel dermatitis. *Contact Dermatitis* 56 (2): 113.

110 Yeo, L., Kuuliala, O., White, I.R., and Alto-Korte, K. (2011). Allergic contact dermatitis caused by solvent orange 60 dye. *Contact Dermatitis* 64 (6): 354–356.

111 Crepy, M.N., Bensefa-Colas, L., Krief, P. et al. (2011). Facial leucoderma following eczema: a new case induced by spectacle frames. *Contact Dermatitis* 65 (4): 243–245.

112 Andersen, K.E., Vestergaard, M.E., and Christensen, L.P. (2014). Triethylene glycol bis(2-ethylhexanoate) – a new contact allergen identified in a spectacle frame. *Contact Dermatitis* 70 (2): 112–116.

113 Ng, W., Kikuchi, Y., Chen, X. et al. (2007). Pseudocysts of the auricle in a young adult with facial and ear atopic dermatitis. *Journal of the American Academy of Dermatology* 56 (5): 858–861.

114 Dessinioti, C. and Katsambas, A. (2013). Seborrheic dermatitis: etiology, risk factors, and treatments: facts and controversies. *Clinics in Dermatology* 31 (4): 343–351.

115 Lava, S.A., Simonetti, G.D., Ragazzi, M. et al. (2013). Juvenile spring eruption: an outbreak report and systematic review of the literature. *British Journal of Dermatology* 168 (5): 1066–1072.

116 Wagner, G., Liefeith, J., and Sachse, M.M. (2011). Clinical appearance, differential diagnoses and therapeutical options of chondrodermatitis nodularis chronica helicis Winkler. *Journal of the German Society of Dermatology* 9 (4): 287–291.

117 Vitale, A., Sota, J., Rigante, D. et al. (2016). Relapsing polychondritis: an update on pathogenesis, clinical features, diagnostic tools, and therapeutic perspectives. *Current Rheumatology Reports* 18 (1): 3.

118 Eismann, R., Gaul, C., Wohlrab, J. et al. (2011). Red ear syndrome: case report and review of the literature. *Dermatology* 223 (3): 196–199.
119 Okon, L.G. and Werth, V.P. (2013). Cutaneous lupus erythematosus: diagnosis and treatment. *Best Practice & Research. Clinical Rheumatology* 27 (3): 391–404.
120 Fernandes, M.S., Girisha, B.S., Viswanathan, N. et al. (2015). Discoid lupus erythematosus with squamous cell carcinoma: a case report and review of the literature in Indian patients. *Lupus* 24 (14): 1562–1566.
121 Wipperman, J. (2014). Otitis externa. *Primary Care* 41 (1): 1–9.
122 Chimenos Kustner, E., Pascual Cruz, M., Pinol Dansis, C. et al. (2006). Lepromatous leprosy: a review and case report. *Medicina Oral, Patología Oral y Cirugía Bucal* 11 (6): E474–E479.
123 Walker, S.L. and Lockwood, D.N. (2007). Leprosy. *Clinics in Dermatology* 25 (2): 165–172.
124 Kaimal, S., Aithal, V., Kumaran, M.S., and Abraham, A. (2013). Cutaneous tuberculosis of the pinna: a report of two cases. *International Journal of Dermatology* 52 (6): 714–717.
125 Morgan, L.G. (1952). Primary tuberculous inoculation of an ear lobe; report of an unusual case and review of the literature. *Journal of Pediatrics* 40 (4): 482–485.
126 Mullegger, R.R. and Glatz, M. (2008). Skin manifestations of Lyme borreliosis: diagnosis and management. *American Journal of Clinical Dermatology* 9 (6): 355–368.
127 Zhao, J., Zhang, X., Chen, Z., and Wu, J.H. (2016). Case report: Bazex syndrome associated with pulmonary adenocarcinoma. *Medicine* 95 (2): e2415.
128 Johansen, J.D., Hald, M., Andersen, B.L. et al. (2011). Classification of hand eczema: clinical and aetiological types. Based on the guideline of the Danish Contact Dermatitis Group. *Contact Dermatitis* 65 (1): 13–21.
129 Boonstra, M.B., Christoffers, W.A., Coenraads, P.J., and Schuttelaar, M.L. (2015). Patch test results of hand eczema patients: relation to clinical types. *Journal of the European Academy of Dermatology and Venereology* 29 (5): 940–947.
130 Cronin, E. (1985). Clinical patterns of hand eczema in women. *Contact Dermatitis* 13 (3): 153–161.
131 Cronin, E. (1972). Clinical prediction of patch test results. *Transactions of the St. John's Hospital Dermatological Society* 58 (2): 153–162.
132 Coenraads, P.J. and Diepgen, T.L. (1998). Risk for hand eczema in employees with past or present atopic dermatitis. *International Archives of Occupational and Environmental Health* 71 (1): 7–13.
133 Gomez-Muga, S., Raton-Nieto, J.A., and Ocerin, I. (2009). An unusual case of contact dermatitis caused by wooden bracelets. *Contact Dermatitis* 61 (6): 351–352.
134 Hoffman, T.E., Hausen, B.M., and Adams, R.M. (1985). Allergic contact dermatitis to "silver oak" wooden arm bracelets. *Journal of the American Academy of Dermatology* 13 (5 Pt 1): 778–779.
135 Colbert, S., Williams, J.V., Mackenzie, N., and Brennan, P.A. (2013). Allergic reaction to a red plastic allergy alert patient identification bracelet: implications for surgical patient safety. *Journal of Perioperative Practice* 23 (7–8): 171–173.
136 Boonchai, W., Maneeprasopchoke, P., Suiwongsa, B., and Kasemsarn, P. (2015). Assessment of nickel and cobalt release from jewelry from a non nickel directive country. *Dermatitis: Contact, Atopic, Occupational, Drug* 26 (1): 44–48.
137 Cronin, E. In: (1980). *Contact Dermatitis*, 714–771. Edinburgh: Churchill Livingstone.
138 Bashir, S.J., Ryan, P.J., McFadden, J.P., and Rycroft, R.J. (2007). Contact dermatitis from dicyclohexylcarbodiimide. *Contact Dermatitis* 56 (3): 151–152.
139 Tan, C., Zhu, W.Y., and Min, Z.S. (2008). Co-existence of contact leukoderma and pigmented contact dermatitis attributed to *Clematis chinensis* Osbeck. *Contact Dermatitis* 58 (3): 177–178.
140 Hawkey, S. and Ghaffar, S. (2015). Neoprene orthopaedic supports: an underrecognised cause of allergic contact dermatitis. *Case Reports in Orthopedics* 2015: 496790.
141 Johnson, R.C. and Elston, D.M. (1997). Wrist dermatitis: contact allergy to neoprene in a keyboard wrist rest. *American Journal of Contact Dermatitis* 8 (3): 172–174.
142 Serrano, P., Medeiros, S., Quilho, T. et al. (2008). Photoallergic contact dermatitis to brosimum wood. *Contact Dermatitis* 58 (4): 243–245.
143 Tanaka, M., Fujimoto, A., Kobayashi, S. et al. (2001). Keyboard wrist pad. *Contact Dermatitis* 44 (4): 253–254.
144 Miller, S., ENS Helms, A., and Brodell, R.T. (2007). Occlusive irritant dermatitis: when is "allergic" contact dermatitis not allergic? *SKINmed: Dermatology for the Clinician* 6 (2): 97–98.
145 Ayres, S. Jr. and Mihan, R. (1970). Wristwatch ringworm. *Archives of Dermatology* 102 (2): 235.
146 Husain, S.L. (1977). Nickel coin dermatitis. *British Medical Journal* 2 (6093): 998.
147 Cronin, E. (1973). Squash ball dermatitis. *Contact Dermatitis* 13: 365.
148 Weinberger, L.N., Seraly, M.P., and Zirwas, M.J. (2006). Palmar dermatitis due to a rubber escalator railing. *Contact Dermatitis* 54 (1): 59–60.
149 Brandão, F.M. (2001). Palmar contact dermatitis due to (meth) acrylates. *Contact Dermatitis* 44 (3): 186–187.
150 Lapière, K., Matthieu, L., Meuleman, L., and Lambert, J. (2001). Primula dermatitis mimicking lichen planus. *Contact Dermatitis* 44 (3): 199.
151 Kumar, B., Saraswat, A., and Kaur, I. (2002). Palmoplantar lesions in psoriasis: a study of 3065 patients. *Acta Dermato-Venereologica* 82 (3): 192–195.
152 Veien, N.K. (2009). Acute and recurrent vesicular hand dermatitis. *Dermatologic Clinics* 27 (3): 337–353, vii.
153 Bryld, L.E., Agner, T., and MennÉ, T. (2003). Relation between vesicular eruptions on the hands and tinea pedis, atopic dermatitis and nickel allergy. *Acta Dermatovenereologica-Stockholm* 83 (3): 186–188.
154 Menné, T., Johansen, J.D., Sommerlund, M., and Veien, N.K. (2011). Hand eczema guidelines based on the Danish guidelines for the diagnosis and treatment of hand eczema. *Contact Dermatitis* 65 (1): 3–12.
155 Brans, R. and John, S. (2016). Clinical patterns and associated factors in patients with hand eczema of primarily occupational origin. *Journal of the European Academy of Dermatology and Venereology* 30 (5): 798–805.
156 Mascarenhas, R., Robalo-Cordeiro, M., Fernandes, B. et al. (2001). Allergic and irritant occupational contact dermatitis from Alstroemeria. *Contact Dermatitis* 44 (3): 196–197.
157 Hassan, I., Rasool, F., Akhtar, S. et al. (2018). Contact dermatitis caused by tulips: identification of contact sensitizers in tulip workers of Kashmir Valley in North India. *Contact Dermatitis* 78 (1): 64–69.
158 Bruynzeel, D.P. (1997). Bulb dermatitis. Dermatological problems in the flower bulb industries. *Contact Dermatitis* 37 (2): 70–77.

159 Kanerva, L., Estlander, T., Jolanki, R., and Tarvainen, K. (1993). Occupational allergic contact dermatitis caused by exposure to acrylates during work with dental prostheses. *Contact Dermatitis* 28 (5): 268–275.

160 Ayadi, M. and Martin, P. (1999). Pulpitis of the fingers from a shoe glue containing 1,2-benzisothiazolin-3-one (BIT). *Contact Dermatitis* 40 (2): 115–116.

161 Monteagudo-Paz, A., Salvador, J.S., Martinez, N.L. et al. (2011). Pulpitis as clinical presentation of photoallergic contact dermatitis due to chlorpromazine. *Allergy* 66 (11): 1503–1504.

162 Temime, P. and Oddoze, L. (1970). Exfoliative cheilitis and recurrent crackled keratotic digital pulpitis can be atopic manifestations. *Bulletin de la Société Française de Dermatologie et de Syphiligraphie* 77 (2): 150–156.

163 Sun, C.C., Guo, Y.L., and Lin, R.S. (1995). Occupational hand dermatitis in a tertiary referral dermatology clinic in Taipei. *Contact Dermatitis* 33 (6): 414–418.

164 Magina, S., Barros, M.A., Ferreira, J.A., and Mesquita-Guimarães, J. (2003). Atopy, nickel sensitivity, occupation, and clinical patterns in different types of hand dermatitis. *American Journal of Contact Dermatiti* 14 (2): 63–68.

165 Wang, B.J., Wu, J.D., Sheu, S.C. et al. (2011). Occupational hand dermatitis among cement workers in Taiwan. *Journal of the Formosan Medical Association* 110 (12): 775–779.

166 Wahlberg, J.E. (1985). Occupational hyperkeratoses in carpet installers. *American Journal of Industrial Medicine* 8 (4–5): 351–353.

167 Bonamonte, D., Foti, C., Vestita, M. et al. (2012). Nummular eczema and contact allergy: a retrospective study. *Dermatitis* 23 (4): 153–157.

168 Wiseman, M.C., Orr, P.H., Macdonald, S.M. et al. (2001). Actinic prurigo: clinical features and HLA associations in a Canadian Inuit population. *Journal of the American Academy of Dermatology* 44 (6): 952–956.

169 Liden, C., Berg, M., Farm, G., and Wrangsjo, K. (1993). Nail varnish allergy with far-reaching consequences. *British Journal of Dermatology* 128 (1): 57–62.

170 Militello, G. (2007). Contact and primary irritant dermatitis of the nail unit diagnosis and treatment. *Dermatologic Therapy* 20 (1): 47–53.

171 Dahdah, M.J. and Scher, R.K. (2006). Nail diseases related to nail cosmetics. *Dermatologic Clinics* 24 (2): 233–239, vii.

172 Moossavi, M. and Scher, R.K. (2001). Nail care products. *Clinics in Dermatology* 19 (4): 445–448.

173 Elmansour, I., Chiheb, S., and Benchikhi, H. (2014). Nail changes in connective tissue diseases: a study of 39 cases. *Pan African Medical Journal* 18: 150.

174 Logan, R.A. and Hawk, J.L. (1985). Spontaneous photo-onycholysis. *British Journal of Dermatology* 113 (5): 605–610.

175 Goncalo, S., Goncalo, M., Matos, J., and Marcues, C. (1992). Contact dermatitis from a billiard cue. *Contact Dermatitis* 26 (4): 263.

176 Schwanitz, H.J. and Uter, W. (2000). Interdigital dermatitis: sentinel skin damage in hairdressers. *British Journal of Dermatology* 142 (5): 1011–1012.

177 Jee, S.H., Wang, J.D., Sun, C.C., and Chao, Y.F. (1986). Prevalence of probable kerosene dermatoses among ball-bearing factory workers. *Scandinavian Journal of Work, Environment & Health* 12 (1): 61–65.

178 Patel, M.R., Bassini, L., Nashad, R., and Anselmo, M.T. (1990). Barber's interdigital pilonidal sinus of the hand: a foreign body hair granuloma. *Journal of Hand Surgery* 15 (4): 652–655.

179 Nguyen, T.A. and Krakowski, A.C. (2016). The "heart sign": an early indicator of dose-dependent doxycycline-induced phototoxicity. *Pediatric Dermatology* 33 (2): e69–e71.

180 Woo, S.M., Choi, J.W., Yoon, H.S. et al. (2008). Classification of facial psoriasis based on the distributions of facial lesions. *Journal of the American Academy of Dermatology* 58 (6): 959–963.

181 Ferry, A.P. and Kaltreider, S.A. (1999). Lichen simplex chronicus of the eyelid. *Archives of Ophthalmology* 117 (6): 829–831.

182 Volden, G., Krokan, H., Kavli, G., and Midelfart, K. (1983). Phototoxic and contact toxic reactions of the exocarp of sweet oranges: a common cause of cheilitis? *Contact Dermatitis* 9 (3): 201–204.

183 Aydin, E., Gokoglu, O., Ozcurumez, G., and Aydin, H. (2008). Factitious cheilitis: a case report. *Journal of Medical Case Reports* 2: 29.

184 Lembo, G., Nappa, P., Balato, N., and Ayala, F. (1985). Hat band dermatitis. *Contact Dermatitis* 13 (5): 334.

185 Ramesh, V. (1991). Foreign-body granuloma on the forehead: reaction to bindi. *Archives of Dermatology* 127 (3): 424.

186 Kumar, A.S., Pandhi, R.K., and Bhutani, L.K. (1986). Bindi dermatoses. *International Journal of Dermatology* 25 (7): 434–435.

187 rorsman, H. (1982). Riehl's melanosis. *International Journal of Dermatology* 21 (2): 75–78.

188 Hughes, O.B., Maderal, A.D., and Tosti, A. (2017). An unusual case of contact dermatitis. *Skin Appendage Disorders* 3 (3): 163–165.

189 Kluger, N. and Le Gallic, G. (2014). Hyperpigmentation of the forehead after baptism: a phototoxic reaction due to chrism. *Annales de Dermatologie et de Vénéréologie* 141 (1): 48–49.

190 McKibben, J. and Smalling, C. (2006). Hailey-Hailey. *Skinmed* 5 (5): 250–252.

191 O'Goshi, K.I., Aoyama, H., and Tagami, H. (1998). Mucin deposition in a prayer nodule on the forehead. *Dermatology* 196 (3): 364.

192 Hansson, C. and Thorneby-Andersson, K. (2001). Allergic contact dermatitis from 2-chloro-p-phenylenediamine in a cream dye for eyelashes and eyebrows. *Contact Dermatitis* 45 (4): 235–236.

193 Ro, Y.S. and Lee, C.W. (1991). Granulomatous tissue reaction following cosmetic eyebrow tattooing. *Journal of Dermatology* 18 (6): 352–355.

194 Giulieri, S., Morisod, B., Edney, T. et al. (2011). Outbreak of *Mycobacterium haemophilum* infections after permanent makeup of the eyebrows. *Clinical Infectious Diseases* 52 (4): 488–491.

195 Ishizaki, S., Sawada, M., Suzaki, R. et al. (2012). Tinea faciei by *Microsporum gypseum* mimicking allergic reaction following cosmetic tattooing of the eyebrows. *Medical Mycology Journal* 53 (4): 263–266.

196 Holden, C.R., Shum, K.W., and Gawkrodger, D.J. (2006). Contact allergy to triphenyl phosphate: probable cross-reactivity to triphenyl phosphite present in an EN46001 system 22 clear oxygen facemask. *Contact Dermatitis* 54 (5): 299–300.

197 Cunha, A.P., Mota, A.V., Barros, M.A. et al. (2003). Corticosteroid contact allergy from a nasal spray in a child. *Contact Dermatitis* 48 (5): 277.

198 Staser, K., Ezra, N., Sheehan, M.P., and Mousdicas, N. (2014). The beak sign: a clinical clue to airborne contact dermatitis. *Dermatitis: Contact, Atopic, Occupational, Drug* 25 (2): 97–98.

199 Shanon, J. and Tas, J. (1958). Dermatitis of the nose due to sniff tobacco. *Annals of Allergy* 16 (2): 156–157.

200 Shah, V., Chaubal, T.V., Bapat, R.A., and Shetty, D. (2017). Allergic contact dermatitis caused by polymethylmethacrylate following intradermal filler injection. *Contact Dermatitis* 77 (6): 407–408.

201 Chang, M.W. and Nakrani, R. (2014). Six children with allergic contact dermatitis to methylisothiazolinone in wet wipes (baby wipes). *Pediatrics* 133 (2): e434–e438.

202 Suzuki, K., Hirokawa, K., Yagami, A., and Matsunaga, K. (2011). Allergic contact dermatitis from carmine in cosmetic blush. *Dermatitis: Contact, Atopic, Occupational, Drug* 22 (6): 348–349.

203 Edman, B. (1985). Sites of contact dermatitis in relationship to particular allergens. *Contact Dermatitis* 13 (3): 129–135.

204 Thyssen, J.P., Menne, T., and Zachariae, C. (2012). Allergic nickel dermatitis caused by shaving: case report and assessment of nickel release from an electric shaver. *Acta Dermato-Venereologica* 92 (1): 95–96.

205 Two, A.M., Wu, W., Gallo, R.L., and Hata, T.R. (2015). Rosacea: Part I. Introduction, categorization, histology, pathogenesis, and risk factors. *Journal of the American Academy of Dermatology* 72 (5): 749–758; quiz 59-60.

206 Noguchi, H., Jinnin, M., Miyata, K. et al. (2014). Clinical features of 80 cases of tinea faciei treated at a rural clinic in Japan. *Drug Discoveries & Therapeutics* 8 (6): 245–248.

207 Schwensen, J.F., Menne, T., Hald, M. et al. (2016). Allergic perioral contact dermatitis caused by rubber chemicals during dental treatment. *Contact Dermatitis* 74 (2): 110–111.

208 Rotstein, E. and Rotstein, H. (1997). The ear-lobe sign: a helpful sign in facial contact dermatitis. *Australasian Journal of Dermatology* 38 (4): 215–216.

209 Hillen, U., Grabbe, S., and Uter, W. (2007). Patch test results in patients with scalp dermatitis: analysis of data of the Information Network of Departments of Dermatology. *Contact Dermatitis* 56 (2): 87–93.

210 Aleid, N.M., Fertig, R., Maddy, A., and Tosti, A. (2017). Common allergens identified based on patch test results in patients with suspected contact dermatitis of the scalp. *Skin Appendage Disorders* 3 (1): 7–14.

211 Sommer, S. and Wilkinson, S.M. (2001). Allergic contact dermatitis caused by a nickel-containing headband. *Contact Dermatitis* 44 (3): 178.

212 Badaoui, A., Bayrou, O., Fite, C. et al. (2015). Allergic contact dermatitis caused by methylisothiazolinone in hair gel. *Contact Dermatitis* 73 (6): 364–366.

213 Torchia, D., Giorgini, S., Gola, M., and Francalanci, S. (2008). Allergic contact dermatitis from 2-ethylhexyl acrylate contained in a wig-fixing adhesive tape and its 'incidental' therapeutic effect on alopecia areata. *Contact Dermatitis* 58 (3): 170–171.

214 Starace, M., Militello, G., Pazzaglia, M. et al. (2007). Allergic contact dermatitis to nickel in a hair clasp. *Contact Dermatitis* 56 (5): 290.

215 Tosti, A., Bardazzi, F., De Padova, M.P. et al. (1985). Contact dermatitis to minoxidil. *Contact Dermatitis* 13 (4): 275–276.

216 La Placa, M., Balestri, R., Bardazzi, F., and Vincenzi, C. (2016). Scalp psoriasiform contact dermatitis with acute telogen effluvium due to topical minoxidil treatment. *Skin Appendage Disorders* 1 (3): 141–143.

CHAPTER 6

Setting up a Patch Test Practice

Elin Dafydd Owen and Mahbub M.U. Chowdhury

CHAPTER CONTENTS

Introduction

Up to 7% of dermatology resources are taken up by contact dermatitis [1]. Those who develop allergic contact dermatitis (ACD) endure both psychological and physical morbidity [2–4] and if wrongly labeled as recalcitrant endogenous eczema, a misdiagnosis will put added pressure on resources through increased follow-up rates and unnecessary prescribing of potentially toxic systemic therapy often with minimal or no symptom resolution.

Occupational skin disease can have a profoundly negative effect on performance and time spent at work, with the potential to make those who suffer susceptible to economic disadvantage [2–6]. Occupational skin disease is a significant problem, accounting for 29% of all work-related illnesses with dermatitis constituting 79% of occupational cutaneous conditions [7].

ACD is thus an important diagnosis and has a poor prognosis unless the allergen is identified and actively avoided [1, 8]. An effective patch test service can have financial value because ascertaining a correct diagnosis has the potential to reduce the burden on an already stretched health service. Designated patch test clinics have been shown to improve pick-up rates of allergens [9] and although perhaps challenging to set up initially, the benefits can be highly rewarding.

So how to set up a patch test clinic? In this chapter we offer some guidance on the basic requirements and resources needed to operate a designated specialist service.

Clinics

Designated and specialist-led patch tests clinics have been shown to yield better diagnostic accuracy [9]. The current annual workload recommended by the British Association of Dermatologists is 100 patch tests per year for a catchment population of 70 000 [1]. Dermatology departments thus have an obligation to allocate sufficient time and space to run regular patch test clinics in concordance with local health demands.

Clinic space

A separate, well-designed, and well-lit room for patch test application and analysis is crucial. Patches should be applied and prepared in the same clinic space where allergens are stored. This will help avoid errors and ensure the clinic is run smoothly.

Designated clinic space is just as vital for post-patch test counseling on the last visit as for the initial history taking. Providing information on the allergen, counseling on avoidance, and treatment planning are basic features of the consultation. Relevant positive patch tests have the potential to significantly influence patients' lives so it is important to allow adequate time and space to support and counsel appropriately.

Common Contact Allergens: A Practical Guide to Detecting Contact Dermatitis, First Edition. Edited by John McFadden, Pailin Puangpet, Korbkarn Pongpairoj, Supitchaya Thaiwat, and Lee Shan Xian.
© 2020 John Wiley & Sons Ltd. Published 2020 by John Wiley & Sons Ltd.
Companion website: www.wiley.com/go/mcfadden/common_contact_allergens

Written information

It is good practice to design comprehensive proformas to avoid vital information being missed (Table 6.1). Clear worksheets listing all allergens in the baseline series with adequate space to document additional batteries should be common practice together with template diagrams to map and number allergens clearly.

Patch testing is a unique *in vivo* test in that it requires at least three visits to a clinical department. Patients need to be informed in advance that attendance requires an exercise in compliance and time management. Information leaflets detailing the logistics and the importance of keeping the back dry throughout the week should be sent out a few weeks in advance. Patients need adequate time to adapt their schedules, inform employees, arrange transport and childcare, and cancel any activities that could potentially thwart results. They should also be instructed to bring personal cosmetic products to the clinic and to contact the department in advance if they are taking oral steroids or immunosuppressive therapy.

This type of approach provides an opportunity to discuss potential issues before the appointment and avoid unnecessary cancelations on the first day.

Written information provided by specialist advisory bodies such as the British Society of Cutaneous Allergy (BSCA) or the American Contact Dermatitis Society (ACDS) are of utmost important and should be provided to all patients with a positive patch test.

Lastly there should be ease of access to reference books to guide and facilitate consultations.

Allergens

There will be local baseline series for your geographical area. For example, the European Baseline Patch Test Series has a detection rate of approximately 80% [10]. It contains both single allergens and mixes, and is currently recommended for all patients by the European Environmental Contact Dermatitis Research Group (EECDRG) [11]. The ACDS has a particularly extensive series.

The efficacy of patch testing is largely determined by adequate selection of allergens and in order to enhance detection it can be desirable to include a number of allergens outside the baseline series. An efficient clinic should have ample selection of additional allergen batteries to fully investigate occupational and lifestyle-related contact allergy. Patch test allergens require regular review and this should be a continuous, dynamic process that coincides with current trends as new allergens emerge and others phase out. Furthermore, all patch test clinics should have means of testing patients' own products safely.

Table 6.1 Work-aids and written material to guide patch test consultations.

Written information on patch test procedure
History sheets
Proforma with baseline series and body map
Patient information leaflets
Textbooks
Skin prick test questionnaires for latex
Proforma for skin prick tests

Suppliers

Chemotechnique Diagnostics (Vellinge, Sweden), FIRMA (Florence, Italy), and SmartPracticeE (Calgary, Canada) are all examples of allergen suppliers. SmartPractice also provides a pre-prepared patch test, the T.R.U.E. Test, where allergens are mixed in with hydrophilic gels which can be applied "as is" on the back.

Most suppliers have the European and International baseline series as well as an alphabetical catalogue of haptens and a clear, comprehensive list of additional screening series.

Allergens are individually supplied in syringes with the name, concentration, and expiry date clearly labeled. As with all scientific and medical investigations, consistency is important and suppliers should be able to provide details on the purity and chemical analysis of all their products. Booklets and catalogues provided by the suppliers should be conveniently on hand in the clinic as they are helpful reference guides on exposure and cross-reactivity. Furthermore, most manufacturers have well-designed websites to simplify stock ordering and facilitate communication between themselves and investigators.

Lastly, patch test accessories such as test chambers, vehicles, and dispensers are conveniently provided by most suppliers, which subsequently ameliorates the process of replenishing stock [12].

Systems

Most clinics standardize their results by adopting and adhering to one test system. It is important therefore to choose a system that functions well and complements available resources.

The systems that are not pre-filled require an individual, usually a nurse or technician, to load haptens onto small discs or chambers that are firmly fixed to bands of adhesive tapes. Several types of discs/chambers are available. These include round aluminum Finn chambers (Epitest, Finland) and square, van der Bend chambers (van der Bend, Netherlands), and IQ chambers (Chemotechnique Diagnostics, Sweden) both of which are made of plastic. The alternative is a pre-prepared system where allergens are mixed in with hydrophilic gels and stuck on immediately.

Storage

Strict storage conditions are imperative and several studies have demonstrated concentration strengths lower than labeled when allergens are stored inadequately [13–15]. Adequate space for storing refrigerators is a basic requirement for a patch test clinic and allergens should be kept at between 2 and 8 °C [11]. Furthermore, due to high evaporation rates, unstable allergens such as fragrances and acrylate chambers should be prepared as close to the time of application as possible to avoid false negatives [16]. Allergens should be stored in the same room or at least in close proximity to where the patients attend for patch application. This reduces the risk of contamination, minimizes human errors, and facilitates the running of a busy clinic.

Training/staffing

Positive sensitization can have significant implications on a person's life [2]. It is therefore essential that the reading of results is carried out at the highest of standards [17]. As with any specialty, maintaining standards is of utmost importance in order to continually optimize services and resources [11].

Adequate staffing alleviates the challenges of running full and time-intensive clinics.

Nursing staff should be fully competent in patch test techniques before they can work independently. Training in allergen profiling, patch test application, mapping, and documentation are all basic requirements.

Inter-individual variation has been demonstrated between techniques used in allergen application [18]. Thus every measure should be taken to ensure as much precision and consistency as possible. Furthermore, stock replenishing in a timely manner should be common practice and every clinic should have a designated staff member to carry out the task.

Personnel should attend updates at scientific conferences (at least 2-yearly for lead specialists and nurses) to assure maintenance of key skills, knowledge, and expertise [11]. Opportunities to visit national or local centers of excellence should be taken.

Clinical governance

Clinical governance is pivotal for any successful service. Audit points outlined by national guidelines should be assessed regularly to ensure standards are met and resources are run at optimum levels. Review of waiting lists, resource demands, and staff capacity is an ongoing process. Clinical practice should be evidence-based and regular multidisciplinary meetings provide an opportunity to discuss allergen trends, new research, guidance, and standards. Furthermore, they provide a platform for all members of staff to vocalize issues and pitfalls within the service. Difficult cases should be discussed and reviewed along with any errors and near misses to address potential safeguarding issues.

Data surveillance

It is common practice for specialist patch test clinics to invest in a specified software system to record patient outcomes. This system should be robust and secure, and allow all information to be entered anonymously. A number of strategies for loading data exist and clinics should choose a method that best fits with their resources [19].

More important perhaps is that large amounts of nationally collected data provide an opportunity for early intervention to reduce sensitization prevalence through regulation, or even withdrawal of known problematic allergens. Furthermore, surveillance can monitor the success of intervention methods by analyzing any decreasing frequencies and identifying persistent and ongoing issues [11, 12].

References

1 Johnston, G.A., Exton, L.S., Mohd Mustapa, M.F. et al. (2017). British Association of Dermatologists' guidelines for the management of contact dermatitis 2017. *British Journal of Dermatology* 176: 317–329.

2 Linn Holness, D. (2001). Results of a quality of life questionnaire in a patch test clinic population. *Contact Dermatitis* 44: 80–84.

3 Cvetkovski, R.S., Zachariae, R., Jensen, H. et al. (2006). Quality of life and depression in a population of occupational hand eczema patients. *Contact Dermatitis* 54: 106–111.

4 Hutchings, C.V., Shum, K.W., and Gawkrodger, D.J. (2001). Occupational contact dermatitis has an appreciable impact on quality of life. *Contact Dermatitis* 45: 17–20.

5 Adisesh, A., Meyer, J.D., and Cherry, N.M. (2002). Prognosis and work absence due to occupational contact dermatitis. *Contact Dermatitis* 46: 273–279.

6 Cvetkovski, R.S., Rothman, K.J., Olsen, J. et al. (2005). Relation between diagnoses on severity, sick leave and loss of job among patients with occupational hand eczema. *British Journal of Dermatology* 52: 93–98.

7 Meyer, J.D., Chen, Y., Holt, D.L. et al. (2000). Occupational contact dermatitis in the UK: a surveillance report from EPIDERM and OPRA. *Occupational Medicine* 50: 265–273.

8 Skoet, R., Zachariae, R., and Agner, T. (2003). Contact dermatitis and quality of life: a structured review of the literature. *British Journal of Dermatology* 149: 452–456.

9 Ormond, P., Hazelwood, E., Bourke, B. et al. (2002). The importance of a dedicated patch test clinic. *British Journal of Dermatology* 146: 304–307.

10 Dillarstone, A. (1997). Cosmetic preservatives. *Contact Dermatitis* 37: 190.

11 Johansen, J.D., Aalto-Korte, K., Agner, T. et al. (2015). European Society of Contact Dermatitis guideline for diagnostic patch testing–recommendations on best practice. *Contact Dermatitis* 73: 195–221.

12 Johansen, J.D., Frosch, P.J., and Lepoittevin, J.P. (2006). *Contact Dermatitis*, 5e. Berlin, Heidelberg: Springer.

13 Goon, A.T., Bruze, M., Zimerson, E. et al. (2011). Variation in allergen content over time of acrylates/methacrylates in patch test preparations. *British Journal of Dermatology* 164: 116–124.

14 Mose, K.F., Andersen, K.E., and Christensen, L.P. (2012). Stability of selected volatile contact allergens in different patch test chambers under different storage conditions. *Contact Dermatitis* 66: 172–179.
15 Siegel, P.D., Fowler, J.F., Law, B.F. et al. (2014). Concentrations and stability of methyl methacrylate, glutaraldehyde, formaldehyde and nickel sulfate in commercial patch test allergen preparations. *Contact Dermatitis* 70: 309–315.
16 Mowitz, M., Svedman, C., Zimerson, E., and Bruze, M. (2014). Fragrance patch tests prepared in advance may give false-negative reactions. *Contact Dermatitis* 71: 289–294.
17 Svedman, C., Isaksson, M., Björk, J. et al. (2012). Calibration' of our patch test reading technique is necessary. *Contact Dermatitis* 66: 180–187.
18 Frick-Engfeldt, M., Gruvberger, B., Isaksson, M. et al. (2010). Comparison of three different techniques for application of water solutions to Finn chambers®. *Contact Dermatitis* 63: 284–288.
19 Uter, W., Amario-Hita, J.C., Balato, A. et al. (2017). European surveillance system on contact allergies (ESSCA): results with the European baseline series, 2013/14. *Journal of the European Academy of Dermatology and Venereology* 31: 1516–1525.

CHAPTER 7
The Role of Providers of Patch Test Products

Bo Niklasson

CHAPTER CONTENTS

Introduction

The role of a provider of patch test products is not solely to be a producer of products but also to be an active partner in the development of new solutions in the field of contact allergy diagnosis. We believe that the production and supply of high-quality diagnostic products is of paramount importance as these products are necessary tools for any physician trying to establish a correct diagnosis of contact allergy, the result of which has a tremendous economic impact in society, i.e. reducing costs related to sick leave, treatment of the disease, and change of jobs [1].

Patch testing and the diagnosis of contact allergy

Contact allergy is manifested by the development of eczema on the skin of an allergic individual after exposure to a causative hapten. While contact allergy cannot be cured (i.e. there is no known treatment analogous to "allergy shots" or specific immunotherapy) it can be diagnosed by patch testing. Patch testing is not to be confused with skin allergy testing (such as skin prick/scratch/injection testing) which is used for the diagnosis of respiratory Type 1 allergies such as allergy to animal hair or pollen.

Patch testing is a challenge procedure of the skin using a patch test device to diagnose delayed reaction, Type 4, allergies. A patch test device consists of a patch test unit (PTU) and one or more test substances. The test substances used in patch testing are known as haptens. The term "allergen" has previously been widely used in the patch testing community when referring to these test substances as they have incorrectly been grouped with the allergens used in prick testing.

Haptens are immunologically incompetent, low molecular (not exceeding 500 Daltons) compounds which are not antigenic by themselves but require binding to a skin protein to become an antigen [2]. Common examples of haptens include nickel, cobalt, fragrances, various preservatives, and formaldehyde.

When performing a patch test, minute amounts (around 20–25 µg) of these haptens are applied, using a syringe or a dropper bottle, into the chambers of a PTU. A PTU is composed of sets of chambers mounted on adhesive tape. The chambers and backing tape can be of various designs and materials but they all serve the same purpose: to create a standardized environment for the hapten to interact with the skin. Some PTUs have additional special features such as waterproof backing tape or adhesive chamber rims to create a closed chamber and cater for a defined dose per area testing. The prepared PTU is thereafter applied onto undamaged areas of the patient's skin (typically the upper back).

The patch test remains on the patient for approximately 48 hours before it is removed. These 48 hours equal the elicitation phase of a contact allergic reaction as the haptens will have permeated the skin and bound to dermal protein, forming

Common Contact Allergens: A Practical Guide to Detecting Contact Dermatitis, First Edition. Edited by John McFadden
Pailin Puangpet, Korbkarn Pongpairoj, Supitchaya Thaiwat, and Lee Shan Xian.
© 2020 John Wiley & Sons Ltd. Published 2020 by John Wiley & Sons Ltd.
Companion website: www.wiley.com/go/mcfadden/common_contact_allergens

antigens. Reading of the skin reaction is performed 24–48 hours after patch test removal. Other subsequent readings may be performed after another 3–5 days [3].

If the body recognizes the complex of haptenated self-peptide + MHC class I and/or II molecules the elicitation phase is initiated, causing a miniature eczema confined to the area (around 1 cm^2) where the chambers have been attached to the skin. If the body does not recognize the complex of haptenated self-peptide + MHC class I and/or II molecules (i.e. there are no appropriate memory T cells present in the patient, i.e. the individual being tested is not sensitized) there will be no reaction on the patient's skin.

In conclusion, two actions are needed: the initial binding of the hapten to a dermal protein followed by the immunological response that shows the altered physiological state of the patient. Patch testing does not diagnose a disease (contact dermatitis/eczema) but rather the immunological condition of the patient (contact allergy).

The importance of the baseline series and relevant standardized testing

In general, the more comprehensive the range of haptens for testing, the higher the yield of positive patch test reactions achieved [4]. To test patients for hundreds of haptens at a time is, however, both impractical and unsuitable since many possible haptens will lack clinical relevance and the physical space available for testing on a patient is limited.

To aid dermatologists in choosing what haptens to test for, national and international contact dermatitis research groups select haptens with high regional relevance to form a patch testing foundation. Such hapten groupings are called standard or baseline series.

An original series was the European Standard (known today as the European Baseline Series, EBS). The European Standard was originally developed by the European Contact Dermatitis Research Group. Since then, the series has been updated continuously and consists today of 30 haptens, and is widely used in European patch testing clinics. The EBS is today governed by the European Society of Contact Dermatitis (ESCD) and its EBS working group – a task force consisting not only of physicians but also industry representatives, myself included, on advisory positions. The EBS will be added to with a hapten extension in 2019 (www.escd.org).

In North America a comprehensive baseline series of 80 haptens, based on research made by the North American Contact Dermatitis Group (NACDG) [4], is often used.

In other regions other baseline series have been developed by regional contact dermatitis research groups to cater for local exposure. Examples of regions where baseline series have been developed as a result of co-operation between industry and research groups include Latin America, Australia, the UK, China, Italy, and Spain. Information on the regional baseline series can be found in the patch test providers' manuals and on the providers' websites [5].

In addition to selecting the proper baseline series, special attention needs to be paid to the patient and the patient history in order to investigate the different sources of exposure that can be related to the patient's symptoms. In such cases the addition of a screening series reflecting occupational or other exposure (i.e. cosmetics, fragrances, medicaments, sunscreens, or acrylics) will help to detect the culprit hapten.

Research and development: creating new haptens

Developing new hapten preparations remains as relevant as ever. The development of new patch test haptens is often initiated by a contact dermatitis research group that suspects a chemical, often unknown to the patch testing community, to be causing allergic contact dermatitis. Initial testing with the suspected hapten might be done with hapten substance compounded at a pharmacy but such substances are not suitable when the relevance of the suspected hapten is to be confirmed on a larger scale. In such cases it is important that testing is coherent and repeatable.

At this stage a pharmaceutical hapten manufacturer producing under good manufacturing practice (GMP), such as Chemotechnique, is approached in order to develop a hapten preparation for a multicenter patient study. The manufacturer then starts the arduous research of developing a manufacturing process for that specific hapten. This research work includes setting up the analytical methods required and creating a practical road map of how to produce the specific hapten in question (following the steps described in the production section). Recent examples of patch test haptens developed after being initiated by studies include hydroperoxides of linalool and limonene [6, 7], photopatch haptens [8], palladium [9], methylisothiazolinone/methylchloroisothiazolinone [10], and sunscreens [11] (Figure 7.1).

Production

Companies producing hapten preparations are typically regulated under pharmaceutical law and as such must be approved as pharmaceutical producers, operating under GMP [12]. This approval requires continuous inspections by health authorities to ensure that the highest standards in terms of quality, efficacy, and safety in production are met. A quality management system ensuring compliance must be in place. The overall responsibility for the quality system is guaranteed by the qualified person (QP) assisted by the quality assurance function (QA), and the quality control function (QC). The production itself involves a number of steps outlined in the following description, which is valid for Chemotechnique production in Vellinge, Sweden (Figure 7.2).

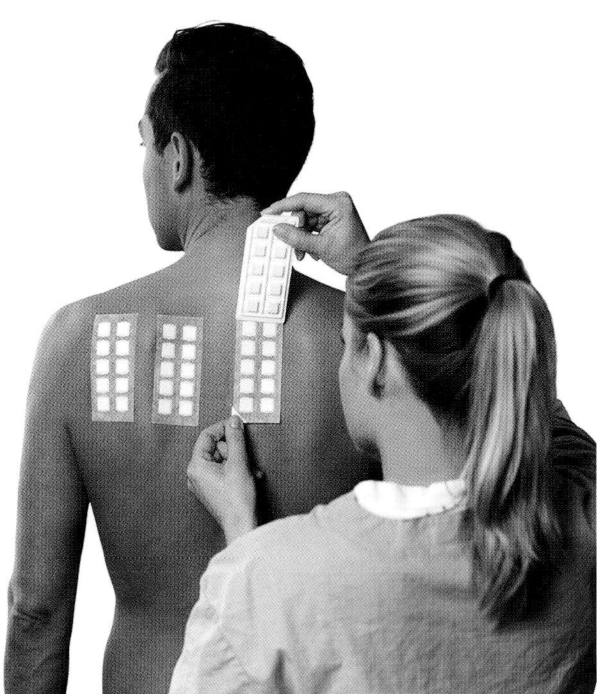

Figure 7.1 Application of patch tests.

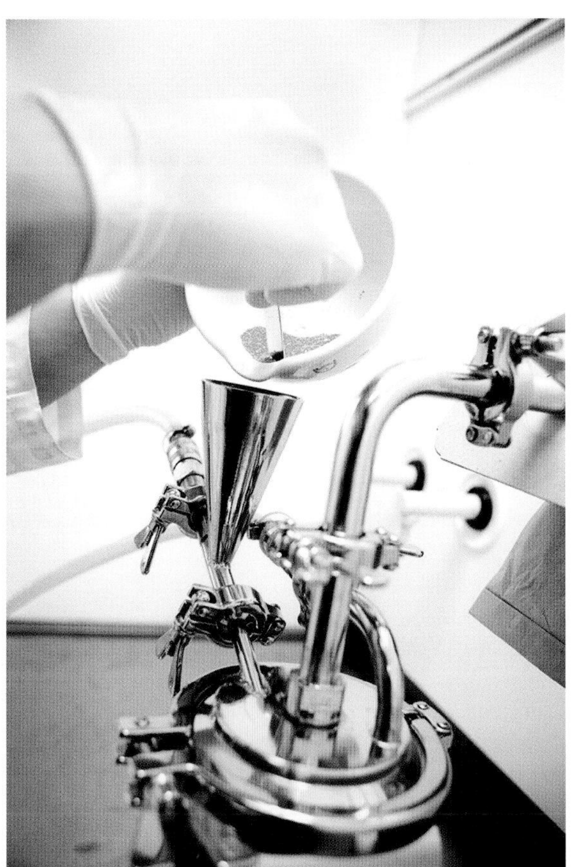

Figure 7.2 Production techniques.

Haptens

The production of hapten test substances is in essence the conversion of solid or liquid high-purity raw material into a semisolid or liquid homogenized dilution of raw material with a specified concentration of hapten.

When producing hapten test substances raw materials are processed using sophisticated equipment to achieve small sized particles. The processed particles are blended and homogenized into a vehicle (most commonly petrolatum for solid haptens or water for liquid haptens) using state-of-the art processes. Depending on the characteristics (purity, quality, and chemical stability) of the raw material, variables such as temperature, moisture, viscosity, and weight are taken into account when setting up the homogenization process and time intervals for the different segments of the processes. The final preparation is dispensed into polypropylene syringes (for semisolid preparations) or polyethylene dropper bottles (for liquid preparations) using custom automated filling and labeling machinery. The entire production is made in such a way that contamination risks are eliminated. Once produced, a batch of hapten preparation must receive a batch release before being cleared for dispatch.

The batch release includes steps such as analysis of color, particle size, chemical identification, physical appearance, air content, and particle distribution in the final hapten preparation to name a few. Tools and methods used in the various steps of physical and chemical analysis include high-performance liquid chromatography (HPLC), Fourier transform infrared spectroscopy (FT-IR), gas chromatography (GC), atomic absorption spectroscopy (AAS), melting point, microscopy, and refractive index of solutions.

Based on the chemical stability of the raw materials (validated by continuous product stability studies) a product expiry is set. Released hapten preparations awaiting dispatch are stored in the dark in temperature-controlled environments at either 2–8 °C or, for a few haptens, in a sub-zero environment depending on hapten requirement.

Patch test units

PTUs that are not sold "pre-filled" with haptens are generally registered as Medical Device Class 1. The Chemotechnique PTUs are manufactured on-site in Sweden following the strict guidelines of the ISO 13485 and ISO 9001 management systems (https://www.iso.org). The PTUs manufactured by Chemotechnique, IQ Ultra™ and the IQ Ultimate™, are created by combining the finest medical grade carrier tape with adhesive foam frames and filter papers with protective covers using proprietary production techniques. Multiple vision systems and high-precision robotics guarantee the quality of the production. Alternative systems used include the Finn Chambers™, which are aluminum discs for holding haptens, mounted on Scanpor™

tape, which is a hypoallergenic surgical tape made of rayon and polyester fibers with a non-latex adhesive.

Skin markers and reading plates are also supplied.

Further developments

Patch testing is not a static discipline and research and development are key. For example, at Chemotechnique research and development form the foundation on which the business is built. New materials, production processes, and compositions are constantly being evaluated in order to improve the various products in our portfolio. The application of our deep understanding of contact allergy extends further than diagnosis. Solutions for the detection of nickel and cobalt in everyday objects help patients suffering from contact allergy to these haptens to identify the causative objects. Venturing into the field of contact allergy protection, an active chelating barrier cream that uses diethylenetriamine penta-acetic acid (DTPA) to immobilize nickel and cobalt ions has been developed, preventing them from entering the epidermis [13, 14].

Legislation, reimbursement, and other challenges

To date there has been no international legislative or regulatory uniformity associated with the practice of the topical diagnostic procedure of patch testing and the haptens used to indicate if an individual patient has an allergic reaction to a particular tested substance. Virtually all substances incorporated into the hapten preparations are readily available and approved for use in consumer products or specific occupations.

Patch testing is practiced primarily by dermatologists. The regulatory tendency has been to incorrectly combine the regulation of patch testing under the "allergy and allergen" classification as practiced by allergists using allergens. Allergy testing involves the invasion of the skin to determine a patient's allergy. These two procedures are completely different and have different levels of patient risk associated with them: patch testing is extremely low risk while allergy testing is higher risk.

Fundamental to establishing a valid scientific basis for accepting the procedural differences between dermatological patch testing and allergist allergy testing is a regulatory understanding of not only the medical procedural differences, but, most importantly, the scientific difference between a hapten, as used in patch testing, and an allergen, as used by an allergist (see the patch testing and the diagnosis of contact allergy section). Because of this, it could be argued that haptens could be regulated as medical devices, while allergens should be regulated as pharmaceuticals.

Today, haptens are generally distributed as unregistered pharmaceutical products on a "named patient" basis, but there are exceptions where haptens are registered, marketed, and sold as Medical Device Class 1. Regulators in Europe and elsewhere are now seemingly striving for a harmonization in regulation regarding the field of patch testing. As a manufacturer of patch test products, we embrace all efforts to clarify the regulation of patch testing. Concerns have arisen, however, around whether or not the progression of this harmonization is heading in a sustainable direction. For instance, some countries do not have legislative exceptions allowing for the distribution of unregistered pharmaceuticals. In such cases pharmaceutical registration for individual haptens is enforced. Due to the very high cost associated with pharmaceutical registrations such regulatory demands will result in one of the following scenarios:

- Comprehensive patch testing will either no longer be offered, as the costs associated with pharmaceutical registration will far exceed what is deemed reasonable to transfer onto hapten pricing, or prices will indeed be transferred to clinics, rendering patch testing an extremely expensive diagnostic method.
- Only specified hapten series with defined concentrations, sold as complete sets with a singular expiry, will be available for purchase. Any adjustment in composition or concentration will demand a new pharmaceutical registration, resulting in hapten series that will not be updated based on patient exposure but rather financial viability.

A recent example of the challenges involved came in 2017 when Chemotechnique was obliged to register the previously unregistered whole range of haptens in Canada [1]. The process not only involved huge costs and a massive strain on our lab department, but major efforts were ultimately spent in confirming that Health Canada, the Canadian health authority, had a correct understanding of the immunological process of contact allergy and allergic contact dermatitis. As a result of this, all of our patch test haptens are now registered pharmaceuticals in Canada.

Moreover, while we see many governments increasing their focus on regulatory compliance, we note that reimbursements for patch testing issued by the very same governments at the same time are being, if not completely removed, reduced from already low levels. We fear that the reduced funding will limit the reach of patch testing, effectively leaving patients underdiagnosed.

Providing patients with hapten information

Moving forward we see the need to not abandon the patient after diagnosis but follow her on her onward journey. A deep understanding of the causative hapten is crucial to ensure patient hapten avoidance post diagnosis. This book and other textbooks and sources such as journals can provide a comprehensive source for hapten information [15]. Other comprehensive sources of hapten information are readily available on the websites of the two major patch test hapten producers (www.chemotechnique.se, www.smartpractice.com). Many clinics are also supplying hapten information sheets to their patients. Information sheets can be useful but the information given to the patients should be tailored to the patient's own circumstances. What I believe could be improved is information not on what is dangerous, but what is safe to use for affected patients. A service provided to the members of the American Contact Dermatitis Society (ACDS) addressing this issue is the Contact Allergen Management Program (or CAMP for short; https://www.contactderm.org/i4a/pages/index.cfm?pageid=3489). CAMP is a database that provides diagnosed patients with information on personal care products that are free of the ingredients that are causing their allergic reactions. I believe that an international version of this service would be most beneficial for patients worldwide. Another service provided for hapten avoidance is the Skinsafe website (https://www.skinsafeproducts.com).

Educational support

Although we see that some countries have difficulties in recruiting physicians interested in contact allergy and performing patch testing, we strive to make patch testing be perceived as relevant. Education is key in order to ensure that there are sufficient numbers of physicians educated to perform patch testing. Providers of patch test products give educational support in the form of sponsoring numerous congress activities and taking part in exhibitions plus arranging their own workshops and sponsoring workshops done by physicians. We particularly look to support the development of patch test services and expertise in countries with rapidly developing manufacturing industries. With joint efforts between providers of patch test products and physicians world-wide, we can together ensure that patch testing remains available for the one-quarter of the general population suffering from contact allergy.

References

1 Improving patch test efficacy: Part 2. Page 21. MA Mcgowan, DJ No, BC Machler, SE Jacob. The Dermatologist, February 2018. www.the-dermatologist.

2 Karlsson, I., Samuelsson, K., Simonsson, C. et al. (2018). The fate of a hapten – from the skin to modification of macrophage migration inhibitory factor (MIF) in lymph nodes. *Scientific Reports* 8: 2895.

3 Johansen, J.D., Aalto-Korte, K., Agner, T. et al. (2015). European Society of Contact Dermatitis guideline for diagnostic patch testing – recommendations on best practice. *Contact Dermatitis* 73(4): 195–221.

4 Schalock, P.C., Dunnick, C.A., Nedorost, S. et al. (2013). American Contact Dermatitis Society core allergen series. *Dermatitis* 24 (1): https://www.contactderm.org/files/public/2013_CoreAllergenList(corrected).pdf.

5 Patch Test Products and Reference Manual. Chemotechnique Diagnostics 2018. www.chemotechnique.se.

6 Deza, G., García-Bravo, B., Silvestre, J.F. et al. and GEIDAC. (2017). Contact sensitization to limonene and linalool hydroperoxides in Spain: a GEIDAC*prospective study. *Contact Dermatitis* 76 (2): 74–80.

7 Björkman, Y.A., Hagvall, L., Siwmark, C. et al. (2014). Air oxidized linalool elicits eczema in allergic patients – a repeated open application test study. *Contact Dermatitis* 70: 129–138.

8 Gonçalo, M., Ferguson, J., Bonevalle, A. et al. (2013). Photopatch testing: recommendations for a European photopatch test baseline series. *Contact Dermatitis* 68 (4): 239–243.

9 Śpiewak, R., Samochocki, Z., Paśnicki, M. et al. (2014). Detection of contact allergy to palladium: sodium tetrachloropalladate is better than palladium chloride. *Allergy* 69: 44–45.

10 Śpiewak, R., Samochocki, Z., Paśnicki, M. et al. (2014). Methylisothiazolinone/methylchloroisothiazolinone and formaldehyde: petrolatum-based patch tests detect more sensitizations. *Contact Dermatitis* 70 (Suppl. 1): 60–61.

11 Kerr, A.C., Niklasson, B., Dawe, R.S. et al. (2009). A double-blind, randomized assessment of the irritant potential of sunscreen chemical dilutions used in photopatch testing. *Contact Dermatitis* 60 (4): 203–209.

12 EudraLex, Volume 4 – Good Manufacturing Practice (GMP) guidelines. https://ec.europa.eu/health/documents/eudralex/vol-4_en.

13 Niklasson, B., Gregorius, A., and Spiewak, R. ESCD Abstracts: Posters, (2016). A novel barrier cream is effective in preventing allergic contact dermatitis from nickel-releasing items. *Contact Dermatitis* 75, S1: 60–106.

14 Niklasson, B. and Isaksson, M.. ESCD Abstracts: Posters, (2016). Allergic contact dermatitis from nickel is prevented using a novel barrier cream. *Contact Dermatitis* 75 (S1): 60–106.

15 de Groot, A.C. (2018). *Monographs in Contact Allergy Vol 1–2. Non-Fragrance allergens in Cosmetics.* CRS Press. ISBN: 13:978-1-138.

SECTION 2

Non-allergic Dermatoses

CHAPTER 8

Elimination or Inclusion of Non-Allergic Skin Diseases

CHAPTER CONTENT

Elimination or inclusion of non-allergic skin diseases is an important part of contact dermatitis practice – as many as 50% of dermatitis patients presenting to the clinic are patch test negative, and in some of those with positive patch tests the allergen identified is either of old or no clinical relevance. Additionally, allergic contact dermatitis (ACD) often coexists alongside non-allergic inflammatory skin disorders. Therefore, it is important to assess for the presence of non-allergic skin diseases. For convenience, eczematous drug reactions are also considered here. The list does not include all other dermatoses, e.g. photodermatoses, which can be found in other textbooks, such as *Rook's Textbook of Dermatology*.

The following is a summary of the more common "non-allergic" conditions to be considered, alongside ACD, which may be referred to a contact dermatitis clinic.

Inflammatory non-dermatitic dermatoses

Psoriasis

- Plaque psoriasis is the most common form and is present in 85–90% of all psoriasis patients [1].
- There is usually loose symmetry, silver and lamellar scaling (may not be present), induration (may not be present), and erythema in well-defined plaques varying from a few millimeters to over 10 cm in size (Figure 8.1).
- Examine the knees, elbows, scalp (areas of scaling and induration interspersed with normal skin, scalp margin often affected), lower back, hands, and feet for evidence of psoriasis.
- Examine the nails – thimble-like pitting, onycholysis, dystrophy, subungual hyperkeratosis, and yellow-brown spots ("oil spots") under the nail plate may be observed.

Common Contact Allergens: A Practical Guide to Detecting Contact Dermatitis, First Edition. Edited by John McFadden, Pailin Puangpet, Korbkarn Pongpairoj, Supitchaya Thaiwat, and Lee Shan Xian.

© 2020 John Wiley & Sons Ltd. Published 2020 by John Wiley & Sons Ltd.

Companion website: www.wiley.com/go/mcfadden/common_contact_allergens

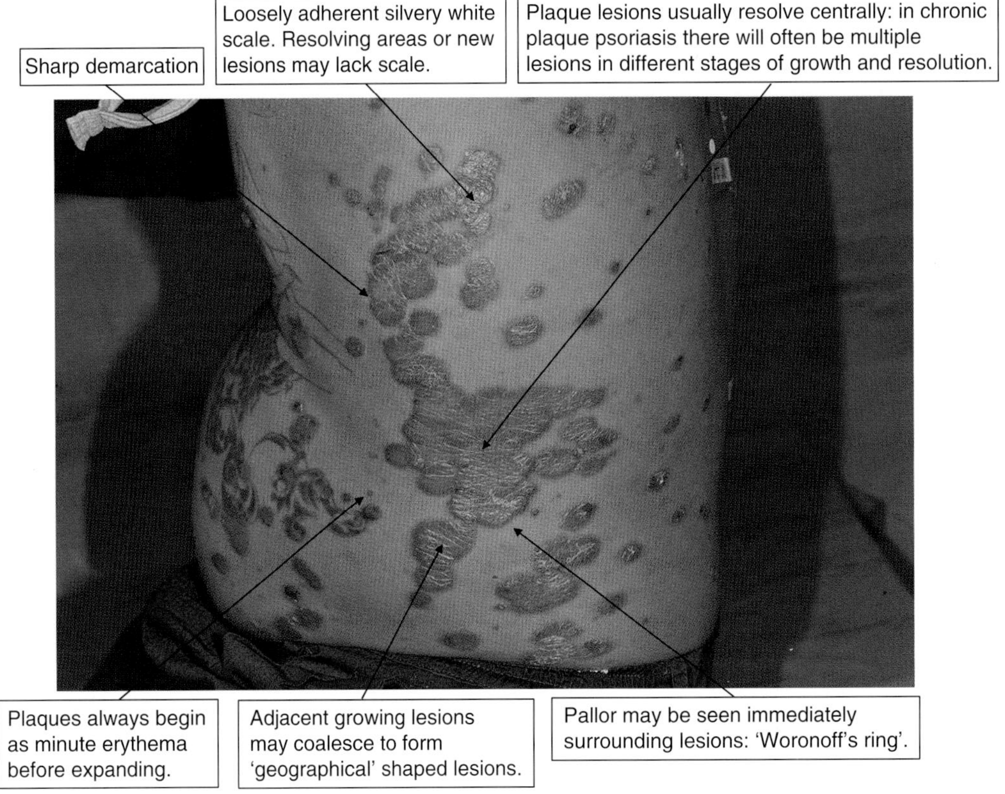
Sharp demarcation
Loosely adherent silvery white scale. Resolving areas or new lesions may lack scale.
Plaque lesions usually resolve centrally: in chronic plaque psoriasis there will often be multiple lesions in different stages of growth and resolution.
Plaques always begin as minute erythema before expanding.
Adjacent growing lesions may coalesce to form 'geographical' shaped lesions.
Pallor may be seen immediately surrounding lesions: 'Woronoff's ring'.

Figure 8.1 Plaque psoriasis.

- Enquire about a family history of psoriasis. Approximately 20% of psoriasis patients will have at least one parent with psoriasis and 15% will have a sibling with psoriasis [2]. In children with psoriasis, there is a positive family history in 70% [3].
- Non-pustular palmar and plantar psoriasis may be difficult to distinguish from irritant contact dermatitis (ICD), ACD or endogenous dermatitis. The characteristic sharp cut-off and silver scales may still be present (Figure 8.2). There may also be evidence of psoriasis elsewhere. If a distinction cannot be made, a diagnosis of psoriasiform dermatitis is sometimes given.
- In a study of 3065 psoriasis patients, 17% (1 in 6) had non-pustular palmar and/or plantar involvement [4]. Of these, 47% had palmoplantar psoriasis, 8% had palmar psoriasis alone and 44% had plantar psoriasis alone. 85% of patients with palmar psoriasis will also have plantar psoriasis.
- In patients with palmar +/− plantar psoriasis, 30% will have typical plaque-like lesions elsewhere on the body [4].
- Four distinct patterns of non-pustular palmar psoriasis have been recorded [4]: involvement confined to the pressure areas (thenar and hypothenar eminences, margins of the hand, and volar aspects of the fingers) in 32% of patients, involvement confined to the non-pressure areas (hollow of the palms) in 29% of patients, discrete lesions over both pressure and non-pressure areas in 22%, and diffuse, keratoderma-like involvement in 17%. Manual workers are twice as likely to have involvement confined to the pressure areas alone compared to non-manual workers.
- Only 4% (10/260) of patients with non-pustular palmar psoriasis had unilateral involvement. All were male with manual duties and the dominant hand was always involved [4].
- Five distinct patterns of non-pustular plantar psoriasis have been recorded [4]: involvement confined to the pressure areas (heels, forefeet, lateral borders of the feet, and plantar aspects of the toes) in 24% of patients, involvement confined to the non-pressure areas (plantar arch) in 30% of patients, discrete lesions over both pressure and non-pressure areas in 33%, diffuse keratoderma-like involvement in 10%, and diffuse involvement with sparing of the instep region in 3%.
- Palmoplantar pustular psoriasis is characterized by yellow sterile pustules as well as brown macules or scale (which the yellow pustules evolve into) (Figure 8.3). Tobacco smokers are over twice as likely to develop palmoplantar pustular psoriasis compared to non-smokers [5].
- Sebopsoriasisis is a combination of seborrheic eczema and psoriasis. The areas that are usually affected are typical for seborrheic eczema (scalp, retroauricular regions, eyebrows, glabella, alae nasi, sternum, axillae, and groin flexures). The scale is often somewhere between the yellow greasy scale of seborrheic eczema and the silver scale of psoriasis. The inflammatory margins are less clear than in plaque psoriasis. Knee and elbow plaques may or may not be present.
- Some studies have indicated an inverse relationship between psoriasis and contact allergy [6]. Other studies have, conversely,

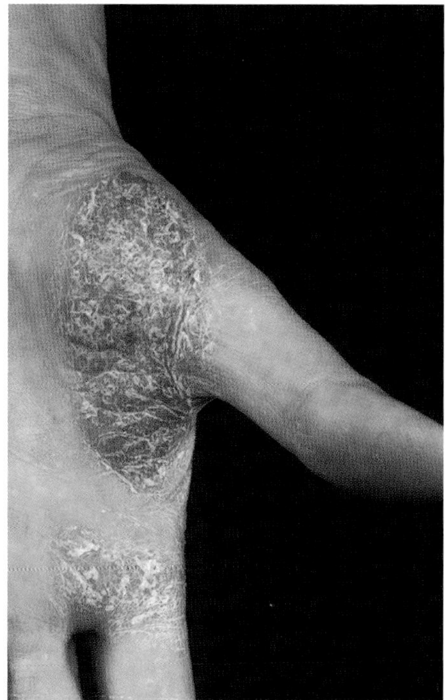
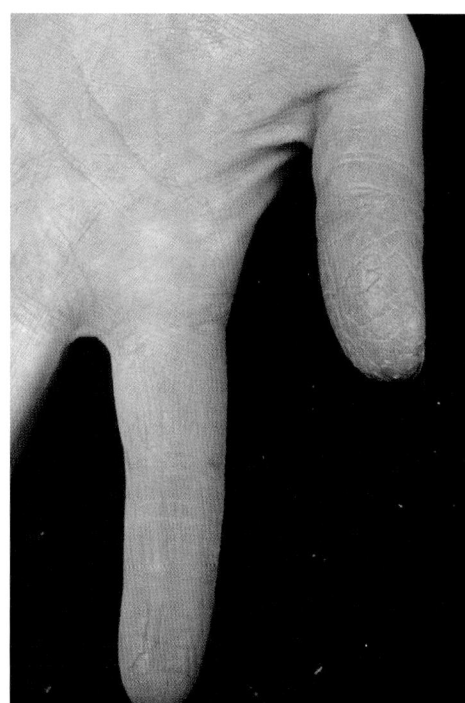

Figure 8.2 Palmar psoriasis versus irritant contact dermatitis.

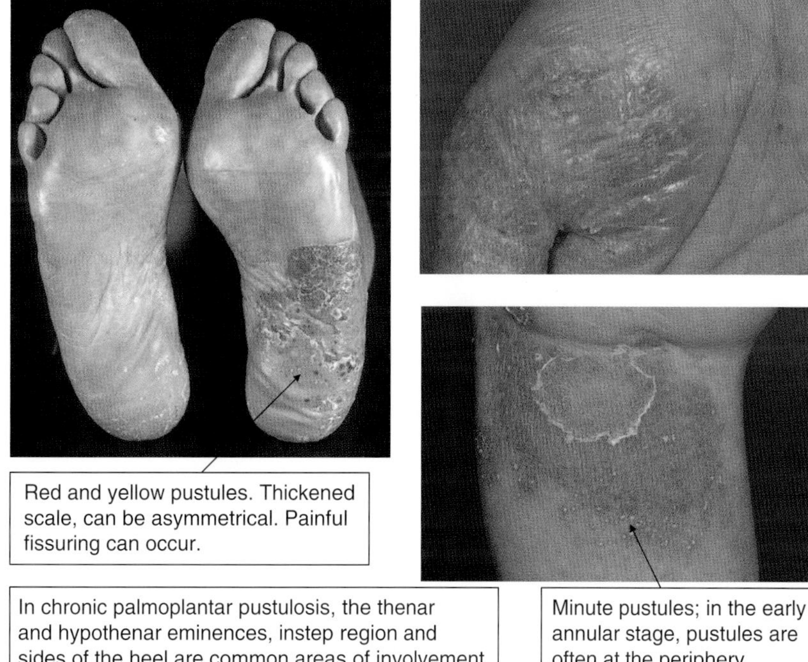

Red and yellow pustules. Thickened scale, can be asymmetrical. Painful fissuring can occur.
In chronic palmoplantar pustulosis, the thenar and hypothenar eminences, instep region and sides of the heel are common areas of involvement.
Minute pustules; in the early annular stage, pustules are often at the periphery.

Figure 8.3 Pustular psoriasis.

shown psoriasis patients with high rates of contact allergy [7]. The largest study to date, a retrospective study of 2104 psoriasis patients, showed patch test positivity rates that were similar to those of dermatitis patients attending the same clinic [8]. However, this is higher than the normal adult population.

- Medicament allergy patch test screening for psoriasis patients should include tar, dithranol, and calcipitriol [9, 10].
- Acute ACD to topical psoralens from topical psoralens-ultraviolet A (PUVA) therapy has been described [11].

- Quaranta et al. found that positive patch tests were delayed in psoriasis patients compared to dermatitis control patients, with a peak reaction at day 7 [12].
- Two cases of ACD to nail hardeners were initially mistaken for pustular psoriasis and nail psoriasis with onycholysis [13].
- ACD affecting the groin/buttocks due to methylisothiazolinone in wet wipes has been misdiagnosed as psoriasis [14].

Tinea

Tinea pedis

- Often (but not always) unilateral or asymmetrical.
- The inflammatory/bullous type (usually caused by *T. mentagrophytes*) has the following characteristics [15]:
  a. hard, tense vesicles, bullae, and pustules on the instep region or mid-anterior plantar surface
  b. vesicles are typically 1–5 mm in diameter
  c. vesicles may coalesce to form herpetiform or serpiginous bullae with an erythematous base
  d. the bullae of *T. interdigitale* occur particularly on the plantar arch and heels, as well as along the sides of the feet, adjacent to the thick part of the plantar stratum corneum. *T. rubrum* may also produce vesicles but these are usually on the thick plantar skin.
- The moccasin type (usually caused by *T. rubrum*) has well-demarcated erythema, fine white scaling, and hyperkeratosis. Usually, this can be differentiated from shoe dermatitis as the instep region is usually involved in moccasin tinea. Hyperkeratotic scaling typically involves the entire plantar surface, with sparing of the dorsa of the feet. Erythema is usually mild. It is not uncommon for both feet and one hand to be involved, and in these cases there is usually also nail involvement [15].
- Approximately one-third of all patients with onychomycosis have concomitant tinea pedis [16].
- The exposure of specific populations to sweating, trauma, occlusive footwear, and communal areas predisposes these groups to an increased incidence of tinea pedis. Up to 72.9% of miners, 58% of soldiers, and 31% of marathon runners examined had mycologically proven tinea pedis. The prevalence of tinea pedis was 29.5% in mosque attendees [15].
- Asymptomatic infections (occult tinea pedis) are common, particularly amongst athletes [15].
- Tinea pedis is uncommon in very young children [17]. However, it is more common in older children. Tinea pedis was reported to have prevalence rates of 6.6% and 1.6% in 11–14-year-old boys and girls, respectively, and 2.2% in 7–10-year-old boys [15, 18].
- Tinea pedis is the most common cause of "id" reactions, a secondary immunological reaction to microbial antigens [19]. The two main types of hand id reactions to tinea pedis are:
  a. a vesicular form, symmetrical with multiple vesicles involving the palms, fingers and interdigital spaces; less commonly, papules and pustules may form at a later stage
  b. a scaly form, which is usually the end result of the vesicular phase, but may also arise as the primary reaction.

Tinea manuum

- Commonly palmar hyperkeratosis and scaling confined to the palmar creases (Figure 8.4).
- Variants include:

Classical variant showing palmar hyperkeratosis and scaling concentrated at the palmar creases.
Variant showing multiple crescentic exfoliating scales.

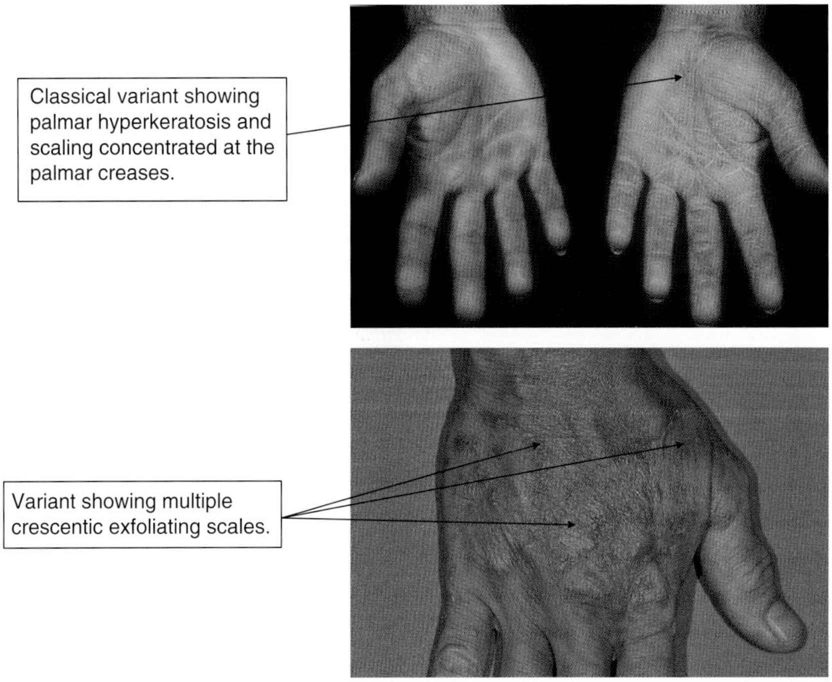

Figure 8.4 Tinea manuum.

a. crescentic exfoliating scales
b. discrete red papules and follicular scaly patches
c. erythematous scaly sheets on the dorsa of the hands – this particular variant is usually zoophilic [20].

- In one Spanish report, tinea manuum was unilateral in 61% of the cases, mostly affecting men (70%) between 11 and 40 years of age. The mean course of the disease was 2 years [21].
- A large survey of 280 patients with tinea manuum [22] classified their cases anatomically as:
  a. unilateral tinea manuum without tinea pedis (33/280 or 12%)
  b. bilateral tinea manuum without tinea pedis (11/280 or 4%)
  c. unilateral tinea manuum with bilateral tinea pedis ("two-foot-one-hand" syndrome) (182/280 or 65%)
  d. bilateral tinea manuum with bilateral tinea pedis (54/280 or 19%)
  e. 60% (169/280) were male.
  f. The mean age was 46 years.
  g. The mean duration of tinea manuum before presentation and diagnosis was 5.4 years.
  h. Altogether, 84% of patients with tinea manuum had associated tinea pedis.
  i. Of those with unilateral tinea manuum, 117/215 or 54.4% involved the right hand.
  j. 59% (165/280) were manual workers.
  k. 54% (152/280) had associated onychomycosis of the hands and/or feet.
  l. Of the cases with associated tinea pedis, 81% (188/232) gave a history of itching/scratching their feet.
- In a retrospective survey, 52/23 624 patients presenting for patch testing at St. John's Contact Dermatitis Clinic from 1982 to 1995 (i.e. approximately four patients per year in a mean yearly total of 1661 new patients assessed) were diagnosed clinically with tinea manuum, confirmed by mycology microscopy and culture. Of these patients:
  a. 90% (47/52) were male
  b. 81% (42/52) were manual workers, of which 39/42 (93%) were male
  c. the five most common occupations in the "tinea manuum" group were car mechanics, machine operators, gas/electricity workers, chemical process workers, and farm workers.
- In one survey, 3/34 subjects had associated tinea barbae [23].
- A unilateral bullous variant has been described [24].
- One case of disuse contracture of the hand from untreated tinea manuum has been described [25].
- Ross syndrome, a rare condition with a tonically dilated pupil which reacts slowly to light but more readily to accommodation, hypotonic reflexes, and segmental hypohidrosis, can have associated dry scaly skin mimicking tinea manuum on the affected palm.

Tinea corporis

- Site of infection typically on exposed skin, unless an extension from pre-existing infection (e.g. groin to buttocks and lower back) [20, 26].
- Lesions may be single or multiple – the latter may remain discrete or coalesce.
- Lesions are characteristically circular and usually sharply marginated with a raised edge. Clearance may occur centrally, but is often incomplete with scattered nodules remaining.
- Usually less inflammatory than tinea capitis and tinea barbae, as tinea-induced inflammation is roughly proportional to the degree of follicular involvement [20].
- In inflammatory lesions, vesicles and pustules may dominate.
- Pruritus is a common symptom.
- As tinea corporis can be zoophilic, ask regarding contact with cats, dogs, horses, cattle, rodents, and hedgehogs (Figure 8.5).
- Tinea corporis can be difficult to differentiate from nummular/discoid eczema. Both are oval or round and itchy, and can occur on the trunk or limbs (discoid being more common on the limbs). The edge in discoid eczema tends to be more vesicular and vivid in color than the edge in tinea corporis, where scaling is a more prominent feature [27]. Discoid eczema shows a variable, fluctuating or intermittent course and evolution, while tinea corporis progresses and spreads steadily until treated. Tinea corporis is usually not symmetrical (Figure 8.6).
- Tinea corporis variants include the following:
  a. Tinea corporis bullosa: tinea corporis may have vesicular and occasionally bullous lesions of up to 2 cm in diameter. This can be misdiagnosed as dermatitis herpetiformis, subcorneal pustulosis, linear IgA disease [28] and bullous pemphigoid [29].
  b. Animal-induced tinea corporis can be very inflamed, pustular, have multiple lesions or form a kerion.
  c. Tinea corporis gladiatorum: common amongst wrestlers. Tinea corporis gladiatorum presents as well-defined,

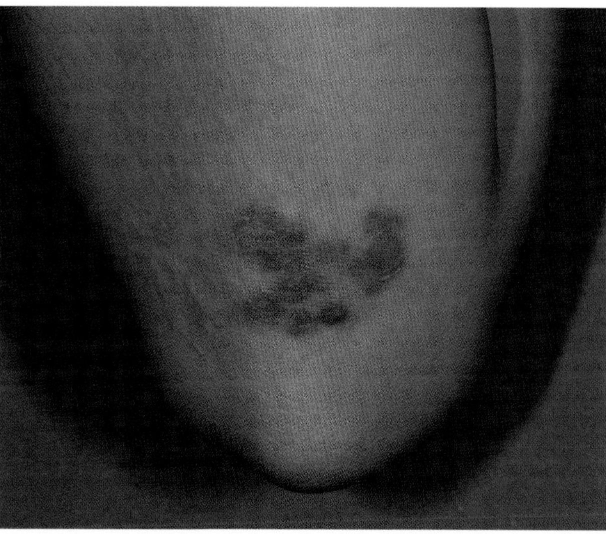

Figure 8.5 Dermatophytosis from a pet cat. Zoophilic dermatophytosis can be very inflamed, may contain pustules and vesicles and can progress rapidly.

Figurate erythema

Tinea corporis often has more prominent scaling of the edge compared to discoid eczema.

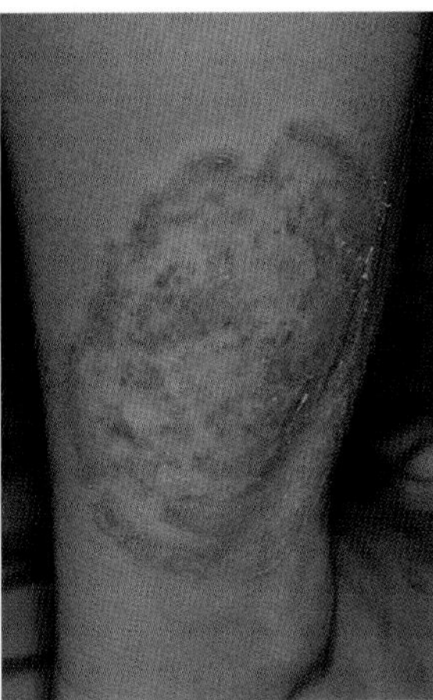

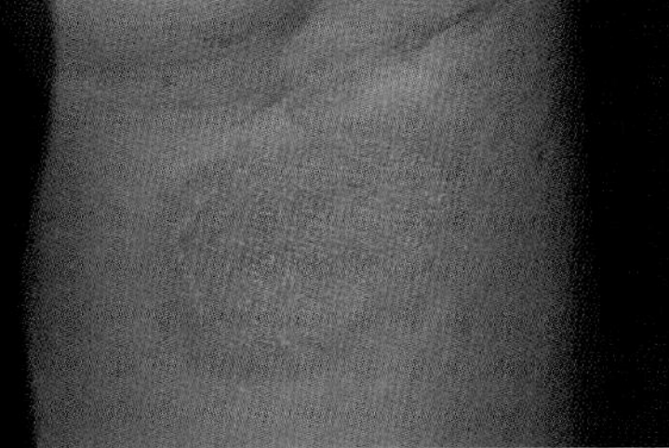

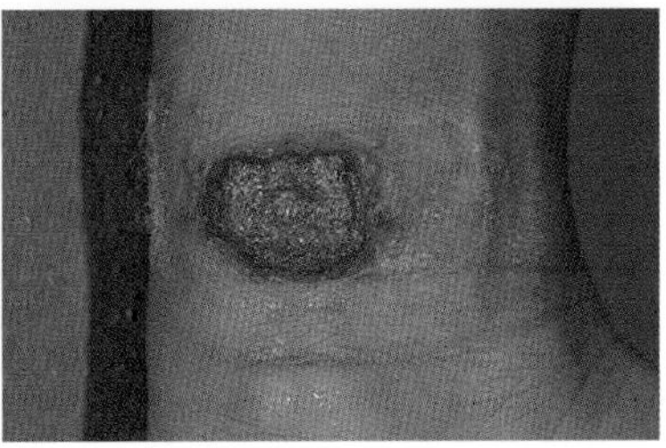

Discoid eczema: the edge often has a more vivid colour and vesiculation compared to tinea corporis.

Figure 8.6 Tinea corporis: the lesion shows an active border that expands gradually. Differential diagnoses include figurate erythema and nummular eczema.

Perifollicular papular form predominates, suggesting lack of immune suppression. Granuloma formation more common in immunocompromised hosts.

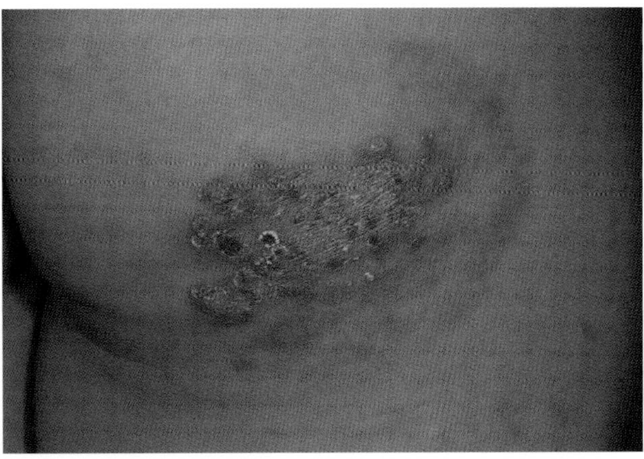

Figure 8.7 Majocchi granuloma on the buttock.

erythematous, and scaly papules and plaques. The annular appearance is not always seen in wrestlers and the lesions are typically found on the head, neck, and arms.

d. Tinea imbricata from *T. concentricum* found in the Pacific islands, Mexico, Southern Asia, and Brazil is characterized by annular lesions with multiple concentric rings.
e. Lichenified psoriasiform plaques on the lower leg caused by *T. rubrum* with perifollicular granulomatous papules of the Majocchi type [20] (Figure 8.7).

Tinea cruris

- During the early stages, the lesions are erythematous with curved lower borders extending from the groin to the thighs [20].
- There is marked pruritus.
- There is variable central clearing but this is usually incomplete with multiple nodules remaining.
- Satellite lesions tend to be few and large.
- Scrotal involvement is common but can be inconspicuous.
- At least one to two pustules can usually be visualized on careful examination.
- Common for tinea cruris to spread to the buttocks, lower back, and abdomen. Occasional spread to the penis can also occur.
- Tinea cruris is commonly associated with tinea pedis; possible transmission could occur when putting on underclothes.
- Tinea cruris can be mistaken for ACD to clothing dye or deodorant. If the clothing dye is from trousers, the inner and posterior thighs are commonly affected with sparing of the areas covered by the undergarment. If the undergarment contains the allergenic dye, the dermatitis then affects the areas of direct contact [30]. ACD to deodorants/feminine hygiene sprays often affects the genitalia and inguinal areas.

Tinea faciei (fungal infection of the non-hair bearing areas of the face)

- Has more atypical forms than tinea corporis [20, 31].
- Often starts as small flat macules that develop a raised border.
- Scaling present in fewer than two-thirds of patients.
- Papules, vesicles, and crusts are (only) sometimes present.

- Complaints of itching, burning, and worsening after sun exposure are common, and as many as half of the patients can be initially misdiagnosed as a photosensitive skin disorder.
- Animals are a common source of contact (zoophilic tinea faciei). The inflammation and induration can be severe (Figure 8.8).
- Periocular tinea is often initially diagnosed as eczema and treated with topical steroids. It is characterized by a diffusely erythematous periocular patch with only limited scale, marked upper eyelid swelling, distortion of the palpebral fissure, and extensive loss of eyelashes [32].

Tinea incognito (steroid modified tinea)

- Degree of alteration is greater with topical rather than oral steroids.
- A raised margin is absent or diminished [20] (Figure 8.9).
- There is reduced inflammation and scaling.
- Nodules (follicular invasion) may be observed.
- Bizarre multiple concentric rings of erythema can occur.
- Typical areas involved are the groin, lower legs, face, and hands.
- Perioral dermatitis with pustulation may occur.
- Periocular infection may resemble a stye.

Tinea from personal appliances

- Tinea can present under a wrist watch and mimic ACD to the watch metal. Clinical differentiation is possible. Tinea tends to start in one small area beneath the watch, then spreads gradually, and the final affected areas may not correspond exactly with the watch site. There is usually evidence of tinea elsewhere [33].
- A rash under a belt was misdiagnosed as ACD to the belt buckle. It transpired to be tinea spreading from the groin [34].
- Tinea on the chin arising from the shared use of a canoe helmet has been observed (McFadden, personal observation).

Scabies

- Characterized by severe chronic pruritus which is more pronounced at night [35, 36] (Figure 8.10).
- Burrows may be observed – these have a long serpiginous brown appearance, with scale at one end and (sometimes) vesicles at the other.
- Burrows are characteristically located on the interdigital spaces of the hand, wrist flexures, scrotum, vulva, penis, elbows, axillae, umbilicus, belt line, nipples, and buttocks.
- There is often a history of preceding travel, visitors staying at the home and/or other members of the family who are scratching.
- Secondary eczematization is common, either from the infestation or post-treatment (post-scabietic treatment dermatitis, often generalized).
- Variants of scabies are:

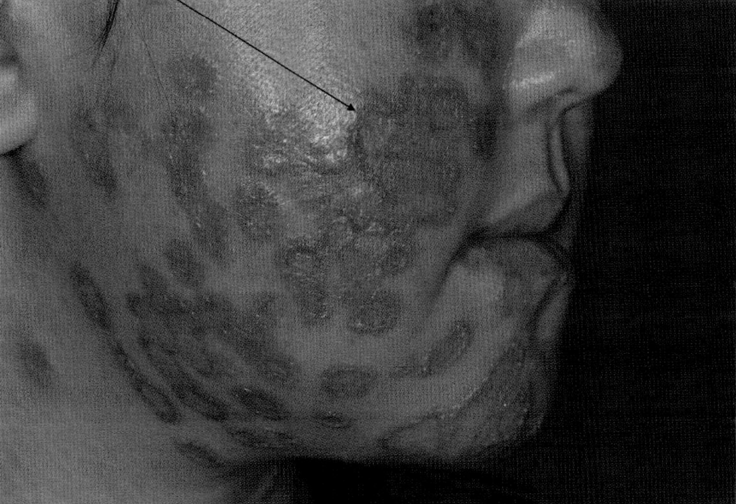

Polycyclic crusted erythematous plaques. Central areas become less scaly. Zoophilic tinea faciei (*Microsporum canis, Trichophyton verrucosum*) tends to present with more severe inflammatory reactions.
Photosensitivity can be a feature.
Multiple lesions can cover large areas.
Atypical features are more common compared to tinea involving other areas of the body.
70% of tinea faciei are initially misdiagnosed. Subsequent steroid treatment will lead to tinea incognito.

Figure 8.8 Zoophilic tinea faciei.

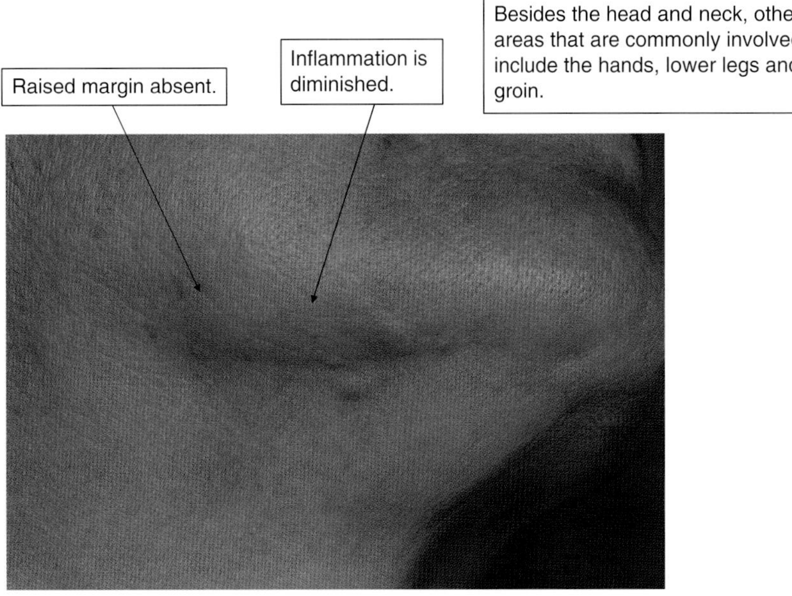

Raised margin absent.
Inflammation is diminished.
Besides the head and neck, other areas that are commonly involved include the hands, lower legs and groin.
Other clinical features can include nodules and multiple concentric rings.
The degree of alteration is usually greater with topical compared to oral steroid use.

Figure 8.9 Tinea incognito after topical corticosteroid application.

a. nodular scabies (7% of cases). This presents with extremely pruritic red-brown nodules 2–20 mm in diameter affecting the genitalia, buttocks, groin, and/or axillae
b. Norwegian scabies in elderly, demented, and immunocompromised individuals but sometimes in individuals with no obvious predisposition. Characteristically, there is a psoriasiform dermatitis affecting the acral areas, white scaling and periungual hyperkeratosis. It may also affect the scalp, neck, face and buttocks.

- A case of ACD to formaldehyde presenting as post-scabies discoid eczema has been reported. The formaldehyde was present in the permethrin cream used to treat the scabies [37].
- In an outbreak of 200 cases of follicular contact dermatitis to chemicals in permanent-pressed sheets, scabies was often considered in the patients' differential diagnosis [38].
- Steroid-modified scabies may lead to extensive lesions and the development of annular and vesiculopustular lesions. Scabies incognito has been reported to mimic dermatitis herpetiformis, urticaria pigmentosa [39], and subcorneal pustular dermatoses [40].

Mycoses fungoides

- During the early stages, mycosis fungoides (MF) often presents on the trunk/non-sun-exposed areas. The breasts and buttocks are in particular favored sites for initial development.
- Classical MF rarely first presents on the face or genitalia.
- Early lesions often show atrophy and scaling.
- One characteristic that may lead to a suspicion of MF is the presence of poikiloderma, especially in sun-protected areas.
- Associated pruritus is usually marked.
- Early stage MF variants include [41]:

a. inflammatory hypopigmented (usually located on non-exposed areas and can also be associated with erythematous lesions/plaques)
b. folliculotropic (with follicular rash, prurigo lesions, acneiform lesions and/or alopecia, especially on the head and neck) (Figure 8.11)
c. poikilodermatous
d. pagetoid reticulosis (solitary psoriasiform/lichenified plaque located on the hands or feet)
e. unilesional MF (single lesion covering less than 5% of the body surface area, usually on a classical site for MF)
f. granulomatous MF (nondescript plaques) and granulomatous slack skin (pendulous folds in flexural areas)
g. MF with ichthyosis (usually a fine scaling eruption resembling ichthyosis vulgaris with either involvement of the lower extremities or widespread involvement)

- As MF progresses, lesions become more obvious, with persistent erythematous plaques. The lesions may become very large, and arcuate or horseshoe-shaped lesions may be present due to areas of regression within individual lesions.
- A long period of chronic dermatitis can precede a diagnosis of MF.
- Fransway and Winklemann [42] reviewed four patients with clinical chronic dermatitis (5–9 years) preceding the diagnosis of MF. In three of the patients, ACD was thought to be the cause of the initial dermatitis. The contact allergens were nickel, chromate, and formaldehyde (editors' note – that ACD can rarely evolve into MF is a controversial view point).
- Pseudolymphomatous dermatitis is a rare form of presentation of ACD. Knackstedt and Zug [43] reviewed the 23 cases published in the literature (searched between 1946 and 2013). Of these:

(a)

A typical burrow is a thread-like scaly line, 3–10 mm long.

The scabies mite can be seen at one end of the burrow as a tiny black speck.

Scabietic burrows are usually found in/on these locations:
- finger webs
- palms
- flexor aspects of wrists
- inner elbows
- axillae
- umbilicus
- areolae (females)
- genitalia (males)
- buttocks
- instep region
- heel

In infants, lesions may be distributed on all body parts, e.g. plantar area of the foot.

(b)

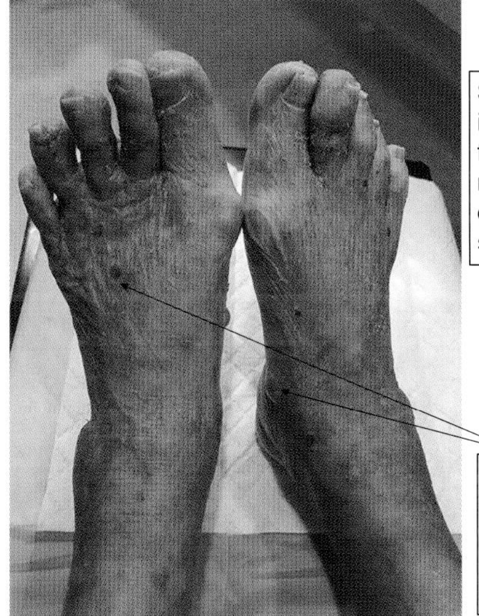

Scabies can present in various atypical forms: papulovesicular, nodular, bullous and crusted (Norwegian) scabies.

Multiple tense bullae and circular erosions post denudation of bullae in bullous scabies.

(c)

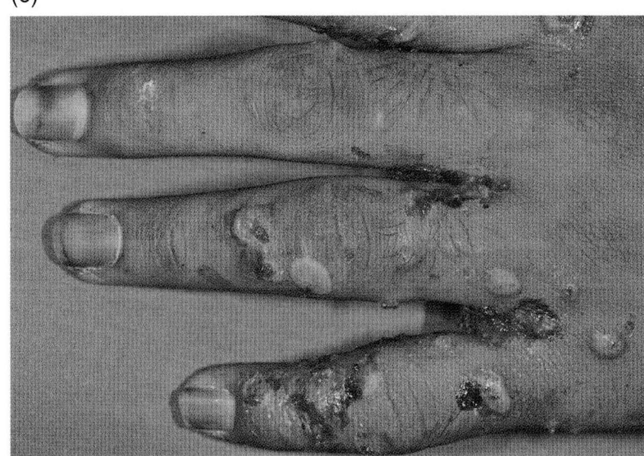

Clinical features of scabies can be obscured by impetiginization, eczematization or steroid treatment (incognito).

Figure 8.10 (a) Dermoscopic picture of a scabietic burrow on a patient's little toe. Courtesy of Dr Chia Chun Ang, Changi General Hospital, Singapore. (b) Bullous scabies. (c) Scabies' burrows masked by impetiginization.

a. 16 (70%) were males
b. the average age was 59 years (range 34–82 years)
c. the three most common areas involved were the thighs (nine cases, 39%), head and neck (nine cases, 39%), and buttocks (five cases, 22%). Many patients had more than one area of involvement or presented with a generalized rash without a distinct distribution.
d. strong patch test reactions were usually observed. The severity of the reactions was quantified in 18 cases: 5 were +++, 11 were ++ and 2 were +.

- The allergens that have been reported to be associated with pseudolymphomatous ACD include [43, 44]:

1. nickel (three cases) – metal frame of spectacles (1), metal necklace (1), gold plated necklace (1)
2. methylisothiazolinone (MI) and/or methylchloroisothiazolinone (MCI) (three cases) – moist wipes (2), airborne from wet paint (1)
3. azo/reactive dyes (three cases) – textile dye in blue overalls (1), elastic band of undergarment (1), trouser cloth (1)
4. gold (two cases) – earrings (2)
5. phosphorous sesquisulphide (two cases) – from "strike anywhere" matches, both direct contact (thigh from box in trouser pocket) and airborne (face) ACD

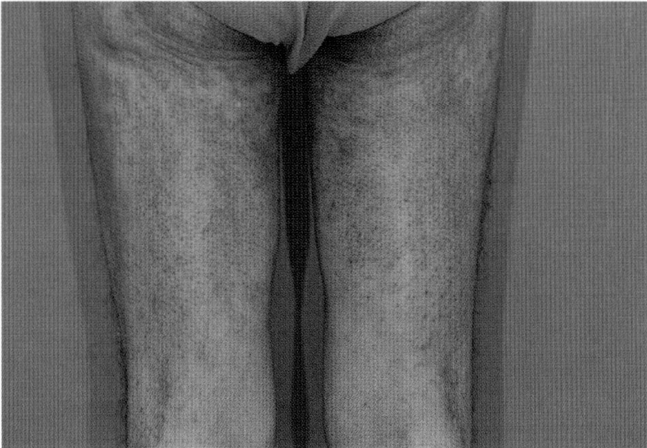

The clinical features of folliculotropic mycoses fungoides can include follicular rashes, prurigo lesions, acneiform lesions and/or alopecia, especially on the head and neck.

Figure 8.11 Folliculotropic mycosis fungoides mimicking follicular eczema.

6. isopropyl-*N*′-phenyl-*p*-phenylenediamine (IPPD) (black rubber) (two cases) – rubber chain on spectacles (1), rubber gloves and automated pedal cables (1)
7. cobalt naphthenate (one case) – marble finishing
8. *p*-phenylenediamine (one case) – black clothing, oil products
9. *p*-tertiary butyl phenol (PTBP) resin (one case) – leather case carrier
10. ethylenediamine dihydrochloride (one case) – kenalog® medicated cream
11. benzydamine hydrochloride (one case) – gynecological cleansing cream.

Eczematous drug reactions

- The most relevant drugs are those that give a systemic contact dermatitis reaction, and are, in at least some cases, a true form of systemic ACD (Figure 8.12). This has also been termed baboon syndrome and systemic drug-related intertriginous and flexural exanthema (SDRIFE).

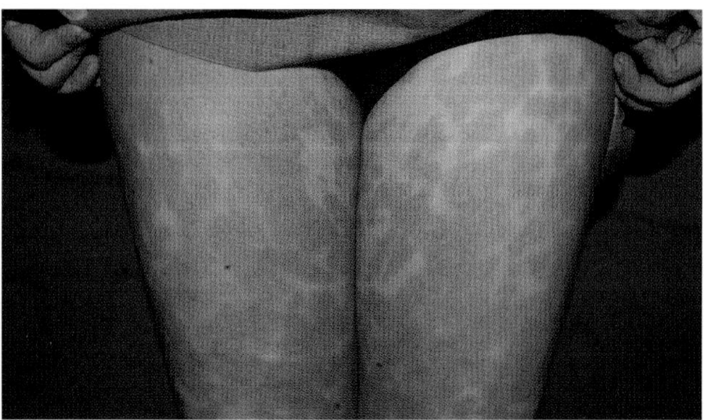

Figure 8.12 Exanthematous drug eruption: erythematous edematous plaques.

- Drugs known to cause SDRIFE [45–59]:
  a. multiple reports – amoxicillin/ampicillin, penicillin, cephalosporins (ceftriaxone, cefuroxime, cephalexin), mitomycin, clindamycin
  b. single reports – erythromycin, roxithromycin, allopurinol, barium sulfate, cimetidine, ranitidine, deflazacort, iv heparin, hydroxyurea, 5-fluorouracil, intravenous immunoglobulin (IVIG), naproxen, nystatin, oxycodone, ketoconazole, hydroxyzine, sulfamethoxazole-trimethoprim, metronidazole, rivastigmine, valacyclovir, telmisartan-hydrochlorothiazide, infliximab, zoledronic acid, paracetamol.
- An unusual case of Symmetrical drug-related intertriginous and flexural exanthema (SDRIFE) which included oral mucosal petechial lesions has been described [60].
- Miyahara et al. proposed reclassifying baboon syndrome/SDRIFE into four subcategories [61]:
  a. classical baboon syndrome caused by systemic (non-drug) ACD
  b. topical drug-induced baboon syndrome (ACD to drug)
  c. systemic drug-induced baboon syndrome (ACD to drug)
  d. SDRIFE – non-contact allergen drug-induced.
- Lichenoid drug reactions (e.g. β-blockers, ACE inhibitors, diuretics) and lichenoid contact dermatitis (e.g. from *p*-phenylenediamine) may be difficult to differentiate.
- An extensive exanthematous rash can be induced both by a reaction to systemic drugs (e.g. penicillin, phenytoin) and systemic chronic actinic dermatitis (CAD) to mercury [62].
- Photosensitive drug reactions (e.g. to amiodarone, tetracycline) may be confused with photocontact dermatitis and other photosensitive dermatoses.
- Pigmented purpuric skin reactions may occur secondary to oral drugs (e.g. carbromal, bromhexine) and as a presentation of ACD (e.g. to rubber).
- Erythroderma can be a presentation of both systemic drug reactions (e.g. acetylsalicylic acid, sulfasalazine, tetracyclines) and ACD (e.g. *Compositae*).

Rosacea

- The American National Rosacea Society Expert Committee developed a classification system for rosacea to help standardize diagnosis [63, 64]. They stated that the presence of one or more major criteria, i.e. flushing (transient erythema), non-transient erythema, papules and pustules, and telangiectasia, gave a diagnosis of rosacea. However, one could argue that other conditions can give, for example, non-transient erythema (psoriasis, Jessner's, lupus), flushing (over 100 different diagnoses can give flushing, e.g. hyperthyroidism), papules and pustules (e.g. acne vulgaris) and telangiectasia (e.g. systemic sclerosis, ataxia telangiectasia).
- The Committee also categorized four subtypes (though patients may have one or more subtypes):

Subtype 1 Erythematotelangiectatic rosacea: Non-transient episodes of flushing and persistent central facial erythema.

There may be erythema involving the peripheral face, ears, neck, and upper aspect of the chest, but periocular skin is usually spared.

Subtype 2 Papulopustular rosacea: In addition to the features of erythematotelangiectatic rosacea, patients experience transient papules and/or pustules in a central facial distribution. In severe cases, these episodes of inflammation can lead to facial edema.

Subtype 3 Phymatous rosacea: Characterized by thickened enlarged skin with irregular surface nodularities. This can occur in any sebaceous facial areas but the nose is the most common site to be affected. Males are more commonly affected.

Subtype 4 Ocular rosacea: Defined by the Committee as having one or more of the following signs/symptoms: watery or bloodshot appearance, foreign body sensation, burning or stinging, dryness, itching, light sensitivity, blurred vision, telangiectasia of the conjunctiva and lid margin, and lid or periocular edema. Other signs include blepharitis, conjunctivitis, and irregularity of the eyelid margin. The diagnosis is one of clinical judgment. Ocular involvement occurs in about 6–50% of patients with cutaneous rosacea and the degree of severity may be independent of the severity of cutaneous involvement. Over half of these patients will have cutaneous rosacea diagnosed first, but in 20% ocular disease is the first presentation.

- Of the diagnostic criteria listed, the presence of flushing, telangiectasia, ocular manifestations, and pustules may usually (but not always) help clinicians differentiate rosacea from ACD.
- Scaling and vesicles are usually absent in rosacea.
- Rosacea can coexist with seborrheic eczema (seborosacea), with the presence of signs from both conditions (e.g. seborrheic eczema also usually present on the scalp).
- Rosacea patients are susceptible to facial sensitive skin, i.e. irritancy and stinging from toiletries. In one study, 24/32 or 66% of rosacea patients (and all 7/7 patients with erythematotelangiectatic rosacea) reacted as "stingers" when 5% lactic acid was applied to their cheeks, compared to 6/32 (19%) healthy controls [65]. Rosacea skin is more readily irritated by sunscreens [66].
- Morbihan's disease is a rare complication of rosacea and is characterized by solid woody non-pitting edema on area(s) of the face, including the periorbital regions, forehead, glabella, nose, and cheeks. It may complicate any stage, early or late, of the disease. Patch testing is usually performed to exclude ACD [67].
- D'erme and Gola report a case of ACD to hydrocortisone-17-butyrate mimicking rosacea with a well-defined papular erythematous rash of the cheeks [68].
- Feser and Mahler [69] reviewed the causes of periocular dermatitis. Although ACD was the most common cause (54% of cases), periorbital rosacea was observed in 4.5% of cases. The presence of multiple periorbital papules and reports of stinging with cosmetics may help in the diagnosis of periocular rosacea.
- ACD to topical antibiotics used to treat rosacea can occur, such as metronidazole, erythromycin [70, 71], and aminoglycosides used to treat ocular rosacea [72]. ACD to arnica, which was being used to treat rosacea as a tincture, has been reported [73]. These may present as a "worsening" of rosacea.
- ACD to brimonidine tartate gel (used to treat the telangiectasia in rosacea) has been reported. This can present as classical ACD or apparent worsening of burning symptoms and erythema [74, 75].
- Rosacea patients were reported to have a significantly higher frequency of contact allergy to propolis compared to other patch test patients [76]. The authors speculated that this may be explained by self-therapy with propolis-containing herbal creams. An increased frequency of contact allergy to fragrance mix 1 and *Myroxylon pereirae* (both of which contain cinnamic chemicals) has been reported [72]. Oral consumption of cinnamon supplements has been reported to cause a flare of rosacea [77].

Lupus

Systemic lupus erythematosus

- In a study of a cohort of 1000 patients with systemic lupus erythematosus, the following cutaneous and oral signs at the onset of disease were observed (in decreasing order of frequency) (Figures 8.13 and 8.14) [78]:
  1. malar rash
  2. photosensitivity
  3. Raynaud's phenomenon
  4. oral ulcers
  5. discoid lesions

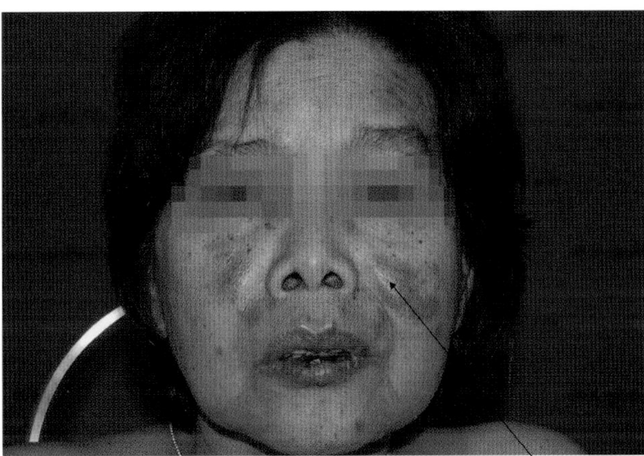

Other signs to look for include Raynaud's phenomenon, livedo reticularis, discoid lesions, oral ulcers, photosensitivity, nail fold erythema/ telangiectasia and nail changes.
The malar rash of lupus usually spares the nasolabial folds.

Figure 8.13 Systemic lupus erythematosus: malar rash, eyebrow, and lip involvement.

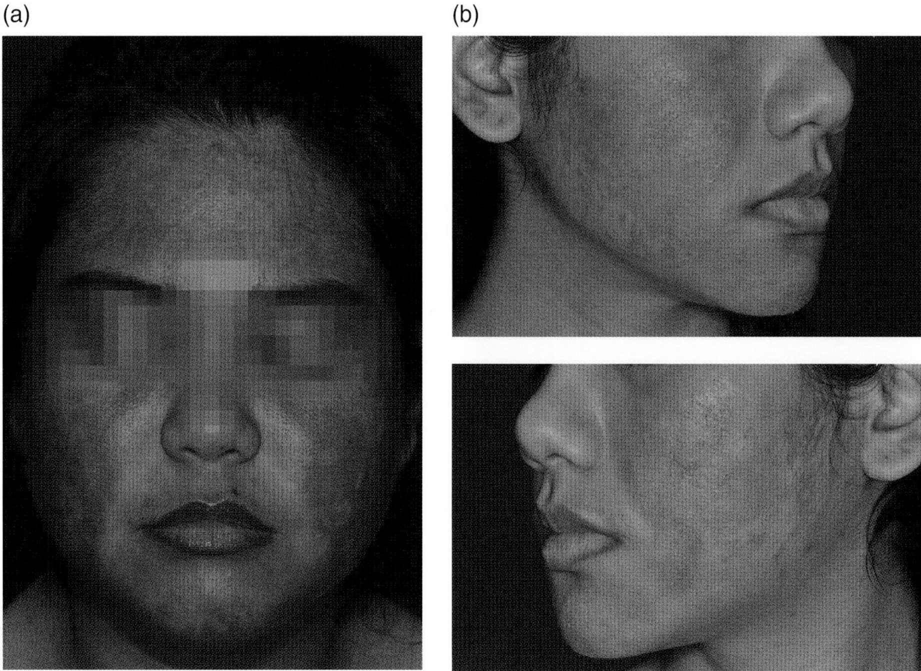

Figure 8.14 (a) Malar rash sparing the nasolabial folds in acute cutaneous lupus erythematosus. (b) Allergic contact dermatitis (parabens, methylisothiazolinones, fragrance) mimicking acute lupus erythematosus.

6. livedo reticularis
7. subacute cutaneous lesions.

Other common signs at presentation were arthritis fever, serositis, nephropathy, and neurological involvement (11%).

- The female/male ratio is 9/1.
- The classic butterfly/malar rash is characterized by erythema and edema and, occasionally, scale which involves the malar areas and the bridge of the nose but not the nasolabial folds (Figures 8.13 and 8.14).
- The lupus maculopapular rash occurs in 5–10% of patients with systemic lupus erythematosus (SLE) and consists of a generalized eruption of symmetrically distributed, small, confluent erythematous spots and papules with a purpuric component.
- The facial dermatoses may resemble contact dermatitis, seborrheic dermatitis (SD) or dermatomyositis.
- Chronic discoid lesions are present in 10%.
- Other cutaneous lesions reported in lupus include bullae, epidermal necrolysis, urticaria and urticarial-like lesions, reticulate telangiectatic lesions on the thenar and hypothenar eminences of the palms and to a lesser extent on the feet, erythromelalgia, hardening, and pigmentation of the skin and face resembling systemic sclerosis, calcinosis (rare), widespread purpura, pyoderma gangrenosum, gangrene, subacute nodules (5%) on the back of the proximal phalangeal joints and wrists, and coarse broken hair/alopecia [79].
- Nail changes may also occur, including hyperkeratotic and ragged nail cuticles, splinter hemorrhages, pitting, ridging, onycholysis, striate leukonychia, and red lunulae [79].
- Kosboth et al. reported a patient with known SLE who developed a rash mimicking the lupus malar rash. This was eventually found to be ACD to nickel in her spectacle frames [80].
- Sanchez-Perez et al. reported a 53-year-old woman who presented with erythematous plaques on the forehead and neck. A diagnosis of lupus was made and histology showed hydropic degeneration and positive immunoflourescence (IMF) with immunoglobulin M (IgM) and C3 deposits at the dermal-epidermal junction. However, the patient was patch test positive to prednicarbate, which she had used topically to treat her head and neck eczema. The patient had negative lupus serology and her rash resolved quickly with avoidance of prednicarbate and alternative treatment of the dermatitis. The diagnosis of ACD presenting with a lupus-like rash was made. The authors noted that this phenomenon had been (rarely) reported previously [81].

Subacute cutaneous lupus erythematosus

- The primary lesion is an erythematous papule/plaque covered with fine scales [82]. These lesions expand and merge in some patients and can mimic those of psoriasis vulgaris (papulosquamous type).
- In a third of patients polycyclic annular lesions are present.
- Vesiculation and crusting can occur at the active border, with pigmentation and telangectasia in the central area.
- The lesions usually occur on sun-exposed areas such as the hands, arms, upper chest, and back.
- There is a lack of scarring.

- Less common types include pityriasiform, vitiligo-like, exfoliative erythroderma-like, toxic epidermal necrolysis (TEN)-like, a variant with generalized poikiloderma, and an acral variant.
- A patient with known SCLE was patch tested as she was complaining of burning mouth. Although initial patch tests were not diagnostic, she returned at day 19 with lesions clinically consistent with SCLE at the patch test sites to spearmint and carvone. Biopsy was confirmatory of SCLE. Retesting showed identical reactions but avoidance of spearmint and carvone in her toothpaste did not lead to symptom resolution. The authors speculate that the patch test agents caused subclinical irritancy which promoted the development of new SCLE lesions at the patch test sites (koebnerization) [83].

Discoid lupus erythematosus

- 70% are localized (usually on the hand or head and neck) (Figure 8.15) [82].
- The lesions are usually annular, erythematous, and well-defined; adherent hyperkeratosis develops later, followed by scarring and atrophy.
- Pigmentary change with central hypopigmentation and peripheral hyperpigmentation is commonly seen, especially in dark-skinned patients.
- Periungual erythema and telangiectasia of the proximal nail folds are commonly seen.
- Guner et al. compared patch test results between patients with discoid lupus erythematosus (DLE) and dermatitis patients. They found that the DLE cohort had a significantly higher positive patch test rate, which was nearly twice that of control dermatitis patients (76% vs 40%). The most significant difference was for *p*-phenylenediamine hair dye (37.5% vs 12.5%). They postulated that ACD could in some cases trigger DLE as a Koebner phenomenon; however, an alternative explanation is that the current inflammation of DLE may promote ACD sensitization [84]. Van Aerde et al. document a case of a marked exacerbation of DLE after a severe hair dye reaction on the head and neck [85].

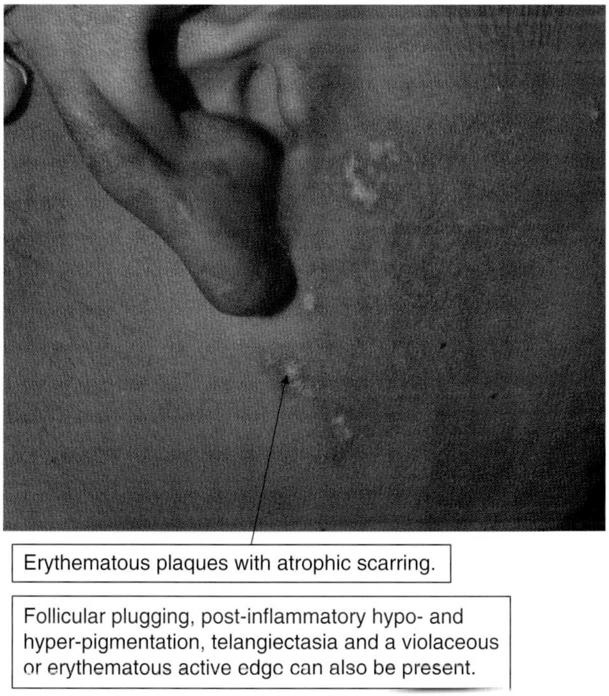

Erythematous plaques with atrophic scarring.
Follicular plugging, post-inflammatory hypo- and hyper-pigmentation, telangiectasia and a violaceous or erythematous active edge can also be present.

Figure 8.15 Discoid lupus erythematosus: erythematous plaque with atrophic scarring.

Sarcoidosis

- Sarcoidosis is known as one of the great imitators in dermatology.
- Cutaneous lesions occur in approximately a third of patients with sarcoidosis. Conversely, over 90% have some form of lung involvement, 20–30% will have eye involvement and 30–40% will have liver involvement. If sarcoidosis is suspected, a detailed clinical examination, chest x-ray (CXR), eye assessment, liver function tests, and blood ACE tests are mandatory.
- Skin signs can be divided into specific (with granulomatous histology) and non-specific (without granulomatous histology).
- Specific signs are:
  1. lupus pernio
  2. skin plaques: purple-red or brown, thickened, circular skin lesions
  3. maculopapular eruptions
  4. subcutaneous nodules (Darier–Roussy disease)
  5. infiltration (thickening) of old scars (scar sarcoidosis).
- Non-specific lesions include:
  a. erythema nodosum; often accompanied by arthritis affecting the ankles, elbows, wrists, and hands (Löfgren syndrome)
  b. nummular eczema
  c. erythema multiforme
  d. calcinosis cutis (deposition of calcium salts within the skin)
  e. pruritus (itch).
- Annular sarcoid lesions are formed by peripheral evolution and central clearing. The central area may become pigmented and scarred. These lesions occur on the back, buttocks, face, and extremities.
- Lupus pernio consists of violaceous nodules situated on the nose (loose symmetrical distribution).
- A woman developed a sarcoidal ACD to palladium after ear piercing [86].
- Two further patients had sarcoidal ACD after ear piercing. Patch testing demonstrated positive reactions to nickel, cobalt, and palladium, and histology demonstrated sarcoidal granulomatous inflammation [87].
- A study of a cohort of erythroderma patients found sarcoidosis to be an uncommon cause [88].
- Sarcoidal reactions to tattoos, such as green tattoos, have been reported [89].

Non-allergic dermatitis

Endogenous dermatitis

Atopic dermatitis

- There are two commonly used or recognized criteria for diagnosing atopic dermatitis (AD), which are usually used in research rather than in clinical practice. The UK working criteria are the best validated (see Table 8.1). Both criteria mention flexural involvement [90–92].
- Flexural inflammation is a key feature of AD (Figure 8.16). Small flexures may be involved as well as the well-recognized larger limb flexures (e.g. the flexural orbital folds and inferior fold between the ear and jawline). Involvement of the philtrum is a classical sign of AD.
- Dry skin is another key feature associated with AD. Poor skin barrier function, defective skin water retention, and increased susceptibility to irritants are common hallmarks.
- Onset is usually, but not always, in childhood. In a recent study the mean age of onset was 3.6 years [93].
- Amongst 100 AD patients, the frequencies of symptoms/signs were as follows [93]:

Xerosis	80%
Hand and foot dermatitis	80%
White dermographism	78%
Food intolerance	72%
Itch when sweating	70%
Anterior neck fold involvement	68%
Intolerance to wool	68%
Course influenced by emotional factors	66%
Tendency toward cutaneous infections	66%
Cheilitis	58%
Ichthyosis/keratosis pilaris	50%
Recurrent conjunctivitis	25%
Nipple eczema (Figure 8.17)	20%
Pityriasis alba	20%

- Associated disease symptoms [93] include:

Exacerbation during winter	70%
History of allergic rhinitis	42%
History of atopy (protein allergy)	36%
History of asthma	37%
Family history of AD	14%
Family history of asthma	43%

- Dennie–Morgan folds, hyperlinear palms, and thinning or absence of the lateral part of the eyebrows (Hertoghe's sign) are useful markers of AD [94].
- There is an association between ichthyosis vulgaris and AD, as both are associated with filaggrin gene deficiency.
- Unusual variants of AD include a nummular distribution associated with heavy Staphylococcal colonization or infection, follicular AD (also termed lichenoid pityriasiform dermatitis), and juvenile papular dermatosis, which is usually located on the knees and elbows and associated with seasonal pollinosis (spring and summer) [95]. A papular form of AD, often on the extensor aspects of the limbs, can occur, especially in African skin.
- AD patients are more prone to irritants. Therefore, hand eczema from ICD is more common in AD patients doing catering, nursing, building, and bar work, for example.
- Exposure to contact irritants and allergens in an occupational setting or from cosmetic use may re-exacerbate or cause a flare of quiescent AD (chemical atopy) [96].
- The association between AD and ACD has been reviewed by Thyssen et al. [97].
  1. There is a significant prevalence of contact sensitization amongst both children and adults with AD, therefore patch testing is a useful investigation.
  2. The prevalence of contact sensitization to some medicament agents (e.g. lanolin and corticosteroids) appears to be higher in patients with AD. Patients with AD should be patch tested to both standard series and, if available, medicament series.
  3. The prevalence of metal contact sensitization may be increased in patients with AD. This may be due to compromised chelation in the stratum corneum.
  4. False positive patch test rates to certain contact allergens, especially nickel, chrome, and cobalt, are higher in patients with AD (possibly due to xerotic skin).
  5. Experimental contact sensitization is marginally reduced in patients with AD.
  6. Patients with AD are immune stimulated by haptens/contact allergens through the Th2 immune pathway as opposed to the Th1 pathway in normal controls. This may explain the previous point as Th2 driven delayed cellular hypersensitivity is less efficient than Th1 systems. This may also explain the phenomenon of chemical atopy/re-exacerbation of AD by contact irritants and allergens (see 8).
  7. Increased exposure to immunomodulatory (hapten/irritant) chemicals at early stages of development may

Table 8.1 UK working party diagnostic criteria for eczema.

Itchy skin condition (required)	
Three of the following:	• Visible flexural eczema, e.g. antecubital and popliteal fossae (or visible dermatitis of the cheeks and extensor surfaces if under 18 months) • Personal history of dermatitis as above • Personal history of dry skin in the last 12 months • Personal history of asthma or allergic rhinitis (or history of eczema in a first-degree relative if <4 years old) • Onset of signs and symptoms under the age of 2 years (this criteria should not be used in children <4 years)

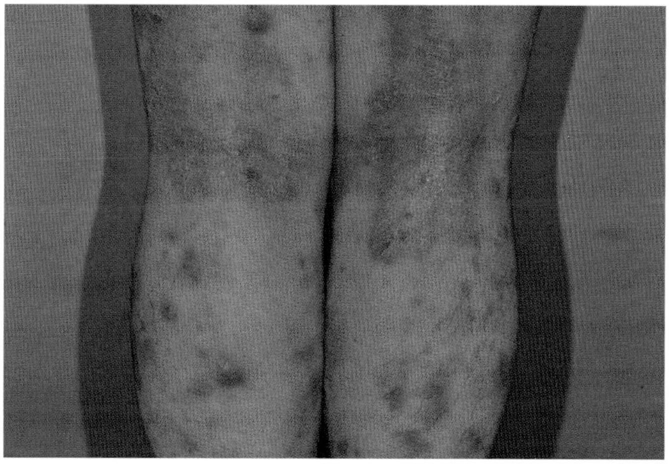

Figure 8.16 (a) Atopic dermatitis showing follicular and large flexural involvement. Both large and small flexures may be involved. (b) Flexural lichenified plaques in atopic dermatitis.

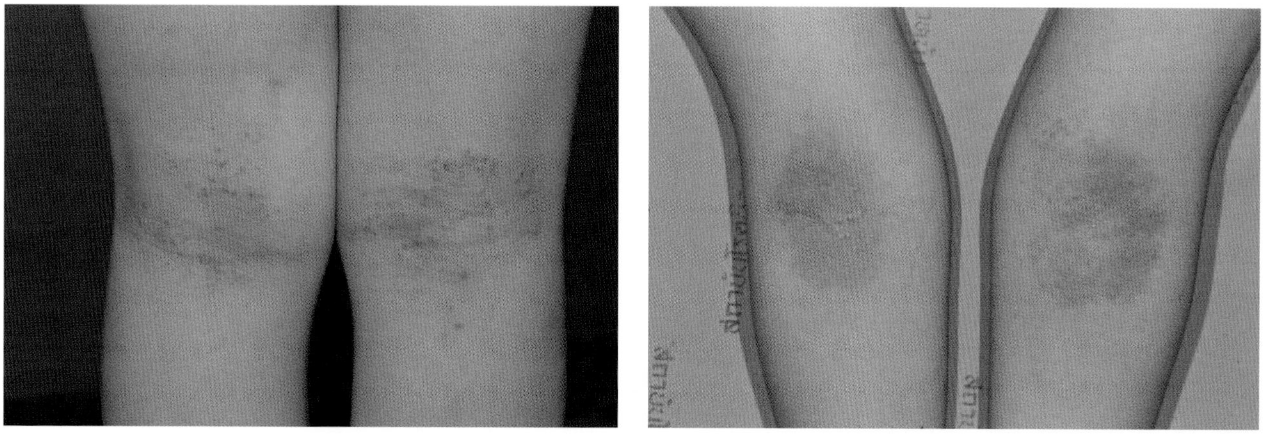

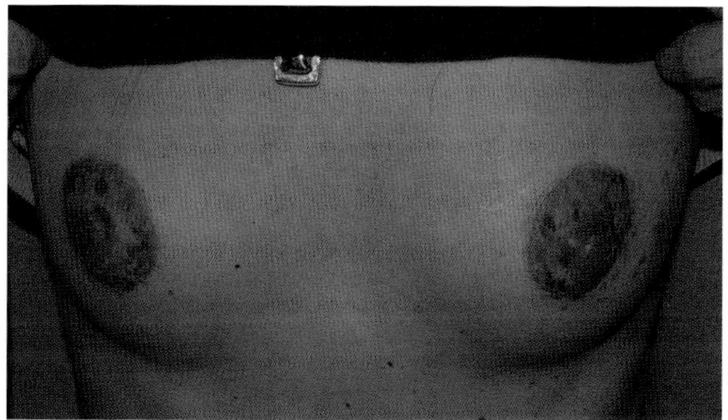

Figure 8.17 Chronic nipple eczema: nipple eczema is one of the minor criteria of Hanifin and Rajka for the diagnosis of atopic dermatitis.

predispose to the development of atopic disease and related atopic allergies.

8. Excessive and prolonged chemical exposure appears to cause a local re-flare and re-exacerbation of quiescent AD.
9. Patients with AD are predisposed to ICD.
10. The observed increased prevalence of some airborne haptens (plants and fragrances) in patients with AD remains unexplained.

Seborrheic dermatitis

- Infantile seborrheic dermatitis (SD) usually occurs within the first 3 months, most characteristically on the scalp with greasy yellow scale but can also involve the nappy area, face and folds such as the retroauricular regions, neck, inguinal and axillary areas. Infantile SD usually resolves by the end of the first year [98].
- In adult SD the lesions consist of macules/thin plaques with well-defined borders that may be pink, light yellow or erythematous, with fine, dry, moist or oily, white, or yellow scales [98].
- Variable degrees of pruritus.
- Areas typically involved in adult SD [98] are:
  a. the face (frequency of involvement 88%): glabella, malar region, nasolabial folds and eyebrows are commonly involved (Figure 8.18). Both blepharitis and beard area involvement can occur.

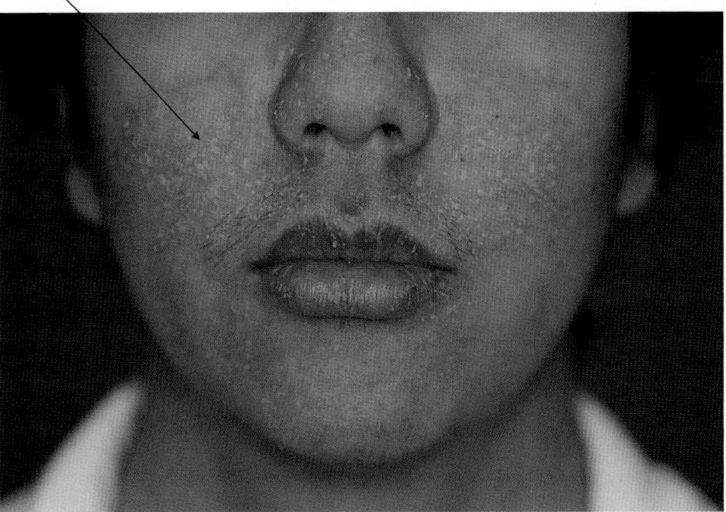

Well-demarcated areas on cheeks involving the nasolabial sulci; loosely symmetrical with greasy scale.
Other sites of involvement include the scalp, other hair-bearing areas, glabella, medial aspects of eyebrows, neck and upper trunk (annular areas), sternum, axilla and groin.
Facial seborrheic eczema may coexist with rosacea: 'seborosacea'.
Pruritus tends to be less marked than in allergic contact dermatitis or atopic dermatitis.
More common in patients with Parkinson's or untreated HIV

Figure 8.18 Seborrheic eczema involving the nasolabial folds and cheeks.

  b. scalp (70%): The severity ranges from mild dandruff/desquamation to thick crusted areas. Scalp SD is usually associated with evidence of SD elsewhere. It may also be associated with annular lesions on the neck and ear involvement.
  c. chest (27%): more scale and erythema, can be psoriasis-like
  d. lower limbs (2.3%)
  e. upper limbs (1.3%)
  f. other areas including flexures (5.5% but could be more): often erythematous rather than scaly, can be moist. Affects the axillary, inguinal, perianal and inframammary regions, as well as the umbilical folds.

- The reported prevalence of SD in human immunodeficiency virus (HIV) patients ranges from 32% to 85%. However, this high rate appears to have been reduced in patients on highly active antiretroviral therapy (HAART) therapy. SD may be a presenting manifestation. SD in HIV patients can be more inflamed and extensive, including the limbs.
- Ear involvement is common. Redness and greasy scaling can occur on the periauricular areas and both sides of the pinna. The posterior earfold may become fissured and can easily become secondarily infected [27].
- A well-characterized variant of ACD to *Parthenium* presents with a seborrheic pattern, with facial rash involving the malar and glabella areas [99]. Airborne ACD can mimic SD, e.g. nail varnish resin [100], methylisothiazolinone (J. McFadden, personal observation).
- Can overlap with psoriasis (see psoriasis section). Involvement of the facial seborrheic areas (eyebrows, glabella, malar region, and nasolabial folds), scalp, sternal area, and flexures. However, scaling, erythema, and induration are more pronounced in psoriasis, and it is less responsive to anti-seborrheic topical therapy. Classical plaque psoriasis (elbows, knees, and body) may or may not be present. SD can also overlap with rosacea (see section 8.1.6).
- 6.3% of 447 patients with eyelid dermatitis had SD overlap [101]. In another study, 11/203 eyelid patients had SD [102]. In a third study of 150 eyelid dermatitis patients, 4% were diagnosed with SD [103].
- Like AD, SD patients may also suffer from sensitive skin syndrome and report stinging on the application of some toiletries, as well as more easily irritated skin [104].
- SD can be complicated by medicament ACD.
  - Facial edema and erythema on the forehead, cheeks, and eyebrows, as well as pruritus 24 hours after applying ketoconazole cream and shampoo. Patch test showed ++ to ketoconazole [105].
  - Exacerbation of vulval dermatitis after application of canesten cream. Patch test showed + to clotrimazole [106].
  - Exacerbation of seborrheic dermatitis at the natal cleft region after application of dermovate NN®. Patch test showed + to nystatin 10% pet. [107].
  - Scrotal SD was treated with budesonide cream. After 3 weeks of initial improvement, the patient represented with extensive vesiculopapular dermatitis on the scrotum and inguinal areas. Patch test showed positive reactions to both the budesonide cream and ointment [108].

Discoid eczema

- Discoid eczema is characterized by acute or chronic morphological eczematous changes shaped as a coin-like plaque.
- Discoid eczema can be:
  a. an endogenous eczema, often associated with dry skin
  b. as part of a spreading AD, often heavily colonized/infected with *S. aureus*
  c. as a form of presentation of primary ACD
  d. as a form of secondary spread of ACD
  e. seborrheic eczema spreading from the scalp can take on an annular morphology, especially on the neck.
- Endogenous discoid eczema can have an acral pattern (hands/forearms/feet/ankles/shins/calves) or central/truncal distribution; the lesions can become secondarily infected.
- In one study, 50 subjects with discoid eczema were patch tested; 28 (56%) reacted to one or more allergens. Potassium dichromate was the most common allergen (20%), followed by nickel (16%), cobalt chloride, and fragrance (12% each). 17 patients (34%) had at least one clinically relevant positive patch test; of these 11 were followed-up at monthly intervals for 5 months and benefited substantially from avoidance of the offending allergens [109].
- In another study, 24/48 patients tested had positive patch tests. The most common were rubber chemicals (10.5%), formaldehyde (4%), neomycin (4%), chromate (4%), and nickel (4%). 13 of 16 patients were followed up by telephone in 1996, and 8113 (61%) stated that they had benefited from patch testing [110].

Varicose eczema

- Erythematous, scaly, and sometimes exudative dermatitis on the lower legs in association with venous hypertension/varicose eczema.
- There is a high incidence of ACD to support elasticated clothing (thiurams), dressings, and topical medicated agents. Most reports of ACD in varicose eczema are included in studies of ACD in leg ulcers.

Endogenous hand eczema

- Endogenous hand eczema can occur with or without foot dermatitis.
- Hand dermatitis is often multifactorial in nature, with frequently more than one element of endogenous, irritant, and ACD involved.
- Patients with a history of AD are more prone to occupational ICD [111].
- Irritant and ACD can re-exacerbate quiescent AD, both locally and distantly (chemical atopy) [96].
- The Danish Contact Dermatitis Group classified hand eczema and studied the frequency of each sub-group in a group of 710 patients with hand eczema [112]. These were:

Vesicular, infrequent eruptions	5.9%
Vesicular, frequent eruptions	31.8%
Dry, fissured	36.1%
Hyperkeratotic palmar	7.4%
Discoid	7.9%
Pulpitis	2.2%
Non-classifiable	8.8%
NB: dorsal interdigital dermatitis could be considered a further subgroup.	

- In the same study, they determined the frequency of ICD and ACD with the possibility of multifactorial elements in some patients:

Vesicular, infrequent eruptions	ICD 27.3%, ACD 24.2%
Vesicular, frequent eruptions	ICD 38.4%, ACD 35%
Dry fissured	ICD 44.3%, ACD 19.4%
Hyperkeratotic palmar	ICD 12.1%, ACD 9.8%
Discoid	ICD 40.9%. ACD 18.2%
Pulpitis	ICD 41.7%, ACD 16.7%

- Boonstra et al. studied the frequency of positive patch test reactions to the European Baseline Series in different subtypes of hand eczema. Of the subtypes, recurrent vesicular eczema had the highest number of patients with at least one contact allergen (52.2%). The frequencies for the other subtypes were: chronic fissured 50.3%, hyperkeratotic 35.3%, pulpitis 33.3%, interdigital 50%, discoid 42.9%, and non-classified 54% [113].
- The most common allergens in recurrent vesicular eczema were nickel (22.6%), MCI/MI (9.8%), cobalt (9.7%), and FM1 (6.7%).
- The most common contact allergens in chronic fissured eczema were nickel (16.5%), MCI/MI (10.4%), cobalt (6.3%), and FM1 (6.1%).
- The most common contact allergens in hyperkeratotic palmar eczema were nickel (12.6%), MCI/MI (6.7%), methyldibromoglutaronitrile (MDBGN) (5.9%), and chromate (5.0%).
- An "apron" pattern, with a semi-circular area of eczema encroaching onto the palm, is indicative of an endogenous component of eczema [114].

Miscellaneous other differential diagnoses

These include photodermatoses (Figure 8.19), vasculitis, connective tissue disease (Figure 8.20), circulatory disease, actinic damage/squamous/basal cell carcinomas (Figure 8.21), other skin infections (Figure 8.22), bullous diseases, other granulomatous disease, acneiform and neutrophilic dermatoses, and factitious disease.

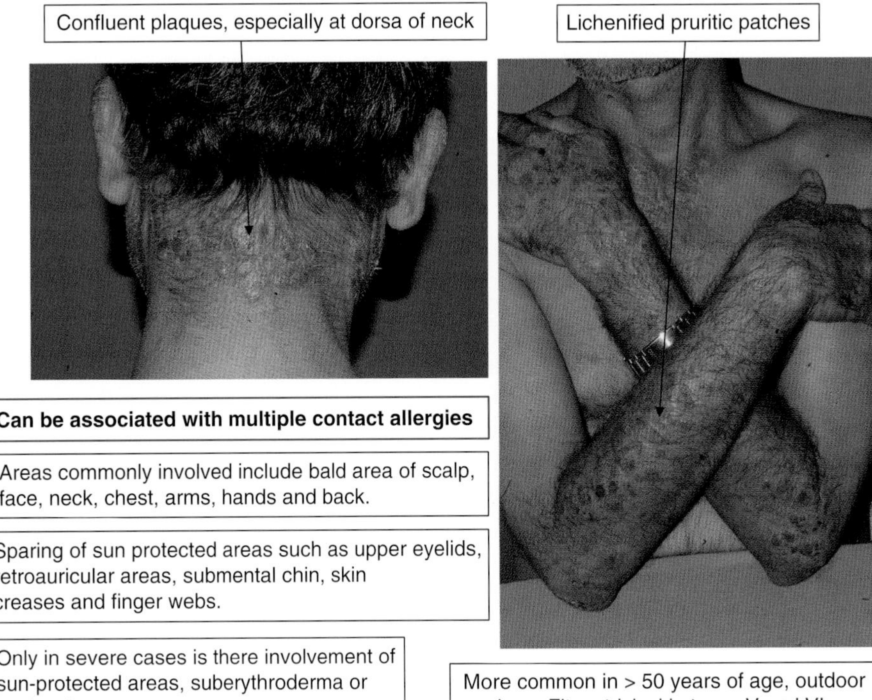

Confluent plaques, especially at dorsa of neck

Areas commonly involved include bald area of scalp, face, neck, chest, arms, hands and back.

Only in severe cases is there involvement of sun-protected areas, suberythroderma or erythroderma.
More common in > 50 years of age, outdoor workers, Fitzpatrick skin types V and VI.

Figure 8.19 Chronic actinic dermatitis on sun-exposed areas.

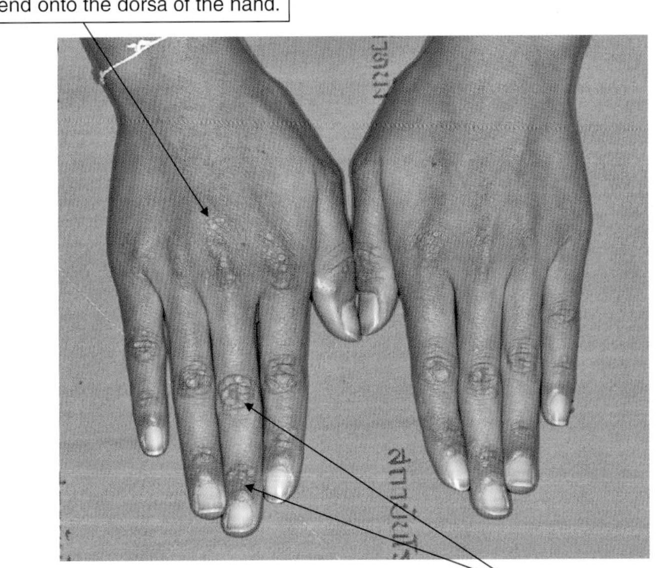

Can extend onto the dorsa of the hand.
Gottron's changes may be macular, papular, plaque or nodular.
As well as affecting the skin over the metacarpophalangeal joints, can also affect the skin over the proximal and distal interphalangeal joints.

Figure 8.20 Gottron's papules in dermatomyositis.

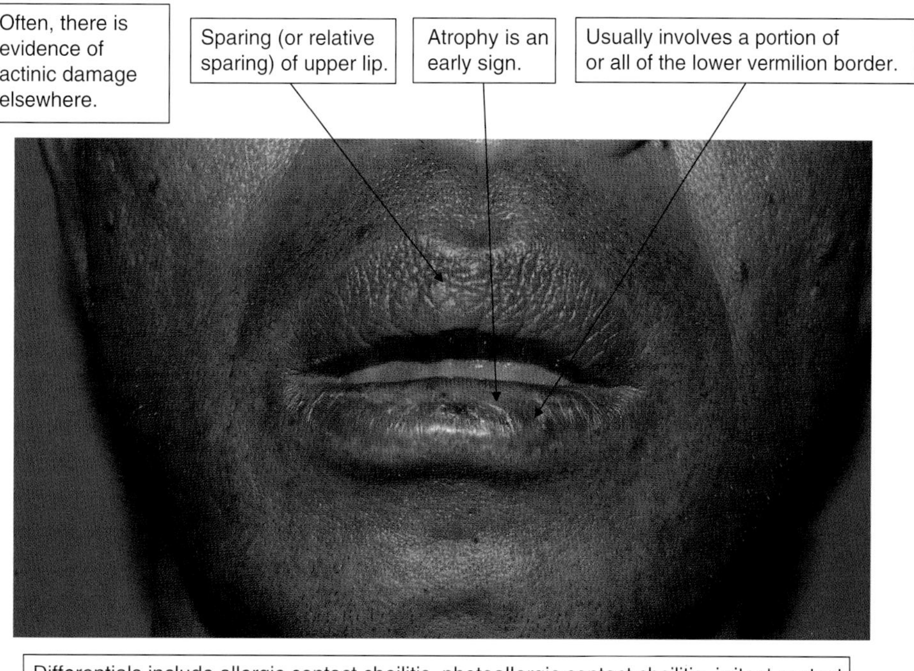

Often, there is evidence of actinic damage elsewhere.
Sparing (or relative sparing) of upper lip.
Atrophy is an early sign.
Usually involves a portion of or all of the lower vermilion border.
Differentials include allergic contact cheilitis, photoallergic contact cheilitis, irritant contact cheilitis, atopic cheilitis, actinic prurigo, lichen planus and discoid lupus.

Figure 8.21 Actinic cheilitis (premalignant): predominantly affects the lower lips.

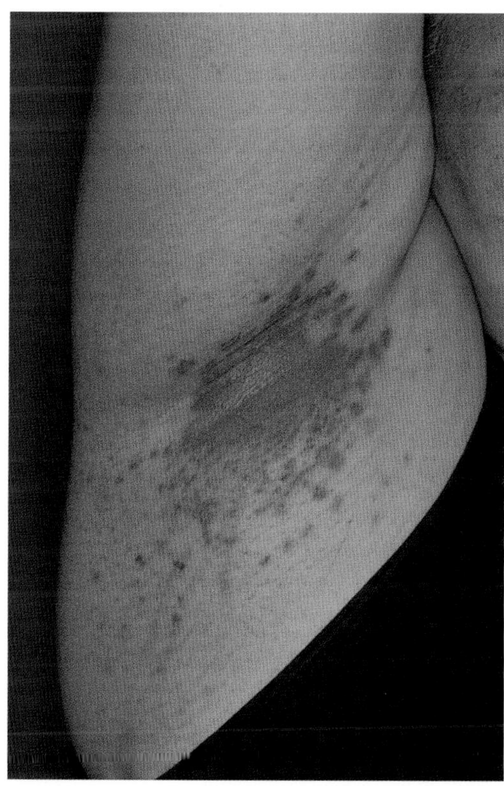

Figure 8.22 Candidal intertrigo showing characteristic satellite lesions.

References

1 Mahil, S.K., Capon, F., and Barker, J.N. (2015). Genetics of psoriasis. *Dermatologic Clinics* 33 (1): 1–11.

2 Naldi, L., Parazzini, F., Brevi, A. et al. (1992). Family history, smoking habits, alcohol consumption and risk of psoriasis. *British Journal of Dermatology* 127 (3): 212–217.

3 Morris, A., Rogers, M., Fischer, G., and Williams, K. (2001). Childhood psoriasis: a clinical review of 1262 cases. *Pediatric Dermatology* 18 (3): 188–198.

4 Kumar, B., Saraswat, A., and Kaur, I. (2002). Palmoplantar lesions in psoriasis: a study of 3065 patients. *Acta Dermato-Venereologica* 82 (3): 192–195.

5 O'Doherty, C.J. and MacIntyre, C. (1985). Palmoplantar pustulosis and smoking. *British Medical Journal* 291 (6499): 861–864.

6 Bangsgaard, N., Engkilde, K., Thyssen, J.P. et al. (2009). Inverse relationship between contact allergy and psoriasis: results from a patient- and a population-based study. *British Journal of Dermatology* 161 (5): 1119–1123.

7 Heule, F., Tahapary, G.J., Bello, C.R., and van Joost, T. (1998). Delayed-type hypersensitivity to contact allergens in psoriasis. A clinical evaluation. *Contact Dermatitis* 38 (2): 78–82.

8 Alwan, W., McFadden, J., White, I.R., and Banerjee, P. (2015). Patch testing in patients with psoriasis: results of a 30-year retrospective cohort study. *British Journal of Dermatology* 173 (Suppl. S1): 171–172.

9 Burden, A.D., Muston, H., and Beck, M.H. (1994). Intolerance and contact allergy to tar and dithranol in psoriasis. *Contact Dermatitis* 31 (3): 185–186.

10 Park, Y.K., Lee, J.H., and Chung, W.G. (2002). Allergic contact dermatitis from calcipotriol. *Acta Dermato-Venereologica* 82 (1): 71–72.
11 Takashima, A., Yamamoto, K., Kimura, S. et al. (1991). Allergic contact and photocontact dermatitis due to psoralens in patients with psoriasis treated with topical PUVA. *British Journal of Dermatology* 124 (1): 37–42.
12 Quaranta, M., Eyerich, S., Knapp, B. et al. (2014). Allergic contact dermatitis in psoriasis patients: typical, delayed, and non-interacting. *PLoS One* 9 (7): e101814.
13 Mestach, L. and Goossens, A. (2015). Allergic contact dermatitis and nail damage mimicking psoriasis caused by nail hardeners. *Contact Dermatitis* 74: 112–114.
14 Chang, M.W. and Nakrani, R. (2014). Six children with allergic contact dermatitis to methylisothiazolinone in wet wipes (baby wipes). *Pediatrics* 133 (2): e434–e438.
15 Ilkit, M. and Durdu, M. (2015). Tinea pedis: the etiology and global epidemiology of a common fungal infection. *Critical Reviews in Microbiology* 41 (3): 374–388.
16 Szepietowski, J.C., Reich, A., Garlowska, E. et al. (2006). Factors influencing coexistence of toenail onychomycosis with tinea pedis and other dermatomycoses: a survey of 2761 patients. *Archives of Dermatology* 142 (10): 1279–1284.
17 Geary, R.J. and Lucky, A.W. (1999). Tinea pedis in children presenting as unilateral inflammatory lesions of the sole. *Pediatric Dermatology* 16 (4): 255–258.
18 English, M.P. and Gibson, M.D. (1959). Studies in the epidemiology of tinea pedis. I. Tinea pedis in school children. *British Medical Journal* 1 (5135): 1442–1446.
19 Ilkit, M., Durdu, M., and Karakas, M. (2012). Cutaneous id reactions: a comprehensive review of clinical manifestations, epidemiology, etiology, and management. *Critical Reviews in Microbiology* 38 (3): 191–202.
20 Hay, R.,.M.M.K. (2004). *Mycology. Rook's Textbook of Dermatology*, 7e. Oxford: Blackwell.
21 Arenas, R. (1991). Tinea manuum. Epidemiological and mycological data on 366 cases. *Gaceta Médica de México* 127 (5): 435–438.
22 Zhan, P., Geng, C., Li, Z. et al. (2013). The epidemiology of tinea manuum in Nanchang area, South China. *Mycopathologia* 176 (1–2): 83–88.
23 Anonymous (1953). Tinea manuum. *Ulster Medical Journal* 22 (Suppl 1): 37.
24 Aste, N., Pau, M., and Aste, N. (2005). Tinea manuum bullosa. *Mycoses* 48 (1): 80–81.
25 Chapel, J. and Chapel, T.A. (1985). Disuse contractures in a patient with tinea manuum and irritant contact dermatitis. *Cutis* 36 (1): 55.
26 Gupta, A.K., Chaudhry, M., and Elewski, B. (2003). Tinea corporis, tinea cruris, tinea nigra, and piedra. *Dermatologic Clinics* 21 (3): 395–400, v.
27 Holden, C. and Berth-Jones, J. (2004). Eczema, lichenification, prurigo and erythroderma. In: *Rook's Textbook of Dermatology*. Oxford: Blackwell Chapter 17: 699–751.
28 Aalfs, A.S. and Jonkman, M.F. (2012). Tinea corporis bullosa due to *Microsporum canis* mimicking linear IgA bullous dermatosis. *European Journal of Dermatology* 22 (6): 805–806.
29 Terragni, L., Marelli, M.A., Oriani, A., and Cecca, E. (1993). Tinea corporis bullosa. *Mycoses* 36 (3–4): 135–137.
30 Cronin, E. (1980). Clothing and textiles. In: *Contact Dermatitis*, 36–92. Edinburgh: Churchill Livingstone.
31 Lin, R.L., Szepietowski, J.C., and Schwartz, R.A. (2004). Tinea faciei, an often deceptive facial eruption. *International Journal of Dermatology* 43 (6): 437–440.
32 Basak, S.A., Berk, D.R., Lueder, G.T., and Bayliss, S.J. (2011). Common features of periocular tinea. *Archives of Ophthalmology* 129 (3): 306–309.
33 Anonymous (1968). Wrist-watch tinea. *British Medical Journal* 1 (5590): 464.
34 Usatine, R. (2001). A belt buckle allergy? *Western Journal of Medicine* 174 (5): 307–308.
35 Hengge, U.R., Currie, B.J., Jager, G. et al. (2006). Scabies: a ubiquitous neglected skin disease. *The Lancet Infectious Diseases* 6 (12): 769–779.
36 Orkin, M. (1975). Today's scabies. *Journal of the American Medical Association* 233 (8): 882–885.
37 Kaminska, R. and Mortenhumer, M. (2003). Nummular allergic contact dermatitis after scabies treatment. *Contact Dermatitis* 48 (6): 337.
38 Panaccio, F., Montgomery, D.C., and Adam, J.E. (1973). Follicular contact dermatitis due to coloured permanent-pressed sheets. *Canadian Medical Association Journal* 109 (1): 23–26.
39 Kim, K.J., Roh, K.H., Choi, J.H. et al. (2002). Scabies incognito presenting as urticaria pigmentosa in an infant. *Pediatric Dermatology* 19 (5): 409–411.
40 Karaca, S., Kelekci, K.H., Er, O. et al. (2015). Scabies incognito presenting as a subcorneal pustular dermatosis-like eruption. *Turkiye parazitolojii dergisi/Turkiye Parazitoloji Dernegi = Acta parasitologica Turcica/Turkish Society for Parasitology.* 39 (3): 244–247.
41 Cho-Vega, J.H., Tschen, J.A., Duvic, M., and Vega, F. (2010). Early-stage mycosis fungoides variants: case-based review. *Annals of Diagnostic Pathology* 14 (5): 369–385.
42 Fransway, A.F. and Winkelmann, R.K. (1988). Chronic dermatitis evolving to mycosis fungoides: report of four cases and review of the literature. *Cutis* 41 (5): 330–335.
43 Knackstedt, T.J. and Zug, K.A. (2015). T cell lymphomatoid contact dermatitis: a challenging case and review of the literature. *Contact Dermatitis* 72 (2): 65–74.
44 Van Steenkiste, E., Goossens, A., Meert, H. et al. (2015). Airborne-induced lymphomatoid contact dermatitis caused by methylisothiazolinone. *Contact Dermatitis* 72 (4): 237–240.
45 Hausermann, P., Harr, T., and Bircher, A.J. (2004). Baboon syndrome resulting from systemic drugs: is there strife between SDRIFE and allergic contact dermatitis syndrome? *Contact Dermatitis* 51 (5–6): 297–310.
46 Morales-Cabeza, C., Caralli Bonett, M.E., Micozzi, S. et al. (2015). SDRIFE-like reaction induced by an intradermal skin test with clindamycin: a case report. *Journal of Allergy and Clinical Immunology: In Practice* 3 (6): 976–977.
47 Bulur, I., Keseroglu, H.O., Saracoglu, Z.N., and Gonul, M. (2015). Symmetrical drug-related intertriginous and flexural exanthema (baboon syndrome) associated with infliximab. *Journal of Dermatological Case Reports* 9 (1): 12–14.
48 Binitha, M.P., Sasidharanpillai, S., John, R., and Sherjeena, P.V. (2014). Symmetrical drug-related intertriginous and flexural exanthema due to ranitidine. *Indian Journal of Pharmacology* 46 (5): 551–552.
49 Sikar Akturk, A., Bayramgurler, D., Salman, S. et al. (2014). Symmetrical drug-related intertriginous and flexural exanthema (SDRIFE) induced by oral metronidazole. *Cutaneous and Ocular Toxicology* 33 (4): 337–338.

50 Gulec, A.I., Uslu, E., Baskan, E. et al. (2014). Baboon syndrome induced by ketoconazole. *Cutaneous and Ocular Toxicology* 33 (4): 339–341.

51 Lugovic-Mihic, L., Duvancic, T., Vucic, M. et al. (2013). SDRIFE (baboon syndrome) due to paracetamol: case report. *Acta Dermatovenerologica Croatica* 21 (2): 113–117.

52 Akkari, H., Belhadjali, H., Youssef, M. et al. (2013). Baboon syndrome induced by hydroxyzine. *Indian Journal of Dermatology* 58 (3): 244.

53 Culav, I., Ljubojevic, S., and Buzina, D.S. (2013). Baboon syndrome/SDRIFE due to sulfamethoxazole-trimethoprim. *International Journal of Dermatology* 52 (9): 1159–1160.

54 Powers, R., Gordon, R., Roberts, K., and Kovach, R. (2012). Symmetrical drug-related intertriginous and flexural exanthema secondary to topical 5-fluorouracil. *Cutis* 89 (5): 225–228.

55 Allain-Veyrac, G., Lebreton, A., Collonnier, C., and Jolliet, P. (2011). First case of symmetric drug-related intertriginous and flexural exanthema (SDRIFE) due to rivastigmine? *American Journal of Clinical Dermatology* 12 (3): 210–213.

56 Ferreira, O., Mota, A., Morais, P. et al. (2010). Symmetrical drug-related intertriginous and flexural exanthema (SDRIFE) induced by telmisartan-hydrochlorothiazide. *Cutaneous and Ocular Toxicology* 29 (4): 293–295.

57 Daito, J., Hanada, K., Katoh, N. et al. (2009). Symmetrical drug-related intertriginous and flexural exanthema caused by valacyclovir. *Dermatology* 218 (1): 60–62.

58 Handisurya, A., Stingl, G., and Wohrl, S. (2009). SDRIFE (baboon syndrome) induced by penicillin. *Clinical and Experimental Dermatology* 34 (3): 355–357.

59 Cohen, P.R. (2015). Zoledronic acid-associated symmetrical drug-related intertriginous and flexural exanthema (SDRIFE): report of baboon syndrome in a woman with recurrent metastatic breast cancer after receiving zoledronic acid. *Dermatology Online Journal* 21 (8): ii.

60 Karadag, A.S., Ozlu, E., Akdeniz, N. et al. (2015). Oral mucosal involvement and petechial lesions: a SDRIFE case with unusual findings. *Cutaneous and Ocular Toxicology* 35: 157–159.

61 Miyahara, A., Kawashima, H., Okubo, Y., and Hoshika, A. (2011). A new proposal for a clinical-oriented subclassification of baboon syndrome and a review of baboon syndrome. *Asian Pacific Journal of Allergy and Immunology* 29 (2): 150–160.

62 Lerch, M. and Bircher, A.J. (2004). Systemically induced allergic exanthem from mercury. *Contact Dermatitis* 50 (6): 349–353.

63 Wilkin, J., Dahl, M., Detmar, M. et al. (2002). Standard classification of rosacea: report of the National Rosacea Society Expert Committee on the classification and staging of rosacea. *Journal of the American Academy of Dermatology* 46 (4): 584–587.

64 Two, A.M., Wu, W., Gallo, R.L., and Hata, T.R. (2015). Rosacea: Part I. Introduction, categorization, histology, pathogenesis, and risk factors. *Journal of the American Academy of Dermatology* 72 (5): 749–758; quiz 59–60.

65 Lonne-Rahm, S.B., Fischer, T., and Berg, M. (1999). Stinging and rosacea. *Acta Dermato-Venereologica* 79 (6): 460–461.

66 Nichols, K., Desai, N., and Lebwohl, M.G. (1998). Effective sunscreen ingredients and cutaneous irritation in patients with rosacea. *Cutis* 61 (6): 344–346.

67 Hu, S.W., Robinson, M., Meehan, S.A., and Cohen, D.E. (2012). Morbihan disease. *Dermatology Online Journal* 18 (12): 27.

68 D'Erme, A.M. and Gola, M. (2012). Allergic contact dermatitis induced by topical hydrocortisone-17-butyrate mimicking papular rosacea. *Dermatitis: Contact, Atopic, Occupational, Drug* 23 (2): 95–96.

69 Feser, A. and Mahler, V. (2010 Mar). Periorbital dermatitis: causes, differential diagnoses and therapy. *Journal der Deutschen Dermatologischen Gesellschaft* 8 (3): 159–166.

70 Valsecchi, R., Pansera, B., and Reseghetti, A. (1996). Contact allergy to erythromycin. *Contact Dermatitis* 34 (6): 428.

71 Madsen, J.T., Thormann, J., Kerre, S. et al. (2007). Allergic contact dermatitis to topical metronidazole – 3 cases. *Contact Dermatitis* 56 (6): 364–366.

72 Jappe, U., Schafer, T., Schnuch, A., and Uter, W. (2008). Contact allergy in patients with rosacea: a clinic-based, prospective epidemiological study. *Journal of the European Academy of Dermatology and Venereology* 22 (10): 1208–1214.

73 Hormann, H.P. and Korting, H.C. (1995). Allergie acute contact dermatitis due to arnica tincture self-medication. *Phytomedicine* 1 (4): 315–317.

74 Rajagopalan, A. and Rajagopalan, B. (2015). Allergic contact dermatitis to topical brimonidine. *Australasian Journal of Dermatology* 56 (3): 235.

75 Swanson, L.A. and Warshaw, E.M. (2014). Allergic contact dermatitis to topical brimonidine tartrate gel 0.33% for treatment of rosacea. *Journal of the American Academy of Dermatology* 71 (4): 832–833.

76 Jappe, U., Schnuch, A., and Uter, W. (2005). Rosacea and contact allergy to cosmetics and topical medicaments–retrospective analysis of multicentre surveillance data 1995–2002. *Contact Dermatitis* 52 (2): 96–101.

77 Campbell, T.M., Neems, R., and Moore, J. (2008). Severe exacerbation of rosacea induced by cinnamon supplements. *Journal of Drugs in Dermatology* 7 (6): 586–587.

78 Cervera, R., Khamashta, M.A., Font, J. et al. (1993). Systemic lupus erythematosus: clinical and immunologic patterns of disease expression in a cohort of 1,000 patients. The European Working Party on Systemic Lupus Erythematosus. *Medicine* 72 (2): 113–124.

79 Rowell, N.R. and Goodfield, M. (1998). The connective tissue diseases. In: *Rook's Textbook of Dermatology*, 8e (eds. R.H. Champion, J.L. Burton, D.A. Burns and S. Breathnach), 2437–2577. Blackwell.

80 Kosboth, M., Chin-Loy, A., Lyons, R. et al. (2007). Malar rash caused by metal allergy in a patient with systemic lupus erythematosus. *Nature Clinical Practice Rheumatology* 3 (4): 240–245.

81 Sanchez-Perez, J., Gala, S.P., Jimenez, Y.D. et al. (2006). Allergic contact dermatitis to prednicarbate presenting as lupus erythematosus. *Contact Dermatitis* 55 (4): 247–249.

82 Fabbri, P., Cardinali, C., Giomi, B., and Caproni, M. (2003). Cutaneous lupus erythematosus: diagnosis and management. *American Journal of Clinical Dermatology* 4 (7): 449–465.

83 Deleuran, M., Clemmensen, O., and Andersen, K.E. (2000). Contact lupus erythematosus. *Contact Dermatitis* 43 (3): 169–170.

84 Guner, E., Kalkan, G., Meral, E., and Baykir, M. (2013). The triggering role of allergic contact dermatitis in discoid lupus erythematosus. *Cutaneous and Ocular Toxicology* 32 (3): 194–199.

85 Van Aerde, E., Kerre, S., and Goossens, A. (2016). Discoid lupus triggered by allergic contact dermatitis caused by a hair dye. *Contact Dermatitis* 74 (1): 61–64.

86 Blum, R., Baum, H.P., Ponnighaus, M., and Kowalzick, L. (2003). Sarcoidal allergic contact dermatitis due to palladium following ear piercing. *Der Hautarzt; Zeitschrift fur Dermatologie, Venerologie, und verwandte Gebiete*. 54 (2): 160–162.

87 Casper, C., Groth, W., and Hunzelmann, N. (2004). Sarcoidal-type allergic contact granuloma: a rare complication of ear piercing. *American Journal of Dermatopathology* 26 (1): 59–62.
88 Yuan, X.Y., Guo, J.Y., Dang, Y.P. et al. (2010). Erythroderma: a clinical-etiological study of 82 cases. *European Journal of Dermatology* 20 (3): 373–377.
89 Kremser, M. (1987). Sarcoid granuloma in green tattooing. *Wiener Klinische Wochenschrift* 99 (1): 14–18.
90 Williams, H.C., Burney, P.G., Pembroke, A.C., and Hay, R.J. (1996). Validation of the UK diagnostic criteria for atopic dermatitis in a population setting. UK Diagnostic Criteria for Atopic Dermatitis Working Party. *British Journal of Dermatology* 135 (1): 12–17.
91 Johnke, H., Vach, W., Norberg, L.A. et al. (2005). A comparison between criteria for diagnosing atopic eczema in infants. *British Journal of Dermatology* 153 (2): 352–358.
92 Hanifin, J. and Rajka, G. (1980). Diagnostic features of atopic dermatitis. *Acta Dermato-Venereologica* 92 (suppl): 44–47.
93 Sehgal, V.N., Srivastava, G., Aggarwal, A.K. et al. (2015). Atopic dermatitis: a cross-sectional (descriptive) study of 100 cases. *Indian Journal of Dermatology* 60 (5): 519.
94 Weidinger, S. and Novak, N. (2016). Atopic dermatitis. *Lancet* 12(387): 1109–1122.
95 Deleuran, M. and Vestergaard, C. (2014). Clinical heterogeneity and differential diagnosis of atopic dermatitis. *The British Journal of Dermatology* 170 (Suppl 1): 2–6.
96 Puangpet, P., Lai-Cheong, J., and McFadden, J.P. (2013). Chemical atopy. *Contact Dermatitis* 68 (4): 208–213.
97 Thyssen, J.P., McFadden, J.P., and Kimber, I. (2014). The multiple factors affecting the association between atopic dermatitis and contact sensitization. *Allergy.* 69 (1): 28–36.
98 Sampaio, A.L., Mameri, A.C., Vargas, T.J. et al. (2011). Seborrheic dermatitis. *Anais Brasileiros de Dermatologia* 86 (6): 1061–1071; quiz 72–4.
99 Sharma, V.K. and Sethuraman, G. (2007). Parthenium dermatitis. *Dermatitis: Contact, Atopic, Occupational, Drug* 18 (4): 183–190.
100 Pongpairoj, K., Morar, N., and McFadden, J.P. (2016). 'Seborrheic dermatitis' of the head and neck without scalp involvement – remember nail varnish allergy. *Contact Dermatitis* 74 (5): 306–307.
101 Ayala, F., Fabbrocini, G., Bacchilega, R. et al. (2003). Eyelid dermatitis: an evaluation of 447 patients. *American Journal of Contact Dermatitis* 14 (2): 69–74.
102 Guin, J.D. (2002). Eyelid dermatitis: experience in 203 cases. *Journal of the American Academy of Dermatology* 47 (5): 755–765.
103 Valsecchi, R., Imberti, G., Martino, D., and Cainelli, T. (1992). Eyelid dermatitis: an evaluation of 150 patients. *Contact Dermatitis* 27 (3): 143–147.
104 Cowley, N.C. and Farr, P.M. (1992). A dose-response study of irritant reactions to sodium lauryl sulphate in patients with seborrheic dermatitis and atopic eczema. *Acta Dermato-Venereologica* 72 (6): 432–435.
105 Liu, J. and Warshaw, E.M. (2014). Allergic contact dermatitis from ketoconazole. *Cutis* 94 (3): 112–114.
106 Cooper, S.M. and Shaw, S. (1999). Contact allergy to clotrimazole: an unusual allergen. *Contact Dermatitis* 41 (3): 168.
107 Cooper, S.M. and Shaw, S. (1999). Contact allergy to nystatin: an unusual allergen. *Contact Dermatitis* 41 (2): 120.
108 Okano, M. (1994). Contact dermatitis due to budesonide: report of five cases and review of the Japanese literature. *International Journal of Dermatology* 33 (10): 709–715.
109 Khurana, S., Jain, V.K., Aggarwal, K., and Gupta, S. (2002). Patch testing in discoid eczema. *Journal of Dermatology* 29 (12): 763–767.
110 Fleming, C., Parry, E., Forsyth, A., and Kemmett, D. (1997). Patch testing in discoid eczema. *Contact Dermatitis* 36 (5): 261–264.
111 Coenraads, P.J. and Diepgen, T.L. (1998). Risk for hand eczema in employees with past or present atopic dermatitis. *International Archives of Occupational and Environmental Health* 71 (1): 7–13.
112 Johansen, J.D., Hald, M., Andersen, B.L. et al. (2011). Classification of hand eczema: clinical and aetiological types. Based on the guideline of the Danish Contact Dermatitis Group. *Contact Dermatitis* 65 (1): 13–21.
113 Boonstra, M.B., Christoffers, W.A., Coenraads, P.J., and Schuttelaar, M.L. (2015). Patch test results of hand eczema patients: relation to clinical types. *Journal of the European Academy of Dermatology and Venereology* 29 (5): 940–947.
114 Cronin, E. (1995). Hand eczema. In: *Textbook of Contact Dermatitis* (eds. R.J.G. Rycroft, T. Menne, P.J. Frosch and C. Benezra), 205–218. Berlin: Springer.

CHAPTER 9

Irritant Contact Dermatitis

CHAPTER CONTENTS

Introduction

Irritant contact dermatitis (ICD) is a dermatitis that occurs in response to an exogenous non-microbial contact agent. Although usually caused by inorganic agents, organic material such as plants can also cause ICD. Unlike allergic contact dermatitis (ACD), the noxious stimulus induces skin inflammation without requiring prior sensitization and this process does not involve immunological memory.

How else does ICD differ from ACD? Clinically, vesiculation is less common in ICD than with ACD. In contrast to ACD, ICD does not have a tendency to spread. ICD appears to be more sensitive with regards to the time and dose of exposure to the causative agent than ACD, although both are affected by these factors. In addition, exposures are more likely to be significant in more than one sphere of activity with a diagnosis of ICD compared to ACD. As an example, a person with a primary diagnosis of ICD of the hands from his or her workplace may also have a hobby with exposure to glues or oils, and may be doing a lot of housework as well.

Different types of irritant contact dermatitis

Several different types of ICD have been described [1]:

1. *Acute ICD.* This usually occurs after exposure to a potent contact irritant with acute vesiculation, erythema, edema, and oozing. Examples of agents which can cause such reactions include industrial solvents, bleaches, and plants, e.g. the sap of euphorbia plants [2]. Sometimes, even with plant irritants, the reaction can be so severe as to resemble a second- or third-degree burn [2]. Caustic agents can cause acute ICD, e.g. cement, which is alkaline, can cause both acute and delayed ICD. Misuse of wash-off products as leave-on products, such as using a shower gel as a leave-on moisturizer [3], is surprisingly common and the prevalence has risen with the trend of using brand names for both leave-on and wash-off personal care products. This misuse may predispose to the development of acute ICD. Some moisturizers with potential irritant agents which are used as "antimicrobials" (e.g. benzalkonium chloride) can also cause acute ICD, especially in the flexural areas where an occlusive effect may increase the potency of the irritant agent [4]. In babies, diaper dermatitis is commonly caused by acute ICD to urine, fecal material, and cleansing agents under occlusive conditions (Figure 9.1) [5].
2. *Delayed acute ICD.* There is an irritant dermatitis with acute signs, but the reaction is delayed after initial contact with the irritant. The lag period can be 8 hours or more. Dithranol, benzalkonium chloride, wet cement, and some acrylates can give this reaction [6].
3. *Cumulative ICD.* The most common form, caused by multiple exposures to weak irritants which have a cumulative effect, causing erythema as well as dryness and leading to scaling and fissuring. The degreasing effects of surfactants play a role. The hands are the most commonly affected site, in particular the dorsal aspects of the fingers and the dorsal interdigital spaces – this pattern is associated with wet work and exposure to detergents (Figure 9.2). Cumulative ICD can also occur under a loose-fitting ring as a result of surfactants getting

Common Contact Allergens: A Practical Guide to Detecting Contact Dermatitis, First Edition. Edited by John McFadden, Pailin Puangpet, Korbkarn Pongpairoj, Supitchaya Thaiwat, and Lee Shan Xian.

© 2020 John Wiley & Sons Ltd. Published 2020 by John Wiley & Sons Ltd.

Companion website: www.wiley.com/go/mcfadden/common_contact_allergens

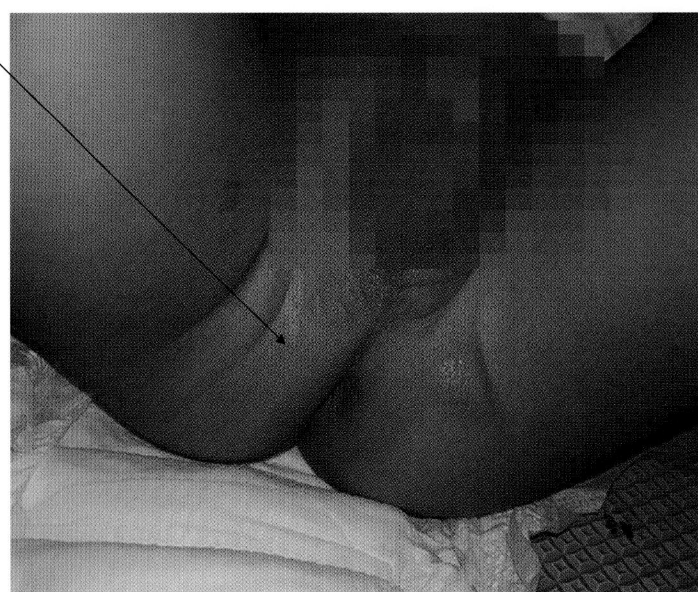

Convexities involved, where the skin is in contact with the diaper. There is no secondary spread.
The differential diagnosis includes atopic dermatitis, seborrheic dermatitis, allergic contact dermatitis, psoriasis, candida and streptococcal/staphylococcal perianal infection. Check for any evidence of atopic or seborrheic dermatitis on the head and neck as well as limbs.
Irritant diaper contact dermatitis and atopic dermatitis may coexist.

Figure 9.1 Diaper dermatitis is commonly caused by acute irritant contact dermatitis to urine, fecal material, and cleansing agents under occlusive conditions.

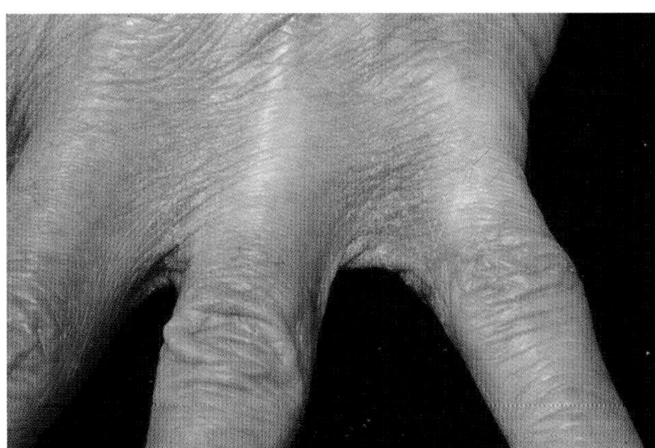

Figure 9.2 The dorsal interdigital spaces are particularly prone to developing cumulative irritant contact dermatitis from liquid soaps/detergents, as the skin here is relatively thin and permeable.

trapped beneath the ring. Holding and using a wet cloth whilst cleaning can give dermatitis affecting the palmar digits and distal palm [7]. It is imperative to keep in mind that hand dermatitis is often multifactorial – apart from ICD, elements of endogenous dermatitis and ACD may be present as well.

4. *Irritant reactions.* These are most commonly found in individuals who are newly engaged in wet work, e.g. bar work, nursing. Chapping and erythema occur on the hands and fingertips, which resolve after the skin adapts.
5. *Pustular/acneiform ICD.* These reactions can occur with oils, metals, tars, and chlorinated compounds. They are most commonly observed in occupational work with oils.
6. *Mechanically induced ICD.* Mechanical shearing forces induce the ICD, and agents such as coarse paper, textiles, plastics, tools, and woods can be involved [8]. Mechanical irritancy can also cause papules and pustules.
7. *Airborne ICD.* This may present with subjective burning sensations alone. Often, however, there is also erythema and scaling affecting the eyelids, cheeks, nasal folds, and neck [9]. Examples of agents causing airborne ICD include acids, alkalis, resins, formaldehyde releasing preservatives (e.g. from paint), slag in metal refineries, mining dust, and sewage sludge [7, 9].
8. *Photoirritant/phototoxic chemicals.* Coal tar, pitch, and some dyes can give burning sensations with erythema on sun exposure. Phytophotodermatitis is a reaction from the activation by long wavelength ultraviolet (UV) radiation of botanical substances called furocoumarins, which are present in some plants and citrus fruits such as lime and lemons. The severity of the rash can range from simple erythema to large bullae, but occurs only at the area of plant contact. The lesions are typically streaky, cause no pruritus but associated pain and often leave post-inflammatory hyperpigmentation which takes several months to fade [10]. Phytophotodermatitis can occur in the following situations: by brushing against rue or hogweed plants whilst walking, squeezing or carrying lemons, using strimmers whilst cutting grass, wearing leis of *Pelea anisata* around the neck in Hawaii, or drinking tequila through lime in Mexico. Reactions are most common during the summer months, when there is more UV light and concentrations of plant furocoumarins are at their highest [10].
9. *Sensitive skin (subjective irritation).* No actual dermatitis is seen, but burning, soreness, and stinging sensations are experienced when the skin is exposed to agents such as cosmetics – exposure to cinnamic chemicals, sodium benzoate, propylene glycol, sorbic acid and benzoic acid can all give rise to stinging symptoms. Sensitive skin may be confined to one region of the body (e.g. face). The stinging agents mentioned can also occasionally cause non-allergic or irritant contact urticaria, characterized by a localized urticarial wheal and flare.

Occupational irritant contact dermatitis

ICD is the most common form of occupational skin disease. In a recent large survey (n = 2177) of occupational skin disorders, ICD was found to be the most common primary diagnosis (44%), followed by ACD (33%) and endogenous eczema (11%) [11]. The most common occupations affected were healthcare workers (24%), skilled manual workers and laborers (23%), food handlers (12%), machine and plant operators (7%), automotive workers (7%), hair and beauty workers (5%), process workers and packers (5%), workers in the engineering industry (4%), and cleaners (3%). People working in the hair and beauty industry were more than three times as likely to have ACD as the primary diagnosis rather than ICD [11]. The most common causes of skin irritation in occupational ICD were water and wet work (38%), soap and detergents (32%), heat and sweating (16%), oils and coolants (15%), solvents (14%), dusts and fibers (10%), as well as acids and alkalis (4%) [11].

Other clinical points

Other important points to note include the following:

- Skin atopy/a history of atopic dermatitis at least doubles the effects of irritant exposure and, therefore, doubles the risk in occupations where hand eczema is a common problem [12].
- Occlusion (e.g. under clothing/gloves or inside boots) significantly enhances the potency of the irritant signal and subsequent inflammation. For instance, diaper, peristomal, and perianal dermatitis are usually ICD caused by a combination of factors (occlusion together with urine, feces, sweat and secondary infection) and may coexist with medicament allergy [7].
- Contact allergens can have irritant properties as well, e.g. epoxy resins, hair dyes, fragrances.
- Cosmetics are not an uncommon cause of ICD. However, this is usually (but not always) transient and mild, and the consumer stops using the particular cosmetic most of the time [7].
- The eyelids are particularly susceptible to ICD from cosmetics – there may be a cumulative etiology [7].
- ICD to sunscreen agents is not uncommon – reactions can sometimes be marked and this is the most common form of reaction to sunscreens in the pediatric age group.
- Clothing contaminated by irritants (e.g. solvents used during the dry-cleaning process) have been reported to cause ICD [13].

General principles of management

The management of ICD is holistic and three-pronged [14]:

1. *Treatment of the inflammation.* This is usually achieved by the use of topical glucocorticosteroids. These should be used for the shortest possible duration to minimize the side effects. Topical calcineurin inhibitors have also been used to treat dermatitis, especially for sites where the skin is thinner and more prone to the side effects of topical glucocorticosteroids (e.g. eyelids/periorbital region). In severe cases, short tapering courses of oral glucocorticosteroids may be required to allow the inflammation to settle more quickly.
2. *Restoration of skin barrier function.* Emollients and moisturizers can help to restore the integrity of the skin's natural epidermal barrier. Although the terms "emollients" and "moisturizers" are sometimes used interchangeably, there are differences between the two. Emollients form a layer on the surface of the skin which prevents water from evaporating, thereby increasing skin hydration [15]. This layer also protects the skin from external noxious stimuli [16]. Moisturizers, however, contain humectants that bind water molecules to hydrate the skin [17]. Mild cases of ICD may respond to emollients and moisturizers alone.
3. *Prevention.* Prevention strategies include avoidance measures, such as the use of personal protective equipment (PPE), both in the workplace and at home. Patient education is critical in this aspect. Diaper dermatitis can be prevented by the use of barrier creams containing zinc oxide, which minimize urine and fecal contact with the skin. The use of emollients and/or moisturizers on a regular basis also helps to maintain an intact skin barrier, which reduces the likelihood of ICD occurrence. The work environment, home environment, and leisure pursuits can all contribute cumulatively to ICD-therefore, resting of the hands away from work should be advised. Full recovery of the skin from acute ICD can take at least 4 weeks [18].

References

1 Harvell, J.D., Lammintausta, K., and Maibach, H.I. (1995). Irritant contact dermatitis. In: *Practical Contact Dermatitis* (ed. J.D. Guin), 7–18. New York: McGraw-Hill.

2 Asilian, A. and Faghihi, G. (2004). Severe irritant contact dermatitis from cypress spurge. *Contact Dermatitis* 51 (1): 37–39.

3 Mose, M., Sommerlund, M., and Koppelhus, U. (2013). Severe acute irritant contact dermatitis presenting as exfoliative erythroderma. *Contact Dermatitis* 69 (2): 119–121.

4 Hann, S., Hughes, T.M., and Stone, N.M. (2007). Flexural allergic contact dermatitis to benzalkonium chloride in antiseptic bath oil. *British Journal of Dermatology* 157 (4): 795–798.

5 Murat-Susić, S. and Husar, K. (2007). Differential diagnosis of skin lesions in the diaper area. *Acta Dermatovenerologica Croatica* 15 (2): 108–112.

6 Slodownik, D., Lee, A., and Nixon, R. (2008). Irritant contact dermatitis: a review. *Australasian Journal of Dermatology* 49 (1): 1–9; quiz 10-1.

7 Wilkinson, S.M. and Beck, M.H. (2010). Contact dermatitis: irritant. In: *Rook's Textbook of Dermatology*, 8e (ed. T. Burns, S. Breathnach, N. Cox and C. Griffiths). Oxford: Wiley-Blackwell.

8 Morris-Jones, R., Robertson, S.J., Ross, J.S. et al. (2002). Dermatitis caused by physical irritants. *British Journal of Dermatology* 147 (2): 270–275.

9 Lachapelle, J.M. (1984). Occupational airborne irritant contact reaction to the dust of a food additive. *Contact Dermatitis* 10 (4): 250–251.
10 Bowers, A.G. (1999). Phytophotodermatitis. *American Journal of Contact Dermatitis* 10 (2): 89–93.
11 Cahill, J.L., Williams, J.D., Matheson, M.C. et al. (2016). Occupational skin disease in Victoria, Australia. *Australasian Journal of Dermatology* 57 (2): 108–114.
12 Coenraads, P.J. and Diepgen, T.L. (1998). Risk for hand eczema in employees with past or present atopic dermatitis. *International Archives of Occupational and Environmental Health* 71 (1): 7–13.
13 Aoki, T. and Kageyama, R. (1989). Three cases of dry cleaning dermatitis. *Nihon Hifuka Gakkai Zasshi* 99 (9): 1035–1038.
14 Lachapelle, J.M., Gimenez-Arnau, A., Metz, M. et al. (2018). Best practices, new perspectives and the perfect emollient: optimizing the management of contact dermatitis. *Journal of Dermatological Treatment* 29 (3): 241–251.
15 Cork, M.J. (1997). The importance of skin barrier function. *Journal of Dermatological Treatment* 8: S7–S13.
16 Zhai, H. and Maibach, H.I. (2002). Barrier creams – skin protectants: can you protect skin? *Journal of Cosmetic Dermatology* 1 (1): 20–23.
17 Lodén, M. (2003). Role of topical emollients and moisturizers in the treatment of dry skin barrier disorders. *American Journal of Clinical Dermatology* 4 (11): 771–788.
18 Lee, J.Y., Effendy, I., and Maibach, H.I. (1997). Acute irritant contact dermatitis: recovery time in man. *Contact Dermatitis* 36 (6): 285–290.

SECTION 3

Common Contact Allergens

Exposure Color Code

- Clothing, jewelry, adornments
- Personal care products, cosmetics/cosmetic procedures
- Household products, domestic environment, including furniture and refurbishment
- Occupational dermatoses, work environment
- Medicines, surgical/dental procedures, herbal/alternative medicines
- Personal appliances/aids
- Leisure activities, sport, travel
- Other exposures (including dietary)
- Not relevant or multiple/general exposure

CHAPTER 10
Nickel

CHAPTER CONTENTS

Common Contact Allergens: A Practical Guide to Detecting Contact Dermatitis, First Edition. Edited by John McFadden, Pailin Puangpet, Korbkarn Pongpairoj, Supitchaya Thaiwat, and Lee Shan Xian.
© 2020 John Wiley & Sons Ltd. Published 2020 by John Wiley & Sons Ltd.
Companion website: www.wiley.com/go/mcfadden/common_contact_allergens

Allergen profiling

- Nickel is a common and ubiquitous element that is present in many metal objects and components. Nickel is the most common cause of contact allergy.

Common sources of exposure

- Ornamentation, e.g. earrings, necklaces, rings, bracelets, bindi.
- Personal appliances, e.g. spectacle frames, coins, scissors, hair pins/grips, pens, keys, key rings/chains, knitting needles, mobile phones, laptop computers, toys, watches.
- Clothing, e.g. jean buttons, belt buckles, studs, clips, hooks, zips, brassieres.
- Medical and dental devices, e.g. prostheses, other metal implants, dental braces/orthodontic appliances, needles.
- Certain occupations, e.g. hairdressers, mechanics, electroplaters, metalworkers, hard metalworkers, office workers.
- Leisure/hobbies, e.g. musicians (multiple), gymnasium equipment.
- Furniture, e.g. chairs.
- Cosmetic/cosmetic appliances, e.g. eyelash curlers.

Potential routes of exposure

Common
- Direct contact, e.g. earrings.

Less Common
- Mucosal, e.g. dental appliances (uncommon).
- Systemic, e.g. prosthesis/medical implants, dietary.

Rare
- Airborne (some occupations).

Theoretical
- Hand-to-face.

Clinical manifestations of contact allergy to nickel

- Direct contact dermatitis (the vast majority of presentations).
- Exacerbation of/mimicking endogenous dermatitis (atopic dermatitis).
- Multifactorial.
- Systemic contact dermatitis.
- Mucosal contact dermatitis (rare).
- Non-eczematous contact dermatitis.
  Lymphomatoid.
  Vitiligo-like.
  Lichenoid.
- Airborne contact dermatitis (rare).
- Rare forms of contact dermatitis – pustular, mimicking basal cell cancer.

Key points

- Nickel allergy is the most common cause of allergic contact dermatitis and occurs up to 10 times more frequently in women than in men.
- The prevalence of nickel allergy in the general population is 9% (men 3%, women 17%).
- The most important cause of nickel sensitization in women is ear piercing, which causes a three-fold increase in nickel allergy risk.
- Perspiration, heat, friction, and sweat increase the risk of nickel allergic contact dermatitis.
- The dimethylglyoxime nickel spot test can detect the release of nickel >0.5 μg/cm²/week. This test has high specificity and moderate sensitivity.
- The EU Nickel directive states that "products which come into direct and prolonged contact with the skin should not release more than 0.5 μg nickel/cm²/week, and piercing posts not more than 0.2 μg nickel/cm²/week."
- Clear nail polish and acrylic spray coating provide a protective shield from nickel-containing items.
- Pustular patch test reactions may occur, especially in atopic individuals.
- Other false positive/irritant reactions can occur in atopic dermatitis patients.
- Ammonium thioglycolate in permanent wave liquids may induce the release of nickel from metal objects and predispose hairdressers to nickel allergic contact dermatitis.
- The significance of dietary nickel as an aggravating factor for dermatitis in nickel-sensitive patients remains uncertain. In some patients who are already highly sensitized to nickel, ingestion of large amounts of dietary nickel may aggravate vesicular hand eczema. However, there is no advantage in avoiding the use of stainless-steel cooking utensils.
- Oral nickel exposure from dental braces at an early age, prior to ear piercing, results in a reduced frequency of nickel allergy.
- Implantation of a prosthesis containing metals to which the patient is sensitized may rarely lead to implant failure or eczema over the operation site. However, the great majority of nickel allergic subjects have prosthesis implants without any problems.
- Concomitant reactions to palladium chloride and nickel occur as cross-reactions; cobalt and nickel concomitantly react as co-sensitizers.
- Non-eczematous nickel contact dermatitis includes lymphomatoid, vitiligo-like, and lichenoid contact dermatitis.
- The potential for nickel dermatitis to undergo secondary spread is underestimated and under-recognized.
- Nickel-allergic patients should avoid jewelry which is less than 18 karat gold.

Introduction

Nickel is a ubiquitous element that surrounds us in most if not all our endeavors. Nickel is present in jewelry, clothes, appliances, accessories, medical, dental, occupational, and recreational pursuits. It is the most common cause of contact allergy.

The most common causes of nickel sensitization in women are through ear piercing and direct contact with nickel-containing jewelry and clothing. There is a highly statistically significant increase in the frequency of nickel allergy amongst women with pierced ears compared to women with unpierced ears ($p < 0.001$) [1, 2]. Perspiration, heat, friction, pressure, and sweat increase the risk of nickel allergic contact dermatitis (ACD).

The dimethylglyoxime nickel spot test

- The dimethylglyoxime nickel spot test is a simple, rapid, and useful test for screening objects for significant nickel release (Figure 10.1). A positive test (pink color) indicates the release of >0.5 μg/cm^2/week of nickel. It can detect nickel in concentrations as low as 10 parts/million (ppm) while most patients have a sensitivity threshold of >11 ppm [3]. Fisher et al. [4] found that 0.44 μg/cm^2 was the elicitation threshold for nickel. This test has high specificity and moderate sensitivity. In Europe (2011), dimethylglyoxime tests were positive in 20–25% of mobile phones, 10–15% of earrings, and up to 80% of children's hair clasps [5].
- The sensitivity of the dimethylglyoxime spot test for nickel at the level not permitted by the EU is 59.3% and the specificity 97.5% [6].

Patch testing

Nickel sulfate hexahydrate 5% in petrolatum is included in the baseline series [7].

- The correlating concentration in the T.R.U.E.® test is 200 μg/cm^2.
- Nickel patch test preparations are, as with other metals, in the salt form, i.e. nickel sulfate.
- Standard (baseline) patch testing does not detect all nickel-sensitive subjects and false-positive reactions can also occur (especially among atopic dermatitis patients).
- Pustular patch test reactions may occur, especially in atopic individuals [8].

Frequency of sensitization

General population

Denmark, 2007 -based on a group of studies	9% (men 3%, women 17%) [9]
Norway, circa 2005, *n* = 1236	17.6% (men 5.1%, women 27.5%, irritant reactions 3.8%) [10]

Europe

Denmark, 1977–2009, *n* = 12 803	10.4% [11]
Sweden, 2003–2004, *n* = 4376	9.9% [12]
Spain, 2005–2010, *n* = 839	25.9% [13]
Spain, 2008, *n* = 1161	25.6% [14]
	Men 9%, women 35%

America

1994–1996, *n* = 3108	14.3%
1996–1998, *n* = 3429	14.2%
1998–2000, *n* = 5827	16.2%
2001–2002, *n* = 4913	16.7%

Relevant: definite 1.6%, probable 10.3%, possible 37.5%, past 33%.

North American Contact Dermatitis Group (NACDG) [15].

Asia

Thailand, 2008–2009, *n* = 157	26.8% [16]
China, 1989–2009, hand eczema, *n* = 366	21.9% [17]

Allergic contact dermatitis to nickel from a belt buckle
The buckle and a clothing stud show a positive 'spot' test to dimethylglyoxime (pink colour).

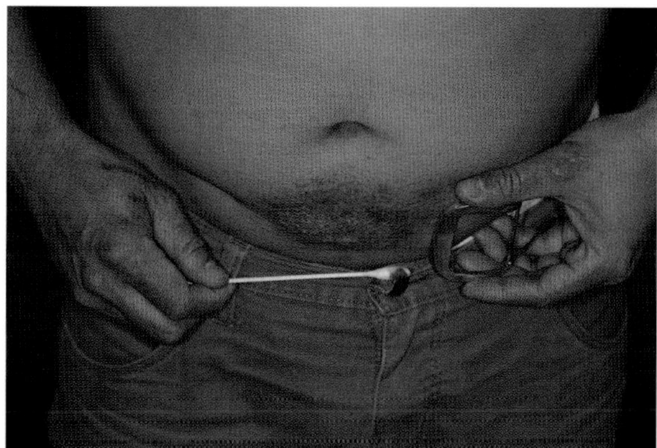

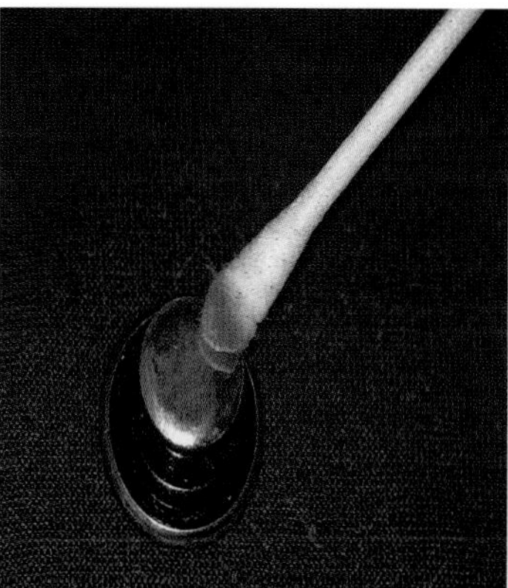

Figure 10.1 The dimethylglyoxime spot test.

Age

- Nickel is the most common contact allergen in children [18].
- Positive patch tests in infants are of dubious clinical relevance and rarely reproducible. Only 2/21 positive nickel patch tests at 12/18 months were reproducible at 3/6 years age and only 1 of these was clinically relevant [19]. Irritant reactions to nickel patch tests are more common in children, so reactions must be interpreted with caution [20].
- Young adults who had been repeatedly patch tested (six times) during the first 3 years of life were found to have a low rate of nickel allergy in their teenage years (1.2%), approximately eight times lower than a comparable group. The authors could not exclude an immunoregulatory effect from repeated patch test challenges in early life [21].

Sex

The prevalence of nickel sensitization is 5–10 times higher in women in most studies.

Clinical disease

It is common for nickel allergy to be detected by patch testing without having any relevance to the presenting cause (Figure 10.2a,b). One must, therefore, guard against over-interpretation of the clinical relevance given to nickel allergy. Although nickel allergy has been extensively reported in the clinical literature, some cases are isolated in the literature (i.e. we could not find further confirmatory reports) and are highlighted as such.

Jewelry

- Patients with contact allergy to nickel should avoid gold that is less than 18 carats. Solid silver and platinum are suitable alternatives. Some "white gold" may contain nickel.

Earring dermatitis

- Earring dermatitis is the most common clinical manifestation of nickel ACD (Figure 10.3). The dermatitis may spread from the primary site to other areas of the ear, neck, scalp, and face. Earring nickel dermatitis can be complicated by split earlobes, fissured granulomas, cysts, and keloid formation [22]. The main differential diagnoses include infection, irritant dermatitis, atopic dermatitis, and ACD from gold, cobalt alone, platinum, and titanium.

Other body piercings

- Other pierced sites (e.g. the nose, umbilicus, and genitals) will increase the risk of both nickel sensitization and local elicitation [23, 24].

Finger ring dermatitis

- Nickel allergy is a common cause of digital ring dermatitis [25], which can often spread. The patient may transfer the ring to the other hand, inducing a further area of dermatitis. Ring dermatitis can be caused by other metals such as gold, palladium ("white gold" may additionally contain nickel and/or palladium), and platinum [26].
- Perhaps the most common cause of "ring dermatitis" is detergent getting trapped under the ring and causing an irritant contact dermatitis from occlusion [27]. Metals such as nickel also have the potential to irritate the skin [28] and have been reported to cause an irritant ring dermatitis [29].

Necklace dermatitis

- Necklace dermatitis from ACD to nickel is also common. There may be accentuation at the sides of the neck or back if the clasp has a high nickel content, or the upper chest if the brooch is nickel-containing. The dermatitis is often chronic and lichenified (Figures 10.4 and 10.5). There may be pigmentary changes. A pseudolymphomatoid variant has been reported. ACD to necklaces can also be caused by other metals, textiles [30], and wood. [31]

Bracelet dermatitis

- Although nickel dermatitis from bracelets is a well-recognized diagnosis, there is surprisingly little in the literature regarding this. The dermatitis may extend along the forearm, especially if the metal bracelets are loose fitting and/or multiple.

Clothing

Jeans buttons

- Friction and sweating may favor the development of nickel ACD to jean buttons (Figure 10.1) [32]. The dermatitis is clinically usually of an annular nature, and can either be small or grow to a large diameter. It is usually located to one side of the umbilicus and may be slightly inferior or superior to the umbilicus (often depending on age, with younger adults wearing the jeans in a lower position).
- In the USA in 2007, 16% of blue jean buttons were positive on dimethylglyoxime (DMG) testing for releasable nickel [33].

Belt buckles

- Byer and Morell [34] contest that belt buckles may be a more common cause of periumbilical dermatitis than jean buttons (Figure 10.6). They found that only 10% of jean buttons they tested were positive for releasable nickel but in contrast 53% of belt buckles were positive.
- Clear nail polish and acrylic spray coating have been shown to provide a protective shield from nickel-containing items without changing the appearance of the objects [3]. These have been used in both jean buttons and earrings to prevent ACD reactions in sensitized individuals.

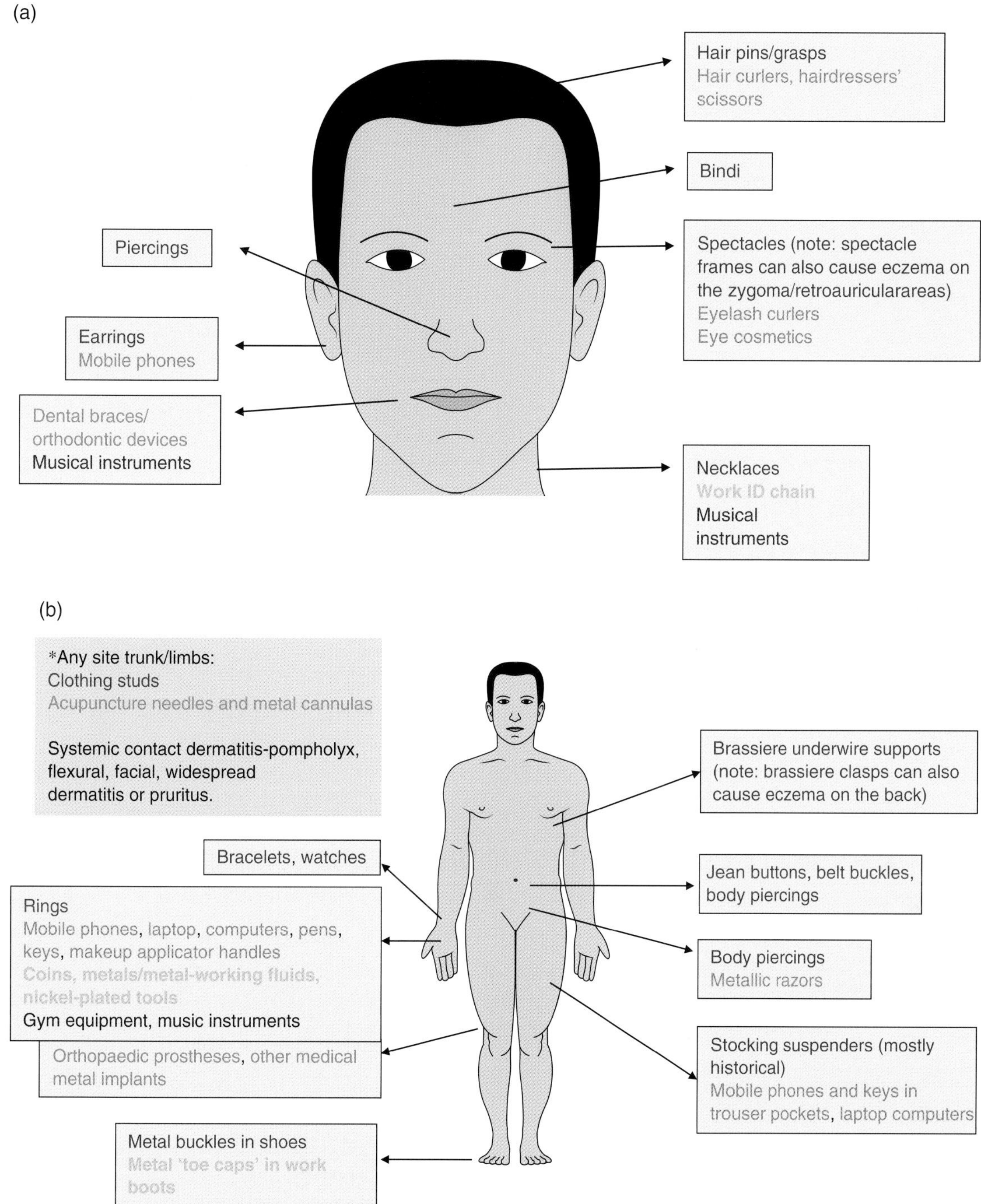

Figure 10.2 Various exposures to nickel causing allergic contact dermatitis.

Brassieres

- Dermatitis from brassiere clasps, with a small area of dermatitis on the mid upper back, has historically been a common form of ACD to nickel though it is less often seen now [35].
- Underwire supports in bras are often positive to dimethylglyoxime spot tests and may cause nickel ACD presenting as plaques of eczema in the inframammary folds [36].
- A sterile pustule developed on the scapular area of the back at the site of a nickel-containing metal ring of a bra shoulder strap, as a manifestation of ACD to nickel [37]. The patch test to nickel was also pustular *(isolated case report).*

Other sources of metal in clothing

- A study from Korea found that 100% of zippers, 66% of studs, 57% of snaps, and 80% of hooks in clothing released significant

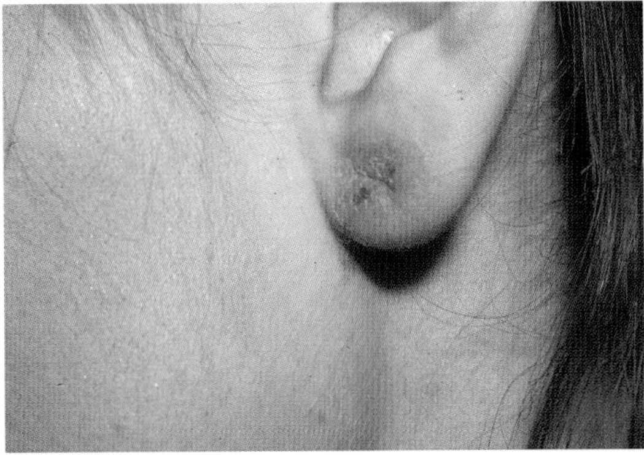

Subtle eczema changes can easily be missed at ear piercing sites without 'microexamination'. Multiple piercings predispose to nickel allergy.

Figure 10.3 Earring dermatitis.

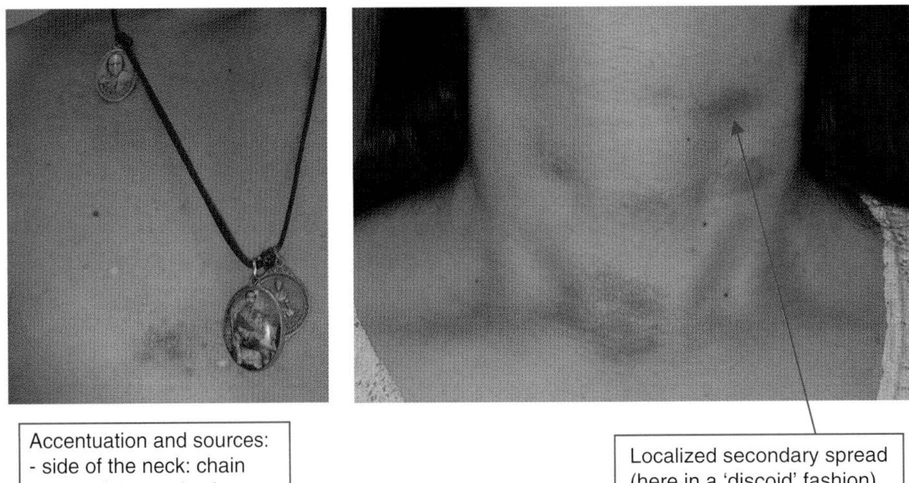

- back of the neck: clasp
- front of the chest: pendant.
Localized secondary spread (here in a 'discoid' fashion).

Figure 10.4 Allergic contact dermatitis to nickel in necklaces.

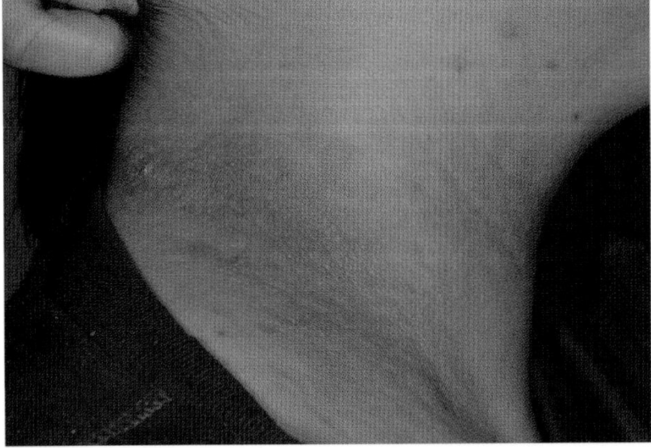

Loose chains can give a wider band of or more scattered dermatitis.

Figure 10.5 Allergic contact dermatitis to nickel in loose-fitting chains.

amounts of nickel [38]. ACD to nickel from these sources will usually present as a dermatitis which can increase in size over time and spread. Metal in children's clothing can also commonly release nickel [39].

- In a large series studying patients with ACD to shoes (n = 165) only a minority (7%) were allergic to nickel; however, the authors note that in some countries (such as Italy) it is fashionable to wear metal buckles in shoes [40]. A case of ACD to nickel and cobalt used as a dye in green plastic shoes presenting as dorsal foot dermatitis was described [41] *(isolated case report).*
- In a survey of 88 eye shadows, five were found to have a nickel content of 40 ppm, which the authors state could be enough to cause nickel ACD [42]. However, a recent large study found no association between nickel allergy and the reporting of dermatitis from mascara or eyeshadow [43]. If there is any suspicion, the patient can perform a ROAT on the wrist to check for any reactions.

Lesions from jean buttons or belt buckles are annular and above, below or to the side but not directly 'on' the umbilicus. The size of the lesion will gradually increase with time.

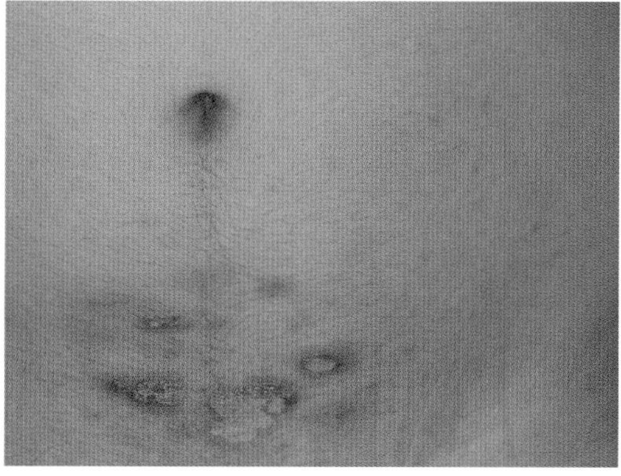
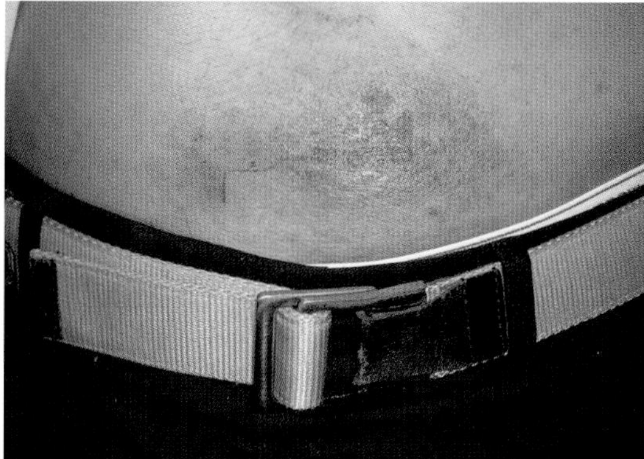

Figure 10.6 Allergic contact dermatitis from jean buttons and belt buckles.

Allergic contact dermatitis to nickel from an eyelash curler. This demonstrates that even short, repeated exposures to nickel can lead to dermatitis.

Predominantly upper eyelid involvement but some lower eyelid involvement is also often observed.

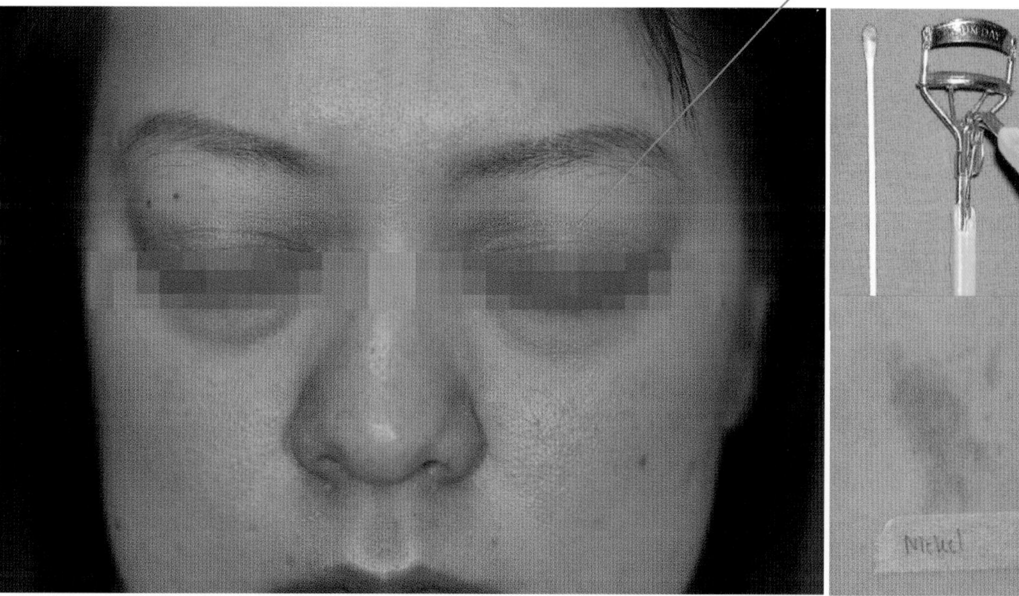

Figure 10.7 Allergic contact dermatitis from an eyelash curler.

Cosmetics

- Nickel at levels of over 300 ppm, with the potential to elicit ACD, was detected in some children's "toy" cosmetic eyeshadow [44].
- Loden et al. [45] investigated 23 nickel-sensitive individuals who were tested to mineral makeup powders containing nickel as an impurity. The results showed that none of the subjects reacted to the products. The authors proposed that the amounts of nickel in powder cosmetics were below the level needed to elicit sensitization reactions.
- ■ ■ ACD to nickel from eyelash curlers is not an uncommon cause of eyelid dermatitis [46, 47]. (Figure 10.7). Both the upper and lower eyelids can be affected. Intermittent short exposures to nickel, such as with eyelash curlers, can evidently build up enough stimulation to elicit a dermatitis reaction. Jacob et al. [48] notes that many handles/ferrules of makeup applicators release nickel (dimethylglyoxime spot test positive). She also points out that hair curlers and hairdressers' scissors may also release nickel.
- ■ Glitter used in cosmetics may be an occult source of metal allergy [49] *(isolated case report of cobalt allergy).*

Bindi

- A 33-year-old woman presented with a 2-year history of recurrent eczema localized to her central forehead where she typically wore her bindi, a common practice amongst Hindus. She had a history of jewelry allergy and was patch test positive to nickel (++) and to the metallic bindi (++), which was also positive on the dimethylglyoxime spot test *(isolated case report)*. The authors also noted that azo dyes such as Brilliant Lake red, paratertiary butyl phenol, kumkum colorants, lead, mercury, and eosin can all cause bindi contact dermatitis [50].

Personal appliances and accessories

Spectacle frame dermatitis

- Smith and Calnan [51] describe the three most common areas of involvement, all correlating with direct contact with the spectacle frames (Figure 10.8). These are, in order of frequency:
  a. retroauricular in association with the ends of the wings
  b. on the sides of the nose under the pads
  c. along the sides of the temples under the wings.

  If the reaction is severe it can spread to involve adjacent areas of the cheeks and eyelids. The differential diagnosis includes airborne ACD, ACD to nail varnish, ACD to hair dye, and ACD to cosmetics. Nickel is used as an alloy in spectacle frames [52]. Free surface nickel was detected in 6.5% of frames claiming to conform to the European Nickel Directive [53].
- Other agents which can cause ACD to spectacle frames include other metals (cobalt, chromate, palladium, and gold), plastic chemicals, dyes, rubber chemicals, and resins [52].

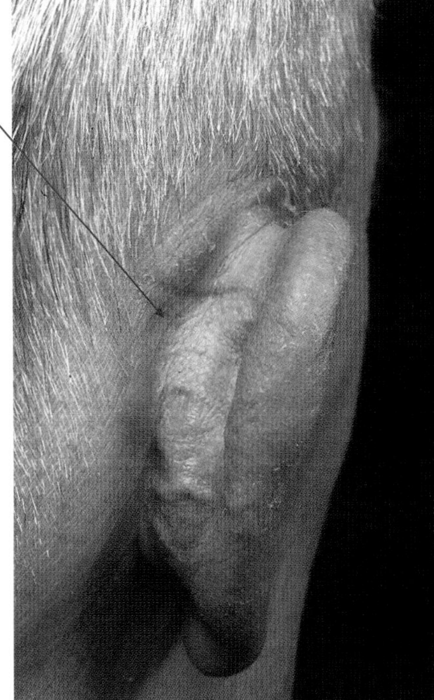

Figure 10.8 Allergic contact dermatitis to spectacle frames.

- Nickel spectacle frame dermatitis may show asymmetry (such as on the maxillary area) if the spectacle frames have been mildly contorted [54].
- Nickel ACD to spectacle frames is associated with fine scratches of the frames which presumably increase with the age of the spectacles [55]. It is perhaps, then, not surprising that when Walsh and Mitchell [56] investigated nickel release from 373 new and 50 used metal spectacle frames they found that 96% of used frames but only 24.5% of new frames were releasing excess nickel.
- An unusual case of nickel ACD from spectacle frames presenting as a pustular acneiform rash which cleared on changing to plastic frames was reported [57] *(isolated case report)*.

Scissors and crochet hooks

- In 2009 in Denmark, two hairdressers were diagnosed with hand eczema from exposure to scissors and crochet hooks, respectively [58]. One case was a 24-year-old hairdresser presenting with unilateral vesicular eczema on the hand using the scissors. She also used a crochet hook, pulling hair through a cap whilst dyeing hair. Both the scissors and hook were dimethylglyoxime spot test positive. This led to extensive spot testing of scissors and crochet hooks in several salons. 1/200 scissors and 7/13 hooks released excess amounts of nickel. Nickel release from scissors appears to be uncommon at present, possibly due to the EU Nickel Directive, although one must keep in mind that thioglycolates can enhance the release of nickel from metal objects [59].

Hair pins/grips

- Hair pins/grasps have long been known to cause nickel ACD locally on the scalp [60]. In a recent study, 24/28 (85%) of hair pins were positive on dimethylglyoxime spot testing [38] and in another study 6/6 (100%) [61].
- A 40-year-old woman complained of an itchy scalp and was found to have active scalp dermatitis. She was patch test positive (++) to nickel, her hair clasp was positive with the dimethylglyoxime spot test, and the area of scalp dermatitis coincided with where she wore the hair clasp. The dermatitis cleared after she stopped wearing the clasp [62] *(isolated case report)*.
- Otitis externa, from the use of a hairpin to assist scratching, has been reported [63] *(isolated case report)*.

Pens, keys, keychains, and knitting needles

- A Danish study DMG tested metallic items obtained from nickel-sensitive patients. They found that the following numbers of items released excess nickel: 5/5 keys, 2/2 keychains, 4/5 knitting needles, and 1/1 pen [61]. Another study found that 44/55 keys were positive with the dimethylglyoxime test [64]. Keys may cause nickel ACD both on the hands and on the thighs if carried in trouser pockets (Figure 10.9).

It is important to view how the patient handles objects. In chronic allergic contact dermatitis of the hands the dermatitis will often spread locally to areas of the hand which do not have primary contact

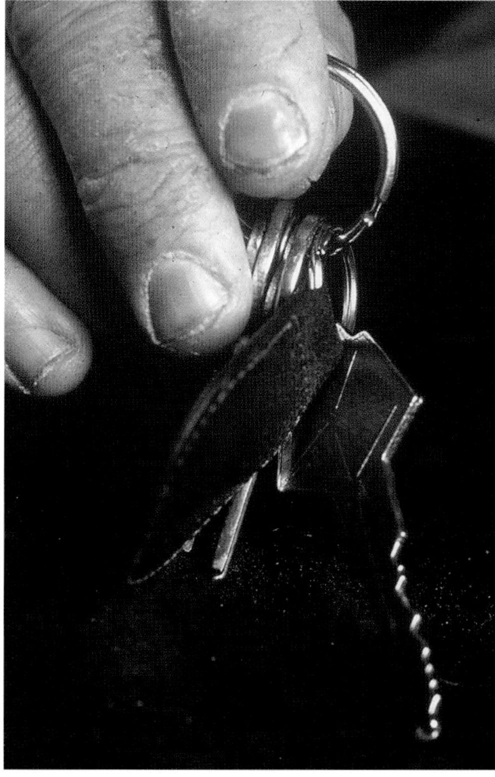

Figure 10.9 Allergic contact dermatitis from keys and keyring.

Mobile phones

- Mobile phone dermatitis was first reported in 2000 [65]. The main affected sites include the preauricular region, ears, lateral cheeks, and the superior and lateral aspects of the chin. Lesions were often unilateral or more pronounced on one side. The characteristic morphology is that of subacute pruritic eczematous papules and plaques and/or vesicles [66]. Carrying mobile phones in trouser pockets can cause dermatitis of the outer thighs [67].
- A survey in 2010 found that 30% of mobile phones released significant amounts of nickel [61]. This may reduce over time with more regulations.
- On reviewing the literature, Richardson et al. (2014) noted that amongst 34 patients whose age was reported with mobile phone ACD, 14 (41.2%) were 8 years or younger and 8 were under 16 years of age with the youngest being 12 years old [68].
- A 25-year-old woman presented with excoriated papular dermatitis of both cheeks and pre-auricular areas, more pronounced on the right side (the phone can be switched to the other hand when a subject uses one hand to write a note) [69]. The right anti-tragus was also involved. It was noted that the patient used the mobile phone for on average 1.5 hours per day, being on an unlimited phone time contract. Another case describes a pruritic lichenoid dermatitis of both the hands and forearms. Examination of the right cheek showed another rectangular-shaped eczematous area on the right preauricular skin and a small sharply demarcated area on the anti-tragus of the ear, in keeping with the contact areas for a mobile phone [70]. A case was reported with widespread involvement of the body including the lower abdomen, extremities, flanks, and face, demonstrating the ability of nickel ACD to undergo secondary spread [71]. In this case, both the mobile phone and headset were positive on the dimethylglyoxime spot test. Another case describes pruritic scaly papules between the breasts, where the patient habitually carried her mobile [72]. There was another case with dermatitis on the superior quadrants of the breasts where the phone was usually carried [73].

Laptop computers

- A 50-year-old non-atopic woman was referred with pruritic vesicular dermatitis on the ulnar surfaces of both hands [74]. She did not have a previous history suggestive of metal allergy. Her dermatitis developed a few weeks after she began using a new laptop computer. The dermatitis was located on skin areas which had been in prolonged contact with metallic parts framing the keyboard. She experienced complete symptom relief after she stopped using the computer. She was patch test positive (++) to nickel and the metallic parts of the laptop were positive on the dimethylglyoxime spot test. Another case was a 7-year-old boy with atopic dermatitis who developed a widespread recalcitrant dermatitis involving his forearms, coming on after he started using a new laptop computer. He was patch test positive to nickel, the computer tested positive on the dimethylglyoxime spot test, and the rash improved with nickel avoidance, including the laptop [75].

Wrist watches

- Nickel ACD from watches is a recognized cause of wrist dermatitis (Figure 10.10). As with rings, the rash may be bilateral if the patient switches the watch from the originally affected wrist. Tinea can mimic wrist watch dermatitis [76].

Toys

- A Danish study found that 73/212 toys purchased in Denmark released significant quantities of nickel [77]. This included a wide array of toys such as spinning tops, skateboards, dolls, tools, purses, and rattles.
- The same group describes three children with nickel ACD from toys [77]. A 1-year-old boy with atopic dermatitis and patch test + to nickel presented with perioral dermatitis which cleared after removal of his favorite sucking toy, a metal key fob. His atopic dermatitis also became more manageable. A 3-year-old with dermatitis of the hands, feet, and

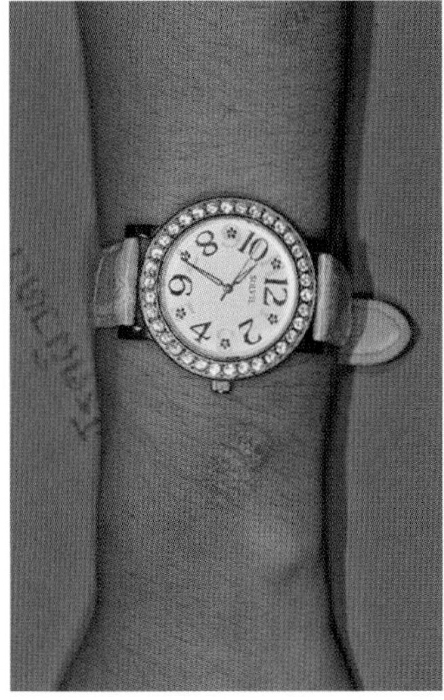

Nickel can be present in many metal objects, including watches.

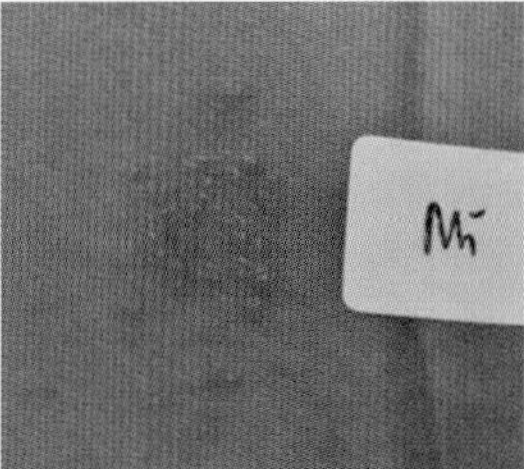

Figure 10.10 Allergic contact dermatitis to wristwatches.

abdomen and patch test + to nickel improved when his metallic toys, e.g. a metal car, were removed. A 2-year-old with atopic dermatitis and eczema on the forearm who was patch test positive (++) to nickel often played with nickel-releasing toy keys. His eczema resolved when the keys were removed.

- Children's hands, tested by the dimethylglyoxime spot test after playing with nickel-containing toys for 30 seconds, revealed the presence of nickel on their fingers [78].

Razors

- A 24-year-old woman presented with a uniform follicular dermatitis on the pubic area 2 days after shaving this area with a metallic razor blade. She had been previously sensitized to nickel from her job. Her patch test reaction to nickel was positive down to a concentration of 0.1% pet [79] *(isolated case report).*

Pistols

- A 42-year-old nickel-allergic man presented with a pruritic erythematous papular eruption on his right flank [37]. He had worked as a bodyguard and wore a pistol in his holster at the site of the dermatitis *(isolated case report).*

Historical stocking-suspender dermatitis

- This is of largely historical interest, as suspender belts are not commonly worn now. In Calnan's study in 1956 [60], however, it was the overwhelmingly most common cause, with over 95% having stocking-suspender dermatitis as their first manifestation of nickel allergy. The posterior suspender sites reacted more frequently than the anterior ones. The other remarkable aspect of this paper is how commonly secondary spread of nickel dermatitis occurred, being recorded in three out of four patients.

Medical- and dental-related nickel allergy

Prostheses and other metal implant devices

- The relationship between metal hypersensitivity and large joint arthroplasties such as the knee was recently reviewed [80]. Several important points were raised:
  a. Metal hypersensitivity after arthroplasty may present as either dermatitis or persistent painful synovitis.
  b. Metal hypersensitivity after arthroplasty is quite rare and should be considered only after eliminating other causes of pain/swelling such as low-grade infection, instability, component loosening or malrotation, referred pain, and chronic regional pain syndrome.
  c. Affected patients may or may not have a history of metal allergy.
  d. Laboratory measurements of inflammation (ESR, CRP) are often negative, as is joint aspiration. The sensitivity and specificity of *in vitro* metal allergy tests (e.g. lymphocyte transformation tests) are not clearly defined.
  e. Surgical revision with replacement of the prosthesis by titanium or zirconium prostheses has been suggested by some reports as symptom relieving. However, the authors suggest that this should only be used as a last resort after non-surgical measures have failed, and patients should be informed that no evidence-based medical guidelines are available to guide decisions regarding revision.
  f. The authors do not recommend routine pre-arthroplasty allergy screening, though this may change in the future with more research.
- Other authors state that implantation of any prosthesis containing metals to which the patient is sensitized may uncommonly/rarely lead to implant failure, prosthesis loosening, in-stent restenosis, pain, inflammation, or allergic contact dermatitis. Nickel, cobalt, and chromium are the three most common allergens involved [81]. Of 72 patients receiving a hip or knee prosthesis with a metal component, five who were previously negative on metal allergy testing developed a positive test a year later [82].
- Of 13 736 foramen ovale closure devices implanted, 38 devices (0.28%) required explantation. The most common reason was severe persistent chest pain (14 cases), thought to be due to nickel allergy [83].
- Allergic nickel dermatitis induced by orthopedic metal implants can (rarely) produce eczema over the operation site, generalized dermatitis, and hand eczema. Bullous, urticarial, or vasculitic eruptions may also occur. Removal of the implant can cure or improve the eczema (but see above: this should only be considered as a last resort and in extenuating circumstances). In some cases, the eczema may relapse or become chronic [84].

Dental braces/orthodontic devices

- Individuals who have had oral exposure to nickel (dental braces) before having their ears pierced have a significantly reduced rate of nickel allergy compared to others who had their ears pierced first [85, 86].

- The rate of nickel hypersensitivity does not appear to be raised in patients who have undergone orthodontic treatment [87].
- A 14-year-old boy presented with crusted vesicles on and around the lips and eczema on the palms and soles after insertion of a stainless steel orthodontic appliance (18% chromium and 8% nickel). The eczema had spread to the scalp, abdomen, and legs. After removal of the appliance, the eczema settled down. Patch testing showed positive reactions to nickel and cobalt [88]. An almost identical case was reported by another group [89].

Needles

- A 19-year-old female had a permanent insulin pump inserted with a butterfly needle into the abdominal subcutaneous layer. A month after its insertion, itchy papules started to appear around the needle site and progressed to form a plaque 10 cm in diameter. The patient was patch test + for nickel and the lesion quickly resolved after removal of the needle [90].
- A 39-year-old woman developed a painful papulonodular dermatitis at the needle site of an infusion pump. The dermatitis subsequently spread over the rest of the abdomen. On patch testing there was a +++ reaction to nickel. The dermatitis resolved when the metallic needle was replaced with a Teflon needle [91] *(isolated case report).*
- A 48-year-old woman presented with an itchy papulovesicular rash on the head, neck, and elbows. She had been receiving acupuncture needle therapy. She was patch test positive (+++) to nickel. Insertion of one of the acupuncture needles resulted in the development of a vesicular plaque. Cessation of acupuncture resulted in complete resolution of her dermatitis [92] *(isolated case report).*

Occupational disease

- Workers potentially exposed to nickel are auto mechanics, bartenders, cashiers, catalyst makers (nickel catalysts), ceramic makers and workers, cleaners, dyers, electronic workers, electroplaters, hairdressers, ink makers, jewelers, metal workers, money handlers, nickel refining and certain chemical processes, production of glass or enamel, production workers (hand tools), spark plug makers, storage battery makers, rubber workers, and textile dyers [93, 94].
- Ammonium thioglycolate in permanent wave liquids can induce the release of nickel from metal objects (e.g. scissors) and cause nickel ACD in hairdressers [59].
- Nickel allergy was found in 8 of 801 car mechanics presenting with hand eczema due to the use of nickel-plated tools [95]. Nickel was released from 5% of 200 unused hand-held work tools for sale in Denmark examined with the dimethylglyoxime spot test. Most of the release was localized to the metal ring at the end of the grip [96].
- Hand eczema in cashiers or other careers who handle coins can be aggravated by nickel release from coins [97]. However, this at present is uncommon in relation to the coin exposure among cashiers and shop assistants, though this may change with the rising nickel content in coins.
- Electroplating involves handling hot nickel salt solutions, exposing workers to nickel absorption through the skin, lungs, and mucous membranes. They consequently have higher urine levels of nickel [98]. Improved hygiene and protective clothing has reduced nickel dermatitis in these workers. Kanerva et al. [98] described one nickel sensitive worker who used protective gloves, shoes, and apron but occasionally developed facial dermatitis.
- Gawkrodger et al. [99] measured the quantities of nickel on the skin of the fingers in different occupations by dimethylglyoxime spot testing. Sufficient amounts of nickel that could induce dermatitis were present on the hands of electroplaters, cashiers, sales assistants, and caterers, which the authors attribute mostly to probable coin handling (see also section below).
- Nickel allergy has been found amongst metalworkers with dermatitis and exposure to cooling oil but the clinical relevance is not always clear. 150 metalworkers exposed to metal and metal-working fluid were assessed and patch tested [100]. 10/150 had work-related dermatitis. 10/150 were patch test positive to metal (all to nickel and most to other metals as well) and 8 of these also had work-related dermatitis. Metal exposure could either occur from direct contact with the metal or through contamination of the cutting oil (metal working fluid). It was not established, however, what the role of nickel allergy was in the dermatitis and the authors comment that most of the minor and major skin problems were irritant in nature.
- Nickel sensitivity was detected in 40 out of 853 hard metal workers [101]. 88% of nickel sensitive individuals had a history of jewelry dermatitis prior to employment in the hard metal industry. In the nickel-sensitized group 40% had severe hand dermatitis, which began 6–12 months after starting employment. Workers with simultaneous nickel and cobalt sensitivity had the most severe hand eczema.

Musicians

These are all isolated case reports.

- A 21-year-old viola player presented with a hyperpigmented lichenified annular plaque on her neck just below the angle of her left mandible and erythematous scaly annular plaques on her left lower neck, where the skin rubbed against a metal fixture on the instrument [102]. She had a positive patch test reaction to nickel. The metallic part of the instrument that contacted the left neck gave a strong positive result on dimethylglyoxime spot testing.
- A 59-year-old professional cellist presented with recurrent eczema on the right hand. The flexor surfaces of the second and third fingers were erythematous, scaly, and vesicular. The location exactly matched the areas of contact with the metal part of the cello bow. He was strongly positive to nickel on patch testing and all the metal parts of the bow were positive on dimethylglyoxime spot testing [103].

- A keen guitarist who played every day developed subacute dermatitis on the middle, ring, and little fingers of the right hand only, with variable involvement of the tips, medial, and lateral aspects [104]. Patch testing to nickel and a short length of guitar string revealed strong positive (++) reactions to both at 2 and 4 days. He changed the guitar strings to gold plated ones and the dermatitis resolved.
- A 19-year-old nickel-allergic female amateur flautist developed eczema on the central area of the chin, just below the lips, 2 months after developing earlobe dermatitis from an earring [105]. She had scaly erythematous plaques on her chin and the location of these plaques exactly matched the areas of contact with the flute.
- A 20-year-old woman presented with episodic perioral dermatitis and wheals on her eyelids and lips after playing the trumpet [106]. She also had reactions to costume jewelry on her finger and neck. She was patch test positive (+) to nickel. On avoiding costume jewelry and applying plastic to the trumpet mouthpiece, her symptoms and rash resolved.
- A 15-year-old boy developed vesicular hand eczema 2 months after starting to play the trombone [107]. He was patch test positive (++) to nickel and the trombone was strongly positive on dimethylglyoxime spot test. The authors suggested that he cover the areas of the trombone in contact with his hand with duct tape.
- There is a single case report of ACD to nickel from a harmonica causing cheilitis [108].
- A case of nickel contact cheilitis from the mouthpiece of a flute is recorded without further details [109].

Sports-related dermatitis

- A Swedish group tested gymnasium equipment which was positive for nickel release (e.g. metallic barbells, weight handles) and then the hands of three men using these gymnasium equipment for an hour [110]. Significant levels of nickel were found on the hands of all three men, the highest level being 1.7 $\mu g/cm^2$. The palms had higher levels than the fingers.

Furniture

- The "school chair" sign is an annular dermatitis on the posterior aspect of the thighs in nickel allergic school girls who are sitting on wooden chairs and whose legs are in contact with the metal screws on the chair seat [111].

Relationship to dyshidrotic eczema and systemic contact dermatitis

- Although there is a significant association between nickel allergy and vesicular/dyshidrotic eczema, the nature of the relationship between nickel allergy and dyshidrotic eczema is controversial. Likewise, many of the reports of systemic contact dermatitis from nickel are single case reports. Some patients with vesicular hand eczema and nickel allergy have been reported to get worse after the ingestion of nickel (see Nickel: E-Supplement chapter). In one study, dietary reduction of nickel led to improvement or remission of eczema [112]. Chelation of nickel with disulfiram 250 mg/day had a beneficial effect in eight of nine subjects in a double-blind, placebo-controlled, crossover study. The reported side effects of disulfiram were fatigue, gastrointestinal symptoms, transient liver enzyme elevation, and increased libido [113].
- A stable nickel isotope, ^{61}Ni, was given in drinking water to 20 nickel-sensitized women and 20 age-matched controls, both groups having vesicular hand eczema of the pompholyx type. Nine of 20 nickel allergic eczema patients experienced aggravation of their hand eczema after nickel administration, and three also developed a maculopapular exanthema. No exacerbation was seen in the control group [114]. The authors also found that more nickel was absorbed from water further away from meals, suggesting that the rates of gastric emptying may play a role.
- An unusual presentation of systemic contact dermatitis was reported from a nickel-containing orthodontic device. A 15-year-old Asian girl presented with persistent unilateral periocular dermatitis without oral lesions. Patch testing showed positive reactions to both nickel (+++) and aluminum chloride (+), which cleared with removal of the orthodontic device [115] *(isolated case report)*.
- The development of "baboon syndrome" (genital and major flexural dermatitis) after insertion of a nickel-containing gynecological sterilization tubal implant was reported [116]. The patient was patch test positive to nickel and there was total clearance of her dermatitis after removal of the implant *(isolated case report)*.

Non-eczematous contact dermatitis

Lymphomatoid

- Lymphomatoid contact dermatitis from nickel in metal frame glasses was diagnosed in a 58-year-old man. He had post-traumatic asymmetry of the nose that resulted in chronic scaly erythematous nodules on the right side of the nose. Histopathology showed a thick lymphohistiocytic infiltrate throughout the dermis. No evidence of malignant lymphoma was found [117].
- A 68-year-old woman presented with a papular rash on the neck after exposure to a nickel-containing gold-plated necklace. Histopathology showed a superficial band-like infiltrate with exocytosis and a Pautrier's microabscess resembling mycosis fungoides. Patch test to nickel was positive [118].

Vitiligo-like depigmentation

- A 40-year-old nickel-allergic man presented with bilateral, symmetrical areas of pea-sized depigmentation correlating with chronic contact with his metal spectacle frames [119].

The authors note a similar case a year earlier where the spectacle metal frame coating had "worn out."

- A 17-year-old female developed periumbilical contact vitiligo occurring 1 month after nickel ACD to her jean button/belt [120].

Lichenoid

- A series of 38 children who presented with periumbilical papules assumed to be due to nickel dermatitis with secondary generalized lichenoid spread was described. Of nine patients patch tested, all were positive to nickel [121].

Erythema multiforme-like dermatitis

- An erythema multiforme-type reaction may occur as either a primary allergic reaction to nickel or secondary spread from an initial reaction [122].

Mimicking sycosis barbae

- A 30-year-old presented with recurrent papular eruptions over his beard area. He had been treated for sycosis barbae several times with antibiotics but with no effect. He was patch test ++ for nickel. The foil on his razor was strongly DMG positive. When he changed to disposable plastic shavers with stainless steel blades, the dermatitis cleared completely within 8 weeks [123] *(isolated case report).*

Secondary spread

- Although not recently commented upon, secondary spread is an underemphasized and relatively under-recognized clinical aspect of nickel ACD. Nickel ACD has a remarkable ability to spread to secondary sites.
- In a series of 312 patients with ACD to nickel, of whom 95% had stocking suspender dermatitis on the thigh as the primary manifestation, Calnan [60] noted secondary spread in three-quarters of the patients. The sites of secondary spread recorded were:

Elbow flexures	79%
Eyelids	26.4%
Sides of neck	25.4%
Generalized	4.7%

- In a separate study Marcussen [124] found that, with the hands as the primary site, there was secondary spread to the face (25% of patients), elbow flexures (35%), and feet (25%). If the face/neck was the primary site, there was secondary spread to the breast in 32%, elbow flexures in 28%, and hands in 10%.

TOACS study and findings regarding nickel allergy

The Odense Adolescence Cohort Study on Atopic Diseases and Dermatitis (TOACS) study originally examined a cohort of Danish adolescents in 1995 to find the prevalence of contact allergy in adolescence and investigate its relationship with atopic dermatitis [85, 125, 126]. This cohort was subsequently reassessed later in life. The main findings with regards to nickel allergy were as follows:

- In the original study of 1501 schoolchildren aged 12–16 years, the most common contact allergy was nickel (8.6%), which was clinically relevant in 69% of cases.
- In the original study there was a significant association between nickel allergy and hand eczema.
- Nickel allergy was found most frequently in girls and the association with ear piercing was confirmed. Application of dental braces (oral nickel exposure) prior to ear piercing (cutaneous nickel exposure) was associated with a significantly reduced prevalence of nickel allergy.
- 442 of the original cohort were patch tested 15 years later. The point prevalence of nickel allergy was 11.8% (clinical relevance 80.8%). The 15-year incidence rate was 6.7%.
- Most new sensitizations were clinically relevant with strong reactions, and many participants reacted to low concentrations. Only a few positive reactions were lost.
- There was a significantly higher prevalence of nickel allergy amongst women who had their ears pierced before the implementation of nickel regulations in Denmark.

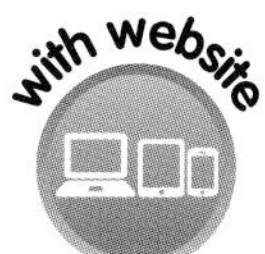

Go to www.wiley.com/go/mcfadden/common_contact_allergens to find the E-supplement for this chapter:

Nickel: E-Supplement

References

1 McDonagh, A.J., Wright, A.L., Cork, M.J., and Gawkrodger, D.J. (1992). Nickel sensitivity: the influence of ear piercing and atopy. *British Journal of Dermatology* 126 (1): 16–18.

2 Nakada, T., Iijima, M., Nakayama, H., and Maibach, H.I. (1997). Role of ear piercing in metal allergic contact dermatitis. *Contact Dermatitis* 36 (5): 233–236.

3 Herro, E.M., Jacob, S.E., and Scheman, A.J. (2012). Nickel exposure from household items: potential method of protection. *Dermatitis* 23 (4): 188–190.

4 Fischer, L.A., Menné, T., and Johansen, J.D. (2005). Experimental nickel elicitation thresholds – a review focusing on occluded nickel exposure. *Contact Dermatitis* 52 (2): 57–64.

5 Thyssen, J.P., Uter, W., Menne, T., and Liden, C. (2011). Revision of the European standard for control of the EU nickel restriction – a probable improvement for European citizens. *Contact Dermatitis* 65 (1): 60–61.

6 Thyssen, J.P., Skare, L., Lundgren, L. et al. (2010). Sensitivity and specificity of the nickel spot (dimethylglyoxime) test. *Contact Dermatitis* 62 (5): 279–288.

7 Shakoor, Z., Al-Mutairi, A.S., Al-Shenaifi, A.M. et al. (2017). Screening for skin-sensitizing allergens among patients with

clinically suspected allergic contact dermatitis. *Saudi Medical Journal* 38 (9): 922–927.

8 Fisher, A.A., Chargin, L., Fleischmajer, R., and Hyman, A. (1959). Pustular patch test reactions; with particular reference to those produced by ammonium fluoride. *Archives of Dermatology* 80: 742–752.

9 Thyssen, J.P., Linneberg, A., Menne, T., and Johansen, J.D. (2007). The epidemiology of contact allergy in the general population – prevalence and main findings. *Contact Dermatitis* 57 (5): 287–299.

10 Dotterud, L.K. and Smith-Sivertsen, T. (2007). Allergic contact sensitization in the general adult population: a population-based study from Northern Norway. *Contact Dermatitis* 56 (1): 10–15.

11 Thyssen, J.P., Ross-Hansen, K., Menne, T., and Johansen, J.D. (2010). Patch test reactivity to metal allergens following regulatory interventions: a 33-year retrospective study. *Contact Dermatitis* 63 (2): 102–106.

12 Fors, R., Persson, M., Bergstrom, E. et al. (2008). Nickel allergy – prevalence in a population of Swedish youths from patch test and questionnaire data. *Contact Dermatitis* 58 (2): 80–87.

13 Aguilar-Bernier, M., Bernal-Ruiz, A.I., Rivas-Ruiz, F. et al. (2012). Contact sensitization to allergens in the Spanish standard series at hospital Costa del Sol in Marbella, Spain: a retrospective study (2005-2010). *Actas Dermo-Sifiliograficas* 103 (3): 223–228.

14 Garcia-Gavin, J., Armario-Hita, J.C., Fernandez-Redondo, V. et al. (2011). Nickel allergy in Spain needs active intervention. *Contact Dermatitis* 64 (5): 289–291.

15 Pratt, M.D., Belsito, D.V., DeLeo, V.A. et al. (2004). North American contact dermatitis group patch-test results, 2001–2002 study period. *Dermatitis* 15 (4): 176–183.

16 Disphanurat, W. (2010). Contact allergy in eczema patients in Thammasat University Hospital. *Journal of the Medical Association of Thailand* 93 (Suppl 7): S7–S14.

17 Ni, C., Dou, X., Chen, J. et al. (2011). Contact sensitization in Chinese patients with hand eczema. *Dermatitis* 22 (4): 211–215.

18 Simonsen, A.B., Deleuran, M., Johansen, J.D., and Sommerlund, M. (2011). Contact allergy and allergic contact dermatitis in children – a review of current data. *Contact Dermatitis* 65 (5): 254–265.

19 Mortz, C.G., Kjaer, H.F., Eller, E. et al. (2013). Positive nickel patch tests in infants are of low clinical relevance and rarely reproducible. *Pediatric Allergy and Immunology* 24 (1): 84–87.

20 Johnke, H., Norberg, L.A., Vach, W. et al. (2004). Reactivity to patch tests with nickel sulfate and fragrance mix in infants. *Contact Dermatitis* 51 (3): 141–147.

21 Christiansen, E.S., Andersen, K.E., Bindslev-Jensen, C. et al. (2016). Low patch test reactivity to nickel in unselected adolescents tested repeatedly with nickel in infancy. *Pediatric Allergy and Immunology* 27 (6): 636–639.

22 Rietschl, R.L. and Fowler, F.J. (1995). *Fisher's Contact Dermatitis*. Chapter 6, 4e. Baltimore: Williams & Wilkins.

23 Fors, R., Persson, M., Bergstrom, E. et al. (2012). Lifestyle and nickel allergy in a Swedish adolescent population: effects of piercing, tattooing and orthodontic appliances. *Acta Dermato-Venereologica* 92 (6): 664–668.

24 Ehrlich, A., Kucenic, M., and Belsito, D.V. (2001). Role of body piercing in the induction of metal allergies. *American Journal of Contact Dermatitis* 12 (3): 151–155.

25 Davies, S.W. (1969). Nickel as cause of wedding-ring dermatitis. *British Medical Journal* 1 (5637): 188.

26 Kawai, K., Zhang, X.M., Nakagawa, M. et al. (1994). Allergic contact dermatitis due to mercury in a wedding ring and a cosmetic. *Contact Dermatitis* 31 (5): 330–331.

27 Paulshock, B.Z. (1969). Wedding ring dermatitis. *Journal of the American Medical Association* 207 (11): 2105.

28 Ermolli, M., Menne, C., Pozzi, G. et al. (2001). Nickel, cobalt and chromium-induced cytotoxicity and intracellular accumulation in human hacat keratinocytes. *Toxicology* 159 (1–2): 23–31.

29 Miller, S., Helms, A., and Brodell, R.T. (2007). Occlusive irritant dermatitis: when is "allergic" contact dermatitis not allergic? *Skinmed* 6 (2): 97–98.

30 Nygaard, U., Kralund, H.H., and Sommerlund, M. (2013). Allergic contact dermatitis induced by textile necklace. *Case Reports in Dermatology* 5 (3): 336–339.

31 Hausen, B.M. (1997). Allergic contact dermatitis from a wooden necklace. *American Journal of Contact Dermatitis* 8 (3): 185–187.

32 Brandrup, F. and Larsen, F.S. (1979). Nickel dermatitis provoked by buttons in blue jeans. *Contact Dermatitis* 5 (3): 148–150.

33 Suneja, T., Flanagan, K.H., and Glaser, D.A. (2007). Blue-jean button nickel: prevalence and prevention of its release from buttons. *Dermatitis* 18 (4): 208–211.

34 Byer, T.T. and Morrell, D.S. (2004). Periumbilical allergic contact dermatitis: blue jeans or belt buckles? *Pediatric Dermatology* 21 (3): 223–226.

35 Calnan, C.D. (1957). Nickel sensitivity in women. *International Archives of Allergy and Applied Immunology* 11 (1–2): 73–80.

36 Jacob, S.E. (2014). Underwire brassieres are a source of nickel exposure. *Pediatric Dermatology* 31 (2): e60.

37 Darlenski, R., Kazandjieva, J., and Pramatarov, K. (2012). The many faces of nickel allergy. *International Journal of Dermatology* 51 (5): 523–530.

38 Cheong, S.H., Choi, Y.W., Choi, H.Y., and Byun, J.Y. (2014). Nickel and cobalt release from jewellery and metal clothing items in Korea. *Contact Dermatitis* 70 (1): 11–18.

39 Jacob, S.E. and Matiz, C. (2011). Infant clothing snaps as a potential source of nickel exposure. *Pediatric Dermatology* 28 (3): 338 339.

40 Angelini, G., Vena, G.A., and Meneghini, C.L. (1980). Shoe contact dermatitis. *Contact Dermatitis* 6 (4): 279–283.

41 Goossens, A., Bedert, R., and Zimerson, E. (2001). Allergic contact dermatitis caused by nickel and cobalt in green plastic shoes. *Contact Dermatitis* 45 (3): 172.

42 Sainio, E.L., Jolanki, R., Hakala, E., and Kanerva, L. (2000). Metals and arsenic in eye shadows. *Contact Dermatitis* 42 (1): 5–10.

43 Thyssen, J.P., Linneberg, A., Menne, T. et al. (2010). No association between nickel allergy and reporting cosmetic dermatitis from mascara or eye shadow: a cross-sectional general population study. *Journal of the European Academy of Dermatology and Venereology* 24 (6): 722–725.

44 Corazza, M., Baldo, F., Pagnoni, A. et al. (2009). Measurement of nickel, cobalt and chromium in toy make-up by atomic absorption spectroscopy. *Acta Dermato-Venereologica* 89 (2): 130–133.

45 Lodén, M., Nilsson, G., Parvardeh, M. et al. (2012). No skin reactions to mineral powders in nickel-sensitive subjects. *Contact Dermatitis* 66 (4): 210–214.

46 Brandrup, F. (1991). Nickel eyelid dermatitis from an eyelash curler. *Contact Dermatitis* 25 (1): 77.

47 Romaguera, C. and Grimalt, F. (1985). Dermatitis from nickel eyelash curler. *Contact Dermatitis* 12 (3): 174.

48 Jacob, S.E., Silverberg, J.I., Rizk, C., and Silverberg, N. (2015). Nickel ferrule applicators: a source of nickel exposure in children. *Pediatric Dermatology* 32 (2): e62–e63.
49 Guarneri, F., Guarneri, C., and Cannavo, S.P. (2010). Nail-art and cobalt allergy. *Contact Dermatitis* 62 (5): 320–321.
50 Baxter, K.F. and Wilkinson, S.M. (2002). Contact dermatitis from a nickel-containing bindi. *Contact Dermatitis* 47 (1): 55.
51 Smith, E.L. and Calnan, C.D. (1966). Studies in contact dermatitis. XVII. Spectacle frames. *Transactions of the St John's Hospital Dermatological Society* 52 (1): 10–34.
52 Walsh, G. and Wilkinson, S.M. (2006). Materials and allergens within spectacle frames: a review. *Contact Dermatitis* 55 (3): 130–139.
53 Walsh, G. and Mitchell, J.W. (2002). Free surface nickel in CE-marked and non-CE-marked spectacle frames. *Ophthalmic & Physiological Optics* 22 (2): 166–171.
54 Scott, K., Levender, M.M., and Feldman, S.R. (2010). Eyeglass allergic contact dermatitis. *Dermatology Online Journal* 16 (9): 11.
55 Kim, I.S., Yoo, K.H., Kim, M.N. et al. (2013). The fine scratches of the spectacle frames and the allergic contact dermatitis. *Annals of Dermatology* 25 (2): 152–155.
56 Walsh, G. and Mitchell, J.W. (1998). The leaching of nickel from new and used metal spectacle frames. *Ophthalmic & Physiological Optics* 18 (4): 372–377.
57 Grimalt, F. and Romaguera, C. (1978). Nickel allergy and spectacle frame contact acne. *Contact Dermatitis* 4 (6): 377.
58 Thyssen, J.P., Milting, K., Bregnhøj, A. et al. (2009). Nickel allergy in patch-tested female hairdressers and assessment of nickel release from hairdressers' scissors and crochet hooks. *Contact Dermatitis* 61 (5): 281–286.
59 Dahlquist, I., Fregert, S., and Gruvberger, B. (1979). Release of nickel from plated utensils in permanent wave liquids. *Contact Dermatitis* 5 (1): 52–53.
60 Calnan, C.D. (1956). Nickel dermatitis. *British Journal of Dermatology* 68 (7): 229–236.
61 Thyssen, J.P., Menne, T., and Johansen, J.D. (2010). Identification of metallic items that caused nickel dermatitis in Danish patients. *Contact Dermatitis* 63 (3): 151–156.
62 Thyssen, J.P., Jensen, P., Johansen, J.D., and Menné, T. (2009). Contact dermatitis caused by nickel release from hair clasps purchased in a country covered by the EU nickel directive. *Contact Dermatitis* 60 (3): 180–181.
63 Ghaffar, S.A. and Todd, P.M. (2009). Chronic recurrent otitis externa secondary to allergic contact dermatitis to nickel and phosphorus sesquisulfide. *Contact Dermatitis* 61 (2): 124–125.
64 Hamann, D., Scheman, A.J., and Jacob, S.E. (2013). Nickel exposure from keys: alternatives for protection and prevention. *Dermatitis* 24 (4): 186–189.
65 Pazzaglia, M., Lucente, P., Vincenzi, C., and Tosti, A. (2000). Contact dermatitis from nickel in mobile phones. *Contact Dermatitis* 42 (6): 362–363.
66 Berk, D.R. and Bayliss, S.J. (2011). Cellular phone and cellular phone accessory dermatitis due to nickel allergy: report of five cases. *Pediatric Dermatology* 28 (3): 327–331.
67 Ozkaya, E. (2011). Bilateral symmetrical contact dermatitis on the face and outer thighs from the simultaneous use of two mobile phones. *Dermatitis* 22 (2): 116–118.
68 Richardson, C., Hamann, C.R., Hamann, D., and Thyssen, J.P. (2014). Mobile phone dermatitis in children and adults: a review of the literature. *Pediatric Allergy, Immunology, and Pulmonology* 27 (2): 60–69.
69 Livideanu, C., Giordano-Labadie, F., and Paul, C. (2007). Cellular phone addiction and allergic contact dermatitis to nickel. *Contact Dermatitis* 57 (2): 130–131.
70 Wohrl, S., Jandl, T., Stingl, G., and Kinaciyan, T. (2007). Mobile telephone as new source for nickel dermatitis. *Contact Dermatitis* 56 (2): 113.
71 Luo, J. and Bercovitch, L. (2008). Cellphone contact dermatitis with nickel allergy. *Canadian Medical Association Journal* 178 (1): 23–24.
72 Suarez, A., Chimento, S., and Tosti, A. (2011). Unusual localization of cell phone dermatitis. *Dermatitis* 22 (5): 277–278.
73 Dannepond, C. and Armingaud, P. (2012). Breast eczema: mobile phones must not be overlooked. *Annales de dermatologie et de venereologie* 139 (2): 142–143.
74 Jensen, P., Jellesen, M.S., Moller, P. et al. (2012). Nickel allergy and dermatitis following use of a laptop computer. *Journal of the American Academy of Dermatology* 67 (4): e170–e171.
75 Jacob, S.E. and Admani, S. (2014). Allergic contact dermatitis to a laptop computer in a child. *Pediatric Dermatology* 31 (3): 345–346.
76 (1968). Wrist-watch tinea. *British Medical Journal* 1 (5590): 464.
77 Jensen, P., Hamann, D., Hamann, C.R. et al. (2014). Nickel and cobalt release from children's toys purchased in Denmark and the United States. *Dermatitis* 25 (6): 356–365.
78 Overgaard, L.E., Engebretsen, K.A., Jensen, P. et al. (2016). Nickel released from children's toys is deposited on the skin. *Contact Dermatitis* 74 (6): 380–381.
79 Kanerva, L. and Estlander, T. (1995). Occupational allergic contact dermatitis associated with curious public nickel dermatitis from minimal exposure. *Contact Dermatitis* 32 (5): 309–310.
80 Lachiewicz, P.F., Watters, T.S., and Jacobs, J.J. (2016). Metal hypersensitivity and total knee arthroplasty. *Journal of the American Academy of Orthopaedic Surgeons* 24 (2): 106–112.
81 Basko-Plluska, J.L., Thyssen, J.P., and Schalock, P.C. (2011). Cutaneous and systemic hypersensitivity reactions to metallic implants. *Dermatitis* 22 (2): 65–79.
82 Frigerio, E., Pigatto, P.D., Guzzi, G., and Altomare, G. (2011). Metal sensitivity in patients with orthopaedic implants: a prospective study. *Contact Dermatitis* 64 (5): 273–279.
83 Verma, S.K. and Tobis, J.M. (2011). Explantation of patent foramen ovale closure devices: a multicenter survey. *JACC: Cardiovascular Interventions* 4 (5): 579–585.
84 Kanerva, L. and Forstrom, L. (2001). Allergic nickel and chromate hand dermatitis induced by orthopaedic metal implant. *Contact Dermatitis* 44 (2): 103–104.
85 Mortz, C.G., Lauritsen, J.M., Bindslev-Jensen, C., and Andersen, K.E. (2002). Nickel sensitization in adolescents and association with ear piercing, use of dental braces and hand eczema. The Odense Adolescence Cohort Study on Atopic Diseases and Dermatitis (TOACS). *Acta Dermato-Venereologica* 82 (5): 359–364.
86 Van Hoogstraten, I.M., Andersen, K.E., Von Blomberg, B.M. et al. (1991). Reduced frequency of nickel allergy upon oral nickel contact at an early age. *Clinical & Experimental Immunology* 85 (3): 441–445.
87 Kolokitha, O.E., Kaklamanos, E.G., and Papadopoulos, M.A. (2008). Prevalence of nickel hypersensitivity in orthodontic patients: a meta-analysis. *American Journal of Orthodontics and Dentofacial Orthopedics* 134 (6): 722 e1–e722. e12; discussion 722–3.

88 Kerosuo, H. and Kanerva, L. (1997). Systemic contact dermatitis caused by nickel in a stainless steel orthodontic appliance. *Contact Dermatitis* 36 (2): 112–113.

89 Pigatto, P.D. and Guzzi, G. (2004). Systemic contact dermatitis from nickel associated with orthodontic appliances. *Contact Dermatitis* 50 (2): 100–101.

90 Romaguera, C., Grimalt, F., and Vilaplana, J. (1985). Nickel dermatitis from an infusion needle. *Contact Dermatitis* 12 (3): 181.

91 Corazza, M., Maranini, C., Aleotti, A., and Virgili, A. (1998). Nickel contact dermatitis due to the needle of an infusion pump, confirmed by microanalysis. *Contact Dermatitis* 39 (3): 144.

92 Romaguera, C. and Grimalt, F. (1979). Nickel dermatitis from acupuncture needles. *Contact Dermatitis* 5 (3): 195.

93 Kanerva, L., Estlander, T., and Jolanki, R. (1993). Occupational allergic contact dermatitis from nickel in bartender's metallic measuring cup. *American Journal of Contact Dermatitis* 4 (1): 39–41.

94 Gawkrodger, D.J., Healy, J., and Howe, A.M. (1995). The prevention of nickel contact dermatitis. A review of the use of binding agents and barrier creams. *Contact Dermatitis* 32 (5): 257–265.

95 Meding, B., Barregard, L., and Marcus, K. (1994). Hand eczema in car mechanics. *Contact Dermatitis* 30 (3): 129–134.

96 Thyssen, J.P., Jensen, P., Liden, C. et al. (2011). Assessment of nickel and cobalt release from 200 unused hand-held work tools for sale in Denmark – sources of occupational metal contact dermatitis? *Science of the Total Environment* 409 (22): 4663–4666.

97 Thyssen, J.P., Gawkrodger, D.J., White, I.R. et al. (2013). Coin exposure may cause allergic nickel dermatitis: a review. *Contact Dermatitis* 68 (1): 3–14.

98 Kanerva, L., Kiilunen, M., Jolanki, R. et al. (1997). Hand dermatitis and allergic patch test reactions caused by nickel in electroplaters. *Contact Dermatitis* 36 (3): 137–140.

99 Gawkrodger, D.J., McLeod, C.W., and Dobson, K. (2012). Nickel skin levels in different occupations and an estimate of the threshold for reacting to a single open application of nickel in nickel-allergic subjects. *British Journal of Dermatology* 166 (1): 82–87.

100 Papa, G., Romano, A., Quaratino, D. et al. (2000). Contact dermatoses in metal workers. *International Journal of Immunopathology and Pharmacology* 13 (1): 43–47.

101 Rystedt, I. and Fischer, T. (1983). Relationship between nickel and cobalt sensitization in hard metal workers. *Contact Dermatitis* 9 (3): 195–200.

102 Jue, M.S., Kim, Y.S., and Ro, Y.S. (2010). Fiddler's neck accompanied by allergic contact dermatitis to nickel in a Viola player. *Annals of Dermatology* 22 (1): 88–90.

103 Macháckvá, J. and Pock, L. (1986). Occupational nickel dermatitis in a cellist. *Contact Dermatitis* 15(1): 41–42.

104 Marshman, G. and Kennedy, C.T. (1992). Guitar-string dermatitis. *Contact Dermatitis* 26 (2): 134.

105 Inoue, A., Shoji, A., and Fujita, T. (1997). Flautist's chin. *British Journal of Dermatology* 136 (1): 147.

106 Nakamura, M., Arima, Y., Nobuhara, S., and Miyachi, Y. (1999). Nickel allergy in a trumpet player. *Contact Dermatitis* 40 (4): 219–220.

107 Jacob, S.E. and Herro, E.M. (2010). School-issued musical instruments: a significant source of nickel exposure. *Dermatitis* 21 (6): 332–333.

108 Fisher, A.A. (1993). Allergic contact dermatitis from musical instruments. *Cutis* 51 (2): 75–76.

109 Freeman, S. and Stephens, R. (1999). Cheilitis: analysis of 75 cases referred to a contact dermatitis clinic. *American Journal of Contact Dermatitis* 10 (4): 198–200.

110 Gumulka, M., Matura, M., Lidén, C. et al. (2015). Nickel exposure when working out in the gym. *Acta Dermato-Venereologica* 95 (2): 247–249.

111 Samimi, S.S., Siegfried, E., and Belsito, D.V. (2004). A diagnostic pearl: the school chair sign. *Cutis* 74 (1): 27–28.

112 Fowler, J.F. Jr. and Storrs, F.J. (2001). Nickel allergy and dyshidrotic eczema: are they related? *American Journal of Contact Dermatitis* 12 (2): 119–121.

113 Fowler, J.F. (1992). Disulfiram is effective for nickel allergic hand eczema. *American Journal of Contact Dermatitis* 3 (4): 175–178.

114 Nielsen, G.D., Soderberg, U., Jorgensen, P.J. et al. (1999). Absorption and retention of nickel from drinking water in relation to food intake and nickel sensitivity. *Toxicology and Applied Pharmacology* 154 (1): 67–75.

115 Cressey, B.D. and Scheinman, P.L. (2012). Periocular dermatitis from systemic exposure to nickel in a palatal expander and dental braces. *Dermatitis* 23 (4): 179.

116 Bibas, N., Lassere, J., Paul, C. et al. (2013). Nickel-induced systemic contact dermatitis and intratubal implants: the baboon syndrome revisited. *Dermatitis* 24 (1): 35–36.

117 Danese, P. and Bertazzoni, M.G. (1995). Lymphomatoid contact dermatitis due to nickel. *Contact Dermatitis* 33 (4): 268–269.

118 Houck, H.E., Wirth, F.A., and Kauffman, C.L. (1997). Lymphomatoid contact dermatitis caused by nickel. *American Journal of Contact Dermatitis* 8 (3): 175–176.

119 Kim, H.I., Kim, D.H., Yoon, M.S. et al. (1991). Two cases of nickel dermatitis showing vitiligo-like depigmentations. *Yonsei Medical Journal* 32 (1): 79–81.

120 Silvestre, J.F., Botella, R., Ramon, R. et al. (2001). Periumbilical contact vitiligo appearing after allergic contact dermatitis to nickel. *American Journal of Contact Dermatitis* 12 (1): 43–44.

121 Sharma, V., Beyer, D.J., Paruthi, S., and Nopper, A.J. (2002). Prominent pruritic periumbilical papules: allergic contact dermatitis to nickel. *Pediatric Dermatology* 19 (2): 106–109.

122 Cook, L.J. (1982). Associated nickel and cobalt contact dermatitis presenting as erythema multiforme. *Contact Dermatitis* 8 (4): 280–281.

123 Goh, C.L. and Ng, S.K. (1987). Nickel dermatitis mimicking sycosis barbae. *Contact Dermatitis* 16 (1): 42.

124 Marcussen, P.V. (1957). Spread of nickel dermatitis. *Dermatologica* 115 (4): 596–607.

125 Mortz, C.G., Bindslev-Jensen, C., and Andersen, K.E. (2013). Nickel allergy from adolescence to adulthood in the TOACS cohort. *Contact Dermatitis* 68 (6): 348–356.

126 Mortz, C.G., Lauritsen, J.M., Bindslev-Jensen, C., and Andersen, K.E. (2002). Contact allergy and allergic contact dermatitis in adolescents: prevalence measures and associations. The Odense Adolescence Cohort Study on Atopic Diseases and Dermatitis (TOACS). *Acta Dermato-Venereologica* 82 (5): 352–358.

CHAPTER 11

Cobalt

CHAPTER CONTENTS

Key points

- Cobalt is present in low-carat jewelry.
- Cobalt can be present in some metal clothing items such as belt buckles and hairpins. It can be present in metal spectacle frames.
- Cobalt can be present in leather items.
- Cobalt allergy is more common in females and in patients under 40 years of age.
- Approximately two-thirds of patients with cobalt allergy will also have nickel allergy.
- Occupational allergic contact dermatitis to cobalt has been reported in construction and cement workers, leather and textile workers, workers using hard metals, pottery painters, money handlers, and machine operatives.
- There have been rare case reports of cobalt allergy and possible prosthesis failure (controversial).
- Cobalt allergy has been reported to cause granulomatous tattoo reactions and a purpuric dermatosis.
- A cobalt spot test exists for identifying significant cobalt release from metal objects and for the presence of cobalt on skin.
- The association of cobalt (and other metal allergies) with both vesicular hand eczema and discoid eczema remains unexplained.

Introduction

The original name for cobalt was "*kobold*," a German word meaning goblin because cobalt ore contains arsenic and so was toxic to early German smelters. The metal's unique properties mean that it is wear resistant, oxidation resistant, ferromagnetic, and conducts electricity. Cobalt is also a bio-essential element and is found in the center of vitamin B12.

It is a component of alloys used in the manufacture of jewelry. "Cobalt blue" is cobalt(II) aluminate ($CoAl_2O_4$) and is widely used in paints and glassware. Cobalt is used in the catalyzation processes of the petroleum and chemical industries, as one of the drying agents for paints, in varnishes, dyes and pigments, and is an essential metal in data recording devices such as hard disk drives and in the manufacture of rechargeable batteries. Its hard wearing properties mean that it is also used in the production of

Common Contact Allergens: A Practical Guide to Detecting Contact Dermatitis, First Edition. Edited by John McFadden, Pailin Puangpet, Korbkarn Pongpairoj, Supitchaya Thaiwat, and Lee Shan Xian.

© 2020 John Wiley & Sons Ltd. Published 2020 by John Wiley & Sons Ltd.

Companion website: www.wiley.com/go/mcfadden/common_contact_allergens

carbides (hard metals) and corrosion- and wear-resistant metal alloys used in heavy industries. Occupational contact dermatitis from cobalt has been reported in hairdressers, barbers, builders and construction workers, checkout operators, machine operatives, and domestic cleaners [1].

Patch testing

- Cobalt chloride 5% pet in the baseline series or the T.R.U.E.® test equivalent.
- False-positive purpuric, follicular, and pustular reactions can occur.
- As with other metal allergens, false-positive reactions frequently occur in patients with atopic eczema or dry skin with macular erythema and scaling but no induration or vesiculation.

Age

- Cobalt allergy is particularly common in individuals under the age of 40, especially amongst women and in conjunction with nickel allergy.

Sex

- More common in females (approximately 3:2), particularly in conjunction with nickel allergy.

Frequency of sensitization

- High prevalence in dermatitis patients, ranging from 4.4% to 10.8% in Europe [2, 3], approximately 10% in America [4], and averaging 3.4% to 8.0% in Asia [5, 6].
- The high rate of false positives on patch testing means that these figures should be interpreted carefully.

Clinical

Common presentations

- Cobalt allergy classically presents as a dermatitis reaction to the metal in jewelry, clothing such as a jean button, stud or belt buckle, and spectacle frames. In this way, common clinical presentations are often both similar to and can be associated with allergic contact dermatitis (ACD) to nickel.

Cobalt allergy and hand dermatitis

- A group of subjects who were cobalt allergic but chromate negative – when compared to a control group who were patch test negative to both – was more likely to have dermatitis affecting the hands and current involvement of the face and arms [7]. The most common sources of cobalt exposure were earrings and leather.
- Cobalt chloride allergy, together with other metal allergies, has been reported to be associated with vesicular hand eczema [8].
- Patients with hand dermatitis due to cement can sometimes have cobalt hypersensitivity in addition to chromium. Although several studies suggest a relationship between oral ingestion of cobalt and vesicular hand eczema in both sensitized and non-sensitized subjects, they have often involved high supra-dietary doses of cobalt and the evidence presented is limited. Low-cobalt diets have neither been a consistently successful nor standardized form of therapy [8–10].

Leather dermatitis

- The first case of ACD to cobalt from leather involved the dorsal aspects of the feet and lower legs from resting the legs on a leather cushion at home [11]. The second case was ACD to cobalt in a leather couch affecting the hands, trunk, and legs. Cobalt levels were identified at 802 ppm (cushion) and 1250 ppm (couch) [11]. The authors note that cobalt may be a potential source of ACD in exposure to leather furniture and clothes.

Discoid eczema

- The most common positive allergens in discoid eczema ($n = 1022$) were nickel sulfate (10.2%), potassium dichromate (7.3%), and cobalt chloride (6.1%). Women had a higher rate of allergy to cobalt chloride [12]. There appears to be a significant association between metal allergy and discoid eczema. However, it has been difficult to prove if metal allergy is a direct cause or if discoid eczema is a manifestation of secondary spread of metal allergy. Potential false-positive patch tests to metal salts should also be considered.

Asthma

- Cobalt-induced asthma is almost exclusively an occupational disease in workers exposed to airborne metal, e.g. welders and metal grinders. Symptoms include wheezing, cough, and shortness of breath. Atopic subjects are more prone. Reactions can be both immunoglobulin-E (IgE) and non-IgE mediated and the majority have positive prick tests to cobalt. Symptoms resolve when the patients are away from work [13].

Non-eczematous contact dermatitis

- Contact with cobalt can trigger both *purpuric lesions* and *sarcoidal-like granulomatous tattoo* reactions [14].

Urticaria

- Type IV hypersensitivity to cobalt is not associated with urticaria. However, there are two single case reports of what was described as urticarial dermatitis that was possibly associated with the insertion of a hip prosthesis in patients with cobalt allergy (positive patch tests) [15, 16].

Case reports

- *Leather couch.* A 66-year-old man developed a chronic generalized dermatitis that was refractory to multiple therapies. He also developed palmoplantar vesicular dermatitis. Patch testing demonstrated a single positive reaction to cobalt (+). He had contact with cobalt from the use of a leather couch for 9 years. After avoidance of the leather couch, the dermatitis improved rapidly and the hand eczema also resolved. However, other unidentified allergens within the leather couch were not excluded with certainty [17].
- A 74-year-old man with severe ischemic cardiomyopathy and paroxysmal atrial fibrillation had a *cardioverter-defibrillator* implanted in the anterior chest wall. Eight months after the implantation, the patient developed a painful and erythematous rash with pruritus over the site of the device. Skin biopsy confirmed the diagnosis of eczema and he was patch tested to cobalt/nickel, epoxy resin, titanium, silicone rubber, and polyurethane. There was a single strong positive reaction to cobalt chloride. The pacemaker and defibrillator leads were made of a metal alloy that consisted of cobalt, nickel, and chromium. The patient was diagnosed with cobalt ACD and responded to corticosteroid therapy [18].
- A single case report describes cobalt allergy to a *dental prosthesis* presenting as a persistent edematous rash of the eyelids and lips [19]. Patch testing revealed a +++ reaction to cobalt chloride and the symptoms were reproduced with a single blind oral provocation test. One week after removal of the dental prosthesis device, the patient's symptoms cleared completely and there was no recurrence on insertion of a new cobalt-free prosthesis.
- A 58-year-old man presented with multiple firm nodules on the right side of the neck and left cheek for 5 years. The nodules appeared after he was accidentally struck with unknown particles whilst sawing. The histopathological results showed lymphoid follicles with germinal center-like structures, with foreign bodies. X-ray microanalysis of the foreign bodies identified tungsten coating small cobalt particles. He was patch tested with a positive reaction to cobalt chloride and a ?+ reaction to tungsten chloride. Lymphocyte transformation tests were positive for cobalt but negative for tungsten. He was diagnosed with *cobalt allergy induced lymphoma cutis* [20].
- Allergic reactions to the cobalt component of *cyanocobalamin* are likely to be exceedingly rare. There are two reports of reactions; in one the injection site becoming red and sore. One patient presented with cheilitis after oral ingestion of B12. Both had positive patch test reactions to cobalt [21].

Occupational dermatitis

- A large retrospective analysis identified that the most common occupations associated with cobalt allergy-related occupational dermatitis were builders, building contractors, retail cash checkout operators, machine operatives, hairdressers, barbers, and domestic cleaners. The authors noted that cobalt-related dermatitis seems to have an early onset and may affect a wide range of occupations [1].
- A large study found that patients with cobalt and chromate co-sensitization were significantly more likely to have occupational skin disease, especially in the construction industry and presumably from cement exposure [22].
- In another large retrospective study, there was a significant association between female patients who had a positive reaction to cobalt and work in the textile and leatherwork industries [23].
- Hard metal workers are more likely to be allergic to cobalt, especially those performing hand etching and hand grinding which are often associated with friction and trauma [21]. Hard metals consist of carbides with cobalt used as a binding agent and they have a high degree of wear resistance. They are used in rock drills, cutting tools, engraving/stamping, and in parts exposed to heavy strain [21].
- A 28-year-old male baker presented with a 6-month history of vesicular hand dermatitis predominantly involving the lateral aspects of the proximal phalanges. He had worked as a baker for 12 years and handled metal baking equipment approximately 100 times in a single working day. He did not use protective gloves and held the baking metal with the lateral aspects of his digits. The dermatitis improved away from work. He was patch tested with a baseline, fragrance, rubber, and baker's series. There was a single + positive reaction to cobalt chloride. A cobalt spot test on the corroded parts of the baker metal sheet was positive [24].

Exposure and release

A handling study of discs showed significant deposition of cobalt after 30 minutes of handling, especially cobalt without the presence of chromium [25].

Jewelry and clothing

- Several studies have looked at the frequency of releasable cobalt from metal jewelry, as adjudged by the percentage that were positive to a cobalt spot test. These are summarized as:

  Study 1 (Korea): 6.2% of 471 items branded jewelry 4.2%, non-branded jewelry 5%, branded belts 40%, branded hairpins 44.4% (more than non-branded belts and hairpins – we speculate that the reason is because cobalt is more expensive), zippers 100%, buttons 10% [26].

  Study 2 (Germany): 38/87 earrings (44% at least one part), posts 22% [27].

  Study 3 (China and Thailand): dark earrings 16% [28].

  Study 4: belts 0.5% from China, 0.9% from America (note large difference from Study 1) [29].

Orthopedic prostheses

Cobalt allergy due to orthopedic devices is only rarely thought to cause clinical problems.

- Cobalt spot tests were performed on 98 cobalt-containing hip implant components removed from patients. 10.2% of these components showed positive reactions and the allergen was detected from the femoral but not from the acetabular components [30].
- Free cobalt, nickel, and chromium (VI) release was assessed in 52 failed hip implants. 3/38 (8%) removed femoral heads and 1/25 (4%) femoral stems – all made from CoCrMo alloys – had positive cobalt spot tests. It is not clear if metal ions released from the prosthetic joints caused sensitization and inflammatory reactions in the surrounding tissue that contributed to implant failure [31].
- 100 patients referred for total hip (48 patients) or total knee (52 patients) arthroplasty, which included metal alloys, were patch tested to metals both preoperatively and 1 year postoperatively. The rate of positive patch test reactions to metals 1 year after surgery increased from 22% to 29% ($p = 0.34$, no statistical significance). Five of 72 patients who had initially tested negative for a metal allergy became positive for metal constituents of the prosthesis. Four were allergic to nickel and one to cobalt. None had a positive reaction to titanium or vanadium. The authors noted that the increase in metal sensitization in 1 year after implantation implied that the prosthesis could be the cause of metal sensitization but this was not associated – albeit in these cases – with joint failure [32].
- The rates of positive patch tests to nickel, chromium, and cobalt were compared between patients with and without revision joint surgery. Revision surgery was not associated with a higher prevalence of metal allergy. However, patients who required two or more surgical revisions demonstrated a higher rate of positive patch tests to cobalt and chromium. Nickel showed a low prevalence of positive reactions whilst cobalt showed a slightly higher rate (4.1% vs 6.3%). No association was found between a previous diagnosis of metal allergy and subsequent failure of an implantation that required revision surgery [33].

Single case reports

- A 54-year-old female had left hip pain after total hip arthroplasty with a conventional polyethylene and cobalt-chromium head. Computed tomography (CT) revealed a cystic lesion at the iliopsoas muscle anterior to the acetabulum; histopathology revealed necrotic tissues and neovascularization with lymphocytic and plasma cell infiltration. She had a positive patch test to cobalt-chromium. The prosthetic joint was removed with debridement of the granulation tissue [34].
- A 53-year-old woman with metal-on-metal (cobalt-chromium-molybdenum) L5–S1 total disc replacement (TDR) developed recurrent back pain, bilateral radicular pain as well as bilateral leg weakness 2 months postoperatively. CT myelography revealed a soft tissue mass within the canal and the foramina. The patient had positive patch tests to cobalt chloride and chromium. On removal of the device, a granulomatous mass with diffuse metallic debris particles was seen on histology. The patient's symptoms improved within 1 year [35].

Dental alloys

While dental alloys and instruments release cobalt, reported clinical reactions are rare and confined to single case reports only.

- 6/8 (75%) dental alloys were positive to cobalt spot testing [30].
- 61 dental instruments and alloys used by dental technicians showed release of cobalt, chromium, and nickel. 23 (38%) had a positive cobalt spot test and 20 (33%) released nickel. Twenty-one instruments and five dental alloys were tested in artificial sweat: all the instruments released cobalt, and all the dental alloys released cobalt with lesser release of nickel and chromium [36].

Metal stents

- Allergy to an everolimus-eluting cobalt chromium stent caused recurrent multi-vessel in-stent restenosis confirmed by positive patch testing to the stent. Oral prednisolone caused resolution of the clinical symptoms [37].

Mobile phones

- 72 mobile phones from different brands in America were spot tested for nickel and cobalt release. The testing areas included buttons, keypads, speakers, and cameras. 24/72 (33%) mobile phones had a positive result to nickel spot test and 10/72 (14%) showed a positive reaction to cobalt spot test. 90.5% of flip phones tested positive for nickel and 52.4% for cobalt [38].

Leather

- Of 15 samples of leather couches, only a single sample of dark-brown colored leather was positive for cobalt detection [17].
- 7/12 leather swatches contained cobalt in excess of 100 ppm with one in excess of 1000 ppm [39].

Polymers, polyesters

- Cobalt is sometimes used in the curing process of polyester [21]. Whether it can be retained in polyester products in concentrations high enough to cause ACD is controversial.

Pottery and paint

- Wet blue and black pottery are potential sources of cobalt exposure. See Cobalt: E-Supplement for a more detailed description.

Cosmetics

- A 37-year-old female presented with dermatitis of the palms and periungual skin. She was patch tested to the baseline series, acrylates, and latex series and had a strongly positive reaction to cobalt chloride (+++). Cobalt was not contained within the nail polish but she had also added a glittering color that contained cobalt. After the patient removed the nail art, the dermatitis cleared completely within 4 weeks [40].

- 66/88 (75%) eye shadows tested contained more than 5 ppm of at least one metallic element. The authors noted that the high concentrations of cobalt and nickel in eye shadow products had the potential to cause ACD [41]. *(Note: controversial.)*

Cobalt spot test

- In 2010, Thyssen et al. reported a screening test for cobalt content in personal or work place objects. The spot test included 0.1% oxalic acid, 0.02% disodium-1-nitroso-2-naphthol-3,6-disulfonate, and 5.0% sodium acetate in deionized water. They reported two types of spot tests: a solution and a gel that could detect the presence of cobalt down to 8.3 ppm. A positive reaction is indicated by the yellow colored solution or gel turning red. Positive results were reported in 8/9 cobalt discs that also gave positive patch tests in cobalt-allergic patients. They did not detect any false-positive reactions to metal discs not containing cobalt [42]. The same authors also note that the cobalt spot test can indicate the presence of available cobalt on skin (0.125 μg/cm^2) as well [43].

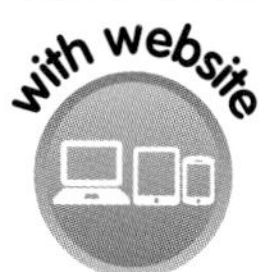

Go to www.wiley.com/go/mcfadden/common_contact_allergens to find the E-supplement for this chapter:

Cobalt: E-Supplement

References

1 Athavale, P., Shum, K.W., Chen, Y. et al. (2007). Occupational dermatitis related to chromium and cobalt: experience of dermatologists (EPIDERM) and occupational physicians (OPRA) in the U.K. over an 11-year period (1993–2004). *British Journal of Dermatology* 157 (3): 518–522.

2 Bordel-Gómez, M.T., Miranda-Romero, A., and Castrodeza-Sanz, J. (2010). Epidemiology of contact dermatitis: prevalence of sensitization to different allergens and associated factors. *Actas Dermo-Sifiliográficas* 101 (1): 59–75.

3 Mahler, V., Geier, J., and Schnuch, A. (2014). Current trends in patch testing – new data from the German Contact Dermatitis Research Group (DKG) and the Information Network of Departments of Dermatology (IVDK). *Journal der Deutschen Dermatologischen Gesellschaft* 12 (7): 583–592.

4 Davis, M.D., Scalf, L.A., Yiannias, J.A. et al. (2008). Changing trends and allergens in the patch test standard series. a mayo clinic 5-year retrospective review, January 1, 2001, through December 31, 2005. *Archives of Dermatology* 144 (1): 67–72.

5 Lim, J.T., Goh, C.L., Ng, S.K., and Wong, W.K. (1992). Changing trends in the epidemiology of contact dermatitis in Singapore. *Contact Dermatitis.* 26 (5): 321–326.

6 Khatami, A., Nassiri-Kashani, M., Gorouhi, F. et al. (2013). Allergic contact dermatitis to metal allergens in Iran. *International Journal of Dermatology* 52 (12): 1513–1518.

7 Bregnbak, D., Thyssen, J.P., Zachariae, C. et al. (2015). Association between cobalt allergy and dermatitis caused by leather articles – a questionnaire study. *Contact Dermatitis* 72 (2): 106–114.

8 Veien, N.K. and Kaaber, K. (1979). Nickel, cobalt and chromium sensitivity in patients with pompholyx (dyshidrotic eczema). *Contact Dermatitis* 5 (6): 371–374.

9 Stuckert, J. and Nedorost, S. (2008). Low-cobalt diet for dyshidrotic eczema patients. *Contact Dermatitis* 59 (6): 361–365.

10 Veien, N.K., Hattel, T., Justesen, O., and Nørholm, A. (1983). Oral challenge with metal salts. (I). Vesicular patch-test-negative hand eczema. *Contact Dermatitis* 9 (5): 402–406.

11 Bregnbak, D., Opstrup, M.S., Jellesen, M.S. et al. (2017). Allergic contact dermatitis caused by cobalt in leather – clinical cases. *Contact Dermatitis* 76 (6): 366–368.

12 Bonamonte, D., Foti, C., Vestita, M. et al. (2012). Nummular eczema and contact allergy: a retrospective study. *Dermatitis* 23 (4): 153–157.

13 Walters, G.I., Robertson, A.S., Moore, V.C., and Burge, P.S. (2014). Cobalt asthma in metalworkers from an automotive engine valve manufacturer. *Occupational Medicine* 64 (5): 358–364.

14 Brandão, M.H. and Gontijo, B. (2012). Contact sensitivity to metals (chromium, cobalt and nickel) in childhood. *Anais Brasileiros de Dermatologia* 87 (2): 269–276.

15 Wong, C.C. and Nixon, R.L. (2014). Systemic allergic dermatitis caused by cobalt and cobalt toxicity from a metal on a metal hip replacement. *Contact Dermatitis* 71 (2): 113–114.

16 Nath, P.I. and Coop, C.A. (2014). Rash and a patch test result positive for cobalt in a patient with a hip replacement. *Annals of Allergy, Asthma & Immunology* 113 (2): 230–232.

17 Thyssen, J.P., Johansen, J.D., Jellesen, M.S. et al. (2013). Consumer leather exposure: an unrecognized cause of cobalt sensitization. *Contact Dermatitis* 69 (5): 276–279.

18 Citerne, O., Gomes, S., Scanu, P., and Milliez, P. (2011). Painful eczema mimicking pocket infection in a patient with an ICD: a rare cause of skin allergy to nickel/cobalt alloy. *Circulation* 123 (11): 1241–1242.

19 Vicente, J. and España, A. (1997). Palpebral oedema associated with sensitization to cobalt in a dental prosthesis. *British Journal of Dermatology* 136 (6): 971–972.

20 Miyamoto, T., Iwasaki, K., Mihara, Y. et al. (1997). Lymphocytoma cutis induced by cobalt. *British Journal of Dermatology* 137 (3): 469–471.

21 Fowler, J.F. Jr. (2016). Cobalt. *Dermatitis: Contact, Atopic, Occupational, Drug* 27 (1): 3–8.

22 Hegewald, J., Uter, W., Pfahlberg, A. et al. (2005). A multifactorial analysis of concurrent patch-test reactions to nickel, cobalt, and chromate. *Allergy* 60 (3): 372–378.

23 Rui, F., Bovenzi, M., Prodi, A. et al. (2010). Nickel, cobalt and chromate sensitization and occupation. *Contact Dermatitis* 62 (4): 225–231.

24 Bregnbak, D., Zachariae, C., and Thyssen, J.P. (2015). Occupational exposure to metallic cobalt in a baker. *Contact Dermatitis* 72 (2): 118–119.

25 Midander, K., Julander, A., Skare, L., and Lidén, C. (2014). Cobalt skin dose resulting from short and repetitive contact with hard metals. *Contact Dermatitis* 70 (6): 361–368.
26 Cheong, S.H., Choi, Y.W., Choi, H.Y., and Byun, J.Y. (2014). Nickel and cobalt release from jewellery and metal clothing items in Korea. *Contact Dermatitis* 70 (1): 11–18.
27 Uter, W., Schmid, M., Schmidt, O. et al. (2014). Cobalt release from earrings and piercing jewellery – analytical results of a German survey. *Contact Dermatitis* 70 (6): 369–375.
28 Hamann, C., Hamann, D., Hamann, K.K., and Thyssen, J.P. (2011). Cobalt release from inexpensive earrings from Thailand and China. *Contact Dermatitis* 64 (4): 238–240.
29 Hamann, D., Hamann, C., Li, L.F. et al. (2012). The Sino-American belt study: nickel and cobalt exposure, epidemiology, and clinical considerations. *Dermatitis* 23 (3): 117–123.
30 Thyssen, J.P., Menné, T., Lidén, C. et al. (2012). Cobalt release from implants and consumer items and characteristics of cobalt sensitized patients with dermatitis. *Contact Dermatitis* 66 (3): 113–122.
31 Jakobsen, S.S., Lidén, C., Soballe, K. et al. (2014). Failure of total hip implants: metals and metal release in 52 cases. *Contact Dermatitis* 71 (6): 319–325.
32 Frigerio, E., Pigatto, P.D., Guzzi, G., and Altomare, G. (2011). Metal sensitivity in patients with orthopaedic implants: a prospective study. *Contact Dermatitis* 64 (5): 273–279.
33 Munch, H.J., Jacobsen, S.S., Olesen, J.T. et al. (2015). The association between metal allergy, total knee arthroplasty, and revision. *Acta Orthopaedica* 86 (3): 378–383.
34 Kosukegawa, I., Nagoya, S., Kaya, M. et al. (2011). Revision total hip arthroplasty due to pain from hypersensitivity to cobalt-chromium in total hip arthroplasty. *Journal of Arthroplasty* 26 (6): 978 e1-3.
35 Zairi, F., Remacle, J.M., Allaoui, M., and Assaker, R. (2013). Delayed hypersensitivity reaction caused by metal-on-metal total disc replacement. *Journal of Neurosurgery. Spine* 19 (3): 389–391.
36 Kettelarij J.A., Lidén C., Axén, E., and Julander, A. (2014). Cobalt, nickel and chromium release from dental tools and alloys. *Contact Dermatitis* 70 (1): 3–10.
37 Nakajima, Y., Itoh, T., and Morino, Y. (2016). Metal allergy to everolimus-eluting cobalt chromium stents confirmed by positive skin testing as a cause of recurrent multivessel in-stent restenosis. *Catheterization and Cardiovascular Interventions* 87 (4): E137–E142.
38 Aquino, M., Mucci, T., Chong, M. et al. (2013). Mobile phones: potential sources of nickel and cobalt exposure for metal allergic patients. *Pediatric Allergy, Immunology, and Pulmonology* 26 (4): 181–186.
39 Hamann, D., Hamann, C.R., Kishi, P. et al. (2016). Leather contains cobalt and poses a risk of allergic contact dermatitis: cobalt indicator solution and X-ray florescence spectrometry as screening tests. *Dermatitis: Contact, Atopic, Occupational, Drug* 27 (4): 202–207.
40 Guarneri, F., Guarneri, C., and Cannavo, S.P. (2010). Nail-art and cobalt allergy. *Contact Dermatitis* 62 (5): 320–321.
41 Sainio, E.L., Jolanki, R., Hakala, E., and Kanerva, L. (2000). Metals and arsenic in eye shadows. *Contact Dermatitis* 42 (1): 5–10.
42 Thyssen, J.P., Menné, T., Johansen, J.D. et al. (2010). A spot test for detection of cobalt release – early experience and findings. *Contact Dermatitis* 63 (2): 63–69.
43 Midander, K., Julander, A., Skare, L. et al. (2013). The cobalt spot test – further insights into its performance and use. *Contact Dermatitis* 69 (5): 280–287.

Exposure Color Code

- Clothing, jewelry, adornments
- Personal care products, cosmetics/cosmetic procedures
- Household products, domestic environment, including furniture, refurbishment
- Occupational dermatoses, work environment
- Medicines, surgical/dental procedures, herbal/alternative medicines, medical
- Personal appliances/aids
- Leisure activities, sport, travel
- Other exposures (including dietary)
- Not relevant or multiple/general exposure

CHAPTER 12

Chromate

CHAPTER CONTENTS

Key points

- The two most common causes of chromate allergic contact dermatitis (ACD) are from exposure to leather and cement.
- The two most commonly affected areas are the feet and hands.
- Chromate hand dermatitis can be severe and has a poor prognosis.
- Chromate ACD can have a detrimental effect on quality of life.
- The frequency of contact allergy in European clinics (1950–2012) has a median average of 6.5% but there has been a gradual reduction over this time and the reported UK clinic rate is 2.1%.
- Chromate is one of the most common causes of occupational contact dermatitis and is particularly prevalent amongst bricklayers/cement workers, other construction workers, leather manufacturers, and chrome platers.
- The hexavalent form of chromate penetrates the skin to a greater extent than the trivalent form and causes more reactions.
- EU legislation has indicated that the concentration of chromium(VI) in cement used on the market should not exceed 2 ppm; this has subsequently led to a reduction in the incidence of cement ACD.
- Occupational asthma due to chromate (e.g. in welders) has been reported.
- Chromate allergic subjects often co-react to other metals.
- ACD to chromate in leather is one of the most common causes of shoe dermatitis. Adults with foot dermatitis and children with either foot dermatitis or juvenile plantar dermatosis have significant rates of footwear contact allergy.
- Other sources of leather exposure leading to chromate ACD include gloves, watchstraps, sofas, jackets, steering wheel covers, hat bands, and tefillin (small leather boxes strapped to the skin for religious purposes).
- Chrome tattoo dermatitis usually involves the green pigment. It can be triggered by ACD to chromate elsewhere, e.g. cement hand dermatitis.
- Orthopedic and dental prostheses are uncommon causes of chromate sensitization.
- As with other metals, false-positive patch test reactions to chromate are common, particularly in patients with atopic dermatitis.
- Approximately 10% of chromate allergic subjects will react to 10 ppm hexavalent chromate (single exposure).

Common Contact Allergens: A Practical Guide to Detecting Contact Dermatitis, First Edition. Edited by John McFadden, Pailin Puangpet, Korbkarn Pongpairoj, Supitchaya Thaiwat, and Lee Shan Xian.

© 2020 John Wiley & Sons Ltd. Published 2020 by John Wiley & Sons Ltd.

Companion website: www.wiley.com/go/mcfadden/common_contact_allergens

Age

- More common in the older age group, e.g. over 40 years (unlike nickel and cobalt).
- There is a significantly high prevalence in children, especially with regards to ACD to footwear.

Sex

- ACD to chromate is traditionally more common in males, with many studies showing a significant difference in frequency between the sexes (unlike nickel and cobalt).
- However, in some areas of the world where cement dermatitis has become less prevalent, leather becomes the most important cause of chromate ACD and the sex ratio shifts away from males toward females.

Atopic dermatitis

- There is a trend towards a higher frequency in atopic dermatitis patients. However, interpreting data regarding metal allergy in relation to atopic dermatitis status can be difficult due to the high rates of false-positive patch test reactions to metals amongst atopic dermatitis patients.

Frequency of sensitization

- General population: median 3%, range 0.5–9.1%.
- European clinics: median 6.5%, range 2.1–17.6%.
- American clinics: median 8%, range 2.4–10.6%.
- Asian clinics: median 7%, range 1.6–35%.
- Note: The highest frequency of sensitization reported may have been influenced by patient recruitment or false-positive readings. The annual prevalence at St John's Institute of Dermatology is usually below 3%.

Patch testing

- Patch testing is usually performed with potassium dichromate 0.5% pet. in Europe and 0.25% in North America. A T.R.U.E.® test equivalent is also available. A study comparing 0.25% and 0.5% potassium dichromate found that 0.25% will miss more true positives but more irritant/false-positive reactions will occur with 0.5% [1]. 0.375% was tried as a compromise but this missed 18% of true positives, whereas reactions at 0.5% were deemed "irritant" [2].
- At St John's Institute of Dermatology, if there is a possibility of a false positive reaction, the patient is retested to potassium dichromate 0.375%.

Clinical disease

Reported sources of exposure causing allergic contact dermatitis to chromate are given in Figure 12.1.

Hand dermatitis

- More common in males (Figure 12.2).
- Often associated with more severe dermatitis.
- Often associated with a poor prognosis.
- Amongst cement workers, the most common sites affected were the palms and dorsal aspects of the hands (near the proximal metacarpophalangeal joints). The most common morphological characteristic noted was hyperkeratosis.
- Relatively low concentrations of chromate can cause vesicular flares in allergic patients.
- 97 cement workers were recruited into a study. 65/97 were suffering from hand dermatitis, 24/97 (24.7%) had a positive patch test to potassium dichromate, 9/97 (9.3%) had allergic reactions to thiuram mix, 9/97 (9.3%) reacted to fragrance mix, and 7/97 (7.2%) were allergic to cobalt chloride. 22 were diagnosed with cement ACD. The most common sites affected were the palms and dorsal aspects of the hands (around the metacarpophalangeal joints). The most common clinical morphology was hyperkeratosis (60%), followed by erythema, dryness, and hyperpigmentation. The authors recommended the use of non-leather gloves to prevent occupational hand dermatitis in cement workers [3].
- A 40-year-old man who had worked in the construction industry for 20 years presented with severe hand dermatitis with fissuring and was patch test positive ++ for potassium dichromate [4]. He presented 11 years later with lymphedema with non-pitting edema of both hands after suffering persistent dermatitis and secondary cellulitis. This case illustrates the potential chronicity and severity of chromate hand dermatitis.

Foot dermatitis

- Caused by leather (Figure 12.3).
- Common in both adults and children.
- Can be associated with multiple shoe allergies.
- Can occasionally present with severe dermatitis.
- 230 foot dermatitis patients were patch tested to a baseline, shoe, and medicament series. 54 (23%) had a positive patch test reaction to one or more allergens, 44 (19%) reacted to baseline allergens, and 13 (6%) reacted to allergens in a shoe series. The most common positive allergens identified were chromate (3.9%), mercapto mix (3.5%), neomycin (3%), and thiuram mix (2.6%). A specific shoe series is ideally added to a baseline series when screening patients with foot dermatitis [5].
- 8483 patients patch tested to a baseline series showed a chromate allergy prevalence of 2.7% (3.0% of women and 2.3% of men). The anatomical locations of the dermatitis were feet (40.3%), hands only (22.2%), arms (15.8%), face/neck (12.7%), and a generalized distribution (13.1%). The hands

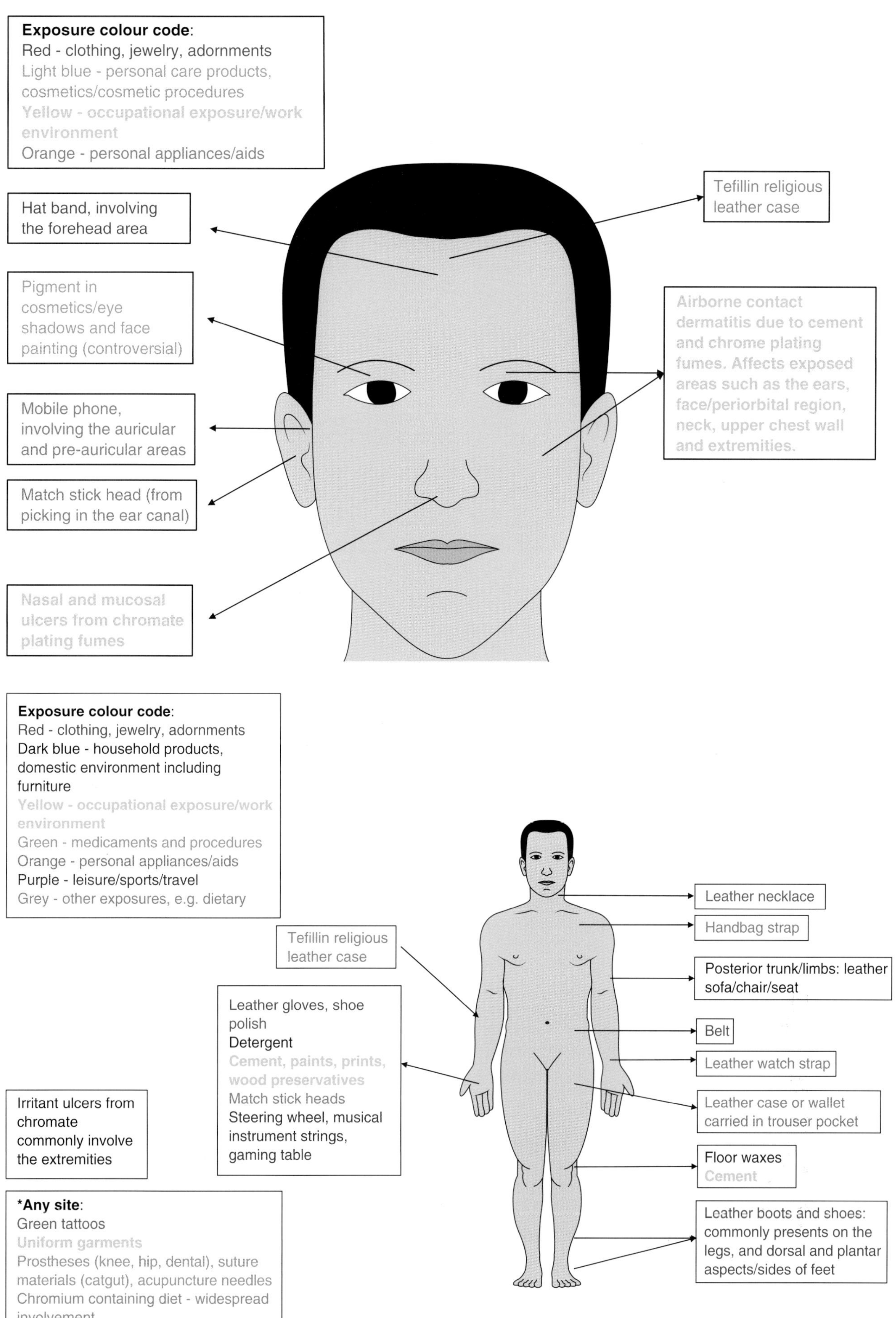
Exposure colour code:
Red - clothing, jewelry, adornments
Light blue - personal care products, cosmetics/cosmetic procedures
Yellow - occupational exposure/work environment
Orange - personal appliances/aids
Hat band, involving the forehead area
Pigment in cosmetics/eye shadows and face painting (controversial)
Mobile phone, involving the auricular and pre-auricular areas
Match stick head (from picking in the ear canal)
Nasal and mucosal ulcers from chromate plating fumes
Tefillin religious leather case
Airborne contact dermatitis due to cement and chrome plating fumes. Affects exposed areas such as the ears, face/periorbital region, neck, upper chest wall and extremities.
Exposure colour code:
Red - clothing, jewelry, adornments
Dark blue - household products, domestic environment including furniture
Yellow - occupational exposure/work environment
Green - medicaments and procedures
Orange - personal appliances/aids
Purple - leisure/sports/travel
Grey - other exposures, e.g. dietary
Tefillin religious leather case
Leather gloves, shoe polish
Detergent
Cement, paints, prints, wood preservatives
Match stick heads
Steering wheel, musical instrument strings, gaming table
Irritant ulcers from chromate commonly involve the extremities
*Any site:
Green tattoos
Uniform garments
Prostheses (knee, hip, dental), suture materials (catgut), acupuncture needles
Chromium containing diet - widespread involvement
Leather necklace
Handbag strap
Posterior trunk/limbs: leather sofa/chair/seat
Belt
Leather watch strap
Leather case or wallet carried in trouser pocket
Floor waxes
Cement
Leather boots and shoes: commonly presents on the legs, and dorsal and plantar aspects/sides of feet

Figure 12.1 Reported exposure sources for allergic contact dermatitis to chromate.

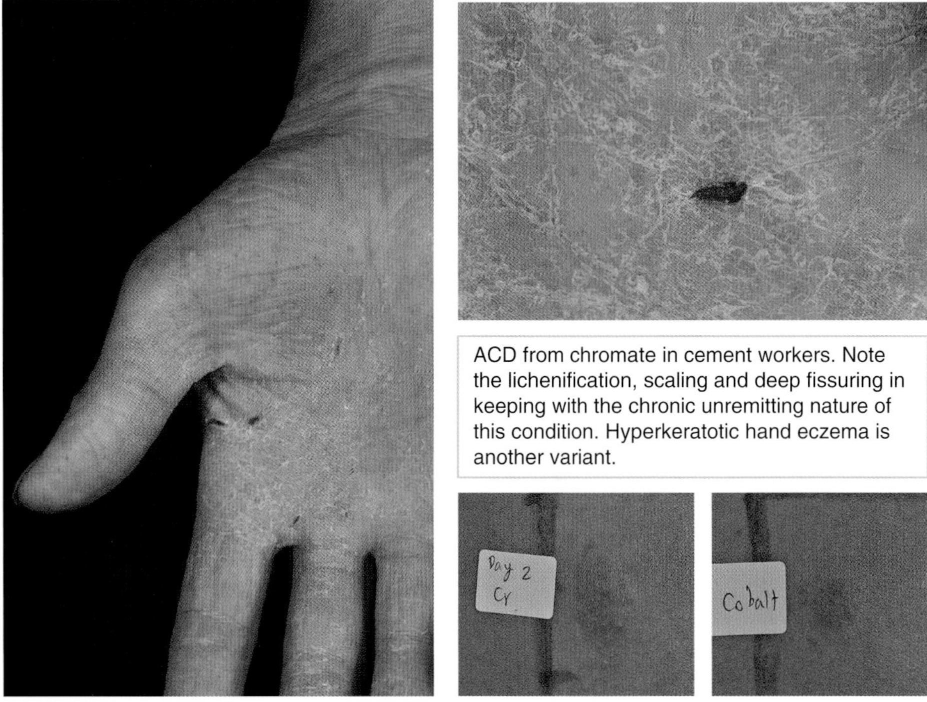

ACD from chromate in cement workers. Note the lichenification, scaling and deep fissuring in keeping with the chronic unremitting nature of this condition. Hyperkeratotic hand eczema is another variant.
Day 2
Cr
Cobalt

Figure 12.2 Cement worker with hand dermatitis. He was positive on patch testing to both chromate and cobalt.

Classical distribution on the dorsal aspects of the feet with spread from the big toe both proximally and laterally. Lichenification and excoriations indicate the chronicity and pruritic nature of the dermatitis.

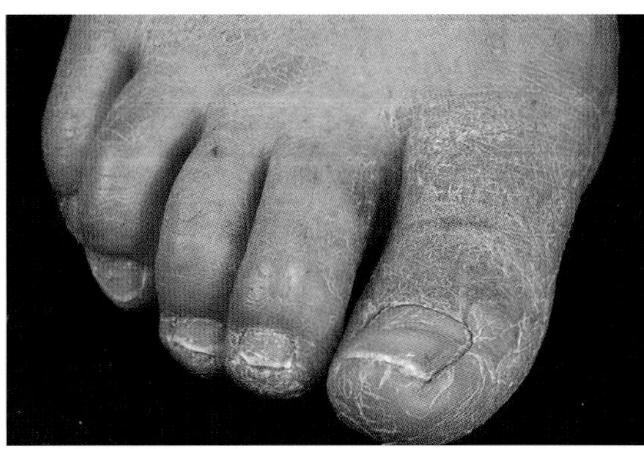

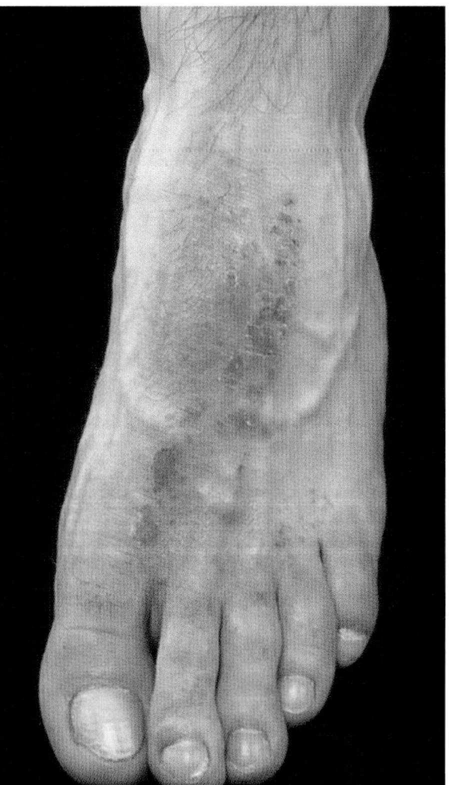

Figure 12.3 Two cases of ACD to chromate in leather (upper component of footwear).

were the only anatomical location which had a significantly higher frequency in men ($p = 0.001$), whilst the feet were significantly more affected in women ($p = 0.03$). The most common sources of exposure were noted to be leather shoes (24.4%), leather gloves (8.6%), and other leather products (3.2%), such as furniture and coats [6].

Other examples of leather exposure

- Leather has now become the principal exposure causing ACD to chromate in Western Europe, exceeding cement in one study by more than 10 times [7].

Gloves

- A 27-year-old professional golfer presented with recurrent erythematous plaques on both hands for several years [8]. The lesions appeared whenever she wore her golf gloves for an extended period of time. She had a ++ reaction to potassium dichromate on patch testing. Analysis of her golf gloves showed a chromate content of 308.91 ppm, sufficient to elicit ACD to chromate.
- Two months after starting work with alkaline coolants and wearing protective leather gloves, a 55-year-old man developed hand dermatitis with hyperkeratosis, scaling, and fissuring [9]. He subsequently also developed foot dermatitis. Patch testing showed a ++ reaction to potassium dichromate. Avoidance of leather and the coolants led to resolution of the dermatitis. Chromium was detected in both the gloves and coolants. The authors suggested that the high alkalinity of the coolants may have facilitated the release of chromate from the leather gloves.

Watch straps, belts, bags, jackets, driving wheel covers

- Although these items do not cause chromate ACD as commonly as shoes or gloves, they are documented as primary sources of exposure in a large survey [7].
- Watch strap dermatitis from allergens in leather may present on one or both wrists, as the patient may switch the strap to the other wrist when inflammation occurs [10].
- ACD to leather allergens in trouser belts can present as a band-like area of dermatitis involving the abdomen, flanks, and back which can then spread across the whole trunk [10].
- Steering wheel dermatitis usually involves the palmar areas [11].

Wallet

- Chromate from wallets carried in trouser pockets can cause ACD (McFadden, unpublished). Dermatitis can develop on the upper outer thigh [12] or buttock, corresponding to the pocket where the wallet is carried.

Sofa dermatitis from chromate

- A 69-year-old woman presented with a severe flare of previously mild eczema affecting her hands, feet, back, calves, and posterior aspects of her arms [13]. She was patch test positive (+++) to potassium dichromate. Two months prior to this exacerbation, she had bought a new leather sofa that she had consistently used for more than 8 hours a day as a bed. After avoiding contact with leather, her dermatitis resolved. A second case was a 40-year-old woman with a long history of pompholyx who presented with worsening hand eczema with new patches affecting the lower back, extensor arms, and legs with a poor response to topical therapy. Patch testing showed positive (++) reactions to both potassium dichromate and a sample of a leather sofa, which she had purchased just prior to the flare of her dermatitis. Her dermatitis improved after leather avoidance.
- More recent cases of leather ACD from sofas have been caused by the desiccant dimethylfumarate rather than chromate [14].

Tefillin

- Two orthodox Jewish men presented with chromate ACD of the left arm to phylacteries/tefillin (a leather box containing holy parchment which is worn during prayer on the left arm and/or the head and is held in place by straps). Case 1 was a 60-year-old male with chronic dermatitis on the left arm and forehead where his skin had been in contact with leather used as part of his orthodox Jewish lifestyle. Case 2 was a 17-year-old with dermatitis located only on his left arm where he wore the tefillin in the same way as the first case. Both patients had corresponding dermatitis at the contact areas. Positive reactions to potassium dichromate and the tefillin were recorded in both patients and their lesions improved after they used chrome-free tefillin [15].

Hat band

- A 55-year-old man presented with a 10-day history of a vesicular itchy rash arranged in a band on the forehead. He was patch test positive (++) to potassium dichromate. Testing his leather hat band with extraction by synthetic sweat found chromium release of 9.66 ppm [16]; testing other parts of the hat revealed only insignificant levels of chromium release.

Potential contact allergens in leather other than chromate

- *p-tert-butylphenol* (PTBP) resin is commonly used as a glue for leather material and can cause ACD from contact with leather, e.g. watchstrap dermatitis [17].
- *Cobalt* has recently been recognized as an important cause of ACD to leather; samples of leather causing ACD have as much as 1250 ppm of cobalt [18]. Leather sources of cobalt causing ACD include cushions, sofas, and footwear [18, 19].
- *Colophonium* used as a tanning/finishing agent for leather (rather than an adhesive in making the shoe) has caused footwear ACD to leather [20].
- *Octylisothiazolinone*, which can be contained in leather, has caused ACD from leather footwear, belts, and watchstraps [10].
- ACD to a leather sofa was reported from exposure to *methylisothiazolinone* used in a leathercare cream product applied to the sofa [21].

- *Formaldehyde* released from leather caused ACD to a leather watchstrap [22].
- ACD to the vegetable tannins *myrabolam* and *quebracho* contained in a leather watch strap has been reported [23].
- A group investigated potential occupational skin hazards in shoe manufacturing workers in Indonesia [24]. They made an extensive list of the materials and chemicals used. They found that the following chemicals were used in the production of leather (though it is not known how much of these agents may be retained in the finished product) (*denotes known contact allergens):
  - tanning agents: potassium dichromate*, 2- mercaptobenzothiazole*, formaldehyde*, glycine, chlorobenzene, glutaraldehyde*
  - preservative/biocide: octylisothiazolinone*, methylchloroisothiazolinone*, metam sodium*, sodium dimethyldithiocarbamate, 2-thiocyanomethyl benzothiazole*
  - dyeing process: disperse orange 3*, acid yellow 36*, *N-N*-isopropyl-*N'*-phenyl-1,4-phenylenediamine (N-IPPD)*, 4-aminobenzene*, benzidine*
  - finishing process: epoxy resin*, polyethylacrylate*, colophonium*.

Orthopedic prostheses

- The role of metal sensitivity from orthopedic prostheses is controversial (see Chapter 10). Patch testing for metal sensitivity often occurs after a localized rash or failure of a joint occurs; however, a positive reaction does not necessarily imply causation by metal allergy, as most metal-sensitive patients can have orthopedic metal implants without risk [25]. In addition, few prospective studies have shown a significant association between the failure of a joint replacement or postoperative eczema and metal allergy [26]. However, it is possible that metal sensitivity can occasionally cause these problems.
- 30 patients presented with local dermatitis occurring 1–3 months after total metal knee replacement. The dermatitis was localized to the outer aspect of the knee, lateral to the anterior midline incision scar. 7/15 who were patch tested reacted to metals: 4 to nickel, 2 to chromate, and 1 to cobalt. However, the dermatitis cleared with topical steroids without recurrence and failure of the joint replacement did not occur. The authors question the clinical relevance of the positive patch tests and speculate that other factors may have played a part [27].
- A 35-year-old man fractured his right ankle and had metal plates (containing nickel and chromate) inserted [28]. A month later, he developed vesicular eczema on the fingers of both hands. Patch tests were positive to both nickel and chromate. The plates and screws were removed and the patient's hand dermatitis improved. However, relapses occurred at a later stage.
- Three patients developed localized dermatitis 3 months after tibial plates were inserted. Two were patch test positive to chromate and one to nickel. The dermatitis resolved in all patients after removal of the plates [29].

Tattoo dermatitis

- Three patients with permanent tattoos (including green color tattoos) presented with chronic generalized dermatitis and pruritus. They were patch tested to a baseline and additional series. All three patients had a strongly positive patch test reaction to potassium dichromate (++). The previously quiescent tattoo also reacted during patch testing, becoming inflamed where it was green (the green color contains chromium oxide). After strict avoidance of chromate in terms of clothing, diet, and cosmetics, both the generalized dermatitis and tattoo inflammation improved [30].
- Two cases of ACD to chromate from cement-activated inflammatory reactions, consisting of itchy papules/nodules, in the green areas of permanent tattoos [31].

Mobile phone dermatitis

- Eight patients had allergic reactions after 9–25 days' use of mobile phones. The clinical presentation was unilateral erythema and papules involving the auricular ($n = 2$) or preauricular ($n = 6$) areas. Three had a previous history of metal allergy. All eight patients had a positive patch test reaction to potassium dichromate: 2/8 showed a strongly positive reaction (++) and 6/8 had a moderate (+) reaction. One patient had a concurrent positive reaction to nickel and another patient to cobalt. The dermatitis disappeared after avoiding mobile phone use. The authors concluded that the mobile phone-induced contact dermatitis in these patients was caused by chromate [32].

Generalized dermatitis

- 1187 patients were patch tested to a baseline series. 208 (17.5%) had positive reactions to at least one metal with positive reactions to nickel 13.1%, cobalt 6.8%, and chromate 3.8%. Those who were sensitized to at least one metal were more likely to have generalized dermatitis [33].

Nummular eczema

- 1022 patients with nummular eczema were patch tested to a baseline and additional series. The upper and lower limbs were the most common sites involved (75.8% and 64.5%, respectively). 332 patients (32.5%) had positive reactions to at least one allergen. The most common positive allergens were nickel sulfate (10.2%), potassium dichromate (7.3%), and cobalt chloride (6.1%). 69.7% of the sensitized patients had a clinically relevant history. Women (54.8%) were more likely to have a positive reaction than men (45.2%) but men had more positive reactions to potassium dichromate than women (6.5% vs 0.8%, respectively). The authors stated that there was a trend at 1–2-year follow-up for the eczema to improve with avoidance of the relevant allergens [34].

Ear

- 66 patients with chronic otitis externa were patch tested. 19/66 (28.8%) of the patients had a positive patch test reaction.

The most common positive allergens were neomycin ($n = 11$), potassium dichromate ($n = 6$), and formaldehyde ($n = 4$). The authors do not comment on the relevance of chromate allergy in this group [35].

- A case series of otitis externa from ACD to chromate in matchstick heads has been described [36]. The authors noted that the patients used chromate-containing matchsticks to pick at their ear canals.

Asthma

- This is an uncommon presentation and has usually been reported in the context of working with metallic salts. Prick and/or patch tests to chromate may be positive.

Systemic contact dermatitis

- Dietary restriction is controversial and not part of standard management.
- 30 patients with a positive reaction to potassium dichromate were orally challenged to 2.5 mg of chromium and a placebo. After ingestion, 17 patients had a reaction to chromate but not to the placebo, two reacted to both chromate and the placebo, and four patients reacted to the placebo but not to chromate. 17/30 (56.7%) of the patients had a flare of their previous dermatitis after the oral challenge with chromate. The specific locations of dermatitis were the hands and/or feet [37]. Another study estimated daily dietary chromate ingestion in Greece to be on average only 0.143 mg/day [38]. However, this may become much higher with mineral supplementation [39].
- A 35-year-old male, with a past history of reacting to a leather wrist watch band, presented with a 2-month history of dermatitis mostly on the lower legs, ankles, hands, and wrists [39]. Several weeks before the onset of dermatitis, he had been taking various vitamin and mineral supplements which included high doses of chromium picolinate. Patch testing showed a ++ reaction to potassium dichromate at 48 and 96 hours. A diagnosis of systemic contact dermatitis to chromate was made.

Occupational allergic contact dermatitis

- Chromate is one of the most common causes of occupational ACD.
- Highest in the construction industry, especially amongst bricklayers/cement workers.
- More frequent in the older age group.
- Can be associated with co-sensitization to rubber chemicals because of the use of protective gloves.
- Electroplaters and tanners are at-risk groups for developing chromate allergy.
- Irritant reactions from chrome fumes may occur in electroplaters.
- Nasal ulcers and chrome leg ulcers are potential irritant effects of chromate.
- Of 22 184 patients diagnosed with occupational contact dermatitis (OCD), 1226 (6%) had chromate induced occupational skin diseases. Chromate OCD was identified more in males than females, with a ratio of 5 : 1. The rates of contact dermatitis increased with age, especially in females over the age of 60. The most common occupations in relation to chromium OCD were *builders and building contractors*, *bricklayers*, *construction workers* and *plasterers*. The authors concluded that chromium-related occupational dermatitis usually has an onset in later working life and often affects those in the building trades [40].
- 472 *tannery workers* were recruited into a questionnaire-based interview and skin examination. 99 had a positive history of occupationally-related dermatitis and 77 were suspected to have OCD. 13/472 (3%) had a positive patch test reaction to at least one tannery allergen. The most common positive allergens were potassium dichromate (9.2%), *N,N*-diphenylguanidine (5.3%), benzidine (3.9%), and sodium metabisulfite (2.6%). The hands, wrists, and forearms were the most common sites involved [41].
- Of 37 *chrome platers* surveyed, 7 had chrome ulcers, 6 had contact dermatitis, and 1 had both (38% in total) [42]. Another 16 (43%) had scars suggestive of previous chrome ulcers. Mucosal irritation was present in 57%, with throat involvement (49%) and/or nasal irritation (41%). A single worker had nasal septal perforation. The chrome ulcers were mostly on the hands, fingers, and wrists. The authors note that only one of the workers with chrome ulcers was allergic to chromate and attribute the etiology of the ulcers to small fissures in the skin and the noxious effects of hexavalent chromate.
- Airborne ACD to chromate fumes from arc welding has been described. A 36-year-old *welder* presented with severe recurrent dermatitis affecting the cheeks, ears, and neck [43]. Just before the eruption began, a new arc welding unit was brought into the work area. The authors note that more fumes are produced in electrical arc welding compared to oxygen welding. Another case reports flares of hand dermatitis as a systemic reaction from inhaling chrome-containing fumes during welding [44].
- Chromate sensitization causing occupational hand dermatitis has been reported in the paper/pulp industry [45].
- A 21-year-old tire fitter developed chromate ACD of the hands from chromate added to the solution used to facilitate sliding tires onto wheel rims. [46] Chromate had been added to prevent rusting.
- A 49-year-old mechanical fitter developed widespread dermatitis starting on the shoulders and lower legs, spreading to the trunk, palms, and soles [47]. This occurred 9 months after starting work (*refitting boiler linings* at a power plant station). Patch testing showed a positive reaction to potassium dichromate. Although the boiler lining had trivalent chromium, the alkalinity and heat from the furnace reaction had caused significant conversion to hexavalent chromium.
- A 44-year-old *sheet metal worker* presented with a recurrence of chromate ACD affecting his hands with vesicular changes, with secondary spread to his arms. He originally had ACD to chromate from working as a bricklayer, but now the source of chromate was the galvanized metal sheets [48].
- Dermatitis from chromate in *cooling oil* has been described. Other cases previously reported have been from *defatting solvents*, *ashes*, *foundry sand*, *television manufacture*, *chrome*

anti-rust paint (still used in the aircraft industry), *diesel oil* (where chrome has been added as a corrosion inhibitor), *timber preservatives* and *magnetic tapes* [49].
- Chromate ACD has occasionally been reported in the *enameling industry*, though dyes are more common causes of allergy in this group [50].
- *Hide glue*, derived from animal skin, including chrome-tanned leather scraps, has traditionally been used as an adhesive in furniture and clockwork. It was a cause of chromate allergy but is not commonly seen now.

Cement

- According to EU legislation, the concentration of chromium(VI) in cement should not exceed 2 ppm. Several studies have shown a beneficial effect from this legislation with a reduction in the number of cases of occupational chromate dermatitis (www.europarl.eu.int/meetdocs/committees/envi/20030219/470365en.pdf).
- Irritant contact dermatitis can occur from exposure to cement due to its alkalinity, especially if trapped inside boots (Figure 12.4).

Orthodontic material

- Although chromate can be contained in orthodontic material, ACD to chromate from exposure to orthodontic material is rarely reported.

Chromate dermatitis and musicians

- A 25-year-old harpist presented with a 5-month history of an eczematous rash on the tips of her fingers of her right hand. Patch testing showed a strong reaction to potassium dichromate. Chromate had been used as a tanning agent for the harp strings [51].
- A 30-year-old professional violinist presented with a 3-year history of hand and foot dermatitis starting on the left ring finger before spreading to both hands and feet. A patch test revealed a strong reaction to potassium dichromate. Chromate was contained in the core of the E-string of his instrument. Changing the string to a type with a stainless or aluminum core resulted in rapid clearing of his dermatitis [52].
- Leather accessories of musical instruments, e.g. *leather handles and straps*, have the potential to cause ACD [52].

Cosmetic/cosmetic procedures

- ACD to chromate in cosmetics should not occur in the EU, which does not allow hexavalent chromium in cosmetics. In one Asian study, analysis of 9 out of 10 eye shadows showed chromium levels of over 10 ppm [53]. However, in their associated report of patients with eyelid dermatitis, the level of chromate sensitivity vs controls (7.5% vs 5.7%) was not significantly different. In another Asian study, 2/22 eye shadows contained levels of hexavalent chromium that were high enough to potentially elicit ACD [54].
- Four cases of allergic chromate granulomas from eyebrow tattooing have been recorded in Asia [55].

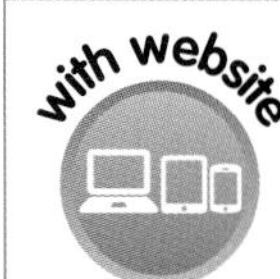

Go to www.wiley.com/go/mcfadden/common_contact_allergens to find the E-supplement for this chapter:

Chromate: E-Supplement

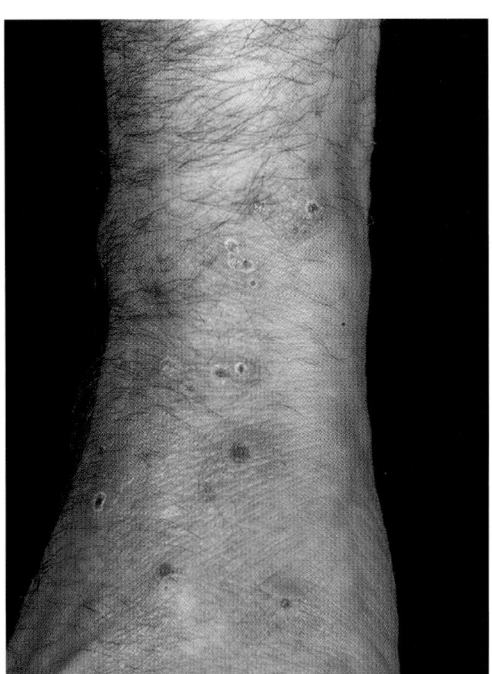

Wet cement is strongly alkaline and can cause a marked, delayed irritant contact dermatitis and sometimes even a burn.

Figure 12.4 Irritant contact dermatitis from wet cement trapped inside work boots.

References

1 Burrows, D. (1987). Comparison of 0.25 and 0.5% potassium dichromate in patch testing. *Boll Dermatol Allergol Profess* 2 (1): 117–20.

2 Burrows, D., Andersen, K.E., Camarasa, J.G. et al. (1989). Trial of 0.5% versus 0.375% potassium dichromate. European Environmental and Contact Dermatitis Research Group (EECDRG). *Contact Dermatitis* 21 (5): 351.

3 Wang, B.J., Wu, J.D., Sheu, S.C. et al. (2011). Occupational hand dermatitis among cement workers in Taiwan. *Journal of the Formosan Medical Association* 110 (12): 775–779.

4 Fitzgerald, D.A. and English, J.S. (1994). Lymphoedema of the hands as a complication of chronic allergic contact dermatitis. *Contact Dermatitis* 30 (5): 310.

5 Holden, C.R. and Gawkrodger, D.J. (2005). 10 years' experience of patch testing with a shoe series in 230 patients: which allergens are important? *Contact Dermatitis* 53 (1): 37–39.

6 Carøe, C., Andersen, K.E., Thyssen, J.P., and Mortz, C.G. (2010). Fluctuations in the prevalence of chromate allergy in Denmark and exposure to chrome-tanned leather. *Contact Dermatitis* 63 (6): 340–346.

7 Thyssen, J.P., Jensen, P., Carlsen, B.C. et al. (2009). The prevalence of chromium allergy in Denmark is currently increasing as a result of leather exposure. *British Journal of Dermatology* 161 (6): 1288–1293.

8 Lim, J.H., Kim, H.S., Park, Y.M. et al. (2010). A case of chromium contact dermatitis due to exposure from a golf glove. *Annals of Dermatology* 22 (1): 63–65.

9 Hedberg, Y.S., Lidén, C., and Lindberg, M. (2016). Chromium dermatitis in a metal worker due to leather gloves and alkaline coolant. *Acta Dermato-Venereologica* 96 (1): 104–105.

10 Aerts, O., Meert, H., Romaen, E. et al. (2016). Octylisothiazolinone, an additional cause of allergic contact dermatitis caused by leather: case series and potential implications for the study of cross-reactivity with methylisothiazolinone. *Contact Dermatitis* 75 (5): 276–284.

11 Jordan, W.P. Jr. (1974). Allergic contact dermatitis in hand eczema. *Archives of Dermatology* 110 (4): 567–569.

12 Evans, A.V., Banerjee, P., McFadden, J.P., and Calonje, E. (2003). Lymphomatoid contact dermatitis to para-tertyl-butyl phenol resin. *Clinical and Experimental Dermatology* 28 (3): 272–273.

13 Patel, T.G., Kleyn, C.E., King, C.M., and Wilson, N.J. (2006). Chromate allergy from contact with leather furnishings. *Contact Dermatitis* 54 (3): 171–172.

14 Lammintausta, K., Zimerson, E., Hasan, T. et al. (2010). An epidemic of furniture-related dermatitis: searching for a cause. *British Journal of Dermatology* 162 (1): 108–116.

15 Friedmann, A.C. and Goldsmith, P. (2008). Tefillin contact dermatitis: a problem in the devout. *Contact Dermatitis* 59 (3): 188–189.

16 Lembo, G., Nappa, P., Balato, N., and Ayala, F. (1985). Hat band dermatitis. *Contact Dermatitis* 13 (5): 334.

17 Ozkaya-Bayazit, E. and Buyukbabani, N. (2001). Non-eczematous pigmented interface dermatitis from para-tertiary-butylphenol-formaldehyde resin in a watchstrap adhesive. *Contact Dermatitis* 44 (1): 45–46.

18 Bregnbak, D., Opstrup, M.S., Jellesen, M.S. et al. (2017). Allergic contact dermatitis caused by cobalt in leather – clinical cases. *Contact Dermatitis* 76 (6): 366–368.

19 Bregnbak, D., Thyssen, J.P., Zachariae, C. et al. (2015). Association between cobalt allergy and dermatitis caused by leather articles – a questionnaire study. *Contact Dermatitis* 72 (2): 106–114.

20 Strauss, R.M. and Wilkinson, S.M. (2002). Shoe dermatitis due to colophonium used as leather tanning or finishing agent in Portuguese shoes. *Contact Dermatitis* 47 (1): 59.

21 Vandevenne, A., Vanden Broecke, K., and Goossens, A. (2014). Sofa dermatitis caused by methylisothiazolinone in a leather-care product. *Contact Dermatitis* 71 (2): 111–113.

22. Kanerva, L., Jolanki, R., and Estlander, T. (1996). Allergic contact dermatitis from leather strap of wrist watch. *International Journal of Dermatology* 35 (9): 680–681.

23 Calnan, C.D. and Cronin, E. (1978). Vegetable tans in leather. *Contact Dermatitis* 4 (5): 295–296.

24 Febriana, S.A., Soebono, H., and Coenraads, P.J. (2014). Occupational skin hazards and prevalence of occupational skin diseases in shoe manufacturing workers in Indonesia. *International Archives of Occupational and Environmental Health* 87 (2): 185–194.

25 Gawkrodger, D.J. (1993). Nickel sensitivity and the implantation of orthopaedic prostheses. *Contact Dermatitis* 28 (5): 257–259.

26 Gawkrodger, D.J. (2003). Metal sensitivities and orthopaedic implants revisited: the potential for metal allergy with the new metal-on-metal joint prostheses. *British Journal of Dermatology* 148 (6): 1089–1093.

27 Verma, S.B., Mody, B., and Gawkrodger, D.J. (2006). Dermatitis on the knee following knee replacement: a minority of cases show contact allergy to chromate, cobalt or nickel but a causal association is unproven. *Contact Dermatitis* 54 (4): 228–229.

28 Kanerva, L. and Förström, L. (2001). Allergic nickel and chromate hand dermatitis induced by orthopaedic metal implant. *Contact Dermatitis* 44 (2): 103–104.

29 Cramers, M. and Lucht, U. (1977). Metal sensitivity in patients treated for tibial fractures with plates of stainless steel. *Acta Orthopaedica Scandinavica* 48 (3): 245–249.

30 Jacob, S.E., Castanedo-Tardan, M.P., and Blyumin, M.L. (2008). Inflammation in green (chromium) tattoos during patch testing. *Dermatitis* 19 (5): E33–E34.

31 Cairns, R.J. and Calnan, C.D. (1962). Green tattoo reactions associated with cement dermatitis. *British Journal of Dermatology* 74: 288–294.

32 Seishima, M., Oyama, Z., and Oda, M. (2003). Cellular phone dermatitis with chromate allergy. *Dermatology* 207 (1): 48–50.

33 Ruff, C.A. and Belsito, D.V. (2006). The impact of various patient factors on contact allergy to nickel, cobalt, and chromate. *Journal of the American Academy of Dermatology* 55 (1): 32–39.

34 Bonamonte, D., Foti, C., Vestita, M. et al. (2012). Nummular eczema and contact allergy: a retrospective study. *Dermatitis* 23 (4): 153–157.

35 Yariktas, M., Yildirim, M., Doner, F. et al. (2004). Allergic contact dermatitis prevalence in patients with eczematous external otitis. *Asian Pacific Journal of Allergy and Immunology* 22 (1): 7–10.

36 Fregert, S. (1962). Otitis externa due to chromate of matches. *Acta Dermato-Venereologica* 42: 473–475.

37 Veien, N.K., Hattel, T., and Laurberg, G. (1994). Chromate-allergic patients challenged orally with potassium dichromate. *Contact Dermatitis* 31 (3): 137–139.

38 Bratakos, M.S., Lazos, E.S., and Bratakos, S.M. (2002). Chromium content of selected Greek foods. *The Science of the Total Environment* 290 (1–3): 47–58.

39 Fowler, J.F. Jr. (2000). Systemic contact dermatitis caused by oral chromium picolinate. *Cutis* 65 (2): 116.
40 Athavale, P., Shum, K.W., Chen, Y. et al. (2007). Occupational dermatitis related to chromium and cobalt: experience of dermatologists (EPIDERM) and occupational physicians (OPRA) in the UK over an 11-year period (1993-2004). *British Journal of Dermatology* 157 (3): 518–522.
41 Febriana, S.A., Jungbauer, F., Soebono, H., and Coenraads, P.J. (2012). Occupational allergic contact dermatitis and patch test results of leather workers at two Indonesian tanneries. *Contact Dermatitis* 67 (5): 277–283.
42 Lee, H.S. and Goh, C.L. (1988). Occupational dermatosis among chrome platers. *Contact Dermatitis* 18 (2): 89–93.
43 Zugerman, C. (1982). Chromium in welding fumes. *Contact Dermatitis* 8 (1): 69–70.
44 Shelley, W.B. (1964). Chromium in welding fumes as cause of eczematous hand eruption. *Journal of the American Medical Association* 189: 772–773.
45 Fregert, S., Gruvberger, B., and Heijer, A. (1972). Sensitization to chromium and cobalt in processing of sulphate pulp. *Acta Dermato-Venereologica* 52 (3): 221–224.
46 Burrows, D. (1981). Chromium dermatitis in a tyre fitter. *Contact Dermatitis* 7 (1): 55–56.
47 Rycroft, R.J. and Calnan, C.D. (1977). Chromate dermatitis from a boiler lining. *Contact Dermatitis* 3 (4): 198–200.
48 Rycroft, R.J. and Calnan, C.D. (1977). Relapse of chromate dermatitis from sheet metal. *Contact Dermatitis* 3 (4): 177–180.
49 Burrows, D. (1984). The dichromate problem. *International Journal of Dermatology* 23 (4): 215–220.
50 Gaddoni, G., Baldassari, L., Francesconi, E., and Motolese, A. (1993). Contact dermatitis among decorators and enamellers in hand-made ceramic decorations. *Contact Dermatitis* 28 (2): 127–128.
51 Nethercott, J.R. and Holness, D.L. (1991). Dermatologic problems of musicians. *Journal of the American Academy of Dermatology* 25 (5 Pt 1): 870.
52 Buckley, D.A. and Rogers, S. (1995). Fiddler's fingers': violin-string dermatitis. *Contact Dermatitis* 32 (1): 46–47.
53 Oh, J.E., Lee, H.J., Choi, Y.W. et al. (2016). Metal allergy in eyelid dermatitis and the evaluation of metal contents in eye shadows. *Journal of the European Academy of Dermatology and Venereology* 30 (9): 1518–1521.
54 Kang, E.K., Lee, S., Park, J.H. et al. (2006). Determination of hexavalent chromium in cosmetic products by ion chromatography and postcolumn derivatization. *Contact Dermatitis* 54 (5): 244–248.
55 Eun, H.C. and Kim, K.H. (1989). Allergic granuloma from cosmetic eyebrow tattooing. *Contact Dermatitis* 21 (4): 276–278.

Exposure Color Code

- Clothing, jewelry, adornments
- Personal care products, cosmetics/cosmetic procedures
- Household products, domestic environment, including furniture and refurbishment
- Occupational dermatoses, work environment
- Medicines, surgical/dental procedures, herbal/alternative medicines
- Personal appliances/aids
- Leisure activities, sport, travel
- Other exposures (including dietary)
- Not relevant or multiple/general exposure

CHAPTER 13

Gold

CHAPTER CONTENTS

Key points

- Due to its stable and inert properties, gold has been used in jewelry, dental fillings, and as components of devices inserted within the human body. It has also been used as pharmacological and homeopathic/alternative therapy.
- Contact allergy to gold can manifest as jewelry dermatitis [1] and inflammatory reactions to dental fillings [2], including oral lichenoid lesions [3].
- Patch test screening with gold thiosulfate can give frequent positive results, but sometimes reactions may be delayed and/or persistent [4, 5].
- Intramuscular injections can induce systemic contact dermatitis in gold allergic patients [6].
- The clinical significance of a positive patch test to gold is not always clear.

Introduction

Gold is a precious metal that is widely used worldwide. Allergic contact dermatitis (ACD) to gold commonly involves direct contact dermatitis from jewelry but granulomatous, oral lichenoid, airborne, systemic, and eyelid contact dermatitis have also been reported [7].

Sex

- The female gender predominates (as much as 90% of patients with gold contact allergy), presumably due to the common wearing of gold jewelry amongst women [8, 9].

Children

- Gold allergy has been identified in children but with overall low clinical relevance. A study showed that 7.7% (30/391) had positive patch test reactions to gold and only 46.7% (14/30) of these gave a relevant history. Furthermore, amongst very young children (aged 0–5 years), clinical relevance was not found [10].

Frequency of sensitization

- The prevalence of contact sensitization to gold in dermatitis patients is usually less than 10% in most dermatitis clinics. However, prevalences of up to 23% from standard and metal series screening have also been reported [11].
- A comparison of gold allergy rates between clinics in two countries found a rate of 23.8% in Lithuania and 13.6% in Sweden [12].
- Among healthy individuals without any skin problems, positive patch test rates to gold of between 4.8 and 12.5% have been observed [6].

Exposure

- Gold was noted to be the second most common sensitizing allergen after nickel in 377 patients who were patch tested to 18 metal allergens. Ear piercing was also noted to be a risk factor for gold sensitization [1].

Common Contact Allergens: A Practical Guide to Detecting Contact Dermatitis, First Edition. Edited by John McFadden, Pailin Puangpet, Korbkarn Pongpairoj, Supitchaya Thaiwat, and Lee Shan Xian.

© 2020 John Wiley & Sons Ltd. Published 2020 by John Wiley & Sons Ltd.

Companion website: www.wiley.com/go/mcfadden/common_contact_allergens

- Jewelry made of gold alloys also contains other metals such as palladium, nickel, cobalt, zinc, cadmium, copper, and tin [13].
- A low-karat gold releases more gold, which may therefore cause more skin reactions than pure/high-karat gold in gold-sensitive patients [14].
- Artificial sweat did not enable the release of gold from alloy jewelry [13], but a study found that a combination of sulfur and the amino acid cysteine, which are found on human skin, promoted the release of gold from alloys [15].
- The presence of gold dental implants was identified as a risk factor for gold sensitization. 33.8% of asymptomatic patients who had gold dental devices had positive patch test reactions to gold compared with 10.8% in the "non-gold dental device" group [2]. The use of gold dental devices has largely been replaced by other metals and alloys in some countries [12].
- A gold hearing aid caused direct contact ACD in a 13-year-old girl with profound sensorineural deafness [16].
- In the past, patients with gold coronary stents had five-fold higher blood levels of gold compared to nickel blood levels in patients with nickel stents. The higher levels of gold in the bloodstream also correlated with stronger patch test and clinical reactions to gold [17, 18].
- High rates of gold sensitization (39%) were found amongst patients who had stents with gold material and the restenosis rate of those with gold stents was 33.8% in the gold-allergic group and 18.6% in the non-allergic group ($p < 0.05$) [19]. Due to the high frequency of restenosis, gold stents are no longer used.
- Gold used as a weight inserted into the upper eyelids has been used to help patients with facial nerve paralysis close their eyelids. Allergy to this gold weight can present with inflammation and edema of the upper eyelids [20].

Clinical presentation

- A study revealed that the most common sites affected were the hands, face, ears, and eyelids (Figure 13.1) [7, 8].
- Perianal and peri-vulval dermatitis were also noted as unusual manifestations of contact allergy to gold [9]. *(Note: Controversial.)*
- Facial involvement where there is only distal direct contact with gold may be hard to explain as relevant [9], though "secondary spread" of metal ACD can occur.
- Gold allergy has been associated not only with oral lichenoid lesions, but with other oral diseases as well. Patch testing to potassium dicyanoaurate was positive in 34.8% and 16.4% of patients with gingivitis and burning mouth syndrome, respectively *(Note: Controversial, association not causation reported.)* [21].
- *Oral lichen planus and lichenoid dermatitis.* A patient with gold dental restoration presented with lacy white patches on his bilateral buccal mucosa, angular cheilitis, and perioral dermatitis. He also complained of temporomandibular joint and oral muscular pain. Patch testing showed positive reactions to gold sodium thiosulfate (++) and potassium dicyanoaurate (++). The patient described no previous problems with gold

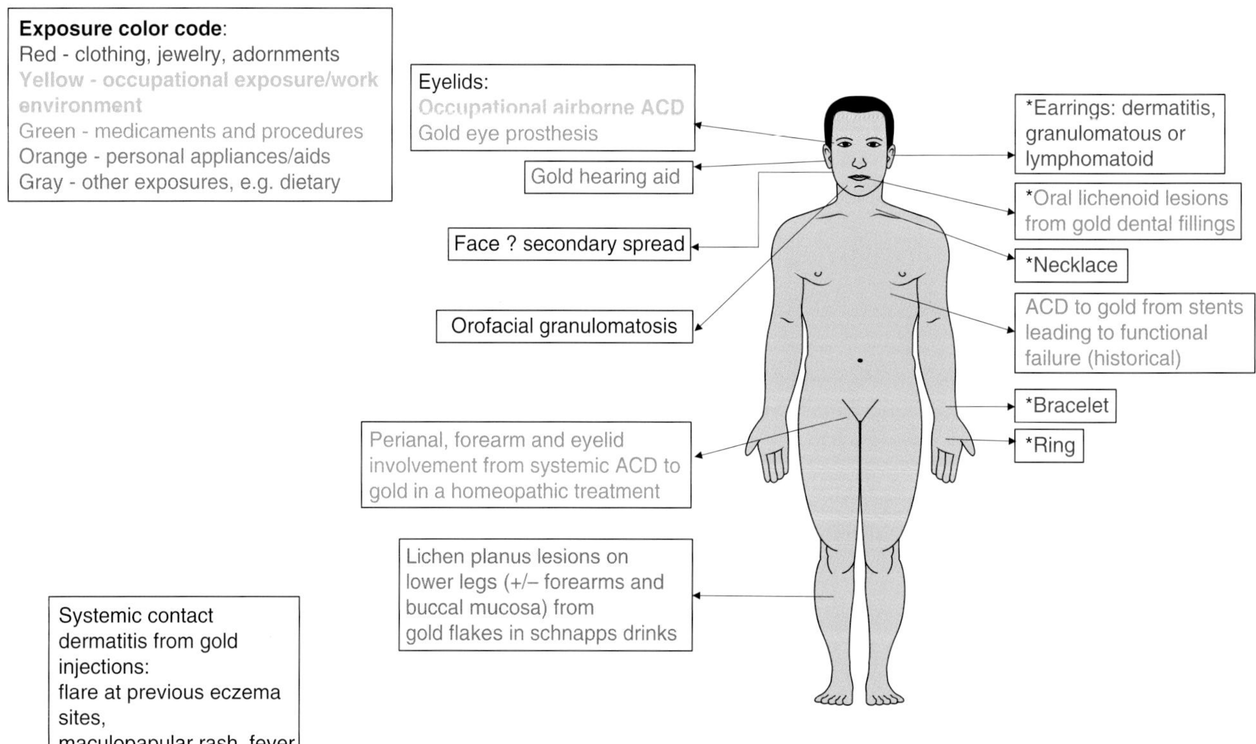

Figure 13.1 Common (*) and uncommon clinical manifestations of contact allergy to gold.

jewelry, but his oral lesions resolved after all the gold dental implants were removed [22].

- Positive patch tests to gold sodium thiosulfate were found in 23.5%, 23.1%, and 20% of patients who suffered from oral lichen planus, genital lichen planus, and cutaneous lichen planus, respectively. Patients were reported to have resolution of their oral lesions after the dental gold was removed [23].
- Eye involvement as a result of airborne contact dermatitis to gold has been reported as an occupational disease in restorers, electronic plating, and laboratory workers [24–26]. The clinical presentations included eyelid dermatitis, chemosis, hyperemia of the tarsal conjunctiva, follicular hypertrophy of the lid, blepharoconjunctivitis, and conjunctival eosinophilia [24–26].
- Another case of ACD to gold from an eyeball prosthesis was reported. The patient developed recurrent seropurulent orbital discharge and eczema of both eyelids and the surrounding skin of the left eye after 5 years of wearing an eye prosthesis made of an alloy from gold, copper, and nickel [27]. Inflammation and edema of the upper eyelids has been reported as an allergic complication of gold weights that were inserted into this area to help patients with facial nerve paralysis (see above) [20].

Systemic contact dermatitis

- A widespread cutaneous rash from systemic contact dermatitis to gold sodium thiomalate was reported [28]. Gold monovalent salt has been used for the treatment of rheumatoid arthritis and is usually administered intramuscularly. The clinical manifestations noted were flare of eczema at the patch test site (80%), flare of eczema at previous sites of dermatitis (26%), toxicoderma or a generalized maculopapular rash (46%) and fever (60%) [29]. Patch testing with gold sodium thiomalate usually showed negative or low-level reactions in gold allergic patients. A higher yield of positive reactions to gold sodium thiomalate was obtained by intracutaneous testing [30]. There were significantly higher serum levels of several cytokines such as tumor necrosis factor-α, soluble tumor necrosis factor receptor 1, interleukin-1 receptor antagonist, and neutrophil gelatinase-associated lipocalin in the patients with gold systemic allergy after systemic provocation [31].
- Systemic contact dermatitis was noted in a 76-year-old female with an eczematous rash involving the perianal region, eyelids, and forearms after 4 months of taking the homeopathic medication Aurocard for heart strengthening. Patch testing gave a strongly positive reaction to 2% gold sodium thiosulfate (+++). The patient had previous gold exposure from gold jewelry and gold dental crowns for many years without any reactions. When she stopped taking the culprit medication, her skin reaction cleared after a few months [32].
- Lesions which were clinically identical to lichen planus were observed in three patients who had been consuming schnapps containing free-floating gold flakes for at least 2 months [33]. In two patients, the lesions were located on the lower legs. In the other patient, the forearms, shins, ankles, and buccal mucosa were affected.

Other case reports

- Orofacial granulomatosis was reported in a 65-year old female who had an upper incisor gold crown for 5 years *(isolated case report)*. She presented with erythema and edema of the upper lip. The histopathology revealed granulomatous areas without any evidence of micro-organisms; there were inflammatory cells surrounding the salivary glands, which may indicate the route of allergen exposure. The clinical presentation resolved completely within 5 months after removal of the gold crown [34].
- Bilateral ear granulomatous contact dermatitis from gold jewelry was reported in a young woman who presented with multiple painless nodules on both ear lobes after wearing her gold earrings. Histopathological examination revealed multiple granulomas with epithelioid histiocytes, multinucleated giant cells, and surrounding lymphocytes with no evidence of caseation or foreign bodies. Patch testing showed a strongly positive reaction to gold sodium thiosulfate (+++), and all laboratory investigations were negative for sarcoidosis. The granulomatous nodules did not subside and persisted after gold avoidance. The authors postulated that sarcoidal granulomatous reactions can be the result of gold-induced production of granulocyte/macrophage colony-stimulating factors (GM-CSF) [35].
- Lymphomatoid contact dermatitis from gold earrings was reported in a 61-year-old female who developed erythematous nodules on the ear lobes for a year. Histopathology revealed dense superficial and deep infiltration, composed of lymphocytes and multinucleated giant cells with birefringent inclusions. Immunohistochemistry showed T-cells (CD45 and CD3 positive, CD20 negative). Patch testing gave a strongly positive reaction to 1% gold sodium thiosulfate and low-level reactions to cobalt and nickel. A biopsy of the patch test reaction showed eczematous dermatitis. The authors postulated that the differing cutaneous reactions for percutaneous (earring) and epicutaneous (patch test) contact with gold were caused by different immunological responses [36].
- A 29-year-old female had eczematous dermatitis on her left arm at the location of a bright yellow colored tattoo. The clinical presentation developed 2 months after the tattoo was inked. Patch testing was performed to a baseline and metal series. Positive reactions to both gold and nickel were found. The authors speculate that gold allergy had caused the tattoo reaction [37].

Clinical relevance

- The clinical relevance of gold sensitization was noted to be relatively low with an estimated rate of between 0 and 54% [14]. The rate of relevance may depend on which patch test allergens were used, the clinical presentation, and a history of previous gold exposure. Sensitization was not considered to be relevant in individuals who never had clinical symptoms or any gold exposure. The clinical relevance of gold allergy should be interpreted with caution [11, 14, 38].

- In a prospective study of patients who were patch test positive to gold, 12/30 reacted to wearing gold containing earrings over an 8-week period compared to 5/30 who wore titanium earrings, illustrating a statistical but low degree of clinical relevance [39].

Patch testing

- Gold sodium thiosulfate is the salt which is commonly used for screening [5]. Gold sodium thiosulfate also gives fewer irritant reactions compared to other gold salts. Delayed positive patch test reactions to gold have been noted at 10 days and up to 3 weeks [40]. Long-lasting patch test reactions to gold sodium thiosulfate were observed in 26% of volunteers who reacted but none of them complained of new or worsening cutaneous problems after re-exposure to gold in a long-term follow-up study [41]. Other gold salts such as gold trichloride and potassium dicyanoaurate have also been used as patch test agents but low elicitation and higher levels of irritant reactions (in particular to gold trichloride) have made these gold salts less popular for patch testing [42, 43].
- Gold sodium thiosulfate is included in most dental series but as patch testing to gold salt can sometimes show strong and persistent reactions with low rates of relevant history, gold is usually not included in the baseline series [44].
- Gold serum levels were significantly higher after patch testing with gold sodium thiosulfate amongst gold allergic patients, but the levels declined quickly and were not any different by days 3 and 7 [45].

Co-sensitization with other metals

Co-sensitization of gold allergic patients with nickel and cobalt has been reported at rates of 33.5% and 18.3%, respectively [8]. Palladium was noted as a potential co-sensitizer – a third of those with palladium allergy also had positive reactions to gold (although this could be a manifestation of palladium cross-reacting with nickel) [46].

Occupational allergic contact dermatitis

- Two restorers presented with airborne contact eczema from gold dust, with eyelid dermatitis and a rash on exposure sites. Patch testing showed strongly positive reactions to gold sodium thiosulfate. The avoidance of exposure to gold dust and gold fumes in the work place environment led to clinical improvement [25].
- An electronic plating worker presented with recurrent dermatitis on his hands and forearms for 8 weeks after contact with gold plates at work. He had positive reactions to aqueous gold chloride 1% (++), 0.5% (++), and 0.25% (++) at 96 hours. The dermatitis resolved without recurrence after gold avoidance [26]. Other clinical manifestations of occupational ACD from exposure to gold plating include eyelid dermatitis and blepharoconjunctivitis [24].

References

1 Nakada, T., Iijima, M., Nakayama, H., and Maibach, H.I. (1997). Role of ear piercing in metal allergic contact dermatitis. *Contact Dermatitis* 36 (5): 233–236.

2 Schaffran, R.M., Storrs, F.J., and Schalock, P. (1999). Prevalence of gold sensitivity in asymptomatic individuals with gold dental restorations. *American Journal of Contact Dermatitis* 10 (4): 201–206.

3 Ahlgren, C., Bruze, M., Möller, H. et al. (2012). Contact allergy to gold in patients with oral lichen lesions. *Acta Dermato Venereologica* 92 (2): 138–143.

4 Davis, M.D., Bhate, K., Rohlinger, A.L. et al. (2008). Delayed patch test reading after 5 days: the Mayo Clinic experience. *Journal of the American Academy of Dermatology* 59 (2): 225–233.

5 Bjorkner, B., Bruze, M., and Möller, H. (1994). High frequency of contact allergy to gold sodium thiosulfate. An indication of gold allergy? *Contact Dermatitis* 30 (3): 144–151.

6 Möller, H. (2010). Contact allergy to gold as a model for clinical-experimental research. *Contact Dermatitis* 62 (4): 193–200.

7 Bruze, M., Edman, B., Björkner, B., and Möller, H. (1994). Clinical relevance of contact allergy to gold sodium thiosulfate. *Journal of the American Academy of Dermatology* 31 (4): 579–583.

8 Fowler, J. Jr., Taylor, J., Storrs, F. et al. (2001). Gold allergy in North America. *American Journal of Contact Dermatitis* 12 (1): 3–5.

9 McKenna, K.E., Dolan, O., Walsh, M.Y., and Burrows, D. (1995). Contact allergy to gold sodium thiosulfate. *Contact Dermatitis* 32 (3): 143–146.

10 Zug, K.A., McGinley-Smith, D., Warshaw, E.M. et al. (2008). Contact allergy in children referred for patch testing: North American contact dermatitis group data, 2001–2004. *Archives of Dermatology* 144 (10): 1329–1336.

11 Davis, M.D., Wang, M.Z., Yiannias, J.A. et al. (2011). Patch testing with a large series of metal allergens: findings from more than 1,000 patients in one decade at Mayo Clinic. *Dermatitis* 22 (5): 256–271.

12 Malinauskiene, L., Bruze, M., and Isaksson, M. (2017). Patch testing with the Swedish baseline series supplemented with a textile dye mix and gold in Vilnius, Lithuania and Malmo, Sweden. *Contact Dermatitis* 77 (3): 189–190.

13 Lidén, C., Nordenadler, M., and Skare, L. (1998). Metal release from gold-containing jewelry materials: no gold release detected. *Contact Dermatitis* 39 (6): 281–285.

14 Chen, J.K. and Lampel, H.P. (2015). Gold contact allergy: clues and controversies. *Dermatitis* 26 (2): 69–77.

15 Svedman, C., Gruvberger, B., Dahlin, J. et al. (2013). Evaluation of a method for detecting metal release from gold; cysteine enhances release. *Acta Dermato Venereologica* 93 (5): 577–578.

16 O'Donoghue, N.B., Rustin, M.H., and McFadden, J.P. (2004). Allergic contact dermatitis from gold on a hearing-aid mould. *Contact Dermatitis* 51 (1): 36–37.

17 Ekqvist, S., Svedman, C., Lundh, T. et al. (2008). A correlation found between gold concentration in blood and patch test reactions in patients with coronary stents. *Contact Dermatitis* 59 (3): 137–142.

18 Ekqvist, S., Lundh, T., Svedman, C. et al. (2009). Does gold concentration in the blood influence the result of patch testing to gold? *British Journal of Dermatology* 160 (5): 1016–1021.
19 Svedman, C., Ekqvist, S., Möller, H. et al. (2009). A correlation found between contact allergy to stent material and restenosis of the coronary arteries. *Contact Dermatitis* 60 (3): 158–164.
20 Björkner, B., Bruze, M., Möller, H., and Salemark, L. (2008). Allergic contact dermatitis as a complication of lid loading with gold implants. *Dermatitis: Contact, Atopic, Occupational, Drug* 19 (3): 148–153.
21 Torgerson, R.R., Davis, M.D.P., Bruce, A.J. et al. (2007). Contact allergy in oral disease. *Journal of the American Academy of Dermatology* 57 (2): 315–321.
22 Tvinnereim, H.M., Lundekvam, B.F., Morken, T. et al. (2003). Allergic contact reactions to dental gold. *Contact Dermatitis* 48 (5): 288–289.
23 Scalf, L.A., Fowler, J.F. Jr., Morgan, K.W., and Looney, S.W. (2001). Dental metal allergy in patients with oral, cutaneous, and genital lichenoid reactions. *American Journal of Contact Dermatitis* 12 (3): 146–150.
24 Estlander, T., Kari, O., Jolanki, R., and Kanerva, L. (1998). Occupational allergic contact dermatitis and blepharoconjunctivitis caused by gold. *Contact Dermatitis* 38 (1): 40–41.
25 Giorgini, S., Tognetti, L., Zanieri, F., and Lotti, T. (2010). Occupational airborne allergic contact dermatitis caused by gold. *Dermatitis* 21 (5): 284–287.
26 Goh, C.L. (1988). Occupational dermatitis from gold plating. *Contact Dermatitis* 18 (2): 122–123.
27 Forster, H.W. Jr. and Dickey, R.F. (1949). A case of sensitivity to gold-ball orbital implant; eczematous contact-type dermatitis due to 14-karat gold. *American Journal of Ophthalmology* 32 (5): 659–662.
28 Möller, H., Larsson, A., Björkner, B. et al. (1996). Flare-up at contact allergy sites in a gold-treated rheumatic patient. *Acta Dermato Venereologica* 76 (1): 55–58.
29 Möller, H. (2000). Clinical response to gold as a circulating contact allergen. *Acta Dermato Venereologica* 80 (2): 111–113.
30 Bruze, M., Björkner, B., and Möller, H. (1995). Skin testing with gold sodium thiomalate and gold sodium thiosulfate. *Contact Dermatitis* 32 (1): 5–8.
31 Möller, H., Ohlsson, K., Linder, C. et al. (1999). The flare-up reactions after systemic provocation in contact allergy to nickel and gold. *Contact Dermatitis* 40 (4): 200–204.
32 Malinauskiene, L., Isaksson, M., and Bruze, M. (2013). Systemic contact dermatitis in a gold-allergic patient after treatment with an oral homeopathic drug. *Journal of the American Academy of Dermatology* 68 (2): e58.
33 Russell, M.A., Langley, M., Truett, A.P. 3rd et al. (1997). Lichenoid dermatitis after consumption of gold-containing liquor. *Journal of the American Academy of Dermatology* 36 (5 Pt 2): 841–844.
34 Lazarov, A., Kidron, D., Tulchinsky, Z., and Minkow, B. (2003). Contact orofacial granulomatosis caused by delayed hypersensitivity to gold and mercury. *Journal of the American Academy of Dermatology* 49 (6): 1117–1120.
35 Armstrong, D.K., Walsh, M.Y., and Dawson, J.F. (1997). Granulomatous contact dermatitis due to gold earrings. *British Journal of Dermatology* 136 (5): 776–778.
36 Conde-Taboada, A., Rosón, E., Fernández-Redondo, V. et al. (2007). Lymphomatoid contact dermatitis induced by gold earrings. *Contact Dermatitis* 56 (3): 179–181.
37 Tammaro, A., Tuchinda, P., Persechino, S., and Gaspari, A. (2011). Contact allergic dermatitis to gold in a tattoo: a case report. *International Journal of Immunopathology and Pharmacology* 24 (4): 1111–1113.
38 Nedorost, S. and Wagman, A. (2005). Positive patch-test reactions to gold: patients' perception of relevance and the role of titanium dioxide in cosmetics. *Dermatitis* 16 (2): 67–70; quiz 55–6.
39 Ahnlide, I., Björkner, B., Bruze, M., and Möller, H. (2000). Exposure to metallic gold in patients with contact allergy to gold sodium thiosulfate. *Contact Dermatitis* 43 (6): 344–350.
40 Bruze, M., Hedman, H., Björkner, B., and Möller, H. (1995). The development and course of test reactions to gold sodium thiosulfate. *Contact Dermatitis* 33 (6): 386–391.
41 Andersen, K.E. and Jensen, C.D. (2007). Long-lasting patch reactions to gold sodium thiosulfate occurs frequently in healthy volunteers. *Contact Dermatitis* 56 (4): 214–217.
42 Fowler, J.F. Jr. (1987). Selection of patch test materials for gold allergy. *Contact Dermatitis* 17 (1): 23–25.
43 Möller, H., Ahnlide, I., Gruvberger, B., and Bruze, M. (2005). Gold trichloride and gold sodium thiosulfate as markers of contact allergy to gold. *Contact Dermatitis* 53 (2): 80–83.
44 Echechipía, S., Villarreal, O., Iriarte, P. et al. (2015). Are all new allergens in TRUE test(R) essential for a baseline set? *Contact Dermatitis* 73 (3): 186–187.
45 Möller, H., Schütz, A., Björkner, B., and Bruze, M. (2004). Percutaneous absorption of gold sodium thiosulfate used for patch testing. *Contact Dermatitis* 51 (2): 63–66.
46 Marcusson, J.A. (1996). Contact allergies to nickel sulfate, gold sodium thiosulfate and palladium chloride in patients claiming side-effects from dental alloy components. *Contact Dermatitis* 34 (5): 320–323.

Exposure Color Code

- Clothing, jewelry, adornments
- Personal care products, cosmetics/cosmetic procedures
- Household products, domestic environment, including furniture and refurbishment
- Occupational dermatoses, work environment
- Medicines, surgical/dental procedures, herbal/alternative medicines
- Personal appliances/aids
- Leisure activities, sport, travel
- Other exposures (including dietary)
- Not relevant or multiple/general exposure

CHAPTER 14

Fragrances Incorporating Fragrance Mix 1, Fragrance Mix 2, Hydroxyisoheyl 3-cyclohexene Carboxaldehyde, Limonene, and Linalool

CHAPTER CONTENTS

Allergen profiling

A profile of allergic contact dermatitis (ACD) to fragrance extracted from case literature and clinical experience is summarized below.

a. *Examples of potential exposure from aspects of daily life*

- Personal care products – 70% are fragranced.
- Home environment – air fresheners, scented candles, partner, sprays for bedding, ironing water
- Occupational – toilet room sprays, catering (cinnamon spice, citrus), health care (scented soap), beautician
- Leisure – gardening – scented plants
- Sports – increased deodorant use
- Travel – room and bed spray, hotel toiletries, car air freshener, insect repellent
- Clothing – fragrance sprayed clothes
- Medicaments – fragranced topical medicaments, suppositories
- Hygiene products – fragranced sanitary towels
- Dental procedures – eugenol in pastes, mouthwash, and toothpaste

Common Contact Allergens: A Practical Guide to Detecting Contact Dermatitis, First Edition. Edited by John McFadden, Pailin Puangpet, Korbkarn Pongpairoj, Supitchaya Thaiwat, and Lee Shan Xian.
© 2020 John Wiley & Sons Ltd. Published 2020 by John Wiley & Sons Ltd.
Companion website: www.wiley.com/go/mcfadden/common_contact_allergens

- Dietary and mucosal – (e.g. flavors citral, cinnamal, geraniol, *Myroxylon pereirae* (MP) chemicals)
- Sexual intercourse/by proxy

b. *Different routes of potential exposure*
- Direct contact
- Airborne
- Hand to face/neck/chest
- Mucosal
- Systemic
- By proxy

c. *Various known clinical manifestations of contact allergy to fragrance*

Minor forms of presentation

- Dermatitis at application site, e.g. on wrists and neck from perfume application, on face and neck from lavender oil on pillow.
- Dermatitis at exposed sites in airborne distribution, e.g. from scented room sprays.
- Mimicking/exacerbating endogenous dermatitis, e.g. generalized atopic dermatitis complicated by ACD from fragrance in emollient.
- Multifactorial dermatitis, e.g. irritant hand dermatitis in an atopic patient worsened by fragrance allergy.

Major forms of presentation

- By proxy ACD, e.g. to partner's aftershave.
- Non-eczematous contact dermatitis – pustular contact dermatitis, granulomatous contact dermatitis – both patterns are more frequent with allergens other than fragrance, e.g. nickel, tattoo pigment.
- Contact urticaria – particularly with cinnamon fragrances.
- Respiratory/mucosal symptoms – frequently reported but poorly documented.
- Oral contact dermatitis, e.g. to cinnamon.

d. *Cross reactions*

Known cross-reactions with chemicals other than fragrances:
- NSAIDs (e.g. ketoprofen)
- sunscreen (octocrylene)
- epoxy resin.

Cross-reactions between fragrances:
- isoeugenol and eugenol
- cinnamal and cinnamyl alcohol
- hydroxycitronellal and geraniol.

Key points

- Fragrances consist of both natural and artificial chemicals that make a pleasant scent. This group represents one of the most ubiquitous chemicals in the personal environment.
- The majority of household and cosmetic products contain fragrance chemicals as an ingredient.
- Fragrance is one of the most common allergens to cause ACD; in most published reports contact allergy to Fragrance Mix 1 (FM1) is second only to nickel in prevalence. Up to 10% of eczema patients patch tested will be positive to one of the fragrance mixes, whilst as many as 14% will be positive when 26 individual fragrances are added to the screening series.
- Fragrance allergy is more common in females and, as with other cosmetic allergens, increases with age, particularly over the age of 40.
- Only approximately one in four patients with contact allergy to fragrance will give a pre-screening history of reacting to fragrances.
- Clinical presentation is varied; it can present as facial, oral and perioral, hand, axillary, perineal or generalized dermatitis.
- Fragrance allergy can also cause pigmented contact dermatitis, immediate hypersensitivity reactions, and systemic contact dermatitis.
- Phototoxic contact dermatitis to fragrance can cause patterned post-inflammatory hyperpigmentation.
- ACD to fragrance often presents as an exacerbation of a pre-existing endogenous dermatitis such as atopic or seborrheic dermatitis.
- Exposure can be through direct contact, airborne, by proxy (connubial), and, occasionally, dietary/oral.
- Common sources of exposure include fine fragrance deodorants, personal care products such as soap, shower gel, and shampoo, dishwashing liquid, medicated and herbal creams/lotions, essential oils, baby care products, cosmetics, air fresheners, scented candles, incense, dental products, and some food/drinks.
- Systemic contact dermatitis from fragrance usually arises from the constituents of MP in spicy food and flavoring.
- Immunological cross-reactions between individual fragrance chemicals and ketoprofen, octocrylene, and epoxy resin have been reported.
- Patch test screening for fragrance allergy in most baseline series includes testing with FM1, Fragrance Mix 2 (FM2), MP, and hydroxyisohexyl 3-cyclohexene carboxaldehyde (HICC). Including individual fragrance chemicals in the baseline screening series will significantly increase the detection rate of fragrance allergy.
- Oxidized linalool (from lavender) and oxidized limonene (from citrus) are emerging new fragrance allergens which are not components of the fragrance mix screening agents and are being included in the baseline/standard series (limonene hydroperoxides 0.3% pet, linalool hydroperoxides 1.0% pet.).
- It may be worth repeating a positive or negative patch test reaction to fragrance if a false-positive or negative result is suspected.

Introduction

Fragrances are chemicals commonly found in many products such as perfume in cosmetics, toiletries, and household products. The screening agents for fragrance allergy in the standard series are FM1 (containing eight fragrance chemicals), FM2 (containing six fragrance chemicals) and MP.

Fragrance sensitization is one of the most common clinical presentations of contact dermatitis. Worldwide studies have found widely varying rates of fragrance allergy, as characterized by positive patch test reactions to FM1 of 6–32%, to FM2 of 1.3–18%, and to MP of 1.5–4%, in patients with eczema attending patch test clinics [1–4]. Although the rates differ considerably between studies and depending on which fragrance markers are used, in eczema patients most report a rate of fragrance allergy of over 4%.

Constituents of fragrance mixes

FM1 constituents

- Cinnamal
- Cinnamyl alcohol

- Amyl cinnamal
- *Evernia prunastri* (formerly known as oak moss)
- Geraniol
- Hydroxycitronellal
- Isoeugenol
- Eugenol

Sorbitan sesquioleate is used as an emulsifier. Initially, the mix was tested at 2% for each agent though now most test the mix with individual agents at 1% concentration in petrolatum.

FM2 constituents

- Citral
- Citronellol
- Coumarin
- Farnesol
- Hexyl cinnamal
- HICC

Myroxylon pereirae

Balsam of Peru, commonly known as *Myroxylon perierae* (MP). Unlike FM1 and FM2, MP is a natural mix of fragrance constituents [5].

- Eugenol
- Vanillin
- Cinnamates
  - cinnamal
  - cinnamyl alcohol
  - benzyl cinnamate
- Benzoates
  - benzoic acid
  - sodium benzoate
- Ferulic acid
- Coniferin
- Note: MP also contains resorcinol monobenzoate, which is used in the production of plastic.

FM1 and FM2 agents are classified by source (Note: some agents could qualify for more than one subgroup).

Spice/herb related: cinnamal, cinnamyl alcohol, amyl cinnamal, isoeugenol, eugenol, hexyl cinnamal, coumarin.

Artificial: HICC, hydroxycitronellal (mostly).

Citrus associated: citral, geraniol, citronellol.

Lichen associated: *E. prunastri*.

Floral: farnesol, isoeugenol, geraniol, citronellol, amyl cinnamal, hexyl cinnamal, hydroxycitronellal, HICC.

Age

- ACD to fragrance can occur at any age and in adults fragrance allergy increases in prevalence with increasing age, as with other cosmetic allergens, and especially over the age of 40 years. Amongst females tested frequency of positive reactions peaked in the 60s and for males it peaked in the 70s [6].
- The North American Contact Dermatitis Group (NACDG) found fragrance to be the most common contact allergen in patients aged 65 and over [7].

Children

- Fragrance is commonly used in children's/infants' toiletries.
- Analyzes of "children's eau de toilette/toy cosmetics" found that several FM1 chemicals were present (geraniol 7/7, hydroxycitronellol 6/7, isoeugenol 2/7). In one cosmetic toy, cinnamyl alcohol was present at a very high concentration (3.7%) [8].
- ACD to fragrances has been reported in very young infants [9].
- Baby wipes and nappy rash creams commonly contain fragrance.

Sex

- Fragrance allergy is up to twice as common amongst females, presumably due to increased exposure.
- This female preponderance to fragrance allergy has been confirmed in the UK, Denmark, and Germany [10–12].
- Older men and the female sex appear to be particularly prone to developing contact allergy to fragrance [6].
- Women have more positive reactions to HICC (2.7 vs 1.6%), cinnamyl alcohol (0.9 vs 0.3%), cinnamal (1.2 vs 0.7%), and eugenol (0.6 vs 0.2%) whilst men have more positive reactions to citral (1.2 vs 0.3%) and coumarin (0.7 vs 0.3%) [13].

Frequency of sensitization

A summary of published studies on the frequency of sensitization (positive patch tests) amongst both the general population and from patch test clinics is given below.

- General population [14–21]
  FM1 range 0.5–6.4%
- Europe [1, 2, 10, 12, 22–28]
  FM1 range 6.0–21%, median 6.7%
  FM2 range 1.3–18.0%, median 4.5%
  MP range 4.0–6.8%, median 5.8%
- America [29–41]
  FM1 range 5.9–11.7%, median 10.4%
  MP range 3.3–11.6%, median 7.6%
- Asia [42–47]
  FM1 range 4–32.4%, median 9.0%
  MP range 1.5–7.3%, median 4.0%

Clinical disease, including case reports

ACD to fragrance is a common cause of dermatitis at various body sites (Figures 14.1–14.6) [48]. Perfumed water is often sprayed on the neck and/or wrist (Figure 14.2).

Periorbital

ACD to fragrance may commonly occur as an airborne dermatitis in the periorbital area or exposed sites (Figure 14.3).

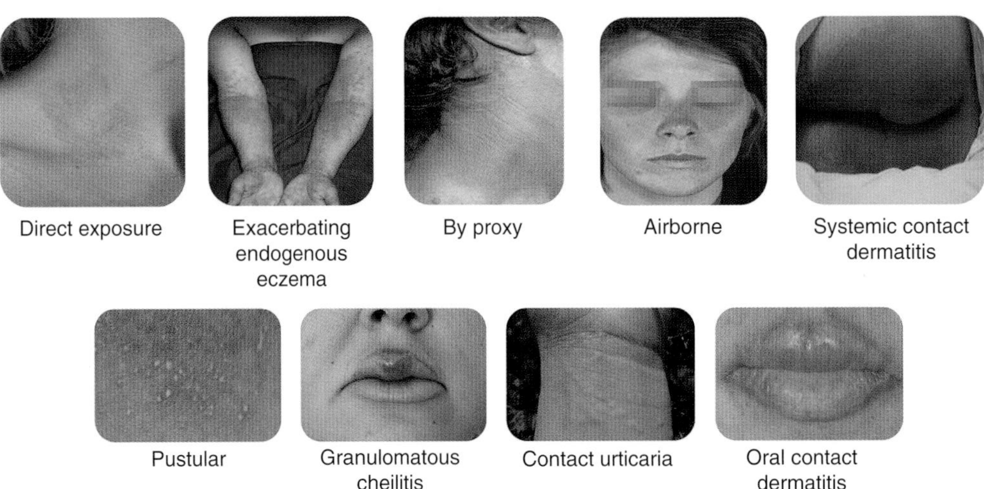

Figure 14.1 Various manifestations of contact allergy to fragrance.

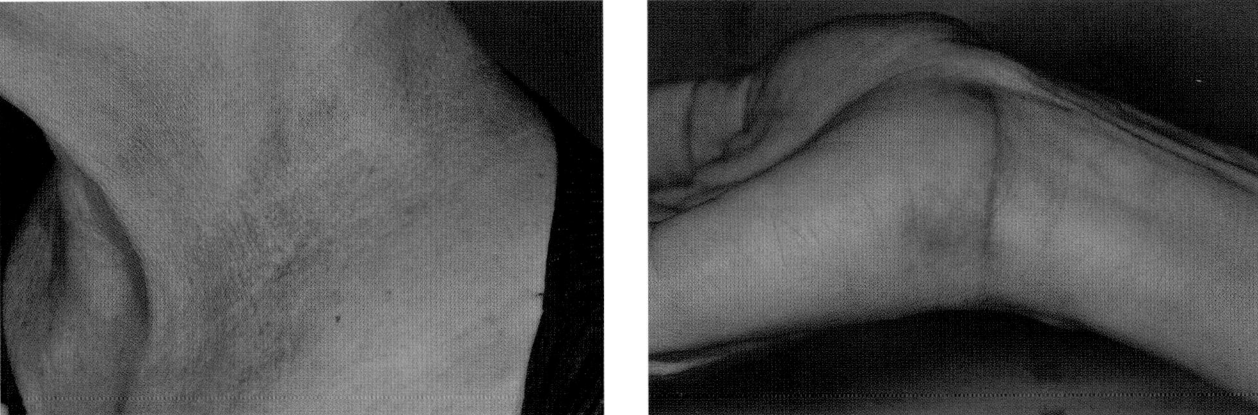

Figure 14.2 ACD from direct contact with fine fragrance spray/touch application. The side of the neck is the most common site of application, followed by the flexor aspect of the wrist. Other common applications include directly onto clothes and spraying a shower to walk through.

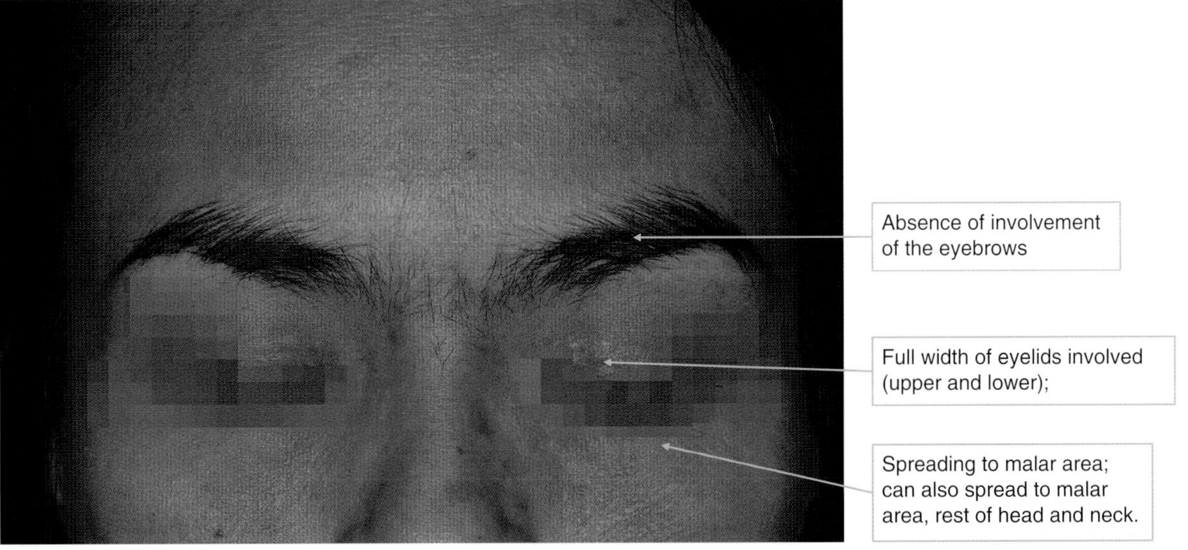

Figure 14.3 Airborne ACD from fragrance – this can involve just the upper eyelids, spread to the malar cheek area, involve the face and neck or involve all exposed areas. Together with resins, plants, and preservatives, fragrance agents are one of the most common causes of airborne ACD.

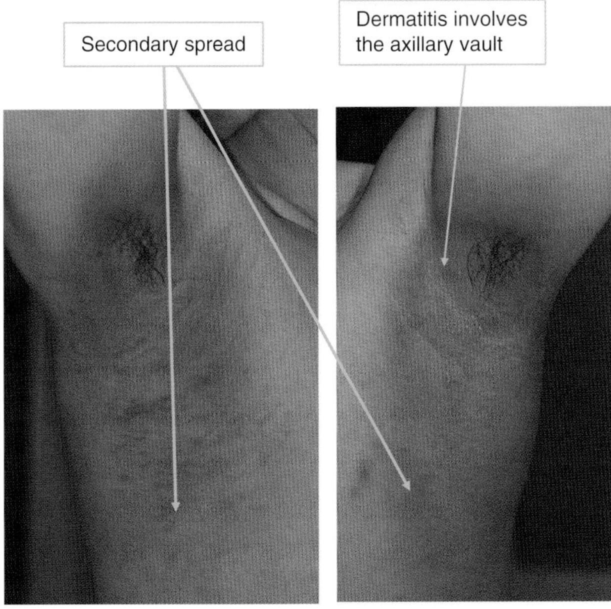
Secondary spread
Dermatitis involves the axillary vault

Figure 14.4 ACD to fragrance from deodorants. The dermatitis involves the vault (unlike clothing dye ACD), is often severe and there can be local secondary spread.

The majority of studies quote fragrance as the most common contact allergen associated with periorbital dermatitis.

- 100 patients with eyelid dermatitis were patch tested. The three most common positive patch test allergens were FM2 (n =19), FM1 (n =17), and MP (n =17). 42 patch tested positive to one or more allergens within an additional fragrance series. 15 (36%) of those allergic to fragrances had no positive reactions to the usual standard series fragrance mixes or components of the mixes such as cinnamal. The most common of these allergens were ylang-ylang (six patients) and sandalwood (four patients). The inclusion of an additional individual fragrance series was suggested when patch testing eyelid dermatitis patients [49].
- A study from Germany (2008) investigated the causes of periorbital dermatitis in over 2000 patients. ACD was the most common cause of periorbital dermatitis (32%). Of those with periorbital ACD, the most common relevant standard allergens were FM1 (19% of periorbital ACD cases) and MP (10%) [50]. The periorbital ACD group was older than the periorbital non-ACD group [51].

Hands

Fragrance is an important allergen related to hand dermatitis, but other contact allergens are also frequently involved.

- Of 658 hand eczema patients who were patch tested to a baseline series and selected fragrance chemicals, 67 (10.2%) had a positive reaction to one or more individual fragrance chemicals. The three most common allergens were citral, HICC, and oxidized limonene. Exposure assessment and the patients' history supported the relevance of fragrances as important allergens associated with hand dermatitis. FM1 would have detected only 45% of these fragrance-allergic individuals [52].

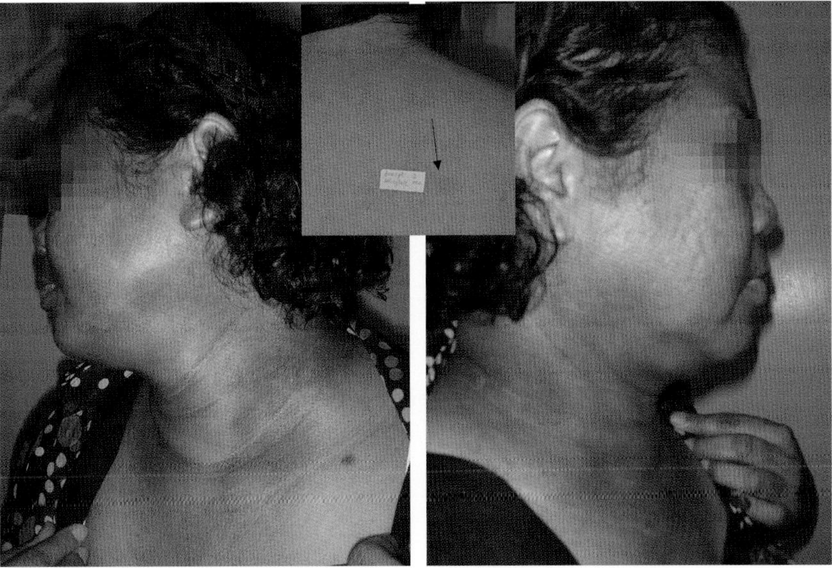
A 55-year-old lady presented with hyperpigmentation of her neck for 1.5 years.
This was pigmented allergic contact dermatitis to the fragrance she was using – the patch test reaction site also became hyperpigmented after 2 months.

Figure 14.5 Pigmented ACD to fragrance. A 55-year-old lady presented with hyperpigmentation of her neck for 1.5 years. This was pigmented ACD to the fragrance she was using – the patch test reaction site also became hyperpigmented after 2 months.

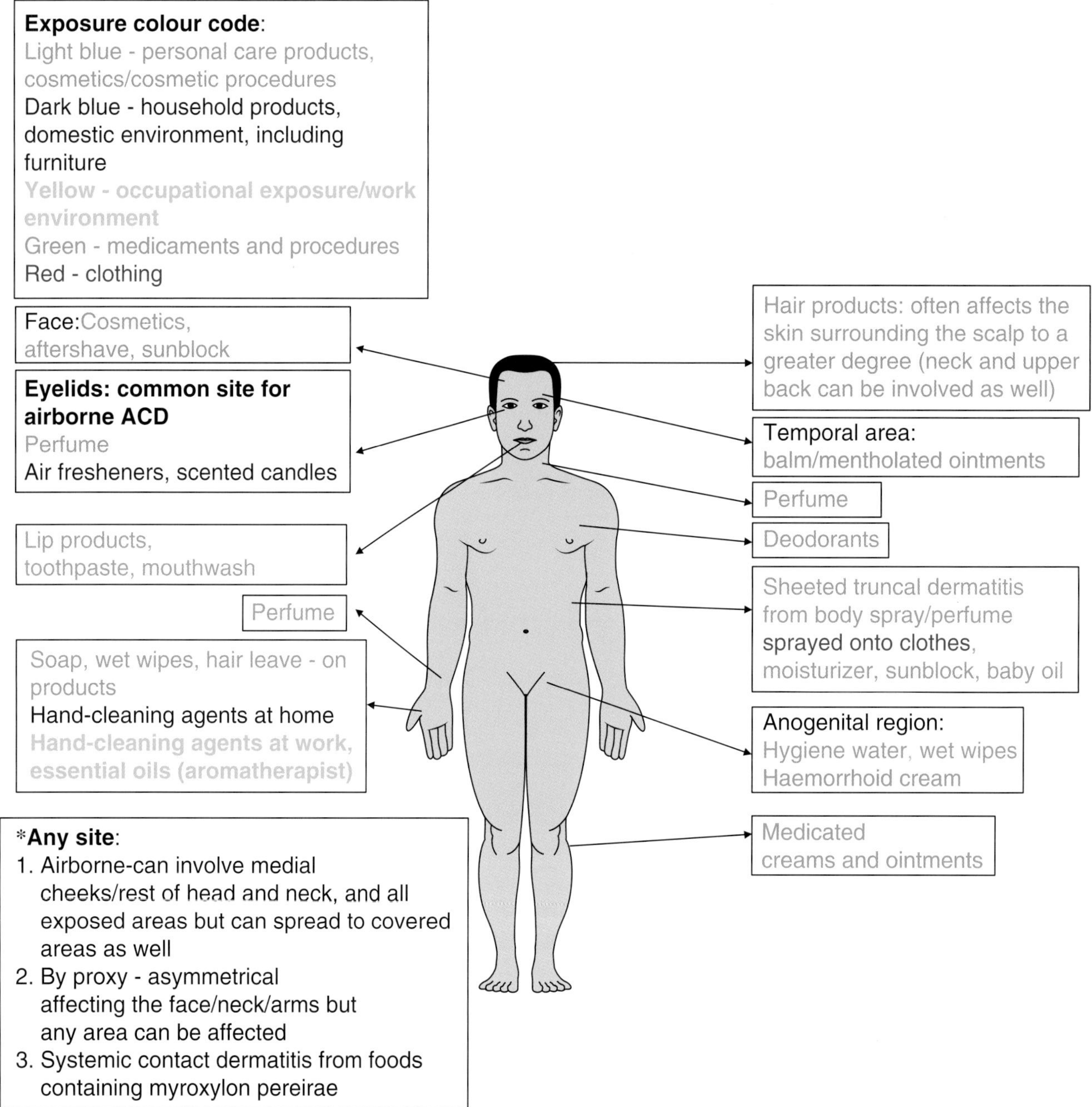

Figure 14.6 Reported exposure sources for ACD to fragrance.

Axillae

Fragrance mix agents are often contained in deodorants and can cause ACD (Figure 14.4). HICC is a common cause of ACD to deodorants. The presence of an astringent such as aluminum salts can act as an adjuvant in promoting allergy to the fragrance chemicals present.

- A survey of 46 deodorants found the most common fragrance chemicals used were limonene, HICC, geraniol and linalool [55].
- Accumulation of fragrance allergens within the axilla by repeated application will predispose to ACD [56]. Of 95 637 eczema patients patch tested to HICC, 2141 had a positive reaction (2.24%). Axillary dermatitis and "multiple positive allergens" were the strongest risk factors for HICC sensitization. The other risk factors for HICC allergy were female sex, previous history of atopic eczema, and age (peak risk between 52 and 67 years, decreasing at over 70 years) [57].
- Axillary dermatitis from fragrance allergy can often be severe due to the "adjuvant" effects of an astringent such as aluminum chloride in the deodorant augmenting the dermatitis reaction.

Oral and perioral dermatitis

- A role for fragrance allergy in "burning mouth syndrome" is controversial and usually hard to prove.
- Fragrance allergy can frequently cause/contribute to cheilitis, e.g. in lipstick.
- ACD to aroma in toothpaste can often cause cheilitis [58].
- Eugenol in mouthwash can cause perioral dermatitis.
- Cinnamal allergy caused by exposure to cola and toothpaste has been reported to cause painful tongue ulceration [59].
- Geraniol allergy caused by exposure to ice cream and sweets has been reported to cause cheilitis [60].
- A study from America reported 196 patients with lips as the sole site of dermatitis (cheilitis) who were subsequently patch tested. Sixty-five (38%) were diagnosed with allergic contact cheilitis. The most common patch test reactions were to FM1 (n = 18) and MP (n = 14). The main sources of relevant fragrance exposure in this study were oral hygiene products followed by lipstick [58].

Orofacial granulomatosis

In one study, immediate reactions to the fragrance chemicals benzoic acid, cinnamal, and cinnamyl alcohol were frequently observed. However, this needs to be interpreted with caution, as type 1 reactions to fragrance/fragrance mix may be non-immunological [61].

In another study, fragrance was found to be one of several contact allergens associated with orofacial granulomatosis. Avoidance was reported as leading to improvement in the majority over the medium term. Again, these results need to be interpreted with caution, as orofacial granulomatosis can fluctuate over the medium term [62].

Ano-genital

Fragrance is one of the most frequently associated contact allergens with dermatitis of the genitalia/anus. Sources of exposure include soaps and douches. MP is contained in some topical medicines for hemorrhoids [63].

- Fragrance is the most common contact allergy associated with vulval dermatitis.
- A study of 575 patients with anogenital symptoms who had undergone patch testing found that FM1 (11.6%) and MP (11.2%) were the most common standard allergens detected. The sources of fragrance exposure were numerous, including soaps and douches. There was a highly significant difference in the rate of relevant positive patch test reactions to cinnamal in the anogenital group (4.9%) compared to the group without anogenital involvement (1.9%), $p = 0.001$ [64].
- Cinnamal is present in MP, a common ingredient in topical therapies for hemorrhoids, which can therefore cause a "medicament" dermatitis in the perianal area [63]. Another study reported an association between allergy to cinnamon fragrances and anogenital dermatitis [65].

Immediate-type hypersensitivity

Fragrance agents, particularly MP and cinnamal/cinnamyl alcohol, can give rise to immediate hypersensitivity/contact urticaria on both an immunological (allergic) and non-immunological basis. A significant role of fragrance allergy in some cases of chronic spontaneous urticaria is unconfirmed and speculative.

- 110 patients were divided into two groups with positive reactions to either (delayed) patch test positive FM1 and/or MP (n = 60) and a negative control group (n = 50). All were closed patch tested to a fragrance series for 30 minutes on the forearm, the three most commonly positive immediate reactions being to MP (58%), cinnamal (38%), and FM1 (12%). No significant difference between the groups was noted, indicating no overall relationship between delayed-type hypersensitivity to fragrance and immediate reactions to fragrance [66].
- Some immediate reactions to fragrances are of a non-allergic nature.

Pigmented contact dermatitis

ACD to fragrance needs to be excluded in cases of undiagnosed chronic head and neck pigmented dermatosis (Figure 14.5) [67, 68].

- A 27-year-old woman presented with hyperpigmented patches on the face. She had positive patch test reactions to lemon oil, geraniol, and hydroxycitronellal, two of those chemicals being present in her face powder. The clinical appearance improved after 6 months of fragrance avoidance [68].

Phototoxic contact dermatitis

- Berloque dermatitis was reported in a case series of Lebanese patients with non-allergic exposure to fragrances containing the chemical bergapten. The pattern of hyperpigmentation corresponded to the pattern of application of the fragrance chemical. Most cases of Berloque dermatitis have hyperpigmented patches on the face and neck [69].

Systemic contact dermatitis

Allergy to fragrance chemicals, particularly constituents of MP, is a potential cause of systemic contact dermatitis (SCD) [70]. Although uncommon, this phenomenon may be underdiagnosed. In a few cases, dietary restriction (a low balsam of Peru diet, Table 14.1) has been reported as being of therapeutic value.

Tomatoes contain the fragrance agents cinnamyl alcohol and coniferyl alcohol but one study reported only a low cross-reactivity between tomatoes and fragrance allergens on patch testing [71, 72].

- SCD can result from exposure to the allergen via oral, intravenous or inhalation routes. SCD can involve the groin/perineum, axilla, face, and hands, or lead to extensive involvement/worsening of an endogenous eczema, or a combination of these. MP is one of the most common allergens to cause SCD. Many of the chemicals found in MP, such as benzyl cinnamate, benzyl benzoate, cinnamin, vanillin, and coumarin, are contained in foods and beverages [73].

Table 14.1 Low *Myroxylon pereirae*/balsam of Peru diet – foods to avoid [70].

Products containing the peel of citrus fruits (oranges, lemons, grapefruit, bitter oranges, tangerines, mandarin oranges, etc.), e.g. marmalade, juice, baked goods, cocktails
Products flavored with essences, e.g. baked goods, candy, chewing gum
Perfumed products, e.g. perfumed teas, tobacco, etc.
Various types of cough medicine and lozenges
Eugenol
Ice cream
Cola and other spiced soft drinks
Spices such as cinnamon, cloves, vanilla, curry (and products made with these spices), e.g. tomato ketchup, chili sauce, chutney, pickled herring, pickled vegetables like beets and cucumbers, baked goods, liver paste, pate, vermouth, bitters, and other similarly spiced beverages

- Of allergic reactions to foods/dietary agents which contain haptens, MP is the most common fragrance agent that has been reported to cause SCD. A trial period of at least a month with avoidance of related chemicals such as citrus fruits, tomatoes, liquors, cinnamon, vanilla, cloves, and ginger (a low balsam of Peru diet) is given to patients with suspected SCD to fragrance [74].
- Long-term (more than 6 months) dietary avoidance of MP-related foods has been reported to lead to improvement in up to 60% of selected patients, but the use of a low-MP diet is controversial, and it is not routinely recommended in patients with positive patch tests to MP [70].

Respiratory airways reactions

At least one study contends that fragrance can cause symptomatic airway irritation, although another study has refuted this [75].

A Danish study reports a higher incidence of airway symptoms on exposure to fragrance chemicals amongst fragrance patch test positive subjects, with the symptoms often starting within minutes of exposure [76].

Further case reports

- ACD to fragrance from citrus peel in cocktail waiters. ACD to lime and FM1 was reported in a 54-year-old bartender with hand dermatitis for the last 18 years. The rash began on her fingerweb spaces, sparing the dorsum of the hand and wrist, then became painful and fissured. The symptoms flared up on working days and improved on holiday. She gave strong patch test positive reactions to lime peel, geraniol, FM1, and FM2. After 2 months of avoidance the dermatitis improved. Geraniol (present in FM1) is contained in citrus oil, as are citral (present in FM 2) and limonene. The patient was diagnosed with relevant work-related contact dermatitis to lime- and citrus-containing chemicals [77].
- Blistering dermatitis from allergic reaction to cinnamon essential oil. A 74-year-old female developed an extensive eczematous and bullous dermatitis on the arms and legs 24 hours after exposure to a mud bath with cinnamon essential oil in a spa. Patch tests were strongly positive to FM1, cinnamon essence, eugenol, cinnamyl alcohol, and cinnamal. After complete cinnamon avoidance there was no recurrence [78].
- Connubial ACD to fragrance presenting as an asymmetrical rash. A 40-year-old female had a refractory eczematous rash involving the lateral aspect of her left forearm and upper arm. Patch tests were positive to FM1 and methychloroisothiazolin one/methyisothiazolinone (MCI/MI); she had already avoided these agents but her dermatitis had not cleared. However, her husband also used a variety of fragranced products – he slept on the left side of the bed and usually had close skin contact with the patient's left arm. The patient's arm dermatitis cleared after her husband stopped using fragranced products. The authors note that connubial (or by proxy) fragrance ACD may be underestimated [79].
- Two patients with ACD to fragrance in Tiger balm were reported. A 48-year-old male suffered from chronic headache after a head injury and started applying "Tiger balm red" for pain relief on his forehead. A few months later he developed eczema of the forehead. He was patch tested to a baseline series and "Tiger balm red" (50% in pet and "as is") with positive reactions to Tiger Balm ++/+++, FM1+, cinnamal ++, and cinnamyl alcohol ++. A 36-year-old female with chronic back pain intermittently applied "Tiger balm red" on the back and eventually developed severe contact dermatitis on the back. She had positive patch tests to Tiger Balm +++, MP +, FM1 ++, cinnamal ++, cinnamyl alcohol ++ and *Cananga odorata* oil (ylang-ylang) ++. The authors note that both patients were sensitized to cinnamal and cinnamyl alcohol by the use of "Tiger balm red" [80].
- ACD to fragrance presenting as ring dermatitis. A 16-year-old girl presented with a pruriginous, vesicular dermatitis on the dorsal and palmar aspects of the index, middle, and ring fingers of both hands for 2 days. The lesions were sharply demarcated under her rings, which were made of rubber and metal. Patch tests were positive to mercury, isoeugenol, geraniol, thimerosal, and to her own eau de toilette and body milk lotion. Ring dermatitis can be a presentation of fragrance allergy from repeated contact with a semi-occluded, mechanically irritated area of skin [81].
- Fragrance ACD after using an electric shaver. A 76-year-old man developed pruritic impetiginized dermatitis on the beard area after 3 weeks of using a new electric shaver. Patch tests were positive to FM1 and MP; he was using a fragranced shaving conditioner. The authors speculate that minimal traumatic abrasions from electric shaving may have facilitated skin penetration of fragrance and the subsequent allergic reaction [82].

Other disease groups and fragrance allergy

The overall fragrance allergy rates amongst patients with and without atopic eczema are similar [83]. Fragrance allergy was found to be common in patients with plaque psoriasis [84].

- Of 34 072 patients who were patch tested with a standard series, 20 700 reported an atopic history such as atopic eczema, hay fever, asthma, and atopy in the family. 7.8% (1046/13 372) of those in the non-atopic group had positive reactions to FM1 while 7.6% (1570/20 700) of atopic patients had fragrance sensitivity (no significant difference) [83].
- Amongst 200 patients with chronic plaque psoriasis, there was a higher rate of sensitivity to both topical medicaments and fragrances compared to those with other dermatologic diseases [84].

Cross-reactions between fragrance chemicals and other allergens

Octocrylene and ketoprofen

Ketoprofen, octocrylene, and cinnamyl alcohol can be viewed as a closely related allergen group [85–89].

- Patients who are allergic or (even more so) photoallergic to ketoprofen have been reported to cross-react with cinnamyl alcohol in varying numbers, but in one study in up to 100% of cases [89]. There is also a high degree of reactions noted to FM1 and MP in these patients as both contain cinnamic chemicals. Lavender and neroli oil reactions were also noted – these were probably co-reactions (though there is a trace of cinnamyl alcohol in lavender oil). Octocrylene is also a common co-reactor with ketoprofen.
- The likelihood of cross-reactivity increases if photoallergy to ketoprofen is present.
- Cross-reactivity may occur because of a shared ketonic group between ketoprofen and cinnamyl alcohol.

Epoxy resin (see also Chapter 26)

- A significant association between contact allergy to epoxy resin and fragrance chemicals (notably isoeugenol and amyl cinnamal) has been reported [90, 91].

Occupational ACD to fragrance

- Fragrance allergy is common in healthcare workers from soap exposure, dentists from eugenol in root canal treatments, mouthwashes, and toothpastes, and machine operators from cutting fluids and skin-protection creams [92, 93].
- Fragrance allergy is common in hairdressers, although this is not consistently reported in series where hairdressers were patch tested [94, 95].
- ACD to cinnamic fragrance chemicals in spices has been reported in bakers, restaurant workers, and food handlers [96].
- Aromatherapists have a high rate of fragrance allergy from exposure to essential oils and should be investigated with an extensive fragrance series [97].
- ACD to *E. prunastri* (formerly oak moss) can be associated with forestry work [98].

Fragrance exposures

See Figure 14.6.

Cosmetic and consumer products

- Approximately two-thirds of all consumer products are fragranced [55, 99–103].
- Geraniol, eugenol, cinnamyl alcohol, hexyl cinnamal, and citronellol are common FM1/FM 2 constituents in deodorants, although HICC, as a potent allergen, has been a more common cause of ACD to deodorants.
- Citronellol, geraniol, hydroxycitronellal, citral, HICC, coumarin, eugenol, hexyl cinnamal, and isoeugenol are common FM1/FM2 constituents of eau de parfum. Deodorants, scented lotions, and fine fragrances are the most common cosmetics identified as causing fragrance ACD.
- Cinnamal is the most common FM1/FM 2 agent found in toothpaste, followed by eugenol. Limonene is another fragrance used very frequently in toothpaste.
- EU legislation introduced in 2005 requires 26 listed individual fragrance chemicals (at concentrations of >10 ppm in leave-on products and >100 ppm in rinse-off products) to be included in the ingredient labeling of cosmetic products while other fragrance chemicals are included within the umbrella label "parfum" as before [104].

Baby personal care products

- Studies report that 84% of baby toiletries and 87% of baby moist tissue paper/wipes contain fragrance [105, 106].

Medicinal products

- Many topical emollients and pharmacological agents are fragranced. Fragrance is often used to mask other odors, e.g. crude lanolin. MP is a common contact allergen in patients with leg ulcers (up to 40%) from fragrance used in topical agents [40]. Cinnamyl alcohol and cinnamal are reported to cause ACD through exposure to "Tiger balm red", which can be used as a topical remedy for wounds [80].

Food products

See section on systemic contact dermatitis.

Notes on patch testing

Studies indicate that routinely testing individual fragrances, in addition to using the fragrance mixes for patch test screening, greatly increases the detection of contact allergy to fragrance (by up to 50%) [107, 108].

A late (day 7) reading will detect more positive fragrance patch tests [109].

Preparation of fragrance allergen patches immediately before testing will optimize the sensitivity of testing [110].

Emerging fragrance allergens

Oxidized linalool

- Tested as linalool hydroperoxides 1% pet./T.R.U.E.® test equivalent
- Linalool is a naturally occurring terpene alcohol chemical found in many flowers and spice plants and is used as an aroma (floral and spicy).
- It is contained in many essential oils: lavender oil, bergamot, ylang-ylang, geranium oil, orange oil, rose oil, rosewood, coriander, petitgrain, ho wood, thyme, clary sage and laurel oil. It is also found in tomatoes.
- (S)-Linalool from coriander oil, sweet orange (*Citrus sinensis*), and tomato has a smell described as sweet lavender with a touch of citrus. The isomer (*R*)-(–)-linalool, found in the oils of rose, neroli, lavender, laurel, and sweet basil (*Ocimum basilicum*), has a more woody lavender smell.
- Linalool is also found in birch trees and some fungi.
- Commercial sources include toiletries, household goods, scented candles, and air fresheners.
- A survey of cosmetic and household products found that linalool was present in the following: 46/70 (66%) personal care products, 47/59 (80%) men's cosmetics, 17/57 (30%) household products, 42/44 (95%) women's fine fragrances, and 12/17 (71%) deodorants. It is not used in oral products (mouthwash, toothpaste) [99].
- Linalool is only a significant allergen when oxidized, so many products containing linalool may not give a reaction.
- Ingestion of linalool in linalool-allergic individuals is not known to cause reactions.
- In a recent British multicentre study, 281/4731 (5.9%) of eczema patients who were patch tested had a positive reaction (i.e. contact allergy) to oxidized linalool [111]. The most commonly affected site was the face, followed by the hands and the "whole body."
- Although linalool is the main allergen in lavender, current patch testing with oxidized linalool only detects approximately half of patients also allergic to lavender oil [112].

Oxidized limonene

- Tested as limonene hydroperoxides 0.3% pet./T.R.U.E.® test equivalent.
- Limonene is a colorless liquid hydrocarbon classified as a cyclic terpene. The more common D-isomer possesses a strong smell of oranges. The less common L-isomer is found in mint oils and has a piney, turpentine-like odor. Limonene takes its name from the lemon, as the rind of the lemon, like other citrus fruits, contains considerable amounts of this compound, which contributes to their odor. It occurs naturally in many essential oils, such as lime, lemongrass, neroli, grapefruit, tangerine, olibanum, peppermint, rose, sage, tea tree, and fennel.
- It is commonly used in toiletries and household products.
- In foods, beverages, and chewing gum, limonene is used as a flavoring (most people who have contact allergy to limonene can still ingest limonene-containing foods without problems).
- Limonene is used as a fragrance, domestic cleaner (solvent), and as an ingredient in water-free hand cleansers. It is a precursor of carvone, an industrial cleaning agent, which is also used as a flavor in toothpaste.
- A UK survey found limonene in the following agents: 43/44 (97%) women's fine fragrances, 29/57 (51%) household products, 45/59 (76%) men's toiletries, 11/17 (65%) deodorants, and 9/14 (64%) dental products [99].
- Limonene is only a significant allergen if it is oxidized by air; products with a long shelf life (e.g. shampoos, perfumes) will be more likely to have their limonene oxidized.
- ACD to limonene is most likely from exposure to limonene-containing toiletries and household goods. However, unusual sources of exposure have been described:
  - A 58-year-old man, whose main pastime was archery, presented with linear eczema on the palmar aspect of his left hand. He was allergic to limonene, which had been a component of a paint stripper applied to his bow [113].
  - Transfer of limonene to the skin of the hand by holding scented candles has been demonstrated after five consecutive 20-second grasps of the candle [114].
  - Occupational limonene allergy was observed in 14 workers who used limonene-containing machine-cleaning detergents and hand cleansers [115].
  - Foti et al. [116] reported hand dermatitis in a laboratory technician from allergy to limonene in a solvent used to dissolve paraffin.
  - A gardener developed ACD of the hand by tending to geraniums, which contain limonene [117].
- Limonene was found to be the most common cause of ACD to tea tree oil [118].
- One recent global audit of limonene allergy in 2900 patients attending patch test clinics found an incidence ranging from 2.5% to 12.1%, with a mean of 5.2% [119]. In a UK study from 13 centers, the mean incidence of patch test positivity to limonene was 5% (range 1.7% to 11.4%) [111].
- 25% of patients reacting to oxidized limonene and linalool will concomitantly react to both, which is probably an indicator of concomitant exposure as they are often both contained in toiletries/household products [120].

Fragrance allergens in essential oils

- Essential oils contain fragrance allergens (data from various intenret sources).
- The most common agents found in 30 essential oils are limonene ($n = 24$), linalool ($n = 22$), geraniol ($n = 13$), citral ($n = 8$), and eugenol ($n = 7$) (McFadden, personal communication).
- For practical purposes, it may be worth advising patients who are allergic to limonene and/or linalool to avoid essential oils.

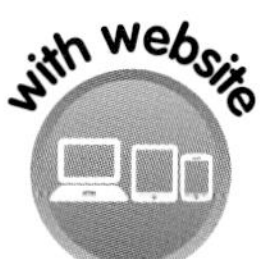

Go to www.wiley.com/go/mcfadden/common_contact_allergens to find the E-supplement for this chapter:

Fragrances: E-Supplement

References

1 Hasan, T., Rantanen, T., Alanko, K. et al. (2005). Patch test reactions to cosmetic allergens in 1995–1997 and 2000–2002 in Finland – a multicentre study. *Contact Dermatitis* 53 (1): 40–45.

2 Bordel-Gomez, M.T., Miranda-Romero, A., and Castrodeza-Sanz, J. (2010). Epidemiology of contact dermatitis: prevalence of sensitization to different allergens and associated factors. *Actas Dermo-Sifiliográficas* 101 (1): 59–75.

3 Salverda, J.G., Bragt, P.J., de Wit-Bos, L. et al. (2013). Results of a cosmetovigilance survey in the Netherlands. *Contact Dermatitis* 68 (3): 139–148.

4 Wang, W.H., Li, L.F., Lu, X.Y., and Wang, J. (2005). Cosmetic dermatitis in Chinese eczema patients patch tested with a modified European standard series of allergens. *Contact Dermatitis* 53 (6): 314–319.

5 Scheman, A., Rakowski, E.M., Chou, V. et al. (2013). Balsam of Peru: past and future. *Dermatitis* 24 (4): 153–160.

6 Buckley, D.A., Rycroft, R.J., White, I.R., and McFadden, J.P. (2003). The frequency of fragrance allergy in patch-tested patients increases with their age. *British Journal of Dermatology* 149 (5): 986–989.

7 Warshaw, E.M., Raju, S.I., Fowler, J.F. Jr. et al. (2012). Positive patch test reactions in older individuals: retrospective analysis from the North American Contact Dermatitis Group, 1994–2008. *Journal of the American Academy of Dermatology* 66 (2): 229–240.

8 Rastogi, S.C., Johansen, J.D., Menne, T. et al. (1999). Contents of fragrance allergens in children's cosmetics and cosmetic-toys. *Contact Dermatitis* 41 (2): 84–88.

9 Nardelli, A., Morren, M.A., and Goossens, A. (2009). Contact allergy to fragrances and parabens in an atopic baby. *Contact Dermatitis* 60 (2): 107–109.

10 Buckley, D.A., Wakelin, S.H., Seed, P.T. et al. (2000). The frequency of fragrance allergy in a patch-test population over a 17-year period. *British Journal of Dermatology* 142 (2): 279–283.

11 Bennike, N.H., Zachariae, C., and Johansen, J.D. (2017). Trends in contact allergy to fragrance mix I in consecutive Danish patients with eczema from 1986 to 2015: a cross-sectional study. *British Journal of Dermatology* 176 (4): 1035–1041.

12 Krautheim, A., Uter, W., Frosch, P. et al. (2010). Patch testing with fragrance mix II: results of the IVDK 2005–2008. *Contact Dermatitis* 63 (5): 262–269.

13 Schnuch, A., Uter, W., Geier, J. et al. (2007). Sensitization to 26 fragrances to be labelled according to current European regulation. Results of the IVDK and review of the literature. *Contact Dermatitis* 57 (1): 1–10.

14 Magnusson, B. and Moller, H. (1979). Contact allergy without skin disease. *Acta Dermato Venereologica Supplementum (Stockholm)* 59 (85): 113–115.

15 Seidenari, S., Manzini, B.M., Danese, P., and Motolese, A. (1990). Patch and prick test study of 593 healthy subjects. *Contact Dermatitis* 23 (3): 162–167.

16 Thyssen, J.P., Linneberg, A., Menne, T. et al. (2009). The prevalence and morbidity of sensitization to fragrance mix I in the general population. *British Journal of Dermatology* 161 (1): 95–101.

17 Schnuch, A., Uter, W., Geier, J., and Gefeller, O. (2002). Epidemiology of contact allergy: an estimation of morbidity employing the clinical epidemiology and drug-utilization research (CE-DUR) approach. *Contact Dermatitis* 47 (1): 32–39.

18 Mortz, C.G., Lauritsen, J.M., Bindslev-Jensen, C., and Andersen, K.E. (2002). Contact allergy and allergic contact dermatitis in adolescents: prevalence measures and associations. The Odense Adolescence Cohort Study on Atopic Diseases and Dermatitis (TOACS). *Acta Dermato-Venereologica* 82 (5): 352–358.

19 Bryld, L.E., Hindsberger, C., Kyvik, K.O. et al. (2003). Risk factors influencing the development of hand eczema in a population-based twin sample. *British Journal of Dermatology* 149 (6): 1214–1220.

20 White, J.M., Gilmour, N.J., Jeffries, D. et al. (2007). A general population from Thailand: incidence of common allergens with emphasis on para-phenylenediamine. *Clinical and Experimental Allergy* 37 (12): 1848–1853.

21 Thyssen, J.P., Menne, T., Linneberg, A., and Johansen, J.D. (2009). Contact sensitization to fragrances in the general population: a Koch's approach may reveal the burden of disease. *British Journal of Dermatology* 160 (4): 729–735.

22 Thyssen, J.P., Carlsen, B.C., Menne, T., and Johansen, J.D. (2008). Trends of contact allergy to fragrance mix I and *Myroxylon pereirae* among Danish eczema patients tested between 1985 and 2007. *Contact Dermatitis* 59 (4): 238–244.

23 Uter, W., Hegewald, J., Aberer, W. et al. (2005). The European standard series in 9 European countries, 2002/2003 – first results of the European Surveillance System on Contact Allergies. *Contact Dermatitis* 53 (3): 136–145.

24 Rudzki, E. and Rebandel, P. (2006). 100 patients positive to balsam of Peru observed in Warsaw (Poland). *Contact Dermatitis* 55 (4): 255.

25 Frosch, P.J., Pirker, C., Rastogi, S.C. et al. (2005). Patch testing with a new fragrance mix detects additional patients sensitive to perfumes and missed by the current fragrance mix. *Contact Dermatitis* 52 (4): 207–215.

26 Uter, W., Geier, J., Frosch, P., and Schnuch, A. (2010). Contact allergy to fragrances: current patch test results (2005–2008) from the Information Network of Departments of Dermatology. *Contact Dermatitis* 63 (5): 254–261.

27 Heisterberg, M.V., Andersen, K.E., Avnstorp, C. et al. (2010). Fragrance mix II in the baseline series contributes significantly to detection of fragrance allergy. *Contact Dermatitis* 63 (5): 270–276.

28 Mahler, V., Geier, J., and Schnuch, A. (2014). Current trends in patch testing – new data from the German Contact Dermatitis Research Group (DKG) and the Information Network of Departments of dermatology (IVDK). *Journal der Deutschen Dermatologischen Gesellschaft* 12 (7): 583–592.

29 Epstein, E., Rees, W.J., and Maibach, H.I. (1968). Recent experience with routine patch test screening. *Archives of Dermatology* 98 (1): 18–22.

30 Lynde, C.W., Warshawski, L., and Mitchell, J.C. (1982). Screening patch tests in 4190 eczema patients 1972–81. *Contact Dermatitis* 8 (6): 417–421.

31 Rudner, E.J., Clendenning, W.E., Epstein, E. et al. (1975). The frequency of contact sensitivity in North America 1972–74. *Contact Dermatitis* 1 (5): 277–280.

32 Nethercott, J.R. (1982). Results of routine patch testing of 200 patients in Toronto, Canada. *Contact Dermatitis* 8 (6): 389–395.

33 Storrs, F.J., Rosenthal, L.E., Adams, R.M. et al. (1989). Prevalence and relevance of allergic reactions in patients patch tested in North America – 1984 to 1985. *Journal of the American Academy of Dermatology* 20 (6): 1038–1045.

34 Nguyen, S.H., Dang, T.P., MacPherson, C. et al. (2008). Prevalence of patch test results from 1970 to 2002 in a multi-centre population in North America (NACDG). *Contact Dermatitis* 58 (2): 101–106.

35 Holness, D.L., Nethercott, J.R., Adams, R.M. et al. (1995). Concomitant positive patch test results with standard screening tray in North America 1985–1989. *Contact Dermatitis* 32 (5): 289–292.

36 Albert, M.R., Gonzalez, S., and Gonzalez, E. (1998). Patch testing reactions to a standard series in 608 patients tested from 1990 to 1997 at Massachusetts General Hospital. *American Journal of Contact Dermatitis* 9 (4): 207–211.

37 Marks, J.G., Belsito, D.V., DeLeo, V.A. et al. (1998). North American Contact Dermatitis Group patch test results for the detection of delayed-type hypersensitivity to topical allergens. *Journal of the American Academy of Dermatology* 38 (6 Pt 1): 911–918.

38 Marks, J.G. Jr., Belsito, D.V., DeLeo, V.A. et al. (2000). North American Contact Dermatitis Group patch-test results, 1996–1998. *Archives of Dermatology* 136 (2): 272–273.

39 Wetter, D.A., Davis, M.D., Yiannias, J.A. et al. (2005). Patch test results from the Mayo Clinic Contact Dermatitis Group, 1998–2000. *Journal of the American Academy of Dermatology* 53 (3): 416–421.

40 Saap, L., Fahim, S., Arsenault, E. et al. (2004). Contact sensitivity in patients with leg ulcerations: a North American study. *Archives of Dermatology* 140 (10): 1241–1246.

41 Belsito, D.V., Fowler, J.F. Jr., Sasseville, D. et al. (2006). Delayed-type hypersensitivity to fragrance materials in a select North American population. *Dermatitis* 17 (1): 23–28.

42 Wang, X.M., Lin, Y.F., Cheng, X.F. et al. (1994). Patch testing with the European standard series in Shanghai. *Contact Dermatitis* 30 (3): 173–174.

43 Sharma, V.K. and Chakrabarti, A. (1998). Common contact sensitizers in Chandigarh, India. A study of 200 patients with the European standard series. *Contact Dermatitis* 38 (3): 127–131.

44 Lu, X., Li, L.F., Wang, W., and Wang, J. (2005). A clinical and patch test study of patients with positive patch test reactions to fragrance mix in China. *Contact Dermatitis* 52 (4): 188–191.

45 Disphanurat, W. (2010). Contact allergy in eczema patients in Thammasat University Hospital. *Journal of the Medical Association of Thailand* 93 (Suppl 7): S7–S14.

46 Minamoto, K. (2010). Skin sensitizers in cosmetics and skin care products. *Nippon Eiseigaku Zasshi* 65 (1): 20–29.

47 An, S., Lee, A.Y., Lee, C.H. et al. (2005). Fragrance contact dermatitis in Korea: a joint study. *Contact Dermatitis* 53 (6): 320–323.

48 Cuesta, L., Silvestre, J.F., Toledo, F. et al. (2010). Fragrance contact allergy: a 4-year retrospective study. *Contact Dermatitis* 63 (2): 77–84.

49 Wenk, K.S. and Ehrlich, A. (2012). Fragrance series testing in eyelid dermatitis. *Dermatitis* 23 (1): 22–26.

50 Feser, A., Plaza, T., Vogelgsang, L., and Mahler, V. (2008). Periorbital dermatitis – a recalcitrant disease: causes and differential diagnoses. *British Journal of Dermatology* 159 (4): 858–863.

51 Herbst, R.A., Uter, W., Pirker, C. et al. (2004). Allergic and non-allergic periorbital dermatitis: patch test results of the Information Network of the Departments of Dermatology during a 5-year period. *Contact Dermatitis* 51 (1): 13–19.

52 Heydorn, S., Johansen, J.D., Andersen, K.E. et al. (2003). Fragrance allergy in patients with hand eczema – a clinical study. *Contact Dermatitis* 48 (6): 317–323.

53 Jain, V.K., Aggarwal, K., Passi, S., and Gupta, S. (2004). Role of contact allergens in pompholyx. *Journal of Dermatology* 31 (3): 188–193.

54 Ni, C., Dou, X., Chen, J. et al. (2011). Contact sensitization in Chinese patients with hand eczema. *Dermatitis* 22 (4): 211–215.

55 Nardelli, A., Drieghe, J., Claes, L. et al. (2011). Fragrance allergens in 'specific' cosmetic products. *Contact Dermatitis* 64 (4): 212–219.

56 Svedman, C., Bruze, M., Johansen, J.D. et al. (2003). Deodorants: an experimental provocation study with hydroxycitronellal. *Contact Dermatitis* 48 (4): 217–223.

57 Uter, W., Geier, J., Schnuch, A., and Gefeller, O. (2013). Risk factors associated with sensitization to hydroxyisohexyl 3-cyclohexene carboxaldehyde. *Contact Dermatitis* 69 (2): 72–77.

58 Zug, K.A., Kornik, R., Belsito, D.V. et al. (2008). Patch-testing North American lip dermatitis patients: data from the North American Contact Dermatitis Group, 2001 to 2004. *Dermatitis* 19 (4): 202–208.

59 Jacob, S.E. and Steele, T. (2007). Tongue erosions and diet cola. *Ear, Nose, & Throat Journal* 86 (4): 232–233.

60 Tamagawa-Mineoka, R., Katoh, N., and Kishimoto, S. (2007). Allergic contact cheilitis due to geraniol in food. *Contact Dermatitis* 56 (4): 242–243.

61 Fitzpatrick, L., Healy, C.M., McCartan, B.E. et al. (2011). Patch testing for food-associated allergies in orofacial granulomatosis. *Journal of Oral Pathology & Medicine* 40 (1): 10–13.

62 Armstrong, D.K., Biagioni, P., Lamey, P.J., and Burrows, D. (1997). Contact hypersensitivity in patients with orofacial granulomatosis. *American Journal of Contact Dermatitis* 8 (1): 35–38.

63 Avalos-Peralta, P., Garcia-Bravo, B., and Camacho, F.M. (2005). Sensitivity to *Myroxylon pereirae* resin (balsam of Peru). A study of 50 cases. *Contact Dermatitis* 52 (6): 304–306.

64 Warshaw, E.M., Furda, L.M., Maibach, H.I. et al. (2008). Anogenital dermatitis in patients referred for patch testing: retrospective analysis of cross-sectional data from the North American Contact Dermatitis Group, 1994–2004. *Archives of Dermatology* 144 (6): 749–755.

65 Buckley, D.A., Rycroft, R.J., White, I.R., and McFadden, J.P. (2000). Contact allergy to individual fragrance mix constituents in relation to primary site of dermatitis. *Contact Dermatitis* 43 (5): 304–305.

66 Tanaka, S., Matsumoto, Y., Dlova, N. et al. (2004). Immediate contact reactions to fragrance mix constituents and *Myroxylon pereirae* resin. *Contact Dermatitis* 51 (1): 20–21.

67 Nakayama, H., Harada, R., and Toda, M. (1976). Pigmented cosmetic dermatitis. *International Journal of Dermatology* 15 (9): 673–675.

68 Serrano, G., Pujol, C., Cuadra, J. et al. (1989). Riehl's melanosis: pigmented contact dermatitis caused by fragrances. *Journal of the American Academy of Dermatology* 21 (5 Pt 2): 1057–1060.

69 Zaynoun, S.T., Aftimos, B.A., Tenekjian, K.K., and Kurban, A.K. (1981). Berloque dermatitis – a continuing cosmetic problem. *Contact Dermatitis* 7 (2): 111–116.

70 Veien, N.K., Hattel, T., Justesen, O., and Norholm, N. (1985). Oral challenge with balsam of Peru. *Contact Dermatitis* 12 (2): 104–107.

71 Paulsen, E., Christensen, L.P., and Andersen, K.E. (2012). Tomato contact dermatitis. *Contact Dermatitis* 67 (6): 321–327.

72 Srivastava, D. and Cohen, D.E. (2009). Identification of the constituents of balsam of Peru in tomatoes. *Dermatitis* 20 (2): 99–105.

73 Kulberg, A., Schliemann, S., and Elsner, P. (2014). Contact dermatitis as a systemic disease. *Clinics in Dermatology* 32 (3): 414–419.

74 Fabbro, S.K. and Zirwas, M.J. (2014). Systemic contact dermatitis to foods: nickel, BOP, and more. *Current Allergy and Asthma Reports* 14 (10): 463.

75 Vethanayagam, D., Vliagoftis, H., Mah, D. et al. (2013). Fragrance materials in asthma: a pilot study using a surrogate aerosol product. *The Journal of Asthma* 50 (9): 975–982.

76 Elberling, J., Linneberg, A., Mosbech, H. et al. (2004). A link between skin and airways regarding sensitivity to fragrance products? *British Journal of Dermatology* 151 (6): 1197–1203.

77 Swerdlin, A., Rainey, D., and Storrs, F.J. (2010). Fragrance mix reactions and lime allergic contact dermatitis. *Dermatitis* 21 (4): 214–216.

78 Garcia-Abujeta, J.L., de Larramendi, C.H., Berna, J.P., and Palomino, E.M. (2005). Mud bath dermatitis due to cinnamon oil. *Contact Dermatitis* 52 (4): 234.

79 Jensen, P., Garcia Ortiz, P., Hartmann-Petersen, S. et al. (2012). Connubial allergic contact dermatitis caused by fragrance ingredients. *Dermatitis* 23 (1): e1–e2.

80 Schliemann, S., Geier, J., and Elsner, P. (2011). Fragrances in topical over-the-counter medicaments – a loophole in EU legislation should be closed. *Contact Dermatitis* 65 (6): 367–368.

81 Cordoba, S., Sanchez-Perez, J., and Garcia-Diez, A. (2000). Ring dermatitis as a clinical presentation of fragrance sensitization. *Contact Dermatitis* 42 (4): 242.

82 Jensen, P., Menne, T., Johansen, J.D., and Thyssen, J.P. (2012). Facial allergic contact dermatitis caused by fragrance ingredients released by an electric shaver. *Contact Dermatitis* 67 (6): 380–381.

83 Buckley, D.A., Basketter, D.A., Kan-King-Yu, D. et al. (2008). Atopy and contact allergy to fragrance: allergic reactions to the fragrance mix I (the Larsen mix). *Contact Dermatitis* 59 (4): 220–225.

84 Malhotra, V., Kaur, I., Saraswat, A., and Kumar, B. (2002). Frequency of patch-test positivity in patients with psoriasis: a prospective controlled study. *Acta Dermato-Venereologica* 82 (6): 432–435.

85 Pigatto, P., Bigardi, A., Legori, A. et al. (1996). Cross-reactions in patch testing and photopatch testing with ketoprofen, thiaprophenic acid, and cinnamic aldehyde. *American Journal of Contact Dermatitis* 7 (4): 220–223.

86 Girardin, P., Vigan, M., Humbert, P., and Aubin, F. (2006). Cross-reactions in patch testing with ketoprofen, fragrance mix and cinnamic derivatives. *Contact Dermatitis* 55 (2): 126–128.

87 Matthieu, L., Meuleman, L., Van Hecke, E. et al. (2004). Contact and photocontact allergy to ketoprofen. The Belgian experience. *Contact Dermatitis* 50 (4): 238–241.

88 Avenel-Audran, M., Dutartre, H., Goossens, A. et al. (2010). Octocrylene, an emerging photoallergen. *Archives of Dermatology* 146 (7): 753–757.

89 Foti, C., Bonamonte, D., Conserva, A. et al. (2008). Allergic and photoallergic contact dermatitis from ketoprofen: evaluation of cross-reactivities by a combination of photopatch testing and computerized conformational analysis. *Current Pharmaceutical Design* 14 (27): 2833–2839.

90 Ponten, A., Bjork, J., Carstensen, O. et al. (2004). Associations between contact allergy to epoxy resin and fragrance mix. *Acta Dermato-Venereologica* 84 (2): 151–152.

91 Andersen, K.E., Christensen, L.P., Volund, A. et al. (2009). Association between positive patch tests to epoxy resin and fragrance mix I ingredients. *Contact Dermatitis* 60 (3): 155–157.

92 Buckley, D.A., Rycroft, R.J., White, I.R., and McFadden, J.P. (2002). Fragrance as an occupational allergen. *Occupational Medicine (London)* 52 (1): 13–16.

93 Tanko, Z., Shab, A., Diepgen, T.L., and Weisshaar, E. (2009). Polyvalent type IV sensitizations to multiple fragrances and a skin protection cream in a metal worker. *Journal der Deutschen Dermatologischen Gesellschaft* 7 (6): 541–543.

94 Tresukosol, P. and Swasdivanich, C. (2012). Hand contact dermatitis in hairdressers: clinical and causative allergens, experience in Bangkok. *Asian Pacific Journal of Allergy and Immunology* 30 (4): 306–312.

95 Guo, Y.L., Wang, B.J., Lee, J.Y., and Chou, S.Y. (1994). Occupational hand dermatoses of hairdressers in Tainan City. *Occupational and Environmental Medicine* 51 (10): 689–692.

96 Ackermann, L., Aalto-Korte, K., Jolanki, R., and Alanko, K. (2009). Occupational allergic contact dermatitis from cinnamon including one case from airborne exposure. *Contact Dermatitis* 60 (2): 96–99.

97 Trattner, A., David, M., and Lazarov, A. (2008). Occupational contact dermatitis due to essential oils. *Contact Dermatitis* 58 (5): 282–284.

98 Aalto-Korte, K., Lauerma, A., and Alanko, K. (2005). Occupational allergic contact dermatitis from lichens in present-day Finland. *Contact Dermatitis* 52 (1): 36–38.

99 Buckley, D.A. (2007). Fragrance ingredient labelling in products on sale in the UK. *British Journal of Dermatology* 157 (2): 295–300.

100 Heisterberg, M.V., Menne, T., Andersen, K.E. et al. (2011). Deodorants are the leading cause of allergic contact dermatitis to fragrance ingredients. *Contact Dermatitis* 64 (5): 258–264.

101 Lysdal, S.H. and Johansen, J.D. (2009). Fragrance contact allergic patients: strategies for use of cosmetic products and perceived impact on life situation. *Contact Dermatitis* 61 (6): 320–324.

102 Uter, W., Yazar, K., Kratz, E.M. et al. (2013). Coupled exposure to ingredients of cosmetic products: I. Fragrances. *Contact Dermatitis* 69 (6): 335–341.

103 Zirwas, M.J. and Otto, S. (2010). Toothpaste allergy diagnosis and management. *Journal of Clinical and Aesthetic Dermatology* 3 (5): 42–47.

104 European Parliament (2003). Directive 200/15/EC of the European Parliament and of the Council of 27 February 2003 amending Council Directive 76/768/EEC on the approximation of the laws of the Member States relating to cosmetic products. *Journal of the European Union* L66: 26–35.

105 White, J.M. and McFadden, J.P. (2008). Exposure to haptens/contact allergens in baby cosmetic products. *Contact Dermatitis* 59 (3): 176–177.

106 Zoli, V., Tosti, A., Silvani, S., and Vincenzi, C. (2006). Moist toilet papers as possible sensitizers: review of the literature and evaluation of commercial products in Italy. *Contact Dermatitis* 55 (4): 252–254.

107 Mann, J., McFadden, J.P., White, J.M. et al. (2014). Baseline series fragrance markers fail to predict contact allergy. *Contact Dermatitis* 70 (5): 276–281.

108 Nardelli, A., Carbonez, A., Ottoy, W. et al. (2008). Frequency of and trends in fragrance allergy over a 15-year period. *Contact Dermatitis* 58 (3): 134–141.

109 Higgins, E. and Collins, P. (2013). The relevance of 7-day patch test reading. *Dermatitis* 24 (5): 237–240.

110 Mowitz, M., Svedman, C., Zimerson, E., and Bruze, M. (2014). Fragrance patch tests prepared in advance may give false-negative reactions. *Contact Dermatitis* 71 (5): 289–294.

111 Audrain, H., Kenward, C., Lovell, C.R. et al. (2014). Allergy to oxidized limonene and linalool is frequent in the UK. *British Journal of Dermatology* 171 (2): 292–297.

112 Hagvall, L. and Christensson, J.B. (2016). Patch testing with main sensitizers does not detect all cases of contact allergy to oxidized lavender oil. *Acta Dermato-Venereologica* 96 (5): 679–683.

113 Tammaro, A., Cortesi, G., Abruzzese, C. et al. (2013). Archer dermatitis: a new case of allergic contact dermatitis. *Occupational and Environmental Medicine* 70 (10): 750.

114 Api, A.M., Bredbenner, A., McGowen, M. et al. (2007). Skin contact transfer of three fragrance residues from candles to human hands. *Regulatory Toxicology and Pharmacology* 48 (3): 279–283.

115 Pesonen, M., Suomela, S., Kuuliala, O. et al. (2014). Occupational contact dermatitis caused by d-limonene. *Contact Dermatitis* 71 (5): 273–279.

116 Foti, C., Zambonin, C.G., Conserva, A. et al. (2007). Occupational contact dermatitis to a limonene-based solvent in a histopathology technician. *Contact Dermatitis* 56 (2): 109–112.

117 Svendsen, M.T., Andersen, K.E., Thormann, H., and Paulsen, E. (2015). *Contact sensitization to Geranium robertianum* L. in an amateur gardener. *Contact Dermatitis* 72 (6): 420–421.

118 Knight, T.E. and Hausen, B.M. (1994). Melaleuca oil (tea tree oil) dermatitis. *Journal of the American Academy of Dermatology* 30 (3): 423–427.

119 Brared Christensson, J., Andersen, K.E., Bruze, M. et al. (2014). Positive patch test reactions to oxidized limonene: exposure and relevance. *Contact Dermatitis* 71 (5): 264–272.

120 Brared Christensson, J., Karlberg, A.T., Andersen, K.E. et al. (2016). Oxidized limonene and oxidized linalool – concomitant contact allergy to common fragrance terpenes. *Contact Dermatitis* 74 (5): 273–280.

Exposure Color Code

- Clothing, jewelry, adornments
- Personal care products, cosmetics/cosmetic procedures
- Household products, domestic environment, including furniture and refurbishment
- Occupational dermatoses, work environment
- Medicines, surgical/dental procedures, herbal/alternative medicines
- Personal appliances/aids
- Leisure activities, sport, travel
- Other exposures (including dietary)
- Not relevant or multiple/general exposure

Preservatives

CHAPTER 15
Formaldehyde

CHAPTER CONTENTS

Key points

- Formaldehyde is a chemical that is widely used across many consumer products and industries.
- Formaldehyde releasing preservatives are important sources of formaldehyde exposure.
- Exposure to formaldehyde-releasing preservatives in liquid soaps, shampoos, and other rinse-off products is common.
- Reactions to formaldehyde-releasing substances are seen in about 50–80% of formaldehyde allergic patients.
- Unlike allergic contact dermatitis to some other preservatives, the hands are often the primary site of presentation. Generalized dermatitis is also not an uncommon form of presentation.
- Nowadays, it is uncommon for formaldehyde resin in clothing to be a problem.
- A significant number of reported allergic cases have occupational relevance.
- Formaldehyde has been reported as the most common relevant allergen amongst domestic cleaners.
- Other workers at increased risk are metalworkers, hairdressers, masseurs, and workers using protective creams, detergents, and liquid soaps.
- Avoidance of formaldehyde can be difficult because of its ubiquitous nature.
- Optimal patch testing using aqueous solutions is achieved with formaldehyde 2% aqueous solution.
- As with other aqueous patch test solutions, false-negative reactions may occur.
- Irritant reactions to formaldehyde can occur (but usually at higher concentrations than used in cosmetic products).
- Quaternium-15 often co-reacts with formaldehyde and reflects its strong formaldehyde-releasing nature. If a quaternium-15 patch test is positive, consider repeating a negative formaldehyde patch test.
- Reported prevalence rates for formaldehyde allergy in patch test clinics vary widely; in Europe 0.5–3% is a common range.

Exposure and use

Figure 15.1 displays the most commonly reported sources of exposure to formaldehyde.

Cosmetics and household goods

- Cosmetics and toiletries, including fingernail polishers and hardeners, antiperspirants, makeup, bubble baths, bath oils, shampoos, creams, and deodorants.
- Household cleansers, disinfectants, air fresheners, dishwashing liquid, and polishes [1].
- Personal care products from two patients with allergic contact dermatitis (ACD) to formaldehyde were analyzed in a dermatology clinic for formaldehyde using a spot test kit [2]. Positive spot test products were then sent for quantitative analysis using gas chromatography-mass spectrometry. Nine out of ten spot test positive products had releasable formaldehyde (5.4–269.4 $\mu g\,g^{-1}$). Of these only two (shampoos) listed a

Common Contact Allergens: A Practical Guide to Detecting Contact Dermatitis, First Edition. Edited by John McFadden, Pailin Puangpet, Korbkarn Pongpairoj, Supitchaya Thaiwat, and Lee Shan Xian.

© 2020 John Wiley & Sons Ltd. Published 2020 by John Wiley & Sons Ltd.

Companion website: www.wiley.com/go/mcfadden/common_contact_allergens

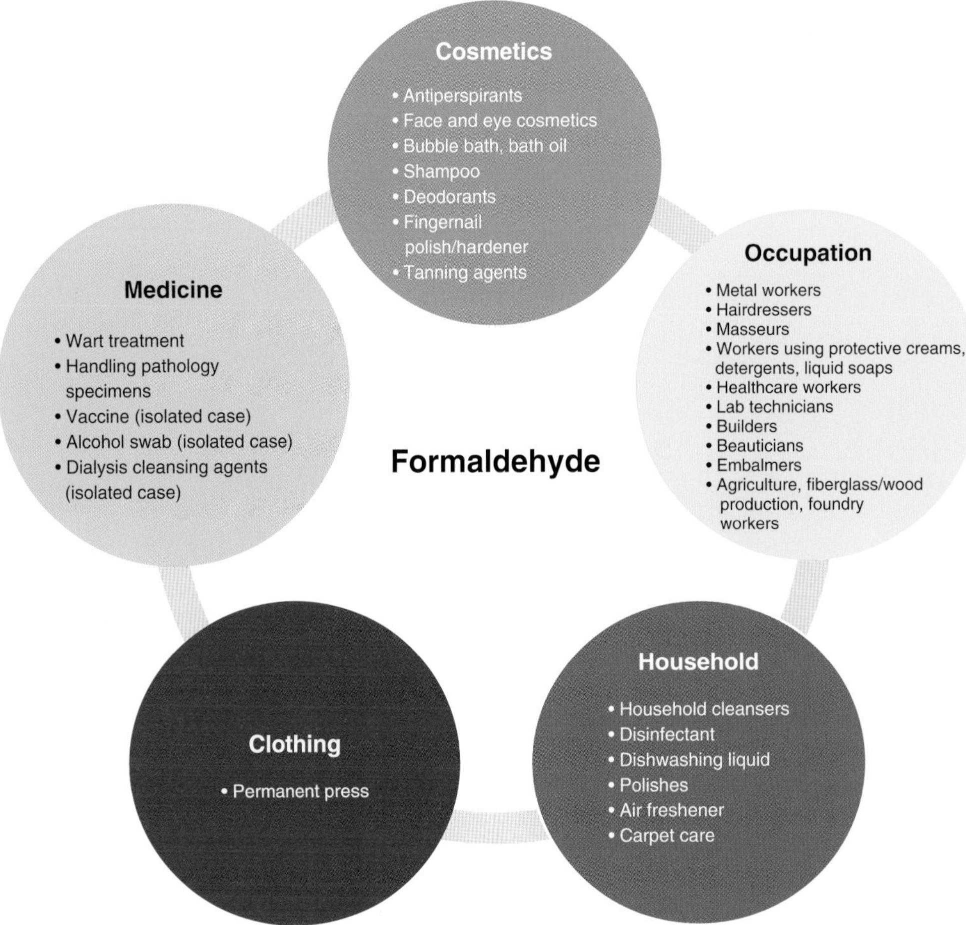

Figure 15.1 Reported sources of formaldehyde exposure.

formaldehyde-releasing product amongst their ingredients. Formaldehyde-positive patients may have to "open test" products if their dermatitis does not resolve on avoiding products containing formaldehyde.

Non-cosmetic exposure and use

- Paper products: water/grease/shrink resistance.
- Pressed wood products, including particle boards, plywood, and medium-density fiberboard (MDF).
- Medications, including wart remedies and medicated creams, orthopedic casts, paints, glues, upholstery, carpeting, plastics, explosives, dyes.
- Clothing, including permanent press, anti-static, anti-wrinkle, and anti-shrink finishes, chlorine-resistant finishes, waterproof finishes, perspiration-proof finishes, moth-proof, and mildew-resistant finishes.
- Embalming fluid and fixatives.
- Preservative for laboratory specimens, smoke from burning wood, coal, charcoal, cigarettes, and vehicle fumes (clinical relevance is not proven), cellulose esters, coatings including melamine, urea, sulfonamide, and phenol resins, photographic plates, rubber cement, tanning agents, toxoids, and vaccines (modified from [1]).

Patch testing

A test concentration of 2% formaldehyde in water (or its T.R.U.E.® test equivalent) is preferable compared to 1% [3] and is currently used in the baseline series at St John's Institute of Dermatology. A test concentration of 2% was formerly used but in the 1980s, some authors argued that patch testing at a concentration of 2% may result in irritation and therefore 1% formaldehyde in water was recommended [4]. In contrast, in recent years it has been evident that patch testing with formaldehyde 2% could detect significantly more formaldehyde-allergic patients compared with 1%, while irritant reactions did not increase [5, 6].

To test for allergic contact urticaria skin exposure for 15 minutes with 1–2% formaldehyde aq. will show a wheal and flare reaction [7].

Frequency of sensitization

The prevalence rates for formaldehyde allergy from patch test clinics have varied widely (from 0% to 15%, see Formaldehyde: E-Supplement), but generally a figure in the low single percentage area is to be expected. In Europe, levels of patch test sensitivity to formaldehyde between 1991 and 2000 remained stable, being in the 2.0–2.5% range. This may be the result of ongoing use of formaldehyde in detergents, formaldehyde-releasing biocides, and other products [8]. Allergy levels to formaldehyde are reported to be higher in North America compared to Europe [9].

Age

Fransway et al. reported that patients between the age of 60 to 69 years were most commonly affected [10], whereas another study showed that the prevalence was markedly higher amongst those aged 41–60 years when compared with patients aged older than 60 years [11]. A higher formaldehyde sensitization rate in children versus adults was reported, which accounted for 4.7% of 412 children (age 4–18 years) [12].

Sex

British and Danish studies showed that women had a significantly higher prevalence of contact allergy to formaldehyde [11, 13].

Clinical disease

- Fransway et al. found that the majority of 300 formaldehyde-sensitive patients experienced chronic dermatitis (duration 1–3 years) and over 70% of cases had received treatment for more than 1 year. Generalized dermatitis was present in 25%, followed by isolated hand dermatitis in 20%, and head and neck dermatitis in 10% [10].
- The hands are usually involved more often than the face in formaldehyde allergy. 'Hands alone' accounted for 51% of formaldehyde allergy, followed by 'face alone' (26%) and generalized dermatitis (10%) [14]. People with hand dermatitis may risk sensitization to formaldehyde through their use of cosmetics and detergents [15].
- A follow-up study of formaldehyde-sensitive patients showed that 35% did 'not pay attention' to their allergy and 25% of products brought for analysis were formaldehyde positive. Patients who 'paid attention' to their allergy had fewer eruptions than those who did not [16].
- Noiesen et al. studied the problems with ingredient label reading. 46% of patients allergic to formaldehyde experienced major difficulties in reading the ingredient labels of cosmetics and toiletries, one factor for this being the different names of formaldehyde releasers needing to be taken into account [17].
- The prognosis of ACD to formaldehyde is generally considered to be less favorable because of widespread exposure to formaldehyde. Flyvholm et al. advised patients to use alternatives to those products containing formaldehyde or formaldehyde releasers. The status of eczema at follow-up was about a third healed, a third improved, and in a third no change [18].
- Dermatitis caused by clothing should be rare now due to restrictive legislation. It tends to affect parts of the body where there is the most friction between the skin and the fabric. For example, "trouser dermatitis" is usually apparent on the inner thighs, gluteal folds, and backs of the knees. Sweating may also be a factor in causing the allergic dermatitis as sweat or sebum appears to bleach free formaldehyde from formaldehyde resins. Individuals sensitive to formaldehyde are not necessarily hypersensitive to formaldehyde resins.

Uncommon cases

- A German bank clerk was diagnosed with occupational contact dermatitis from formaldehyde in banknote paper. His dermatitis was located to the tips of his right thumb and index finger. Banknote paper may contain formaldehyde and its resins to prevent mildew and to improve its wet strength and water resistance [19].
- Exposure to hidden formaldehyde can cause ACD. A 49-year-old woman developed a recurrent rash related to alco-swabs used for disinfecting venepuncture sites. Her patch tests showed positive reactions to formaldehyde, colophonium, 4-tert-butylcatechol, 2-tert-butyl-4-methoxyphenol, chlorhexidine diacetate, hydrogen peroxide, different alco-swabs containing chlorhexidine, and alco-swabs containing only ethanol and water. Despite the fact that the labeled ingredients were only 82% ethanol and water, formaldehyde was detected in the alco-swabs by both the chromotropic acid method and high-performance liquid chromatography (HPLC) [20].
- Finch et al. reported a patient who developed an airborne ACD from MDF containing melamine-formaldehyde resin. Patch tests to both formaldehyde and melamine-formaldehyde resin were positive. The rash had appeared the day after sawing and sanding a MDF door in his home [21].
- Systemic contact dermatitis was reported in a 48-year-old man following an injection of formaldehyde-containing influenza vaccine. The patch testing results showed strongly positive reactions to formaldehyde and formaldehyde releasers [22]. In addition, systemic allergic dermatitis from formaldehyde derived from aspartame as a component of food and drink, artificial sweetener, and montelukast tablets was suspected in three case reports [23–25].

Occupational disease

- Occupational formaldehyde allergy is common and occurs in metalworkers, hairdressers, masseurs, and workers using protective creams, detergents, and liquid soaps [15].
- In occupational environments, workers may be exposed through contact with formaldehyde solutions or liquid resins with the skin or eyes. Occupational exposure to formaldehyde is highly variable and can occur in numerous industries, including the manufacture of formaldehyde and formaldehyde-based resins, wood composite and furniture production, plastic production, embalming,

foundry operations, fiberglass production, construction, agriculture, firefighting, and histology/pathology/biology laboratories.

- A study from Germany found that formaldehyde was the most common occupationally relevant sensitizer amongst female cleaners. The patients often used medical examination gloves for single use. These gloves are suitable only for protection against infections and are not resistant to chemicals. Formaldehyde can penetrate gloves made from natural rubber within a few minutes up to hours, depending on the material thickness. Material safety data sheets for formaldehyde recommend the use of gloves made from nitrile (0.4 mm), chloroprene (0.5 mm), fluorinated rubber (0.7 mm) or butyl rubber (0.5 mm) [26].
- Chang et al. [1] reviewed formaldehyde exposure at work. Those with significant exposure included nurses and physicians (disinfectants), builders (wood and insulation), painters (paints), laboratory technicians (formalin as a specimen preservative), beauticians/hairdressers (cosmetics), domestic cleaners (cleaning fluids/disinfectants), and morticians (embalming fluid).
- Short-term exposure to high levels of formaldehyde has been reported with embalmers, pathologists, and paper workers. Lower levels of exposure have usually been reported for the manufacture of synthetic vitreous fibers, abrasives, and rubber, and in formaldehyde production [27].
- Occupational exposure can be reduced by identifying potential sources of exposure (material safety data sheets should be made available to the employers and workers) and taking precautions to minimize exposure by wearing suitable protective garments.

Formaldehyde-releasing substances

The most commonly encountered commercial names associated with formaldehyde-releasing substances are [15]:

quaternium-15
imidazolidinyl urea
diazolidinyl urea
DMDM hydantoin
tris-(hydroxymethyl) nitromethane
2-bromo-2-nitropropane-1,3-diol
methenamine.

DMDM hydantoin contains 0.5–2.0% free formaldehyde and is used in cosmetics in concentrations of 0.1–1.0%, which can result in up to 200 ppm of formaldehyde [18].

In one study reactions to formaldehyde-releasing substances were seen in 79% of formaldehyde-allergic patients [15]. Contact allergy to the formaldehyde releaser itself, without allergy to free formaldehyde, is less frequent [28, 29].

Most aqueous solutions of formaldehyde releasers contain free formaldehyde. Petrolatum-based patch test materials with formaldehyde releasers do not contain free formaldehyde, but probably start releasing it upon contact with sweat [30].

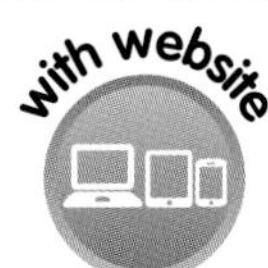

Go to www.wiley.com/go/mcfadden/common_contact_allergens to find the E-supplement for this chapter:

Formaldehyde: E-Supplement

References

1 Chang, C.C. and Gershwin, M.E. (1992). Perspectives on formaldehyde toxicity: separating fact from fantasy. *Regulatory Toxicology and Pharmacology* 16 (2): 150–160.

2 Ham, J.E., Siegel, P., and Maibach, H. (2018). Undeclared formaldehyde levels in patient consumer products: formaldehyde test kit utility. *Cutaneous and Ocular Toxicology* 1–18.

3 Ponten, A., Goossens, A., and Bruze, M. (2013). Recommendation to include formaldehyde 2.0% aqua in the European baseline patch test series. *Contact Dermatitis* 69 (6): 372–374.

4 De Groot, A.C. (2011). Contact allergy to formaldehyde. *British Journal of Dermatology* 164 (3): 463.

5 Isaksson, M., Brared-Christensson, J., Engfeldt, M. et al. (2014). Patch testing with formaldehyde 2.0% in parallel with 1.0% by the Swedish Contact Dermatitis Research Group. *Acta Dermato-Venereologica* 94 (4): 408–410.

6 Ponten, A., Aalto-Korte, K., Agner, T. et al. (2013). Patch testing with 2.0% (0.60 mg/cm^2) formaldehyde instead of 1.0% (0.30 mg/cm^2) detects significantly more contact allergy. *Contact Dermatitis* 68 (1): 50–53.

7 Imbus, H.R. (1985). Clinical evaluation of patients with complaints related to formaldehyde exposure. *Journal of Allergy and Clinical Immunology* 76 (6): 831–840.

8 Wilkinson, J.D., Shaw, S., Andersen, K.E. et al. (2002). Monitoring levels of preservative sensitivity in Europe. A 10-year overview (1991–2000). *Contact Dermatitis* 46 (4): 207–210.

9 Deza, G. and Gimenez-Arnau, A.M. (2017). Allergic contact dermatitis in preservatives: current standing and future options. *Current Opinion in Allergy and Clinical Immunology* 17 (4): 263–268.

10 Fransway, A.F. and Schmitz, N.A. (1991). Formaldehyde and formaldehyde-releasing biocides: incidences of cross-reactivity and the significance of the positive response to formaldehyde. *American Journal of Contact Dermatitis* 2 (2): 78–88.

11 Thyssen, J.P., Engkilde, K., Lundov, M.D. et al. (2010). Temporal trends of preservative allergy in Denmark (1985–2008). *Contact Dermatitis* 62 (2): 102–108.

12 Kuljanac, I., Knezevic, E., and Cvitanovic, H. (2011). Epicutaneous patch test results in children and adults with allergic contact dermatitis in Karlovac county: a retrospective survey. *Acta Dermatovenerologica Croatica* 19 (2): 91–97.

13 Jong, C.T., Statham, B.N., Green, C.M. et al. (2007). Contact sensitivity to preservatives in the UK, 2004–2005: results of multicentre study. *Contact Dermatitis* 57 (3): 165–168.

14 Jacobs, M.C., White, I.R., Rycroft, R.J., and Taub, N. (1995). Patch testing with preservatives at St John's from 1982 to 1993. *Contact Dermatitis* 33 (4): 247–254.

15 Aalto-Korte, K., Kuuliala, O., Suuronen, K., and Alanko, K. (2008). Occupational contact allergy to formaldehyde and formaldehyde releasers. *Contact Dermatitis* 59 (5): 280–289.
16 Agner, T., Flyvholm, M.A., and Menné, T. (1999). Formaldehyde allergy: a follow-up study. *American Journal of Contact Dermatitis: Official Journal of the American Contact Dermatitis Society* 10 (1): 12–17.
17 Noiesen, E., Munk, M.D., Larsen, K. et al. (2007). Difficulties in avoiding exposure to allergens in cosmetics. *Contact Dermatitis* 57 (2): 105–109.
18 Flyvholm, M.A. and Menné, T. (1992). Allergic contact dermatitis from formaldehyde. A case study focussing on sources of formaldehyde exposure. *Contact Dermatitis* 27 (1): 27–36.
19 Koch, P. (1995). Occupational contact dermatitis from colophony and formaldehyde in banknote paper. *Contact Dermatitis* 32 (6): 371–372.
20 Friis, U.F., Dahlin, J., Bruze, M. et al. (2014). Hidden exposure to formaldehyde in a swab caused allergic contact dermatitis. *Contact Dermatitis* 70 (4): 258–260.
21 Finch, T.M., Prais, L., and Foulds, I.S. (1999). Allergic contact dermatitis from medium-density fibreboard containing melamine-formaldehyde resin. *Contact Dermatitis* 41 (5): 291.
22 Kuritzky, L.A. and Pratt, M. (2015). Systemic allergic contact dermatitis after formaldehyde-containing influenza vaccination. *Journal of Cutaneous Medicine and Surgery* 19 (5): 504–506.
23 Veien, N.K. and Lomholt, H.B. (2012). Systemic allergic dermatitis presumably caused by formaldehyde derived from aspartame. *Contact Dermatitis* 67 (5): 315–316.
24 Hill, A.M. and Belsito, D.V. (2003). Systemic contact dermatitis of the eyelids caused by formaldehyde derived from aspartame? *Contact Dermatitis* 49 (5): 258–259.
25 Castanedo-Tardan, M.P., Gonzalez, M.E., Connelly, E.A. et al. (2009). Systematized contact dermatitis and montelukast in an atopic boy. *Pediatric Dermatology* 26 (6): 739–743.
26 Liskowsky, J., Geier, J., and Bauer, A. (2011). Contact allergy in the cleaning industry: analysis of contact allergy surveillance data of the Information Network of Departments of Dermatology. *Contact Dermatitis* 65 (3): 159–166.
27 National Toxicology Program. 12th Report on Carcinogens: National Toxicology Program; 2011. Available from: http://ntp.niehs.nih.gov/index.cfm?objectid=72016262-BDB7-CEBA-FA60E922B18C2540.
28 de Groot, A.C., White, I.R., Flyvholm, M.A. et al. (2010). Formaldehyde-releasers in cosmetics: relationship to formaldehyde contact allergy. Part 1. Characterization, frequency and relevance of sensitization, and frequency of use in cosmetics. *Contact Dermatitis* 62 (1): 2–17.
29 de Groot, A., White, I.R., Flyvholm, M.A. et al. (2010). Formaldehyde-releasers in cosmetics: relationship to formaldehyde contact allergy. Part 2. Patch test relationship to formaldehyde contact allergy, experimental provocation tests, amount of formaldehyde released, and assessment of risk to consumers allergic to formaldehyde. *Contact Dermatitis* 62 (1): 18–31.
30 Emeis, D., de Groot, A.C., and Brinkmann, J. (2010). Determination of formaldehyde in formaldehyde-releaser patch test preparations. *Contact Dermatitis* 63 (2): 57–62.

Exposure Color Code

- Clothing, jewelry, adornments
- Personal care products, cosmetics/cosmetic procedures
- Household products, domestic environment, including furniture and refurbishment
- Occupational dermatoses, work environment
- Medicines, surgical/dental procedures, herbal/alternative medicines
- Personal appliances/aids
- Leisure activities, sport, travel
- Other exposures (including dietary)
- Not relevant or multiple/general exposure

CHAPTER 16

Quaternium-15

CHAPTER CONTENTS

Key points

- Quaternium-15 is a preservative found in many cosmetics such as moisturizers, shampoos, hair rinses, eye makeup, emollient lotions and creams, shaving cream, nail hardeners, and some brands of talcum powder.
- Its use in products may be more common in the USA than in Europe.
- Typical cosmetic use levels range between 0.05% and 2.0%.
- Diverse use in non-cosmetic products, including cooling oils, insulation products, pressed woods, paints, and in the construction industry.
- European studies showed a prevalence of 0.6–1.9% for + patch tests to quaternium-15 in eczema patients, though another report gave a figure of 4%.
- The prevalence rate has been consistently higher in USA patch test clinics.
- There is approximately half to two thirds "clinical relevance" for positive patch tests to quaternium-15.
- The most common clinically relevant sources of exposure were moisturizers, hair preparations, and facial cosmetics.
- Allergic contact dermatitis (ACD) to quaternium-15 increases with age in adults.
- ACD to quaternium-15 is approximately twice as common in females.
- ACD to quaternium-15 is a common and important cause of facial, hand, and vulval dermatitis.
- Quaternium-15 is an important allergen in hairdressers and beauticians.
- Quaternium-15 is a significant formaldehyde releaser. Patients who are allergic to formaldehyde should also avoid quaternium-15 and other formaldehyde releasing preservatives.
- Approximately half of patients with a positive patch test to formaldehyde will also have a positive patch test to quaternium-15, and approximately half of patients with a positive patch test to quaternium-15 will have a positive patch test to formaldehyde.
- Patients allergic to quaternium-15 should also avoid methenamine as there is significant co-reactivity between quaternium-15 and methenamine, probably due to a similar chemical structure.

Exposure and use

Quaternium-15 is used in a wide variety of both cosmetic and non-cosmetic goods [1–8].

Cosmetics and household goods

Quaternium-15 has wide and diverse uses in toiletries, household goods, and consumer products, including:

- Cosmetics such as foundation, concealers, blushers, bronzers, mascara, eye shadows, eyeliners and pencils, nail hardeners, and some talcum powders.
- Skincare products such as creams, moisturizing lotions [1], makeup remover, sunscreens, and Oilatum® cream (historical – no longer used in Oilatum® products) [2].
- Personal hygiene items such as soaps, cleansers, shampoos, hair rinses, shaving cream, and disinfectants.

Common Contact Allergens: A Practical Guide to Detecting Contact Dermatitis, First Edition. Edited by John McFadden, Pailin Puangpet, Korbkarn Pongpairoj, Supitchaya Thaiwat, and Lee Shan Xian.

© 2020 John Wiley & Sons Ltd. Published 2020 by John Wiley & Sons Ltd.

Companion website: www.wiley.com/go/mcfadden/common_contact_allergens

- Durable press (wrinkle-resistant) fabrics.
- Cleaning products, waxes, polishes, and paints.
- Tobacco and cigarette smoke.
- Smoke from wood, coal, kerosene, or charcoal fires.

The use of quaternium-15 in products may be more common in the USA than in Europe.

Non-cosmetic exposure and use

- Diverse use in non-cosmetic products, including cooling oils, insulation products, pressed woods, paints, and in the construction industry.
- Used as an antimicrobial agent in water-based metalworking fluids [3, 4].
- Electrode attachment gels used in healthcare, e.g. electroencephalography skin preparation gel [5], embalming and preserving fluids, pressed woods such as particle board manufacturing facilities [6], medium-density fiberboard (MDF), plywood, oriented strand boards (OSBs), urea-formaldehyde resins, metalworking fluids/coolants, adhesives, water-based inks, floor wax and polish, industrial cutting fluid, jointing cement, paper and pulp, paperboard, construction materials, laundry starch, printing pastes, textile finishing solutions, spinning emulsions, photocopier toner [7].

Patch testing

- Quaternium-15 is included in the baseline series in the USA and in Europe. One percent quaternium-15 in petrolatum/T.R.U.E.® test equivalent is the recommended concentration.

Frequency of sensitization

- Average 0.6–1.9% in European patch test clinics but higher in the USA. This may be because quaternium-15 was previously tested at 2% in pet. in the USA versus 1% in Europe and there is a higher exposure of the US population to formaldehyde releasers [8].

Age

- As with other common cosmetic contact allergens, contact allergy to quaternium-15 increases with age (over 65 years prevalence 11.9%, 19–64 years 8.4%, 18 years and under 3.2%) [9].
- In a retrospective chart review of 100 children aged 4–18 years, positive reactions to quaternium-15 were recorded in 4% of children with eczema [10].

Sex

- Quaternium-15 allergy is approximately twice as common in females [11, 12].

Clinical disease

- ACD to quaternium-15 is a common and important cause of *facial*, *hand*, and *vulval* dermatitis [8, 13–16].
- In another study, quaternium-15 was reported as a common cause of preservative-induced contact dermatitis, with a clinical relevance of 89% [13].
- A 1999 review of ACD causing hand dermatitis reported quaternium-15 to be the most commonly associated preservative contact allergy [14] (currently, it is methylisothiazolinone).
- There are numerous case reports of individuals developing contact dermatitis from products containing quaternium-15 such as *soaps*, *shampoos*, *conditioners*, and *moisturizers* [13]. Quaternium-15 can be a relevant allergen in patients with atopic dermatitis, along with the other formaldehyde releasers [16].
- A 21-year-old smoker presented with dermatitis on the opposing areas of the second and third fingers of both hands for 3 years. Patch testing showed a ++ positive reaction to formaldehyde and a + positive reaction to quaternium-15. Although she did not react to the smoked and unsmoked components of her roll-your-own cigarettes, using a cigarette holder improved her symptoms [17].

Occupational disease

- Quaternium-15 can be an allergen in *healthcare workers*, *hairdressers*, and *beauticians* [18, 19].
- One study from the USA reported that 29% of clinically relevant contact allergies among healthcare workers tested were due to quaternium-15 and attributed this to preservatives in skin cleaning and washing products [20]. *(Note: Likely to be much less in Europe and probably less so now in America.)*
- Quaternium-15 was contained in Microshield™ moisturizing lotion, a product that used to be commonly used in Australian hospitals. ACD of the hands to Microshield has been reported in a nurse. The formulation, however, has recently been changed [1].
- Mose et al. [21] reviewed occupational contact dermatitis amongst *painters* in Denmark. They found a significant increase in positive patch tests to quaternium-15 amongst painters compared to other groups, 6/219 (3%) vs 7/1095 (0.5%, $p = 0.004$). However, as quaternium-15 is not used in paints, they attributed this finding to the formaldehyde-releasing properties of this preservative.
- Quaternium-15 was found to be the fifth most common clinically relevant allergen amongst hairdressers, though this has not been reported elsewhere [19].

Other areas of interest

Concomitant sensitization to formaldehyde

- Approximately half of patients with a positive patch test to formaldehyde will also have a positive patch test to quaternium-15, and approximately half of patients with a positive patch test to quaternium-15 will have a positive patch test to formaldehyde.

- Quaternium-15 has been purported to release formaldehyde in aqueous formulations. It is one of the highest formaldehyde-releasing preservatives [22].

Cross-reactivity to methenamine

- Patients allergic to quaternium-15 should also avoid the preservative methenamine, as there is significant co-reactivity between quaternium-15 and methenamine.
- Data from Finland showed that a third of quaternium-15 sensitive patients also reacted to methenamine. The simultaneous reactions are probably more related to their close chemical structures – quaternary ammonium compounds – than to their common formaldehyde-releasing capacity [23].

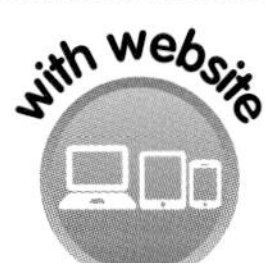

Go to www.wiley.com/go/mcfadden/common_contact_allergens to find the E-supplement for this chapter:

Quaternium-15: E-Supplement

References

1 Cahill, J. and Nixon, R. (2005). Allergic contact dermatitis to quaternium 15 in a moisturizing lotion. *Australasian Journal of Dermatology* 46 (4): 284–285.

2 Boffa, M.J. and Beck, M.H. (1996). Allergic contact dermatitis from quaternium 15 in Oilatum cream. *Contact Dermatitis* 35 (1): 45–46.

3 Rossmoore, H.W. (1981). Antimicrobial agents for water-based metalworking fluids. *Journal of Occupational Medicine* 23 (4): 247–254.

4 Marks, J.G. Jr. and DeLeo, V.A. (1997). Standard allergens. In: *Contact and Occupational Dermatology*, 61–132. St. Louis, MO: Mosby.

5 Finch, T.M., Prais, L., and Foulds, I.S. (2001). Occupational allergic contact dermatitis from quaternium-15 in an electroencephalography skin preparation gel. *Contact Dermatitis* 44 (1): 44–45.

6 Saary, M.J., House, R.A., and Holness, D.L. (2001). Dermatitis in a particleboard manufacturing facility. *Contact Dermatitis* 44 (6): 325–330.

7 Zina, A.M., Fanan, E., and Bundino, S. (2000). Allergic contact dermatitis from formaldehyde and quaternium-15 in photocopier toner. *Contact Dermatitis* 43 (4): 241–242.

8 de Groot, A.C., White, I.R., Flyvholm, M.A. et al. (2010). Formaldehyde-releasers in cosmetics: relationship to formaldehyde contact allergy. Part 1. Characterization, frequency and relevance of sensitization, and frequency of use in cosmetics. *Contact Dermatitis* 62 (1): 2–17.

9 Warshaw, E.M., Raju, S.I., Fowler, J.F. Jr. et al. (2012). Positive patch test reactions in older individuals: retrospective analysis from the North American Contact Dermatitis Group, 1994–2008. *Journal of the American Academy of Dermatology* 66 (2): 229–240.

10 Hogeling, M. and Pratt, M. (2008). Allergic contact dermatitis in children: the Ottawa hospital patch-testing clinic experience, 1996 to 2006. *Dermatitis* 19 (2): 86–89.

11 Jacobs, M.C., White, I.R., Rycroft, R.J., and Taub, N. (1995). Patch testing with preservatives at St John's from 1982 to 1993. *Contact Dermatitis* 33 (4): 247–254.

12 Schnuch, A., Lessmann, H., Geier, J., and Uter, W. (2011). Contact allergy to preservatives. Analysis of IVDK data 1996–2009. *British Journal of Dermatology* 164 (6): 1316–1325.

13 Burkemper, N.M. (2015). Contact dermatitis, patch testing, and allergen avoidance. *Missouri Medicine* 112 (4): 296–300.

14 Maier, L.E., Lampel, H.P., Bhutani, T., and Jacob, S.E. (2009). Hand dermatitis: a focus on allergic contact dermatitis to biocides. *Dermatologic Clinics* 27 (3): 251–264, v–vi.

15 O'Gorman, S.M. and Torgerson, R.R. (2013). Allergic contact dermatitis of the vulva. *Dermatitis* 24 (2): 64–72.

16 Shaughnessy, C.N., Malajian, D., and Belsito, D.V. (2014). Cutaneous delayed-type hypersensitivity in patients with atopic dermatitis: reactivity to topical preservatives. *Journal of the American Academy of Dermatology* 70 (1): 102–107.

17 Carew, B. and Muir, J. (2014). Patch testing for allergic contact dermatitis to cigarettes: smoked/unsmoked components and formaldehyde factors. *Australasian Journal of Dermatology* 55 (3): 225–226.

18 Kadivar, S. and Belsito, D.V. (2015). Occupational dermatitis in health care workers evaluated for suspected allergic contact dermatitis. *Dermatitis* 26 (4): 177–183.

19 Warshaw, E.M., Wang, M.Z., Mathias, C.G. et al. (2012). Occupational contact dermatitis in hairdressers/cosmetologists: retrospective analysis of North American Contact Dermatitis Group data, 1994 to 2010. *Dermatitis* 23 (6): 258–268.

20 Suneja, T. and Belsito, D.V. (2008). Occupational dermatoses in health care workers evaluated for suspected allergic contact dermatitis. *Contact Dermatitis* 58 (5): 285–290.

21 Mose, A.P., Lundov, M.D., Zachariae, C. et al. (2012). Occupational contact dermatitis in painters: an analysis of patch test data from the Danish Contact Dermatitis Group. *Contact Dermatitis* 67 (5): 293–297.

22 Latorre, N., Borrego, L., Fernandez-Redondo, V. et al. (2011). Patch testing with formaldehyde and formaldehyde-releasers: multicentre study in Spain (2005–2009). *Contact Dermatitis* 65 (5): 286–292.

23 Aalto-Korte, K. (2000). Simultaneous allergic contact dermatitis to quaternium 15 and methenamine. *Contact Dermatitis* 42: 365.

CHAPTER 17

Diazolidinyl Urea and Imidazolidinyl Urea

CHAPTER CONTENTS

Key points

- Imidazolidinyl urea (IU) and diazolidinyl urea (DU) are formaldehyde-releasing agents, used as antimicrobial preservatives in the formulation of many cosmetics, skincare products, household detergents, and (a few) pharmaceutical creams and ointments.
- There is a high degree of cross-reactivity between IU and DU; patients allergic to one should avoid the other.
- As a result of their high water solubility, they can be incorporated into a wide range of water-based cosmetics, toiletries, and household goods. Allergic contact dermatitis (ACD) can therefore present as reactions to many different products.
- ACD to DU and/or IU has been reported from exposure to hair gel, day and night creams, body lotion, a hospital antimicrobial hand gel, eyeliner, facial moisturizer, and ultrasonic gel.
- As general classes of cosmetics, skincare products are the most common cause of ACD to DU and/or IU, followed by haircare products, facial cleansers, suncare products, makeup, body cleansing products, and intimate hygiene products.
- Incidence of contact allergy from patch test clinics: DU: Europe 0.5–1.4%, USA 2.4–3.7%; IU: Europe 0.3–1.4%, America 1.3–3.3%.
- Occupational disease: hairdressers and cosmetic workers are at risk.
- Although an effective microbicidal agent, activity against fungi is limited. DU/IU is therefore often combined with parabens for antifungal activity.
- DU appears to be a stronger sensitizer than IU.
- Patients allergic to formaldehyde should avoid IU, DU, and other formaldehyde-releasing substances such as quaternium-15 and DMDM hydantoin.
- In the EU, IU and DU are permitted in cosmetics at up to 0.6% and 0.5%, respectively.

Diazolidinyl urea

Exposure and use

Cosmetics

- Some studies suggest that DU is present in more American than European cosmetics [1, 2] (Figure 17.1).

Non-cosmetic use

- DU is used as a preservative in multiple products and can be found in cleansers, liquid soaps, cleaning agents, and other household products, and in pet shampoos.

Patch testing

2% DU in petrolatum is the recommended concentration.

Common Contact Allergens: A Practical Guide to Detecting Contact Dermatitis, First Edition. Edited by John McFadden, Pailin Puangpet, Korbkarn Pongpairoj, Supitchaya Thaiwat, and Lee Shan Xian.

© 2020 John Wiley & Sons Ltd. Published 2020 by John Wiley & Sons Ltd.

Companion website: www.wiley.com/go/mcfadden/common_contact_allergens

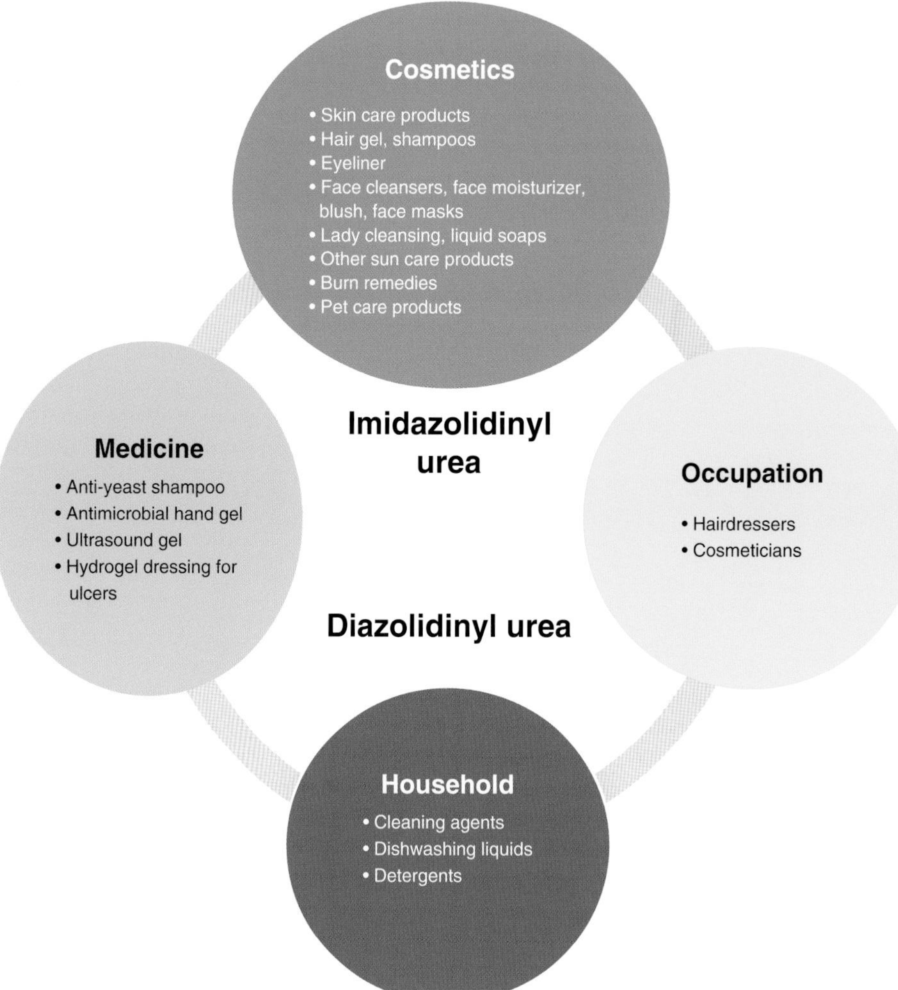

Figure 17.1 Exposure sources for diazolidinyl and imidazolidinyl urea.

Frequency of sensitization

The prevalence varies from approximately 1% to 3%.

Clinical disease and case reports

- *Hair gel*: The first case of ACD to DU was from a hair gel [3].
- *Day cream, night cream, and body lotion*: The first case series of ACD to DU reported four cases – eyelid dermatitis from DU in day and night creams, an exacerbation of atopic dermatitis of the eyelids and face from DU in day and night creams, dermatitis of the neck, hands, arms, and legs after using a trio of day cream, night cream, and body lotion all containing DU, and a patient with multiple cosmetic reactions, all containing DU [4].
- *Hand dermatitis*: DU (1% pet.) tested positive in 5.9% of hand-only dermatitis cases in the North American Contact Dermatitis Group (NACDG) hand dermatitis study [5].
- A 14-year-old atopic girl reported persistent eczematous lesions for 3 months prior to presentation, primarily located on her hands with intermittent spread to the face and neck. She had been using two cosmetic creams (same brand) to treat her atopic hand eczema; she also used a *body cream* from the same brand. She was patch test positive to DU (+++) and IU (++), and to the three creams. The *hand creams* contained both DU and IU, while the body cream contained only DU [6].
- *Hydrogels*: Hydrogels are colorless transparent aqueous gels which contain modified carboxymethylcellulose polymer together with propylene glycol as known components. They are commonly used to treat leg ulcers. Carvalho et al. reported an 84-year-old man and 77-year-old woman who developed allergy to hydrogel dressings but were patch test negative to propylene glycol. As they were both patch test positive to DU and IU, they suspected that these preservatives may have been contained in the hydrogel dressings [7].
- *Varied distribution of dermatitis in DU allergic patients*: Hectorne and Fransway [8] reported on 58 patients with contact allergy to DU. They noted that the most common distribution was generalized dermatitis (21%), then generalized

without facial involvement (19%), face only (12%), hands only (12%), trunk and legs (5%), trunk and arms (3%), arms and legs (3%), arms and face (3%), hands and feet (3%), hands and forearms (3%), legs and hands (3%), and other locations (10%). Correlations between exposure to specific DU-containing agents and exacerbations of dermatitis were hard to confirm. Correlations were identified less than 10% of the time. DU-containing agents implicated included facial cosmetics as well as haircare and handcare products. 78% of the DU + patients were also patch test + to formaldehyde, and 30% also reacted to IU on patch testing [8].

- *Antimicrobial hand gel*: A 44-year-old female nurse with a 4-year history of hand dermatitis was referred to an occupational dermatology clinic in Melbourne. In 2009, her hand dermatitis had worsened when she started working in a neonatal intensive care unit, where she used antimicrobial hand gel more frequently. Her hands improved when she spent time away from work but worsened again within 2 days of returning. She was patch test + to DU, which was contained in the hand gel [9].
- *The most common cosmetic source of ACD to DU is from skincare products*: Over a 10-year period (2000–2010) Travassos et al. recorded specific cosmetic agents, as well as the implicated cosmetic ingredients in them, causing cases of ACD. DU was implicated 29 times: in skincare products (14/29), haircare products (3/29), suncare products (4/29), facial cleansers (6/29), and makeup (2/29). IU was implicated 22 times: in skin care products (12/22), haircare products (6/22), body cleansing products (1/22), facial cleansers (2/22), and intimate hygiene products (1/22) [10].

Formaldehyde release

- The primary mode of sensitization to DU is via formaldehyde release. Ideally, patients allergic to formaldehyde should avoid using products that contain either DU or IU. Less optimally, patients reacting to formaldehyde should be advised to perform a repeated open application test (ROAT) before using a cosmetic containing DU as a preservative [11]. A significant minority of patients reacted to DU without reacting to formaldehyde and/or other formaldehyde releasers [8]. As DU breaks down to numerous components, a number of contact allergic reactions to DU may be caused by the release of formaldehyde and other components in the biocide [2]. Jordan induced sensitization to 2% DU in 19 of 150 patients; approximately 50% of these sensitized patients also became sensitive to IU [12].
- The closed container diffusion method for the quantification of free formaldehyde in the presence of formaldehyde donors demonstrated significant levels of free formaldehyde in creams containing DU [13].

How often are patients reacting to DU also allergic to formaldehyde?

USA	69–81%
Europe	12–55%

How often are patients reacting to formaldehyde also allergic to DU?

USA	24.5%
Europe	4–30%

How often are patients reacting to DU also allergic to IU?

USA	29%
UK	60–75% [14]

Dooms-Goossens et al. found that of all DU-sensitized subjects, 50% will react to IU [15].

Imidazolidinyl urea

Exposure and use

Cosmetics

- This preservative has been one of the most widely used in the world [16, 17] (Figure 17.1). IU is more active against bacteria than fungi. The concentration of IU in cosmetics is typically 0.1–0.3%, although it has been used as high as 5%. It is often combined with methyl and propyl parabens for optimal antifungal activity [18].
- Due to its high water solubility, IU can be incorporated into most water-based cosmetics [6]. It is present in a wide range of liquid and powder products such as baby lotions, skin cream, sunscreens, shampoos (including anti-yeast), eyeliners, blushers, perfumes, deodorants, hair dyes, shaving cream, and face masks [17, 19, 20]. IU appears to exert its preservative effect mainly through inhibition of protein and DNA syntheses [21].
- The frequency of use of IU in 33 212 cosmetics and toiletries in the USA from the FDA Voluntary Cosmetic Registration Database in 2008 was 7% (stay-on 7.8% vs rinse-off 4.7%) [2].

Non-cosmetic exposure and use

- IU is used as a preservative in multiple products and can be found in cleaning agents, burn remedies, medicated shampoos, ultrasound gels, moisturizing lotions and creams, and petcare products.

Patch testing

- 2% IU in petrolatum is the recommended concentration. A patch test concentration of 600 mg/cm[2] in a hydrophilic dried-in vehicle (T.R.U.E.® test) was found to be adequate and safe for both IU and DU [22].

Frequency of sensitization

Overall, a prevalence rate of between 1% and 3% is typical.

Case reports (see also DU case reports)

- *Eye liner, face moisturizer*: The first case reports of ACD to IU (previously referred to as Germall 115) were from exposure to an eyeliner and a face moisturizer [23].
- *Ultrasonic gel*: An adult woman had a painful shoulder treated with ultrasound. 12 hours after treatment, she experienced intense pruritus and acute dermatitis on the exact areas where the ultrasonic gel had been applied. The gel contained IU [24].

Clinical disease

- The face and hands were the sites of IU allergy for 69% and 19% of patients, respectively [25].
- Hand dermatitis data from the NACDG for 1994 to 2004 revealed that 3.8% of their hand dermatitis patients had clinically relevant allergy to IU [5].

Occupational disease

- Hairdressers, cosmetologists, machinists and production workers can all be exposed to both IU and DU [26,27]. Cleansing agents at work can also be a potential source of exposure.

Formaldehyde release

- IU releases formaldehyde into cosmetics at temperatures above 10 °C. A 1974 study found that formaldehyde release occurred at the non-physiological conditions of 60 °C and a pH of 6. In water-containing cosmetics like shampoos, formaldehyde release increased with a rise in the pH and temperature of the solution, as well as a longer storage period [28].
- A Taiwanese study revealed that eight domestic and imported cosmetic products, labeled as containing IU and purchased between 1995 and 1996, had total and free formaldehyde contents of 50–390 ppm and 7–79 ppm, respectively [29].
- Patients allergic to formaldehyde should avoid IU, DU, and other formaldehyde-releasing substances such as quaternium-15 and DMDM hydantoin.

How often are patients reacting to IU also allergic to formaldehyde?

USA	46–63%
Europe	11–53%

How often are patients reacting to formaldehyde also allergic to IU?

USA	10–17%
Europe	4–23%

How often are patients reacting to IU also allergic to DU?

UK	44–75% [14]

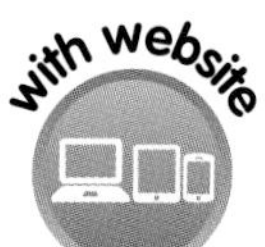

Go to http://www.wiley.com/go/mcfadden/common_contact_allergens to find the E-supplement for this chapter:

Diazolidinyl Urea and Imidazolidinyl Urea: E-Supplement.

References

1 Flyvholm, M.-A. (2005). Preservatives in registered chemical products. *Contact Dermatitis* 53: 27–32.

2 de Groot, A.C., White, I.R., Flyvholm, M.A. et al. (2010). Formaldehyde-releasers in cosmetics: relationship to formaldehyde contact allergy. Part 1. Characterization, frequency and relevance of sensitization, and frequency of use in cosmetics. *Contact Dermatitis* 62 (1): 2–17.

3 Kantor, G.R., Taylor, J.S., Ratz, J.L., and Evey, P.L. (1985). Acute allergic contact dermatitis from diazolidinyl urea (Germall II) in a hair gel. *Journal of the American Academy of Dermatology* 13 (1): 116–119.

4 de Groot, A.C., Bruynzeel, D.P., Jagtman, B.A., and Weyland, J.W. (1988). Contact allergy to diazolidinyl urea (Germall II). *Contact Dermatitis* 18 (4): 202–205.

5 Warshaw, E.M., Ahmed, R.L., Belsito, D.V. et al. (2007). Contact dermatitis of the hands: cross-sectional analyses of North American Contact Dermatitis Group data, 1994–2004. *Journal of the American Academy of Dermatology* 57 (2): 301–314.

6 García-Gavín, J., González-Vilas, D., Fernández-Redondo, V., and Toribo, J. (2010). Allergic contact dermatitis in a girl due to several cosmetics containing diazolidinyl-urea or imidazolidinyl-urea. *Contact Dermatitis* 63 (1): 49–50.

7 Carvalho, R., Maio, P., Amaro, C. et al. (2011). Hydrogel allergic contact dermatitis and imidazolidinyl urea/diazolidinyl urea. *Cutaneous and Ocular Toxicology* 30 (4): 331–332.

8 Hectorne, K.J. and Fransway, A.F. (1994). Diazolidinyl urea: incidence of sensitivity, patterns of cross-reactivity and clinical relevance. *Contact dermatitis.* 30 (1): 16–19.

9 Cahill, J.L. and Nixon, R.L. (2011). Allergic contact dermatitis in health care workers to diazolidinyl urea present in antimicrobial hand gel. *Medical Journal of Australia* 194 (12): 664–665.

10 Travassos, A.R., Claes, L., Boey, L. et al. (2011). Non-fragrance allergens in specific cosmetic products. *Contact Dermatitis* 65 (5): 276–285.

11 Perret, C.M. and Happle, R. (1989). Contact sensitivity to diazolidinyl urea (Germall II). *Archives of Dermatological Research* 281 (1): 57–59.

12 Jordan, W.P. (1984). Human studies that determine the sensitizing potential of haptens: experimental allergic contact dermatitis. *Dermatologic Clinics* 2: 533–538.

13 Karlberg, A.T., Skare, L., and Lindberg, I. (1998). Nyhammar E. A method for quantification of formaldehyde in the presence of formaldehyde donors in skin-care products. *Contact dermatitis.* 38 (1): 20–28.

14 de Groot, A., White, I.R., Flyvholm, M.A. et al. (2010). Formaldehyde-releasers in cosmetics: relationship to formaldehyde contact allergy. Part 2. Patch test relationship to formaldehyde contact allergy, experimental provocation tests, amount of formaldehyde released, and assessment of risk to consumers allergic to formaldehyde. *Contact Dermatitis* 62 (1): 18–31.

15 Dooms-Goossens, A., de Boulle, K., Dooms, M., and Degreef, H. (1986). Imidazolidinyl urea dermatitis. *Contact Dermatitis* 14 (5): 322–324.

16 Block, S.S. (1993). Disinfectants and antiseptics. In: *Kirk-Othmer Encyclopedia of Chemical Technology*, 4e, vol. 8 (eds. J.I. Kroschwitz and M. Howe-Grant), 252–268. New York: Wiley.

17 Imidazolidinyl urea - National Toxicology Program - NIH. https://ntp.niehs.nih.gov/ntp/htdocs/chem_background/exsumpdf/imidazolidinylurea_508.pdf.

18 Cosmetic Ingredients Review Expert Panel (1980). Final report of the safety assessment for imidazolidinyl urea. In: *In Cosmetic Ingredients: Their Safety Assessment*, vol. 1980 (ed. R. Elder), 133–146. Pathotox Publishers.

19 Pepe, R.C., Wenninger, J.A., and McEwen, G.N. (2001). *International Cosmetic Ingredient Dictionary and Handbook*, 796. Washington, DC: The Cosmetic, Toiletry, and Fragrance Association.

20 Lv, C., Hou, J., Xie, W., and Cheng, H. (2015). Investigation on formaldehyde release from preservatives in cosmetics. *International Journal of Cosmetic Science* 37 (5): 474–478.

21 Amouroux, I., Pesando, D., Noel, H., and Girard, J.P. (1999). Mechanisms of cytotoxicity by cosmetic ingredients in sea urchin eggs. *Archives of Environmental Contamination and Toxicology* 36 (1): 28–37.

22 Agner, T., Andersen, K.E., Björkner, B. et al. (2001). Standardization of the TRUE test imidazolidinyl urea and diazolidinyl urea patches. *Contact Dermatitis* 45 (1): 21–25.

23 Fisher, A.A. (1975). Allergic contact dermatitis from Germall 115, a new cosmetic preservative. *Contact Dermatitis* 1 (2): 126.

24 Ando, M., Ansótegui, J., Muñoz, D., and Fernández de Corrès, L. (2000). Allergic contact dermatitis from imidazolidinyl urea in an ultrasonic gel. *Contact Dermatitis* 42 (2): 109–110.

25 Jacobs, M.C., White, I.R., Rycroft, R.J., and Taub, N. (1995). Patch testing with preservatives at St John's from 1982 to 1993. *Contact Dermatitis* 33 (4): 247–254.

26 Aalto-Korte, K., Kuuliala, O., Suuronen, K., and Alanko, K. (2008). Occupational contact allergy to formaldehyde and formaldehyde releasers. *Contact Dermatitis* 59 (5): 280–289.

27 Higgins, C.L., Palmer, A.M., Cahill, J.L., and Nixon, R.L. (2016). Occupational skin disease among Australian healthcare workers: a retrospective analysis from an occupational dermatology clinic, 1993–2014. *Contact Dermatitis* 75 (4): 213–222.

28 The Scientific Committee on Cosmetic Products and Non-Food Products Intended for Consumers Opinion Concerning the Determination of Certain Formaldehyde Releasers in Cosmetic Products [https://ec.europa.eu/health/ph_risk/committees/sccp/documents/out188_en.pdf].

29 Wu, P.W., Chang, C.C., and Cheng, S. (2003). Determination of formaldehyde in cosmetics by HPLC method and acetylacetone method. *Journal of Food and Drug Analysis* 11 (1): 8–15.

Exposure Color Code

- Clothing, jewelry, adornments
- Personal care products, cosmetics/cosmetic procedures
- Household products, domestic environment, including furniture and refurbishment
- Occupational dermatoses, work environment
- Medicines, surgical/dental procedures, herbal/alternative medicines
- Personal appliances/aids
- Leisure activities, sport, travel
- Other exposures (including dietary)
- Not relevant or multiple/general exposure

CHAPTER 18

2-Bromo-2-nitropropane-1,3-diol

CHAPTER CONTENTS

Key points

- 2-Bromo-2-nitropropane-1,3-diol is a very effective preservative used in cosmetics and toiletries with broad-spectrum microbicidal properties, especially against *Pseudomonas*.
- Allergic contact dermatitis (ACD) often presents on the face and/or hands.
- Patch tested at St. John's Institute of Dermatology using a concentration of 0.5% pet. Positive reactions are usually of clinical relevance; irritant patch test reactions are uncommon.
- Patch test positivity rates in patients are lower in Europe compared with North America (0.5–1% vs 2–3%). Positivity rates have remained approximately the same over several years.
- Occupational relevance in hairdressers, farmers, paper mill workers, blue-collar workers, and healthcare workers (HCWs).
- Co-reactivity with formaldehyde is less common when compared with other formaldehyde releasing agents such as quaternium-15; 2-bromo-2-nitropropane-1,3-diol releases lower levels of formaldehyde in comparison.
- There are reports of allergy in the context of reactions to topical medicaments, but these are now mainly of historical interest.

Exposure and use

Sources of exposure are given in Table 18.1.

Cosmetics and household goods

- 2-Bromo-2-nitropropane-1,3-diol was invented by The Boots Company PLC, Nottingham, England, in the early 1960s and its first application was as a preservative for pharmaceuticals.
- 2-Bromo-2-nitropropane-1,3-diol is commonly present in skincare products [1, 2]. The largest group consists of makeup bases, followed by hair conditioners, blushers, cleansing preparations, wet wipes, and eyebrow pencils.

Cosmetic legislation

- 2-Bromo-2-nitropropane-1,3-diol is permitted in cosmetics in the EU up to a level of 0.1%. Most products contain it at concentrations of 0.02–0.1%.

Non-cosmetic exposure and use

- Water treatment, cooling tower water, water baths, air-conditioning/humidification systems, oil field mud.
- Gas and oil operations.
- Pulp, paper mills (pulping operations), wet-end additives.
- Water-based paints, inks, and adhesives.
- Metalworking fluids (not allowed in the EU).
- Others: binding agents, coloring agents, milk processing plants, paints/lacquers, pharmaceutical products, slurries, surface treatment for paper, cardboard and other non-metals, viscosity-adjustors, and washing detergents [3, 4].
- In a Danish registry of chemical products, 2-bromo-2-nitropropane-1,3-diol was found in all categories except for cutting fluids, hardeners, and printing inks [2]. Although not uncommonly found in impregnating agents (12.13%), polishes (3.72%), and paints/lacquers (2.82%), it is less commonly present in cleaning agents (1.83%), flooring agents (1.5%), adhesives/glues (0.56%), construction materials (0.41%), and filling agents (0.3%).

Common Contact Allergens: A Practical Guide to Detecting Contact Dermatitis, First Edition. Edited by John McFadden, Pailin Puangpet, Korbkarn Pongpairoj, Supitchaya Thaiwat, and Lee Shan Xian.

© 2020 John Wiley & Sons Ltd. Published 2020 by John Wiley & Sons Ltd.

Companion website: www.wiley.com/go/mcfadden/common_contact_allergens

Table 18.1 Sources of 2-bromo-2-nitropropane-1,3-diol.

Shampoos, hair conditioners, soaps, and moisturizers
Makeup bases, blushers, eyebrow pencils, and mascaras
Cleansing lotions, moist towels, and baby wipes
Washing detergents and fabric conditioners
Topical medications
Textile, paints, humidifiers, adhesives, paper, and pesticides
Water-cooling towers
Preservatives for milk samples
Additives in simulated silage

Frequency of sensitization

As with many contact allergens, the rates vary within and between countries, but typically the rate is around 1%, with results generally falling in the range of 0.2–3%.

Age

The results of studies by the North American Contact Dermatitis Group (NACDG) showed that the incidence of positive reactions to 2-bromo-2-nitropropane-1,3-diol between 1994 and 2008 was 3.0% overall [5].

Adults	2.9%, clinically relevant 2.0%
Elderly ≥65 years	3.9%, clinically relevant 2.6%
Children ≤18 years	2.3%, clinically relevant 1.4%

Sex

Allergy rates to 2-bromo-2-nitropropane-1,3-diol are similar in men and women [6, 7].

Patch testing

- The test concentration of 2-bromo-2-nitropropane-1,3-diol at St. John's Institute of Dermatology is 0.5% pet. Irritant reactions occur frequently at 1% pet. according to the results of Ford and Beck, Maibach and Rudner [8–10].
- Irritant reactions may occur even with 0.5% pet., albeit at a low and acceptable incidence. In doubtful cases, re-testing with 0.25% pet. or a repeated exposure test, according to the suggestions of Storrs and Bell [11], is recommended. Highly sensitive patients may still react to a patch test with 2-bromo-2-nitropropane-1,3-diol 0.1% pet., as Frosch and Weickel have described in their series [12].
- Both 0.25% pet. and 0.5% pet. 2-bromo-2-nitropropane-1,3-diol preparations have been used for patch testing.
- At St. John's between 1982 and 1993, the rate of positivity to 2-bromo-2-nitropropane-1,3,-diol fluctuated between 0.3% and 1.0%. Logistic regression analysis revealed no significant change in prevalence over this time [7]. In the USA, frequencies of sensitization ranged from 2.1% to 3.3% (mean, adjusted for sample size 2.8%). In studies performed in European countries, prevalence rates were consistently lower, ranging from 0.4% to 1.2% (mean, adjusted for sample size 0.9%). Relevance was established or considered "probable" in up to 80% of the positive patients [3].
- Active sensitization to 2-bromo-2-nitropropane-1,3-diol has not, to our knowledge, been reported.
- As a positive reaction to 2-bromo-2-nitropropane-1,3-diol is mostly relevant and significant, it is often included in the baseline series.

Clinical disease

- ACD is most commonly seen as a reaction to a cosmetic. In one study from 1990, 38/8149 patients patch tested were positive (prevalence 0.47%); 17/33 were of current clinical relevance. Of these 17 cases 6 had contact dermatitis of the hands, 4 had facial dermatitis and 2 had generalized eczema [4].
- 2-Bromo-2-nitropropane-1,3-diol allergy has been associated with leg dermatitis in one study [6].
- A survey found that 60% of 20 allergic cases were of clinical relevance [8].
- Patients with atopic dermatitis were significantly associated with contact hypersensitivity to 2-bromo-2-nitropropane-1,3-diol compared with non-atopic patients [13].
- Allergy to 2-bromo-2-nitropropane-1,3-diol is one of the more common causes of contact dermatitis to wet wipes, which can affect, in order of frequency, the anal/genital area, hands, face, and eyelids [14].
- In a retrospective study of preservative allergy from St. John's, of 32 patients allergic to 2-bromo-2-nitropropane-1,3-diol, 60% involved the face and 29% involved the hands [7].
- Eucerin® moisturizer contained this preservative in the past and, consequently, cases of dermatitis caused by 2-bromo-2-nitropropane-1,3-diol were more common before it was replaced [11]. There is a single case report of ACD from 2-bromo-2-nitropropane-1,3-diol in a topical metronidazole agent [15]. However, the preservative is not currently listed by the British National Formulary as being contained within topical medications.
- In both a Thai study to evaluate patch testing and histopathology in Thai patients with erythema dyschromicum perstans, lichen planus pigmentosus, and pigmented contact dermatitis [16], and a pilot study from India to evaluate cosmetic contact sensitivity in melasma patients [17], 2-bromo-2-nitropropane-1,3-diol was one of the allergens which showed positive patch test reactions. However, the association does not infer causality.

Occupational disease

- ACD caused by 2-bromo-2-nitropropane-1,3-diol is more common in certain occupations such as hairstylists, janitorial services, farmers, painters, printers, blue-collar workers, and HCWs (Figure 18.1). Furthermore, machinists dealing with cutting fluids and spin oil, paper mill workers in contact with slimicides, and textile workers who dye fabrics are at increased risk. Cutting fluids may induce more allergies because they have a higher pH, which increases the release of formaldehyde [18].

- Allergy was observed in an occupational setting in 18% of 2-bromo-2-nitropropane-1,3-diol ACD cases in one large German study [6].
- There was a single case report of a worker at a polyester yarn manufacturing plant developing ACD to 2-bromo-2-nitropropane-1,3-diol from handling yarn containing this preservative [19].
- There was a single case report of forearm dermatitis in a veterinary surgeon due to ACD to 2-bromo-2-nitropropane-1,3-diol contained in a lubricant jelly [20].
- Three cases of allergic vesicular hand dermatitis in "milk recorders" were reported, where 2-bromo-2-nitropropane-1,3-diol was used as a preservative in the process of testing dairy milk [21].
- Two cases of ACD from 2-bromo-2-nitropropane-1,3-diol manifested as chronic hand dermatitis in two machinists working with coolant oil [22].
- 2-Bromo-2-nitropropane-1,3-diol was one of the important occupational contact allergens with a statistically significant association with blue-collar workers [23].
- HCWs had significantly more work-related ACD to 2-bromo-2-nitropropane-1,3-diol than non-HCWs [24, 25].

Concomitant sensitization to formaldehyde

- 2-Bromo-2-nitropropane-1,3-diol can degrade to formaldehyde,2-(hydroxymethyl)-2-nitropropane-1, 3-diol (Tris nitro, a formaldehyde releaser used in metalworking fluids) and bromonitroethanol. Heat and alkaline conditions hasten this process. As the product gets older, the formaldehyde levels continue to increase [10, 25, 26].

How often are patients reacting to 2-bromo-2-nitropropane-1, 3-diol also allergic to formaldehyde?

- Reports of concomitant reactions vary [27, 28]. Less than 25% (range 2–25%, median 17%) of 2-bromo-2-nitropropane-1,3-diol-sensitive patients co-react to formaldehyde [28]. This suggests that most patch test reactions to 2-bromo-2-nitropropane-1,3-diol indicate sensitivity to this preservative per se and are not related to formaldehyde allergy.

How often are patients reacting to formaldehyde also allergic to 2-bromo-2-nitropropane-1,3-diol?

- Less than 10% (range 1–10%, median 4%) of patients allergic to formaldehyde react to 2-bromo-2-nitropropane-1,3-diol [28]. In a Spanish study, 0.74% of formaldehyde allergic patients reacted to 2-bromo-2-nitropropane-1,3-diol [27]. Therefore, 2-bromo-2-nitropropane-1,3-diol releases little formaldehyde and the association with formaldehyde, though statistically significant, is weak. Concomitant ("dual") sensitization to formaldehyde and the parent molecule may also contribute to these associations in a number of cases.
- A survey of shampoos and cosmetics showed that no agents containing 2-bromo-2-nitropropane-1,3-diol had detectable levels of formaldehyde (detection limit 0.001%) [29].
- Concomitant sensitization was found in about a third of cases in three studies [4, 30, 31]. An emulsion containing 0.02% 2-bromo-2-nitropropane-1,3-diol has been reported to release up to 15 ppm formaldehyde [11]. Jordan et al. determined that the threshold for a clinical reaction in formaldehyde-sensitive patients was 30 ppm formaldehyde [32]. Therefore, formaldehyde-sensitive patients may or may not react to a product containing

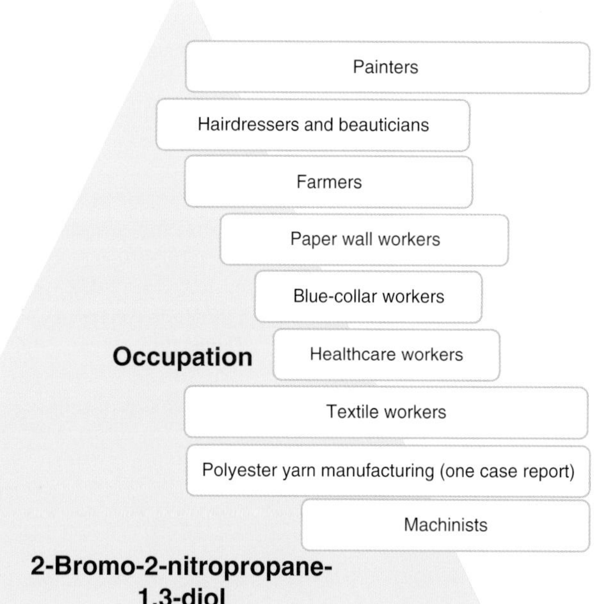

Figure 18.1 Occupations associated with allergic contact dermatitis to 2-bromo-2-nitropropane-1, 3-diol.

2-bromo-2-nitropropane-1,3-diol, depending on the concentration of the preservative, the type of product (leave-on or wash-off), the length of exposure and the status of the skin.

References

1 de Groot, A.C. and Veenstra, M. (2010). Formaldehyde-releasers in cosmetics in the USA and in Europe. *Contact Dermatitis* 62 (4): 221–224.

2 Flyvholm, M.A. (2005). Preservatives in registered chemical products. *Contact Dermatitis* 53 (1): 27–32.

3 de Groot, A.C., White, I.R., Flyvholm, M.A. et al. (2010). Formaldehyde-releasers in cosmetics: relationship to formaldehyde contact allergy. Part 1. Characterization, frequency and relevance of sensitization, and frequency of use in cosmetics. *Contact Dermatitis* 62 (1): 2–17.

4 Frosch, P.J., White, I.R., Rycroft, R.J. et al. (1990). Contact allergy to Bronopol. *Contact Dermatitis* 22 (1): 24–26.

5 Warshaw, E.M., Raju, S.I., Fowler, J.F. Jr. et al. (2012). Positive patch test reactions in older individuals: retrospective analysis from the North American Contact Dermatitis Group, 1994–2008. *Journal of the American Academy of Dermatology* 66 (2): 229–240.

6 Schnuch, A., Lessmann, H., Geier, J., and Uter, W. (2011). Contact allergy to preservatives. Analysis of IVDK data 1996–2009. *British Journal of Dermatology* 164 (6): 1316–1325.

7 Jacobs, M.C., White, I.R., Rycroft, R.J., and Taub, N. (1995). Patch testing with preservatives at St John's from 1982 to 1993. *Contact Dermatitis* 33 (4): 247–254.

8 Ford, G.P. and Beck, M.H. (1986). Reactions to Quaternium 15, Bronopol and Germall 115 in a standard series. *Contact Dermatitis* 14 (5): 271–274.

9 Maibach, H.I. (1977). Dermal sensitization potential of 2-bromo-2-nitropropane-1,3-diol (Bronopol). *Contact Dermatitis* 3 (2): 99.

10 Rudner, E.J. (1977). North American Group results. *Contact Dermatitis* 3 (4): 208–209.

11 Storrs, F.J. and Bell, D.E. (1983). Allergic contact dermatitis to 2-bromo-2-nitropropane-1,3-diol in a hydrophilic ointment. *Journal of the American Academy of Dermatology* 8 (2): 157–170.

12 Frosch, P.J. and Weickel, R. (1987). *Hautarzt* [Contact allergy to the preservative bronopol] 38 (5): 267–270. In German.

13 Shaughnessy, C.N., Malajian, D., and Belsito, D.V. (2014). Cutaneous delayed-type hypersensitivity in patients with atopic dermatitis: reactivity to topical preservatives. *Journal of the American Academy of Dermatology* 70 (1): 102–107.

14 Warshaw, E.M., Aschenbeck, K.A., Zug, K.A. et al. (2017). Wet wipe allergens: retrospective analysis from the North American Contact Dermatitis Group 2011–2014. *Dermatitis: contact, atopic, occupational, drug* 28 (1): 64–69.

15 Choudry, K., Beck, M.H., and Muston, H.L. (2002). Allergic contact dermatitis from 2-bromo-2-nitropropane-1,3-diol in Metrogel. *Contact Dermatitis* 46 (1): 60–61.

16 Tienthavorn, T., Tresukosol, P., and Sudtikoonaseth, P. (2014). Patch testing and histopathology in Thai patients with hyperpigmentation due to erythema dyschromicum perstans, lichen planus pigmentosus, and pigmented contact dermatitis. *Asian Pacific Journal of Allergy and Immunology* 32 (2): 185–192.

17 Prabha, N., Mahajan, V.K., Mehta, K.S. et al. (2014). Cosmetic contact sensitivity in patients with melasma: results of a pilot study. *Dermatology Research and Practice* 2014: 316219.

18 Maier, L.E., Lampel, H.P., Bhutani, T., and Jacob, S.E. (2009). Hand dermatitis: a focus on allergic contact dermatitis to biocides. *Dermatologic Clinics* 27 (3): 251–264, v–vi.

19 Podmore, P. (2000). Occupational allergic contact dermatitis from both 2-bromo-2-nitropropane-1,3-diol and methylchloroisothiazolinone plus methylisothiazolinone in spin finish. *Contact Dermatitis* 43 (1): 45.

20 Wilson, C.L. and Powell, S.M. (1990). An unusual case of allergic contact dermatitis in a veterinary surgeon. *Contact Dermatitis* 23 (1): 42–43.

21 Grattan, C.E., Harman, R.R., and Tan, R.S. (1986). Milk recorder dermatitis. *Contact Dermatitis* 14 (4): 217–220.

22 Robertson, M.H. and Storrs, F.J. (1982). Allergic contact dermatitis in two machinists. *Archives of Dermatology* 118 (12): 997–1002.

23 Schwensen, J.F., Menne, T., Veien, N.K. et al. (2014). Occupational contact dermatitis in blue-collar workers: results from a multicentre study from the Danish Contact Dermatitis Group (2003–2012). *Contact Dermatitis* 71 (6): 348–355.

24 Kadivar, S. (2015). Belsito DV. Occupational dermatitis in health care workers evaluated for suspected allergic contact dermatitis. *Dermatitis: contact, atopic, occupational, drug* 26 (4): 177–183.

25 Molin, S., Bauer, A., Schnuch, A., and Geier, J. (2015). Occupational contact allergy in nurses: results from the Information Network of Departments of Dermatology 2003–2012. *Contact Dermatitis* 72 (3): 164–171.

26 Sasseville, D. (2004). Hypersensitivity to preservatives. *Dermatologic Therapy* 17 (3): 251–263.

27 Latorre, N., Borrego, L., Fernandez-Redondo, V. et al. (2011). Patch testing with formaldehyde and formaldehyde-releasers: multicentre study in Spain (2005–2009). *Contact Dermatitis* 65 (5): 286–292.

28 de Groot, A., White, I.R., Flyvholm, M.A. et al. (2010). Formaldehyde-releasers in cosmetics: relationship to formaldehyde contact allergy. Part 2. Patch test relationship to formaldehyde contact allergy, experimental provocation tests, amount of formaldehyde released, and assessment of risk to consumers allergic to formaldehyde. *Contact Dermatitis* 62 (1): 18–31.

29 Rastogi, S.C. (1992). A survey of formaldehyde in shampoos and skin creams on the Danish market. *Contact Dermatitis* 27 (4): 235–240.

30 Peters, M.S., Connolly, S.M., and Schroeter, A.L. (1983). Bronopol allergic contact dermatitis. *Contact Dermatitis* 9 (5): 397–401.

31 Frosch, P.J. and Weickel, R. (1987). Contact allergy to the preservative bronopol. *Der Hautarzt; Zeitschrift fur Dermatologie, Venerologie, und verwandte Gebiete* 38 (5): 267–270. (Kontaktallergie auf das Konservierungsmittel Bronopol).

32 Jordan, W.P. Jr., Sherman, W.T., and King, S.E. (1979). Threshold responses in formaldehyde-sensitive subjects. *Journal of the American Academy of Dermatology* 1 (1): 44–48.

CHAPTER 19

Methylchloroisothiazolinone/Methylisothiazolinone

CHAPTER CONTENTS

Key points

- Methylchloroisothiazolinone/methylisothiazolinone (MCI/MI) is the International Nomenclature of Cosmetic Ingredients (INCI) name for the preservative and this is the name that must appear on cosmetic ingredient listing in the European and US markets if a product contains it.
- The legislation on cosmetics and household products regarding permitted levels is stricter than the legislation on industrial products.
- MCI/MI is frequently used in cosmetics and toiletries, paints, industrial lacquers, metal-working fluids, cutting oils, cleaning and polishing agents, inks and glues.
- Workers affected with allergic contact dermatitis (ACD) include painters, hairdressers, perfumers, metal workers, batch mixers in paint or chemical plants, laboratory technicians, printers, carpet makers, paper makers, paper hangers, painters, bricklayers, and potters.
- MCI/MI is not a good screening agent in the assessment of contact sensitivity to the other isothiazolinones because cross-reactions are uncommon and unpredictable.
- The recent epidemic of ACD to MI also witnessed a significant rise in patch test positivity to MCI/MI.

Exposure and use

Cosmetics

- MCI/MI is the tenth most frequently used preservative, being found in approximately 5% of cosmetic products in 2008 [1]. In Switzerland, it has been estimated that the total number of chemical products preserved with MCI/MI was about 6000 [2]. A review in 2011 noted that MI had started to be used as a 'stand alone' preservative in cosmetics [3].
- MCI/MI is permitted in concentrations of up to 15 ppm in rinse-off cosmetics in the EU and in the USA.

Non-cosmetic exposure and use

MCI/MI is frequently used in paints, wood stains, latex emulsions, cooling tower water, lacquers, metal-working fluids, cutting oils, cleaning products, polishing agents, wood and leather preservatives, printing inks, glues, cellulose solutions, polymer emulsions, fillers, pottery glazes, and slime-control agents in paper mills [4, 5]. Up to 80% of water-based paints currently contain MCI/MI. Treatment of painted walls with the inorganic sulfur salt sodium bisulfite can lead to the inactivation of MCI/MI's allergenic properties by opening its ring [6].

Patch testing

In the European Standard Series, it is recommended that testing is with 200 ppm MCI/MI (0.02% aq.) or the T.R.U.E.® test equivalent.

Concomitant positive reactions to MCI/MI were seen in 41–67.3% of MI allergic patients, whereas 39.5% of MCI/MI positives react to MI [7, 8]. The explanations are not conclusive between exposure to MI in MCI/MI and contact allergy to MCI with cross-reactivity to MI. MI-allergic patients were more likely to react to more than three different allergens ('polysensitisers').

Common Contact Allergens: A Practical Guide to Detecting Contact Dermatitis, First Edition. Edited by John McFadden, Pailin Puangpet, Korbkarn Pongpairoj, Supitchaya Thaiwat, and Lee Shan Xian.
© 2020 John Wiley & Sons Ltd. Published 2020 by John Wiley & Sons Ltd.
Companion website: www.wiley.com/go/mcfadden/common_contact_allergens

Sensitization

Over the last 10 years there has been a noticeable increase in sensitization, usually above 3% in clinics, as a consequence of the 'isothiazolinone' epidemic.

Age

Italy (2002–2008) age 3–36 months	MCI/MI	4.4% [9]
UK (2005–2014) age ≤ 16 years	MCI/MI	6% [10]

Common in children and over the age of 40 years.

Sex

MCI/MI sensitization seems to be more common amongst women. Cronin et al. reported that the frequency of contact sensitivity to MCI/MI ranged from 0.6% to 3.3% in females and from 0% to 1.4% in males [11].

Clinical disease

- The typical patient is a woman who presents with hand or facial eczema. Lesions may involve only the eyelids even though the causative cosmetic has been applied to the entire face. Unusual presentations include scaly, urticarial or infiltrated plaques mimicking seborrheic dermatitis, follicular ACD [12], photodermatitis, and photoaggravated contact dermatitis [13].
- MCI/MI in moist toilet paper was a cause of perianal, perineal, or gluteal ACD in adults (its use in moist toilet tissue should have been discontinued by now) [14]. Guimaraens et al. described the first woman with hand dermatitis from using moist toilet paper for her baby [15]. De Groot reported another case of vesicular hand eczema secondary to perianal ACD caused by moistened toilet tissues. The vesicular dermatitis was considered to be an id reaction [16]. *(Note: MCI/MI should not be contained in wet tissue paper anymore.)*
- Other unexpected sources of exposure include carpet shampoos, fabric softeners [5], and grinding dust [17].
- There have been some reports of airborne ACD due to isothiazolinones contained in wall paints and glues. Even limited and indirect exposure is sufficient to elicit a severe allergic reaction [3, 6, 18, 19]. MCI/MI can provoke acute dermatitis or respiratory symptoms after an individual stays in a freshly painted room [6]. Concentrations of MCI/MI in the air a few days after painting may be high enough to elicit airborne reactions in sensitized patients.

Occupational disease

- Isothiazolinone contact allergy was significantly associated with occupational dermatitis ($p = 0.03$) when compared with other patch-tested patients. Exposure to isothiazolinones in occupational products was found in 30% of allergic cases [7]. The affected workers include hairdressers, perfumers, metal workers, machinists, batch mixers in paint or chemical plants, laboratory technicians, radiology technicians [20], healthcare workers, beauty workers [21], repairmen, café workers [22], restaurant workers, printers, carpet makers, paper makers, paper hangers, painters, bricklayers, potters, and furniture restorers [20–23]. Four of nine machinists in a jet turbine plant were reported to have ACD to MCI/MI, whilst five had irritant contact dermatitis [24].
- In the flax-spinning mill industry, MCI/MI was introduced in 1995. The first spinners with contact allergy were seen 2 months later. 20 out of 100 spinners were reported as having a new rash, with blistering of the fingers of both hands and patchy forearm rashes. The prevalence was about 6–8% each year [4]. An additional report showed a case of occupational hand eczema due to MI in coating oil (spin finish) from the yarn [25].
- A diesel mechanic presented with vesicular hand eczema, thereafter evolving into hyperkeratotic and fissured hand eczema. He had a positive patch test to MCI/MI (++). During the course of his work, he came into contact with diesel oil containing Kathon FP (MCI/MI in dipropylene glycol) [26].

Other areas of interest

Chemical burns

Exposure to concentrated solutions of MCI/MI can be severely irritating in an occupational setting and can probably induce sensitization. A patient with severe irritant contact dermatitis due to MCI/MI (1.15%) was reported from Singapore. Workers should wear protective clothing and all containers should be leak tested [27]. Three workers with contact allergy after chemical burns from MCI/MI were subsequently reported from the USA [28]. Sodium bisulfite can instantly deactivate MCI/MI. It prevents corrosive skin reactions and decreases the elicitation of ACD [29]. However, sodium bisulfite has potentially hazardous effects. 2% glutathione-containing emollients were found to inactivate up to 2400 ppm of MCI/MI [30].

Active sensitization

Active sensitization to MCI/MI has previously been reported. The patient had negative initial patch test reactions. On day 25, she noticed two itchy eczematous lesions, each the size and shape of a positive patch test reaction, on her back. Repeat patch testing showed a +++ reaction to MCI/MI 200 ppm [31].

Willi et al. reported primary sensitization to isothiazolinone in a cooling tower cleaner 10 days after first exposure. Previous studies have found the persistence of radioactively labeled MCI in the skin over several days – isothiazolinone was assumed to persist in the skin of this patient [32].

Cross-reactivity

Other members of the isothiazolinone family, octylisothiazolinone and 1,2-benzisothiazoline-3-one (1,2-BIT; Proxel), can be found in paints, dyes, photographic solutions, plastic emulsions, air fresheners, and mold-releasing oils in the pottery industry [5]. Although they share a similar chemical structure, true cross-sensitivity was thought to be unlikely [33]. They were found not to cross-react by Schubert [19]. MCI/MI is, therefore, not a good screening agent in the assessment of contact sensitivity to the other isothiazolinones.

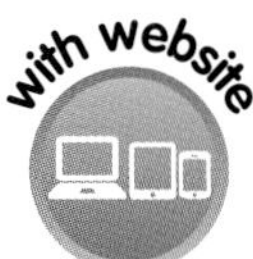

Go to http://www.wiley.com/go/mcfadden/common_contact_allergens to find the E-supplement for this chapter:

Methylchloroisothiazolinone and Methylsiothiazolinone: E-Supplement

References

1 Steinberg, D.C. (2008). Voluntary registration of cosmetics and 2007 frequency of preservative use. *Cosmet Toiletries Magazine* 123: 47–52.
2 Reinhard, E., Waeber, R., Niederer, M. et al. (2001). Preservation of products with MCI/MI in Switzerland. *Contact Dermatitis* 45 (5): 257–264.
3 Lundov, M.D., Krongaard, T., Menne, T.L., and Johansen, J.D. (2011). Methylisothiazolinone contact allergy: a review. *British Journal of Dermatology* 165 (6): 1178–1182.
4 Podmore, P. (1998). An epidemic of isothiazolinone sensitization in a flax spinning mill. *Contact Dermatitis* 38 (3): 165–166.
5 Sasseville, D. (2004). Hypersensitivity to preservatives. *Dermatologic Therapy* 17 (3): 251–263.
6 Bohn, S., Niederer, M., Brehm, K., and Bircher, A.J. (2000). Airborne contact dermatitis from methylchloroisothiazolinone in wall paint. Abolition of symptoms by chemical allergen inactivation. *Contact Dermatitis* 42 (4): 196–201.
7 Lundov, M.D., Thyssen, J.P., Zachariae, C., and Johansen, J.D. (2010). Prevalence and cause of methylisothiazolinone contact allergy. *Contact Dermatitis* 63 (3): 164–167.
8 Schnuch, A., Lessmann, H., Geier, J., and Uter, W. (2011). Contact allergy to preservatives. Analysis of IVDK data 1996–2009. *British Journal of Dermatology* 164 (6): 1316–1325.
9 Fortina, A.B., Romano, I., Peserico, A., and Eichenfield, L. (2011). Contact sensitization in very young children. *Journal of the American Academy of Dermatology* 65: 772–779.
10 Smith, V.M., Clark, S.M., and Wilkinson, M. (2016). Allergic contact dermatitis in children: trends in allergens, 10 years on. A retrospective study of 500 children tested between 2005 and 2014 in one UK centre. *Contact Dermatitis* 74 (1): 37–43. .
11 Cronin, E., Hannuksela, M., Lachapelle, J.M. et al. (1988). Frequency of sensitisation to the preservative Kathon CG. *Contact Dermatitis* 18 (5): 274–279.
12 Concha-Garzon, M.J., Solano-Lopez, G., Montes, A. et al. (2015). Follicular allergic contact dermatitis due to methylchloroisothiazolinone/methylisothiazolinone (MCI/MI) in a rinse-off soap product. *Clinical and Experimental Dermatology* 40 (6): 690–691.
13 Pirmez, R., Fernandes, A.L., and Melo, M.G. (2015). Photoaggravated contact dermatitis to Kathon CG (methylchloroisothiazolinone/methylisothiazolinone): a novel pattern of involvement in a growing epidemic? *British Journal of Dermatology* 173 (5): 1343–1344.
14 Gardner, K.H., Davis, M.D., Richardson, D.M., and Pittelkow, M.R. (2010). The hazards of moist toilet paper: allergy to the preservative methylchloroisothiazolinone/methylisothiazolinone. *Archives of Dermatology* 146 (8): 886–890.
15 Guimaraens, D., Conde-Salazar, L., and Gonzalez, M.A. (1996). Allergic contact dermatitis on the hands from chloromethylisothiazolinone in moist toilet paper. *Contact Dermatitis* 35 (4): 254.
16 de Groot, A.C. (1997). Vesicular dermatitis of the hands secondary to perianal allergic contact dermatitis caused by preservatives in moistened toilet tissues. *Contact Dermatitis* 36 (3): 173–174.
17 Isaksson, M. and Persson, L. (2015). Occupational contact dermatitis caused by methylchloroisothiazolinone/methylisothiazolinone through exposure to filler dust containing this preservative and with a positive patch test reaction to the dust. *Contact Dermatitis* 73 (2): 119–120.
18 Garcia-Gavin, J., Vansina, S., Kerre, S. et al. (2010). Methylisothiazolinone, an emerging allergen in cosmetics? *Contact Dermatitis* 63 (2): 96–101.
19 Schubert, H. (1997). Airborne contact dermatitis due to methylchloro- and methylisothiazolinone (MCI/MI). *Contact Dermatitis* 36 (5): 274.
20 Pazzaglia, M., Vincenzi, C., Gasparri, F., and Tosti, A. (1996). Occupational hypersensitivity to isothiazolinone derivatives in a radiology technician. *Contact Dermatitis* 34 (2): 143–144.
21 Urwin, R., Warburton, K., Carder, M. et al. (2015). Methylchloroisothiazolinone and methylisothiazolinone contact allergy: an occupational perspective. *Contact Dermatitis* 72 (6): 381–386.
22 Vauhkala, A.R., Pesonen, M., Suomela, S. et al. (2015). Occupational contact allergy to methylchloroisothiazolinone/methylisothiazolinone and methylisothiazolinone. *Contact Dermatitis* 73 (3): 150–156.
23 Corazza, M., Mantovani, L., Bacilieri, S., and Virgili, A. (2001). A child with "occupational" allergic contact dermatitis due to MCI/MI. *Contact Dermatitis* 44: 53.
24 Madden, S.D., Thiboutot, D.M., and Marks, J.G. Jr. (1994). Occupationally induced allergic contact dermatitis to methylchloroisothiazolinone/methylisothiazolinone among machinists. *Journal of the American Academy of Dermatology* 30 (2 Pt 1): 272–274.

25 Podmore, P. (2000). Occupational allergic contact dermatitis from both 2-bromo-2-nitropropane-1,3-diol and methylchloroisothiazolinone plus methylisothiazolinone in spin finish. *Contact Dermatitis* 43 (1): 45.
26 Bruynzeel, D.P. and Verburgh, C.A. (1996). Occupational dermatitis from isothiazolinones in diesel oil. *Contact Dermatitis* 34 (1): 64–65.
27 Tay, P. and Ng, S.K. (1994). Delayed skin burns from MCI/MI biocide used in water treatment. *Contact Dermatitis* 30 (1): 54–55.
28 Primka, E.J. 3rd and Taylor, J.S. (1997). Three cases of contact allergy after chemical burns from methylchloroisothiazolinone/methylisothiazolinone: one with concomitant allergy to methyldibromoglutaronitrile/phenoxyethanol. *American Journal of Contact Dermatitis: Official Journal of the American Contact Dermatitis Society* 8 (1): 43–46.
29 Gruvberger, B. and Bruze, M. (1998). Can chemical burns and allergic contact dermatitis from higher concentrations of methylchloroisothiazolinone/methylisothiazolinone be prevented? *American Journal of Contact Dermatitis* 9 (1): 11–14.
30 Gruvberger, B. and Bruze, M. (1998). Can glutathione-containing emollients inactivate methylchloroisothiazolinone/methylisothiazolinone? *Contact Dermatitis* 38 (5): 261–265.
31 Isaksson, M. and Gruvberger, B. (2003). Patch test sensitization to methylchloroisothiazolinone + methylisothiazolinone and 4,4′-diaminodiphenylmethane. *Contact Dermatitis* 48 (1): 53–54.
32 Willi, R., Pfab, F., Zilker, T. et al. (2011). Danger from the workplace: allergic contact dermatitis from the first exposure to isothiazolinones. *Contact Dermatitis* 64 (6): 361–362.
33 Damstra, R.J., van Vlotten, W.A., and van Ginkel, C.J. (1992). Allergic contact dermatitis from the preservative 1,2-benzisothiazolin-3-one (1,2-BIT; Proxel): a case report, its prevalence in those occupationally at risk and in the general dermatological population, and its relationship to allergy to its analogue Kathon CG. *Contact Dermatitis* 27 (2): 105–109.

Exposure Color Code

- Clothing, jewelry, adornments
- Personal care products, cosmetics/cosmetic procedures
- Household products, domestic environment, including furniture and refurbishment
- Occupational dermatoses, work environment
- Medicines, surgical/dental procedures, herbal/alternative medicines
- Personal appliances/aids
- Leisure activities, sport, travel
- Other exposures (including dietary)
- Not relevant or multiple/general exposure

CHAPTER 20

Methylisothiazolinone

CHAPTER CONTENTS

Key points

- MI has caused an epidemic of ACD.
- MI is now banned by the EU in leave-on cosmetic products.
- MI can cause ACD through its use in toiletries and household goods, as well as in an occupational setting.
- Occupational at-risk groups include painters, pottery workers, glass makers, and beauticians.
- There is a limited but clinically important potential for cross-reactivity between the isothiazolinones.
- Can present as pseudoangioedema from airborne contact with wall paint.
- Wheezing can occur with airborne contact dermatitis.

Exposure and uses

In 2007, the US Food and Drug Administration estimated that MI was used in 1125 cosmetic agents, including shampoos, shower gels, face/hand/body creams, hand soaps, and deodorants. The ban on leave-on products and severe restrictions on wash-off products coming into place regarding cosmetic agents will continue to impact the use profile.

MI is used in industry as an antimicrobial in pulp/mills, cooling water systems, and the oil industry. It is also used as a preservative in adhesives, coatings, fuels, metal-working fluids, resin emulsions, and paints (Figures 20.1 and 20.2) [1].

Clinical risk factors associated with methylisothiazolinone (MI) contact sensitization

Uter et al. [2] looked at clinical risk factors for MI allergy. They found associations with age >40 years old, female sex, facial (and to a lesser extent hand) dermatitis, anogenital involvement and the use of cosmetics. McFadden et al. also found that facial involvement, female sex, and age >40 years were associated with MI allergy [3].

Common Contact Allergens: A Practical Guide to Detecting Contact Dermatitis, First Edition. Edited by John McFadden, Pailin Puangpet, Korbkarn Pongpairoj, Supitchaya Thaiwat, and Lee Shan Xian.

© 2020 John Wiley & Sons Ltd. Published 2020 by John Wiley & Sons Ltd.

Companion website: www.wiley.com/go/mcfadden/common_contact_allergens

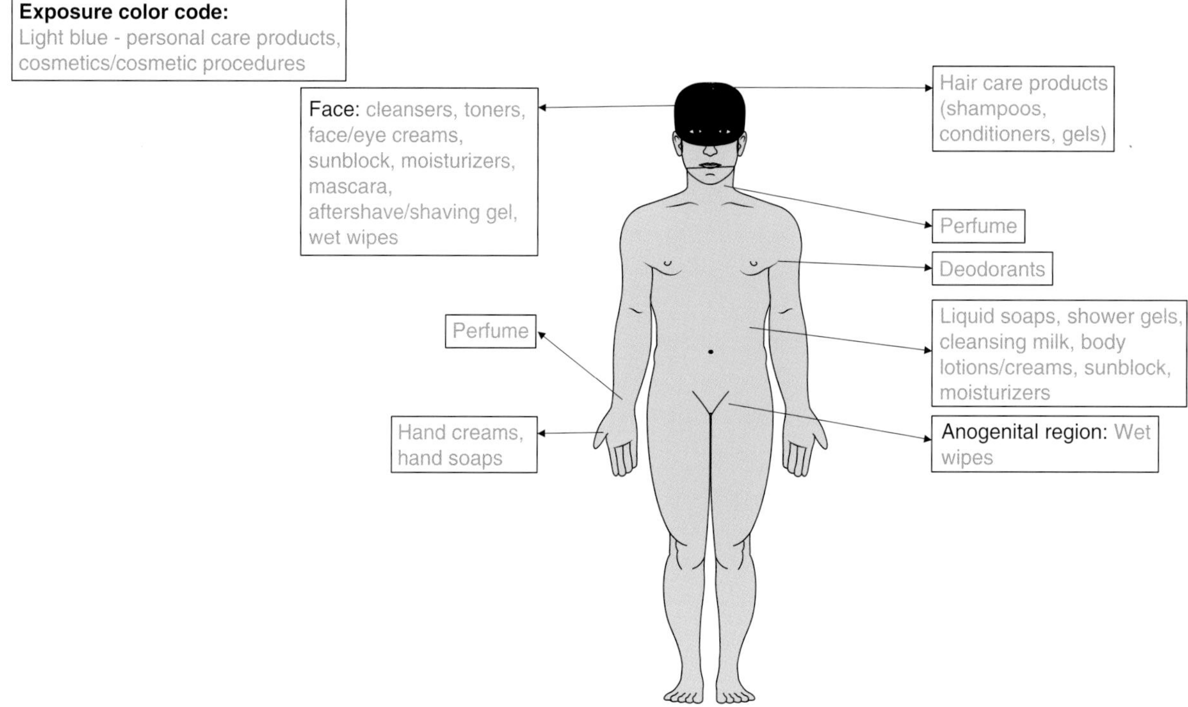

Figure 20.1 Cosmetic sources of isothiazolinone exposure. Note: Since the EU ban on MI in leave-on cosmetic products these should now not be relevant for the EU (they are still allowed in wash-off products).

Occupational exposure and MI allergy

- Uter et al. found that MI allergy was most associated with the following occupations: painters, pottery workers, glass makers, and cosmetologists [2]. The first cases of MI allergy in 2004 and 2006 were associated with paint exposure, one in painters (Isakson 2004) and one in workers in a paint factory (Figure 20.2) [4].
- A retrospective study from Finland between 2002 and 2013 showed that the most at-risk occupational groups were hairdressers, beauticians, mechanics, repairmen, and machinists. In addition, painters, paint factory workers, as well as cafe and restaurant workers were also at risk [5].

Patch testing concentration used

- It has now been generally accepted that the optimal concentration for testing for MI sensitization is with MI aq. 0.2% (2000 ppm) [6].

Frequency of sensitization

Although patch testing for MI allergy has been performed at different concentrations (see above), there has been a largely consistent rising trend in the incidence of MI allergy reported from patch test clinics over the 4 years after 2010. The Gentofte group started testing for MI allergy alone as early as 2006 [7]. Between 2006 and 2009, there was an MI allergy rate of between 1.1% and 1.7%. However, from 2010 to 2012 there was a significant upward trend to 3.7% [8]. In multiple centers in the UK there was a 6.4-fold increase in the detection of MI allergy between 2010 and 2013, with over half the centers reporting a frequency of MI allergy in over 10% of patients tested [9].

With awareness of an epidemic of MI allergy and reduction in the use of MI in leave-on products, levels of sensitization have started to reduce (6% in European clinics in 2015 [10]).

Patch testing and relevance

- In a recent Belgian series, current (certain or probable) relevance was found in 75.6% (2010), 81.6% (2011), and 80.6% (2012) of cases [11].

Patch testing: strength of reaction

- Of positive patch test reactions to MI in 2012/2013 in Finland, 279/416 (67%) were ++ or +++ reactions [12].
- A report from Denmark (2006–2010) found that MI allergic patients were more likely than other patch test + patients to have

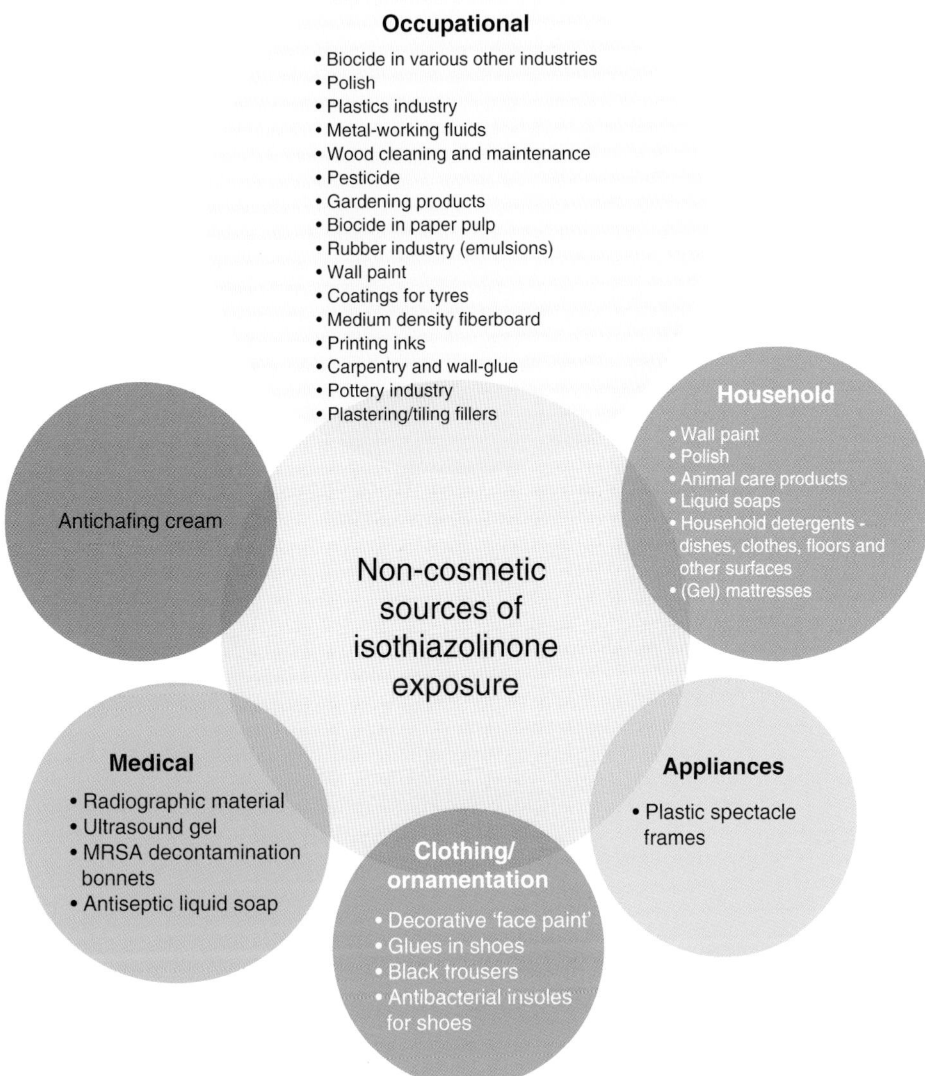

Figure 20.2 Non-cosmetic sources of isothiazolinone exposure.

concomitant reactions to three or more allergens ($p < 0.001$) [7]. Thus, MI allergic patients are more likely to be **polysensitizers**.

- The repeated open application test (ROAT) in MI allergic patients found that 18% reacted to 20 times lower concentration than the then permitted concentration (100 ppm) of MI in cosmetics [13]. In the same study, 64% reacted to creams containing 100 and 50 ppm.

Clinically relevant exposures

The main sources of clinically relevant exposures reported with MI allergy are (i) leave-on cosmetic products (MI should no longer be contained in these in the EU), (ii) wash-off cosmetic products, (iii) wet wipes (MI should no longer be contained in these in the EU), (iv) household products, and (v) paint. Furthermore, there is a trend for multiple rather than isolated sources of exposure (Figure 20.1).

Cross-reactivity between MI and other isothiazolinones

- Limited cross-reactivity or co-reactivity may occur.

Clinical disease

Cosmetics and household goods

Cosmetics and household goods represent the majority of cases. There are often multiple sources of exposure. Hair care products, dishwashing agents and liquid soaps are common sources.

Allergic contact dermatitis (ACD) from paint, respiratory symptoms, and pseudoangioedema

- ■ A 36-year-old man presented with recurrent severe dermatitis of the face and neck, which resolved on holiday. He had recently had his apartment refurbished. The patch test to methylchloroisothiazolinone/MI (MCI/MI) was weakly +. His dermatitis had first started when he was working in a casino which had its walls repainted with paint containing MCI/MI. The rash occurred when he frequented his flat at the weekend. After 3 months, the facial dermatitis resolved. Another 57-year-old man known to be allergic to MI and MCI/MI developed severe facial dermatitis with burning of the face and dyspnea necessitating oral prednisolone. This started after his wife began painting their house with an emulsion containing MI, MCI, and benzisothiazolinone [14].
- ■ ■ An Australian case of airborne ACD after exposure to MI-containing wall paint was reported. A 24-year-old woman developed periorbital edema and acute dermatitis of her face, neck, and upper chest. Nocturnal cough and wheeze were also present [15]. ACD to MI, either airborne from wet wall paint or from decorative face paint, can present as "pseudoangioedema" (Figure 20.3).

Wet-wipe tissues

The use of MI in wet-wipe tissues should have been discontinued. Dermatitis has been noted in the perianal area, hands, and/or face (periorbital, cheeks, and/or perioral area).

Eczema-mimicking photodermatosis

- ■ A patient presented with eczema of the face, neck, and proximal arms similar to a photodermatosis after using a MI-containing facial ointment [16]. Whether photoexacerbation of ACD to MI can occur is a subject of ongoing debate.

Children

- ■ Patel et al. [17] reported their series of 310 children patch tested to a modified baseline series between January 2011 and September 2013. Thirteen (4.2%) were found to be allergic to MCI/MI. They had patch tested 18 children since August 2013 with 0.2% MI and identified two patients with allergy to MI. They attributed all their pediatric cases of isothiazolinone allergy to the use of wet wipes and cosmetics/toiletries.

Ineffectiveness of rubber gloves as protection against MI

- ■ A 55-year-old nurse presented with a 20-year history of chronic hand eczema. A previous patch test showed contact allergy to MCI/MI. Despite using nitrile gloves at work and rubber latex gloves at home, her hand dermatitis persisted. Further patch testing showed ++(+) reactions to MI. Testing with skin occluded by nitrile and rubber latex gloves showed a negative reaction with nitrile but a + reaction with rubber latex. This study appears to indicate that rubber latex gloves may not fully protect against the penetration of MI [18].

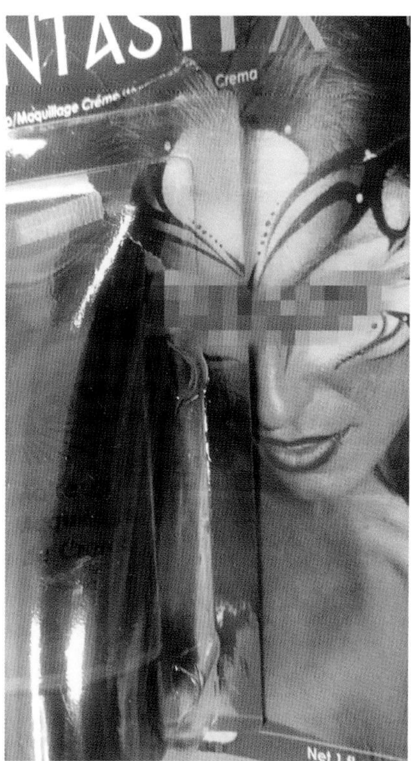

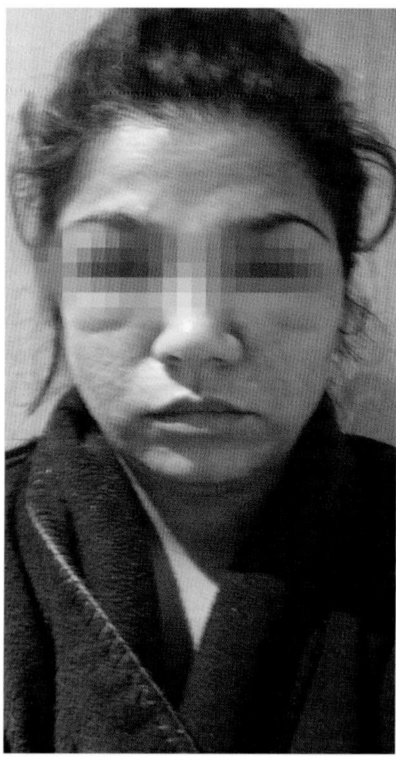

Figure 20.3 Acute ACD from MI in decorative "facepaint" presenting as "pseudoangioedema," with rapid onset and edema as a prominent sign. Other cases reported to present as "pseudoangioedema" include acute ACD to p-phenylenediamine, inhaled budesonide, propolis, castor oil, benzoyl peroxide, diphenylcyclopropenone, and cinnamon.

Waist-reduction belt

- A 68-year-old man with longstanding perianal dermatitis and recurrent hand eczema presented with erythematous and pruritic patches on the abdomen [19]. These corresponded to the areas in contact with the electrodes of a waist-reduction belt. Skin contact with the belt was enhanced by a contact gel supplied with the belt. Resolution of dermatitis was achieved with potent topical steroids. Patch testing revealed doubtful reactions to MCI/MI and a ++ reaction to MI 0.05% aq. The ingredient labeling of the contact gel showed that it contained both MI and MCI.

Deodorant

- A case of axillary dermatitis was attributed to MI in the deodorant the patient was using [20].

Leather sofa

- ACD to MI used in a leather care product applied to a sofa was described. There was generalized dermatitis with accentuation on the posterior aspects of the thighs [21].

Spectacle frame dermatitis

- A patient presented with a dermatitis on the temples where spectacle frame sidebars touched the skin, consistent with ACD to spectacle frames. Patch testing was positive to MI and mass spectrometry analysis revealed the presence of MI in the spectacle frame, even in the center of the plastic [22].

Shoe glue

- A case of foot dermatitis from MI in a glue used to adhere three parts of an upper component of a work shoe was reported [23].

Other cosmetic and non-cosmetic sources of isothiazolinone exposure

- These have recently been summarized by Aerts et al. (Figures 20.1 and 20.2) [24].

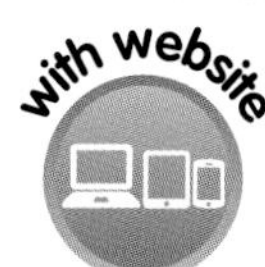

Go to http://www.wiley.com/go/mcfadden/common_contact_allergens to find the E-supplement for this chapter:

Methylisothiazolinone: E-Supplement.

References

1 Burnett, C.L., Bergfeld, W.F., Belsito, D.V. et al. (2010). Final report of the safety assessment of methylisothiazolinone. *International Journal of Toxicology* 29 (4 Suppl): 187S–213S.

2 Uter, W., Geier, J., Bauer, A., and Schnuch, A. (2013). Risk factors associated with methylisothiazolinone contact sensitization. *Contact Dermatitis* 69 (4): 231–238.

3 McFadden, J.P., Mann, J., White, J.M. et al. (2013). Outbreak of methylisothiazolinone allergy targeting those aged >/=40 years. *Contact Dermatitis* 69 (1): 53–55.

4 Thyssen, J.P., Sederberg-Olsen, N., Thomsen, J.F., and Menne, T. (2006). Contact dermatitis from methylisothiazolinone in a paint factory. *Contact Dermatitis* 54 (6): 322–324.

5 Vauhkala, A.R., Pesonen, M., Suomela, S. et al. (2015). Occupational contact allergy to methylchloroisothiazolinone/methylisothiazolinone and methylisothiazolinone. *Contact Dermatitis* 73 (3): 150–156.

6 Engfeldt, M., Brared-Christensson, J., Isaksson, M. et al. (2015). Swedish experiences from patch testing Methylisothiazolinone separately. *Acta Dermato-Venereologica* 95 (6): 717–719.

7 Lundov, M.D., Thyssen, J.P., Zachariae, C., and Johansen, J.D. (2010). Prevalence and cause of methylisothiazolinone contact allergy. *Contact Dermatitis* 63 (3): 164–167.

8 Lundov, M.D., Opstrup, M.S., and Johansen, J.D. (2013). Methylisothiazolinone contact allergy--growing epidemic. *Contact Dermatitis* 69 (5): 271–275.

9 Johnston, G.A. (2014). Contributing members of the British Society for Cutaneous A. The rise in prevalence of contact allergy to methylisothiazolinone in the British Isles. *Contact Dermatitis* 70 (4): 238–240.

10 Schwensen, J.F., Uter, W., Bruze, M. et al. (2017). The epidemic of methylisothiazolinone: a European prospective study. *Contact Dermatitis* 76 (5): 272–279.

11 Aerts, O., Baeck, M., Constandt, L. et al. (2014). The dramatic increase in the rate of methylisothiazolinone contact allergy in Belgium: a multicentre study. *Contact Dermatitis* 71 (1): 41–48.

12 Lammintausta, K., Aalto-Korte, K., Ackerman, L. et al. (2014). An epidemic of contact allergy to methylisothiazolinone in Finland. *Contact Dermatitis* 70 (3): 184–185.

13 Lundov, M.D., Zachariae, C., and Johansen, J.D. (2011). Methylisothiazolinone contact allergy and dose-response relationships. *Contact Dermatitis* 64 (6): 330–336.

14 Lundov, M.D., Mosbech, H., Thyssen, J.P. et al. (2011). Two cases of airborne allergic contact dermatitis caused by methylisothiazolinone in paint. *Contact Dermatitis* 65 (3): 176–179.

15 Wright, A.M. and Cahill, J.L. (2015). Airborne exposure to methylisothiazolinone in paint causing allergic contact dermatitis: an Australian perspective. *The Australasian Journal of Dermatology*.

16 Gabelein-Wissing, N., Lehmann, P., and Hofmann, S.C. (2015). Allergic contact eczema to a long-used cosmetic: Methylisothiazolinon, a type IV-allergen. *Der Hautarzt; Zeitschrift fur Dermatologie, Venerologie, und Verwandte Gebiete* 66 (6): 462–464.

17 Patel, A.N., Wootton, C.I., and English, J.S. (2014). Methylisothiazolinone allergy in the paediatric population: the epidemic begins? *The British Journal of Dermatology* 170 (5): 1200–1201.

18 Espasandin-Arias, M. and Goossens, A. (2014). Natural rubber gloves might not protect against skin penetration of methylisothiazolinone. *Contact Dermatitis* 70 (4): 249–251.

19 Uter, W., Uter, M., Steen-Schuberth, B., and Schnuch, A. (2012). Allergic contact dermatitis caused by methylisothiazolinone from a 'waist reduction belt'. *Contact Dermatitis* 66 (6): 347–348.

20 Amaro, C., Santos, R., and Cardoso, J. (2011). Contact allergy to methylisothiazolinone in a deodorant. *Contact Dermatitis* 64 (5): 298–299.

21 Vandevenne, A., Vanden Broecke, K., and Goossens, A. (2014). Sofa dermatitis caused by methylisothiazolinone in a leather-care product. *Contact Dermatitis* 71 (2): 111–113.
22 El-Houri, R.B., Christensen, L.P., Persson, C. et al. (2016). Methylisothiazolinone in a designer spectacle frame – a surprising finding. *Contact Dermatitis* 75 (5): 310–312.
23 Silva, C.A., El-Houri, R.B., Christensen, L.P., and Andersen, F. (2017). Contact allergy caused by methylisothiazolinone in shoe glue. *Contact Dermatitis* 77 (3): 175–176.
24 Aerts, O., Goossens, A., Lambert, J., and Lepoittevin, J.P. (2017). Contact allergy caused by isothiazolinone derivatives: an overview of non-cosmetic and unusual cosmetic sources. *European Journal of Dermatology: EJD* 27 (2): 115–122.

Exposure Color Code

- Clothing, jewelry, adornments
- Personal care products, cosmetics/cosmetic procedures
- Household products, domestic environment, including furniture and refurbishment
- Occupational dermatoses, work environment
- Medicines, surgical/dental procedures, herbal/alternative medicines
- Personal appliances/aids
- Leisure activities, sport, travel
- Other exposures (including dietary)
- Not relevant or multiple/general exposure

CHAPTER 21

Parabens

CHAPTER CONTENTS

Key points

- Parabens are weak sensitizers.
- Contact allergy is uncommon.
- Paraben esters including methylparaben, ethylparaben, propylparaben, benzylparaben, and butylparaben are the most widely used preservatives in cosmetic products.
- Popular because of their low irritant potential, non-toxicity, stability, bioavailability, broad antimicrobial activity, and low cost.
- Multiple parabens in one product are used to extend antimicrobial coverage.
- A typical paraben preservative system contains methyl and propylparaben.
- Parabens can be found in pharmaceuticals, shampoos, commercial moisturizers, shaving gels, personal lubricants, topical/parenteral spray tanning solutions, toothpaste, and food additives.
- Common in topical medicaments; labeled in medicines as "hydroxybenzoates."
- Most cases of paraben contact allergy are caused by topical creams applied to leg ulcers or chronic dermatoses.
- Sensitized individuals may be able to use products containing parabens on non-inflamed skin, a phenomenon called "the paraben paradox."

Exposure and use

Cosmetics and household goods

- The antimicrobial effects of parabens and their use as preservatives was first established in 1924 [1]. Parabens are the most common preservatives used in *cosmetics, skincare products, medications* and *foods* (Figure 21.1). They are popular because of their low irritant potential, non-toxicity, stability, bioavailability, broad antimicrobial activity, and low cost [2]. A typical paraben preservative system contains methyl and propylparaben. Rastogi et al. found that 77% of investigated cosmetics contained 0.01–0.87% parabens. The frequency of use of parabens has been ranked: methyl > ethyl > propyl > butyl > benzyl. In paraben-containing cosmetics, the maximum concentrations were 0.32% methyl and propylparaben, 0.19% ethylparaben, and 0.07% butyl and benzylparaben. An individual may, therefore, have multiple sources of exposure to parabens [3].
- A Swedish survey of 100 moisturizers (1998) found that parabens were the most commonly used preservative [4].

Products that can contain parabens

- *Sunscreens; skin creams, lotions, ointments;*
- *Moisturizers*: present in 170/276 (62%) of moisturizers available from pharmacies in Chicago (2008) [5];
- *Topical medications* for skin pain or infections, hemorrhoid treatments, ear and nose drops, rectal and vaginal medications, and local anesthetics; Unna's boot *bandages*; [6]
- *Cosmetics* such as foundation and powders, blushers, mascaras, eye shadows, eyeliners and pencils, lipsticks, quick-dry nail products, bronzers and makeup removers;
- *Soaps, cleansers and hygiene products* [7];
- *Shaving products*, e.g. foam;
- *Hair care products*, e.g. shampoo;
- *Antiperspirants and deodorants*;
- *Toothpastes*;
- *Pet care and grooming products.*

Common Contact Allergens: A Practical Guide to Detecting Contact Dermatitis, First Edition. Edited by John McFadden, Pailin Puangpet, Korbkarn Pongpairoj, Supitchaya Thaiwat, and Lee Shan Xian.
© 2020 John Wiley & Sons Ltd. Published 2020 by John Wiley & Sons Ltd.
Companion website: www.wiley.com/go/mcfadden/common_contact_allergens

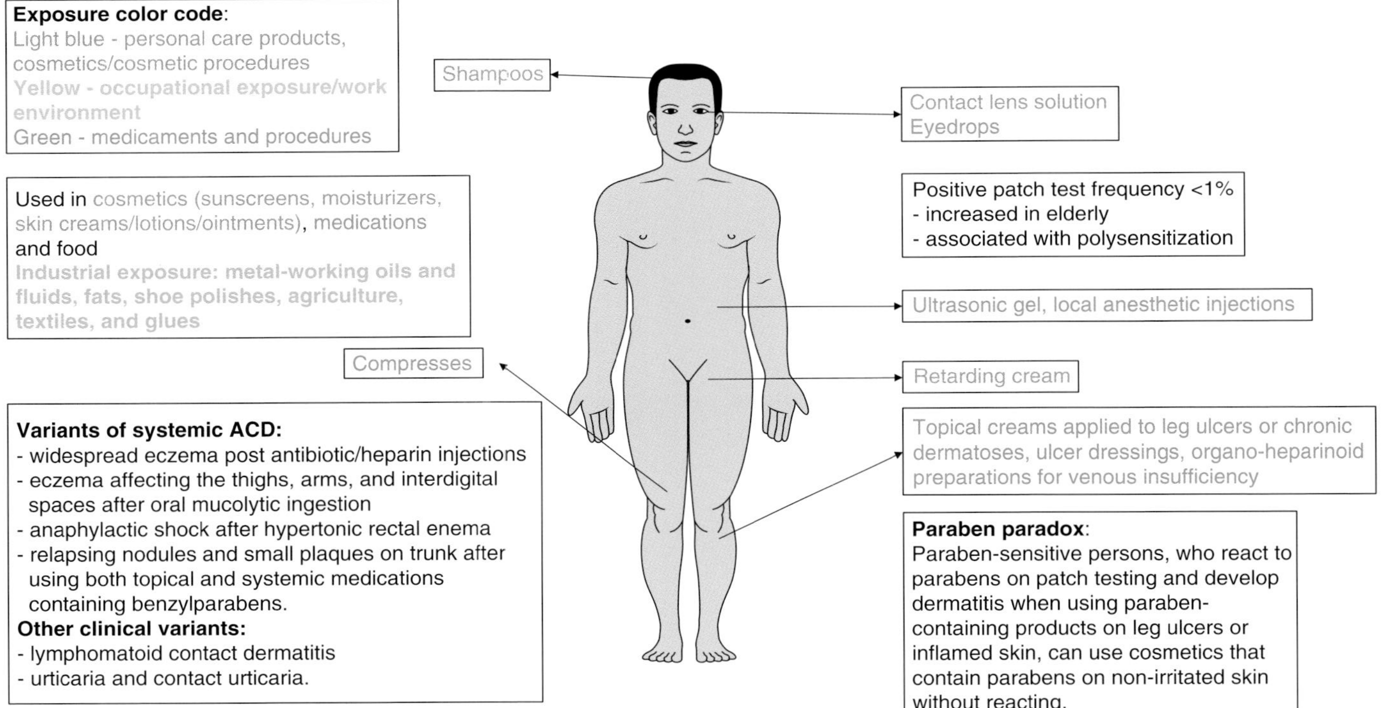

Exposure color code:
Light blue - personal care products, cosmetics/cosmetic procedures
Yellow - occupational exposure/work environment
Green - medicaments and procedures
Shampoos
Contact lens solution
Eyedrops
Used in cosmetics (sunscreens, moisturizers, skin creams/lotions/ointments), medications and food
Industrial exposure: metal-working oils and fluids, fats, shoe polishes, agriculture, textiles, and glues
Positive patch test frequency <1%
- increased in elderly
- associated with polysensitization
Ultrasonic gel, local anesthetic injections
Compresses
Retarding cream
Variants of systemic ACD:
- widespread eczema post antibiotic/heparin injections
- eczema affecting the thighs, arms, and interdigital spaces after oral mucolytic ingestion
- anaphylactic shock after hypertonic rectal enema
- relapsing nodules and small plaques on trunk after using both topical and systemic medications containing benzylparabens.
Other clinical variants:
- lymphomatoid contact dermatitis
- urticaria and contact urticaria.
Topical creams applied to leg ulcers or chronic dermatoses, ulcer dressings, organo-heparinoid preparations for venous insufficiency
Paraben paradox:
Paraben-sensitive persons, who react to parabens on patch testing and develop dermatitis when using paraben-containing products on leg ulcers or inflamed skin, can use cosmetics that contain parabens on non-irritated skin without reacting.

Figure 21.1 Reported clinical features and exposure sources for allergic contact dermatitis to parabens.

Non-cosmetic exposure and use

- In industry, parabens can be found in metal-working oils and fluids, fats, shoe polishes, agriculture, textiles, and glues.

Use in food

- Allergic reactions to orally ingested paraben-containing foods are rare. It is not usually necessary for paraben-sensitive patients to avoid these diets. Contact with foods preserved with parabens rarely causes hand eczema in cooks and food handlers [8]. The relevant E numbers are E209 and E214–219.

Patch testing

- Parabens are generally tested as a mix of 15% in petrolatum (3% each of methyl, ethyl, propyl, butyl and benzyl-parahydroxybenzoate). Paraben mix is routinely present in all baseline series. The patch test paraben mix is near irritation threshold. Weak reactions should be interpreted carefully. If there is a ?+ reaction at the first reading, then it is suggested that the individual parabens are then tested for reading on the final day.
- Patch testing to a steroid cream with low paraben concentrations may give a false-negative reaction. Interestingly, parabens have high positivity in "angry backs"/excited skin; 9/39 "angry backs" had a positive patch test reaction to paraben mix, but only three of these were positive on retesting [9].
- Cross-reactions exist between the paraben esters [7]. Other reported potential cross-reactions are with benzocaine, para-aminobenzoic acid (PABA) esters, paraphenylenediamine, and sulfonamide (but not commonly observed) [8].

Frequency of sensitization

As with many contact allergens, the frequency varies quite widely, but is typically in the range of 0.2–2.0%. Except where data derive from selected patient studies, higher rates should be interpreted with caution. Interestingly, the ratio of allergy prevalence in the general population and patch test clinics has been calculated to be equivalent [7, 10].

Age

- Paraben mix is an allergen that showed an increased sensitization rate in elderly patients compared with adult patients [11]. Onder and Oztas found that 4% of patients older than 56 years gave positive patch test reactions to paraben mix [12]. Paraben allergy has been described in a baby [13].
- A Danish study showed age-related differences in prevalence (0–18 years 0.3%, 19–40 years 0.3%, 41–60 years 0.5%, >60 years 0.9%; p trend 0.001) [14].

Sex

From most of the epidemiology reports, paraben contact allergy is most common in men.

Clinical and occupational disease (Figure 21.1)

- Paraben hypersensitivity is uncommon despite its widespread use. It appears that repeated applications of relatively low concentrations of parabens in medications and cosmetics may lead to sensitivity. At the usual concentrations of 0.1–0.3% in cosmetics, parabens rarely cause adverse reactions.
- Most cases of paraben contact allergy are caused by continual contact with *topical creams applied to leg ulcers or chronic dermatoses* [15]. Patients can present with worsening of an existing rash or failure to respond to treatment [16]. Paraben allergy should be suspected in any patients with recalcitrant dermatitis which has not responded to treatment [17]. A study from Onder et al. showed that 2 of 40 patients diagnosed with *chronic otitis externa* with recalcitrant ear itching had positive patch tests to parabens [18].
- Angelini et al. report a prevalence of 2.4% for paraben allergy in patients with foot dermatitis [19].
- *Systemic allergic contact dermatitis* has been seen in a patient who had been sensitized to parabens from topical medicaments for her leg ulcer. She had a widespread eczematous eruption after an intramuscular injection of paraben-containing ampicillin [20].
- Contact allergy to parabens is significantly *associated with polysensitization* (contact allergy to three or more unrelated allergens) [21].
- Foti et al. report a case of severe *genital dermatitis* after the use of a retarding cream for men during sexual intercourse. The patient was allergic to the parabens contained within the cream [22].
- Sánchez-Pérez et al. report a 72-year-old man with a history of rashes affecting the interdigital spaces, thighs, and arms, which were related to the oral ingestion of a mucolytic. Patch testing to the ingredient methylparaben 3% pet. was positive at day 2 and day 4. Oral administration of 200 mg of methylparaben activated the patient's inflammatory truncal plaques and reactivated the patch test site [23].
- Sato et al. describe "heparin" allergy in a 24-year-old woman undergoing chronic dialysis therapy. She presented with an acute widespread rash after an intracatheter injection of heparin. Both parabens and benzocaine showed a + leukocyte migration inhibition test. Patch testing was not employed [24]. Kajimoto et al., by observing a significant increase in *in vivo* reactions to prilocaine in the presence of methylparabens, postulated that the frequency of anaphylactoid reactions was related to the presence of methylparabens [25].
- A 9-year-old child presented with life-threatening anaphylactic shock after hypertonic rectal enema administration. Methylparaben/sodium methylparaben were suspected to be the causative allergens [26].

- Hirudoid® cream is an organoheparinoid preparation widely used in Portugal in the 1980s for chronic venous insufficiency. Pecegueiro et al. report a series of 31 cases with allergic contact dermatitis to this cream. 6/31 had a positive patch test to methylparaben [27].
- Fisher describes a single case report of allergic contact dermatitis to parabens in contact lens solution [28].
- A 62-year-old man had been using *eyedrops* containing methyl and propylparabens for 1 year. Over the previous month, he had developed conjunctivitis and eyelid dermatitis. On patch testing, he had ++ reactions to the eyedrops (Clarvisan®), methylparaben, and propylparaben [29]. *(Note: Parabens at present are only occasionally used as a preservative in eyedrops.)*
- A 62-year-old man developed localized dermatitis 24 hours after the application of an *ultrasonic gel* to his right leg. He had a history of stasis dermatitis and intolerance to some cosmetics. On patch testing, there were positive reactions to the gel and paraben mix. The gel contained methylparaben and propylparaben (both <3%) [30].
- There is a single case report of paraben allergic contact dermatitis from a tar *shampoo* [31].
- There are two separate case reports of paraben allergic contact dermatitis from *child's clay* [32, 33].
- Fine and Dingman report a single case of severe allergic contact dermatitis from methylparabens contained within a *local anesthetic* involving the abdomen and thighs, following suction-assisted lipectomy of these areas [34].
- Tosti et al. report a single case of a 43-year old woman who presented with a 3-year history of *relapsing nodules and small plaques* on her trunk. Skin biopsy showed a superficial and deep perivascular lymphohistiocytic infiltrate in the dermis with no spongiosis, suggestive of Jessner's benign lymphohistiocytic infiltrate. Patch testing revealed a ++ reaction to benzylparaben at 72 hours. Just before the aggravation of her condition, she had been using topical and systemic drugs containing benzylparabens. Avoiding further contact with the preservative led to full resolution within a few weeks. They postulate that this case supports "Epstein's concept," that a deeply located allergen may cause a "dermal" type of allergic contact dermatitis [35, 36].
- A different case of dermatitis from systemic allergy to parabens was reported by Carradori et al. [20]. A 65-year-old woman presented with a *generalized eczematous eruption after administration of an intramuscular injection* of ampicillin. The patient had suffered from leg ulcers for 2 years. Patch testing revealed positive reactions to both methyl and ethylparabens. They were both contained within the systemic ampicillin preparation.
- *Lymphomatoid contact dermatitis* caused by methylchloroisot hiazolinone/methylisothiazolinone (MCI/MI) and paraben mix has been reported [37].
- *Urticaria and contact urticaria* have occasionally been reported [38].

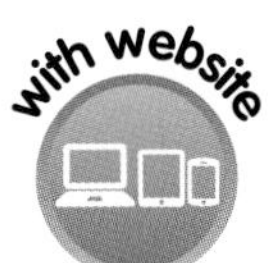

Go to www.wiley.com/go/mcfadden/common_contact_allergens to find the E-supplement for this chapter:

Parabens: E-Supplement

References

1 Fransway, A.F. (1991). The problems of preservation in the 1990s. II. Agents with preservative function independent of formaldehyde release. *American Journal of Contact Dermatitis* 2: 145–174.

2 Soni, M.G., Burdock, G.A., Taylor, S.L., and Greenberg, N.A. (2001). Safety assessment of propyl paraben: a review of the published literature. *Food and Chemical Toxicology* 39 (6): 513–532.

3 Rastogi, S.C., Schouten, A., de Kruijf, N., and Weijland, J.W. (1995). Contents of methyl-, ethyl-, propyl-, butyl- and benzylparaben in cosmetic products. *Contact Dermatitis* 32 (1): 28–30.

4 Gruvberger, B., Bruze, M., and Tammela, M. (1998). Preservatives in moisturizers on the Swedish market. *Acta Dermato-Venereologica* 78 (1): 52–56.

5 Zirwas, M.J. and Stechschulte, S.A. (2008). Moisturizer allergy: diagnosis and management. *Journal of Clinical and Aesthetic Dermatology* 1 (4): 38–44.

6 Praditsuwan, P., Taylor, J.S., and Roenigk, H.H. Jr. (1995). Allergy to Unna boots in four patients. *Journal of the American Academy of Dermatology* 33 (5 Pt 2): 906–908.

7 Mowad, C.M. (2000). Allergic contact dermatitis caused by parabens: 2 case reports and a review. *American Journal of Contact Dermatitis* 11 (1): 53–56.

8 Sasseville, D. (2004). Hypersensitivity to preservatives. *Dermatologic Therapy* 17 (3): 251–263.

9 Duarte, I., Lazzarini, R., and Bedrikow, R. (2002). Excited skin syndrome: study of 39 patients. *American Journal of Contact Dermatitis* 13 (2): 59–65.

10 Mirshahpanah, P. and Maibach, H.I. (2007). Relationship of patch test positivity in a general versus an eczema population. *Contact Dermatitis* 56 (3): 125–130.

11 Balato, A., Balato, N., Di Costanzo, L., and Ayala, F. (2011). Contact sensitization in the elderly. *Clinics in Dermatology* 29 (1): 24–30.

12 Onder, M. and Oztas, M.O. (2003). Contact dermatitis in the elderly. *Contact Dermatitis* 48 (4): 232–233.

13 Nardelli, A., Morren, M.A., and Goossens, A. (2009). Contact allergy to fragrances and parabens in an atopic baby. *Contact Dermatitis* 60 (2): 107–109.

14 Thyssen, J.P., Engkilde, K., Lundov, M.D. et al. (2010). Temporal trends of preservative allergy in Denmark (1985–2008). *Contact Dermatitis* 62 (2): 102–108.

15 Fisher, A.A. (1993). The parabens: paradoxical preservatives. *Cutis* 51 (6): 405–406.

16 Evans, S. (1970). Epidermal sensitivity to "lanolin" and "parabens": occurrence in pharmaceutical and cosmetic products. *British Journal of Dermatology* 82 (6): 625.

17 Schorr, W.F. (1968). Paraben allergy. A cause of intractable dermatitis. *Journal of the American Medical Association* 204 (10): 859–862.

18 Onder, M., Onder, T., Ozünlü, A. et al. (1994). An investigation of contact dermatitis in patients with chronic otitis externa. *Contact Dermatitis* 31 (2): 116–117.

19 Angelini, G., Vena, G.A., and Meneghini, C.L. (1980). Shoe contact dermatitis. *Contact Dermatitis* 6 (4): 279–283.

20 Carradori, S., Peluso, A.M., and Faccioli, M. (1990). Systemic contact dermatitis due to parabens. *Contact Dermatitis* 22 (4): 238–239.

21 Carlsen, B.C., Menné, T., and Johansen, J.D. (2008). Associations between baseline allergens and polysensitization. *Contact Dermatitis* 59 (2): 96–102.

22 Foti, C., Bonamonte, D., Antelmi, A. et al. (2004). Allergic contact dermatitis to condoms: description of a clinical case and analytical review of current literature. *Immunopharmacology and Immunotoxicology* 26 (3): 481–485.

23 Sánchez-Pérez, J., Diez, M.B., Pérez, A.A. et al. (2006). Allergic and systemic contact dermatitis to methylparaben. *Contact Dermatitis* 54 (2): 117–118.

24 Sato, K., Kazama, J.J., Wada, Y. et al. (2002). Hypersensitivity to paraoxybenzoic acid esters (parabens) in a dialysis patient. *Nephron* 92 (3): 728–729.

25 Kajimoto, Y., Rosenberg, M.E., Kytta, J. et al. (1995). Anaphylactoid skin reactions after intravenous regional anaesthesia using 0.5% prilocaine with or without preservative – a double-blind study. *Acta Anaesthesiologica Scandinavica* 39 (6): 782–784.

26 Raulin-Gaignard, H., Berlengi, N., Gatin, A. et al. (2013). Severe allergic reaction due to a rectal enema. *Archives de Pediatrie: Organe Officiel de la Societe Francaise de Pediatrie* 20 (12): 1329–1332.

27 Pecegueiro, M., Brandão, M., Pinto, J., and Conçalo, S. (1987). Contact dermatitis to Hirudoid cream. *Contact Dermatitis* 17 (5): 290–293.

28 Fisher, A. (1985). Allergic reactions to contact lens solutions. *Cutis* 36 (3): 209–211.

29 Vilaplana, J. and Romaguera, C. (2000). Contact dermatitis from parabens used as preservatives in eyedrops. *Contact Dermatitis* 43 (4): 248.

30 Eguino, P., Sánchez, A., Agesta, N. et al. (2003). Allergic contact dermatitis due to propylene glycol and parabens in an ultrasonic gel. *Contact Dermatitis* 48 (5): 290.

31 Cooper, S.M. and Shaw, S. (1998). Allergic contact dermatitis from parabens in a tar shampoo. *Contact Dermatitis* 39 (3): 140.

32 Downs, A.M., Sansom, J.E., and Simmons, I. (1998). Let Rip! Fun Pot dermatitis. *Contact Dermatitis.* 38 (4): 234.

33 Verhaeghe, I. and Dooms-Goossens, A. (1997). Multiple sources of allergic contact dermatitis from parabens. *Contact Dermatitis* 36 (5): 269–270.

34 Fine, P.G. and Dingman, D.L. (1988). Hypersensitivity dermatitis following suction-assisted lipectomy: a complication of local anesthetic. *Annals of Plastic Surgery* 20 (6): 573–575.

35 Tosti, A., Fanti, P.A., and Pileri, S. (1989). Dermal contact dermatitis from benzylparaben. *Contact Dermatitis* 21 (1): 49–51.

36 Epstein, S. (1956). Contact dermatitis due to nickel and chromate; observations on dermal delayed (tuberculin-type) sensitivity. *AMA Archives of Dermatology* 73 (3): 236–255.

37 Knackstedt, T.J. and Zug, K.A. (2015). T cell lymphomatoid contact dermatitis: a challenging case and review of the literature. *Contact Dermatitis* 72 (2): 65–74.

38 Henry, J.C., Tschen, E.H., and Becker, L.E. (1979). Contact urticaria to parabens. *Archives of Dermatology* 115 (10): 1231–1232.

Exposure Color Code

- Clothing, jewelry, adornments
- Personal care products, cosmetics/cosmetic procedures
- Household products, domestic environment, including furniture and refurbishment
- Occupational dermatoses, work environment
- Medicines, surgical/dental procedures, herbal/alternative medicines
- Personal appliances/aids
- Leisure activities, sport, travel
- Other exposures (including dietary)
- Not relevant or multiple/general exposure

CHAPTER 22
para-Phenylenediamine

CHAPTER CONTENTS

Allergen profile

A profile of allergic contact dermatitis (ACD) to *para*-phenylenediamine (*p*-phenylenediamine, PPD) from case literature and clinical experience.

a. Examples of potential exposure from aspects of daily life
- Personal care products – hair dye
- Occupational – hairdressers
- Travel – temporary "black henna" beach tattoo
- Clothes – shoes (rare)

Note: May cross-react with disperse dyes (clothing), black rubber (occupational, travel, leisure, home), and caines (medicaments).

b. Routes of potential exposure
- Direct exposure
- By proxy

c. Various known clinical manifestations of contact allergy to PPD

Major forms of presentation
- Direct contact
- Exacerbation of endogenous eczema
- By proxy contact dermatitis
- Mimicking angioedema

Minor forms of presentation
- Non-eczematous forms of contact dermatitis

Lichenoid
Pigmented
Depigmented
Pseudolymphomatoid
Purpuric
Erythema multiforme-like
Neutrophilic and eosinophilic dermatoses
- Contact urticaria
- Other reported forms of presentation

Primary sensitization (henna beach tattoo)
Bullous
Prurigo nodularis-like
Lichen simplex chronicus

Reported cross-reactions
- Other aromatic amine hair dyes, e.g. toluenediamine
- Azo/disperse dyes
- Black rubber
- Benzocaine
- Some epoxy hardeners

Common Contact Allergens: A Practical Guide to Detecting Contact Dermatitis, First Edition. Edited by John McFadden, Pailin Puangpet, Korbkarn Pongpairoj, Supitchaya Thaiwat, and Lee Shan Xian.
© 2020 John Wiley & Sons Ltd. Published 2020 by John Wiley & Sons Ltd.
Companion website: www.wiley.com/go/mcfadden/common_contact_allergens

Key points

- *Aromatic amine use dominates the hair dye industry*. PPD is, like other commonly used hair dye agents, a member of the aromatic amine family. The hair dye process involves oxidation and polymerization. However, the oxidation process is also involved in the allergenicity of the chemicals. PPD is classified as an extreme sensitizer.
- *Hair dyeing is a standard cosmetic practice*. In Europe, it is estimated that 75% of adult women and 18% of adult men dye their hair. Hair dye use often starts in the teenage years.
- *ACD to PPD is more common in females*. The female-to-male ratio is 2 : 1 except in communities where males commonly dye their facial hair, where the ratio trends toward a male majority.
- *The prevalence of ACD to PPD in adults increases with age*, as with allergy to other cosmetic agents.
- *Hair dye allergy is common in both dermatitis patients and the general adult population*. The most comprehensive literature review of PPD sensitization amongst dermatitis patients found a median prevalence of 4.3% in Asia, 4% in Europe, and 6.2% in America. Amongst the normal adult population, a prevalence of 1% in Europe and 2.7% in Asia has been reported.
- *ACD to hair dye often involves inflammation and swelling of the areas of skin around the scalp, such as the forehead, neck, and ears*. Periorbital involvement can also commonly occur. The scalp is often less inflamed, presumably because the scalp hairs absorb a significant amount of chemical, reducing the dose delivered locally.
- *First hair dye allergic reactions often occur after a change in "dose"*. Sensitization to PPD, as with other cosmetic allergens, is usually "silent" initially. The first episode of ACD (elicitation) to PPD often occurs after a change in the patient's hair dyeing habits, such as change to a darker shade, time hair dye is left on, and frequency of application, i.e. a change in dose applied. In some cases, the periorbital area can be involved.
- *Mistaken for angioedema*. ACD to PPD can be severe and mistreated as angioedema. Acute severe cases should be treated with oral as well as topical steroids.
- *Hair dye allergy is a great "mimicker" of dermatological diseases*. There are a wide variety of *alternative* ways in which ACD to hair dye can occur. These include lichenoid reactions, pruritus, bullous dermatitis, hyperpigmentation, hypopigmentation, depigmentation/vitiligoid achromia, erythema multiforme-like reactions, pseudolymphomatoid reactions, neutrophilic dermatitis, nummular dermatitis, prurigo nodularis, lichen simplex, dermatitis-by-proxy, and facial dermatitis from beard/mustache/eyebrow/eyelash dyeing. Erythema multiforme-like reactions can occur both locally and distally (e.g. arms).
- *Contact urticaria to PPD is rare but can occasionally present as an acute medical emergency*.
- *Henna tattoos*. Sensitization through exposure to a temporary "henna" beach tattoo usually presents in young children/adults with a severe sensitization reaction occurring 10–24 days after application. The tattoo agents are usually impregnated with high doses of PPD or other aromatic agents.
- *A common occupational disease*. ACD to PPD is a common disease in hairdressers and beauticians, and commonly presents with hand dermatitis.
- *PPD is an effective screening test for hair dye allergy*. Patch testing to PPD is the usual screening test for hair dye allergy employed in most patch test standard screens. Although it acts as a relatively effective screen, one out of every six patients allergic to the second most commonly used hair dye chemical, *p*-toluenediamine, will not react to PPD.
- *Reduce PPD patch test concentrations for patients who have had clinically severe allergic reactions*. Patients with a history of severe ACD to PPD or who have a history of a henna tattoo reaction should be tested at a reduced concentration of PPD (0.1% for severe hair dye reactions, 0.01% for henna tattoo reactions). If this patch test is negative, the patch test concentrations applied may then be increased by gradation.
- Patch test reactions to PPD can occasionally become positive on day 7 or later. *Active sensitization to PPD* through patch testing may occasionally occur.
- *Cross-reactions to clothing (azo) dyes* as identified by patch testing are common, being observed in 80% of patients with strong patch test reactions (++, +++) to PPD. However, only a minority of PPD allergic patients will experience clothing dye reactions clinically.
- *Cross-reactions to benzocaine and* IPPD (isopropyl-*N*′-phenyl-*p*-phenylenediamine) are also observed, but at a much lower rate.
- *Many patients diagnosed with ACD to PPD will continue to attempt to dye their hair*. Patients who are strongly sensitized (patch test +++) almost always have to cease dyeing their hair.

Epidemiology

Frequency of sensitization

In 2008, Thyssen et al. reported that the median prevalence of PPD sensitization among dermatitis patients was 4.3% in Asia, 4% in Europe, and 6.2% in North America [1].

Age

- A study to evaluate the association between age and PPD sensitization found that allergy was significantly higher in the 46–55-year-old age group in both sexes [2].
- Almeida et al. found a clinical correlation between patients' age and the origin of sensitization to PPD. The source of sensitization in older age groups is hair dyes, whereas the source of exposure in children is often henna tattoos [3].
- The prevalence of positive patch test reactions to PPD in children aged 14 years or younger was 2.36%, which was lower than other age groups. A study in children aged 1–14 years old showed a strikingly higher proportion of +++ patch test reactions to PPD (43% of all positive PPD reactions) compared to other age groups. No difference was observed with respect to other contact allergens. The main suspected exposures associated with extreme reactions to PPD in children were hair dyes and henna tattoos. Extremely strong positive patch test reactions to PPD were associated with head and neck dermatitis, exposure to hair dyes or tattoos, and dermatitis of the arms [4]. Subjects sensitized through henna tattoos may go on to develop severe reactions when they start dyeing their hair.

Sex

- Studies on the prevalence of PPD sensitization between women and men showed conflicting results. There were some reports of PPD sensitization being more common in women than men (1.3–1.8 : 1) [2, 5, 6]. In contrast, some studies found a higher prevalence in men than women (1.6–2.2 : 1) [7, 8].

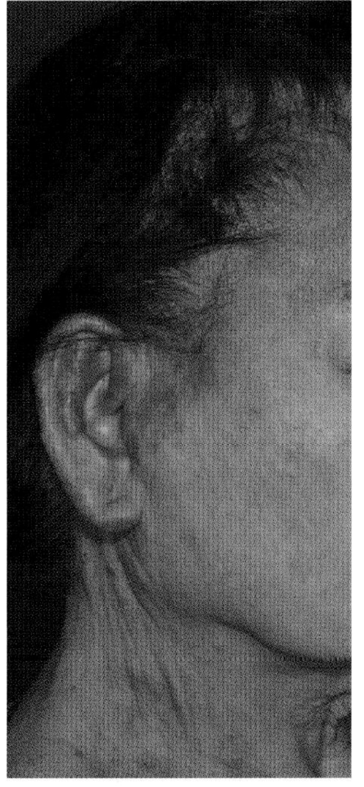

Figure 22.1 ACD to PPD/hair dye most prominently affecting the skin surrounding the scalp.

ACD to PPD/hair dye; the skin surrounding the scalp (forehead, neck, ears, temple) is usually more severely affected than the scalp. The periorbital area can also be affected.

- Several studies of patch test populations from Asian and Middle Eastern centers found the sex ratio reversed with males in the majority. This could be explained by both an increased use of hair dye and dyeing of facial hair amongst males.

Clinical (including case reports)

In one large survey, hair dyes were the commonest allergens associated with dermatitis of the scalp and surrounding skin (Figure 22.1) [9]. A separate study from India to evaluate patients with suspected facial contact dermatitis from cosmetic products indicated that PPD was the most common positive patch test allergen [10].

Hair dye reactions

The dermatitis caused by PPD in hair dyes usually extends beyond the scalp to the forehead, around the hairline, neck, eyelids, and face. The dermatitis is usually more severe on the skin margin surrounding the scalp rather than the scalp skin itself as scalp hair absorbs much of the allergen (Figure 22.1). The duration of both clinical and patch test reactions may last several weeks due to the persistence of the allergen in the skin [11].

Mustache, beard, and sideburn allergic reactions

- Individuals who dye their mustache and/or sideburns usually dye their facial hair every week. As a result, they tend to be more readily sensitized by PPD because of a much larger cumulative dose [12]. Beard dermatitis from PPD allergy may present with pruritic erythematous papules [13] and prurigo nodularis-like eruptions [14]. Distant sites may be involved [15].

Allergic contact dermatitis due to eyelash and eyebrow coloring

- The clinical presentations of allergic reactions following eyelash or eyebrow dyeing include severe blepharoconjunctivitis [16–18], centrofacial edema [16], eyelid edema [19], loss of eyelashes [20], and xanthelasma palpebrarum [21]. Periorbital eczema may also be present [22]. The usual agent involved is 2-chloro-PPD, but patch testing with PPD is usually positive [23]. ACD from *p*-toluenediamine in a cream dye for eyelashes and eyebrows has also been reported [24].

Diverse variety of clinical presentations

PPD allergy may present in a large variety of ways other than dermatitis. Indeed, the clinical presentation of PPD allergy is more varied than for most other common contact allergens. Presentations include:

- *Immediate-type reactions: contact urticaria syndrome [25, 26], contact anaphylaxis [27]*

  This is an uncommon clinical picture of PPD allergy. The patient may present with sneezing, conjunctivitis, runny nose, dry cough, dyspnea, facial swelling, and generalized urticaria. The clinical signs and symptoms appear immediately, mostly within 5–20 minutes, after contact with the causative agent. The diagnosis is confirmed by skin-prick testing with PPD solutions.
- *Pruritus, erythema*

  A 35-year-old man presented with redness, vesicles, and weeping on a temporary holiday tattoo which was applied 2 weeks before onset of the rash. Around the pruritic tattoo there was an erythematous maculopapular rash. There was no previous history of hair dye exposure. Patch testing showed a ++ positive reaction to PPD [28].

- *Vesicles and bullous dermatitis*
  A 33-year-old woman developed sharply demarcated erythematous, itchy, and papulovesicular swellings distributed at the sites of her "black henna tattoos" after she took part in a "mehndi" ritual on her friend's wedding day [29]. Another case was a 20-year-old lady who presented with hand swelling and painful vesicles and bullae along her black henna tattoo sites. The eruption appeared 24 hours after application. Patch testing showed a positive reaction to PPD [30].
- *Hyperpigmentation*
  Two sisters developed long-lasting hyperpigmentation 10 days after receiving temporary "henna" tattoos. Patch testing showed positive reactions to PPD in both patients. One girl also had positive results to IPPD/black rubber, toluenediamine, nitro-phenylenediamine, Direct Orange 34, and disperse dyes, including Blue 124/106 mix, Orange 1, Red 1, and Yellow 3, in keeping with a high degree of cross-reactivity to azo dyes in patients highly sensitized to PPD [31].
- *Long-lasting hypopigmentation*
  There are reports of long-lasting hypopigmentation after PPD exposure. Lesions were reported to persist for more than 6–12 months [32–35]. This is in contrast to prolonged hyperpigmentation, which has also been noted [36].
- *Depigmentation: chemical leukoderma, vitiligoid achromia, and some patients with a diagnosis of vitiligo*
  PPD can cause skin depigmentation and graying of the hair. PPD has a chemical structure similar to tyrosine and its metabolite compounds can be toxic to melanocytes [37]. A 16-year-old female developed depigmentation (which the authors termed "vitiligoid achromia") 5 days after temporary tattooing with PPD-containing hair dye; the achromia appeared only in the tattoo areas, including the eyebrows, glabella, left hand, and both feet. Some eyebrow hairs then developed depigmentation [38]. Another two cases of contact vitiligo were also reported. The depigmentation developed a few weeks after exposure to PPD in tattoos. The lesions had persisted for more than 2 years at the time of reporting [39].

  A Korean study in 125 patients with vitiligo in specific locations, onset in the elderly, and/or previous inflammation or itch showed that 78.4% of the patients had positive patch test reactions to at least one contact allergen. In addition, there was a significant association between lesions located on the scalp and/or hairline and patch test reactivity to PPD ($p = 0.002$, odds ratio = 3.06). A positive correlation between allergen avoidance and improvement of vitiligo was also demonstrated ($p = 0.03$) [40].
- *Lichenoid reactions*
  There are several case series and reports of lichenoid contact dermatitis from PPD allergy. All cases developed reactions within 2 weeks of PPD exposure [41–43].
- *Erythema multiforme-like eruption*
  There are several reports of both generalized and localized erythema multiforme-like eruptions occurring in patients with PPD allergy. The sources of PPD exposure in these cases were "henna" tattoos, rubber products and hair dyes [33, 44–50]. Erythema multiforme-like reactions can occur locally, around the scalp, or distally.

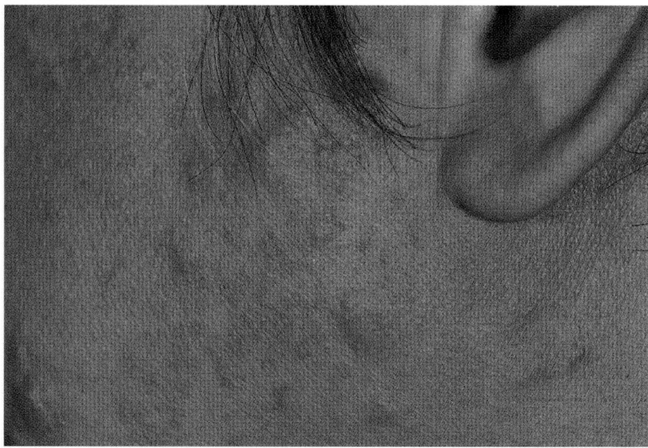

Figure 22.2 ACD to PPD presenting as pseudolymphoma of the head and neck. Other non-eczematous manifestations of ACD to PPD include erythema multiforme, lichenoid, pigmented and hypopigmented dermatosis, urticaria, neutrophilic and eosinophilic dermatoses, and pururitic dermatoses.

- *Pseudolymphomatoid reaction [51] (Figure 22.2)*
  A 4-year-old girl developed dermatitis and an erythema multiforme-like eruption on her face and hands. Her earlobes showed a pseudolymphoma-like morphology. The patient had a recent history of having a "henna" tattoo. Patch testing showed a +++ positive reaction to 0.05% PPD after 24 hours. There was also a positive reaction to azo dyes [48]. Another case was a 37-year-old man who presented with consort contact dermatitis to PPD in his partner's hair dye. The rash usually flared up when his partner dyed her hair. The patient initially had an itchy facial rash for 3 months. He then developed widespread erythematous tumid papules and plaques on his cheeks, upper limbs, and body. Skin biopsy was consistent with a pseudolymphomatoid dermatitis. Patch testing indicated a positive reaction to PPD [52].
- *Angioedema-like/pseudoangioedema (but delayed type hypersensitivity reaction) (Figure 22.3)*
  A 22-year-old woman presented with an angioedema-like reaction 2 days after she dyed her hair for the first time. Testing with the European standard series showed a positive reaction to PPD. The patient had a black henna tattoo 2 years ago [53]. A 34-year-old woman presented with edema and erythema of her forehead, both cheeks, and periorbital areas 2 days after she dyed her eyelashes. Severe and persistent blepharoconjunctivitis was also evident. Patch testing showed a ++ positive reaction to 0.5% PPD in pet. at day 1 [16]. A 33-year-old pregnant woman presented with severe facial swelling 3 days after using hair dye. Patch testing showed +++ positive reactions to PPD and 4-toluenediamine, and +++ positive reactions to 4-aminophenol and 3-aminophenol [54]. A Danish study in 55 cases of severe acute ACD to PPD found that most patients presenting to the emergency department were wrongly treated as angioedema [55].

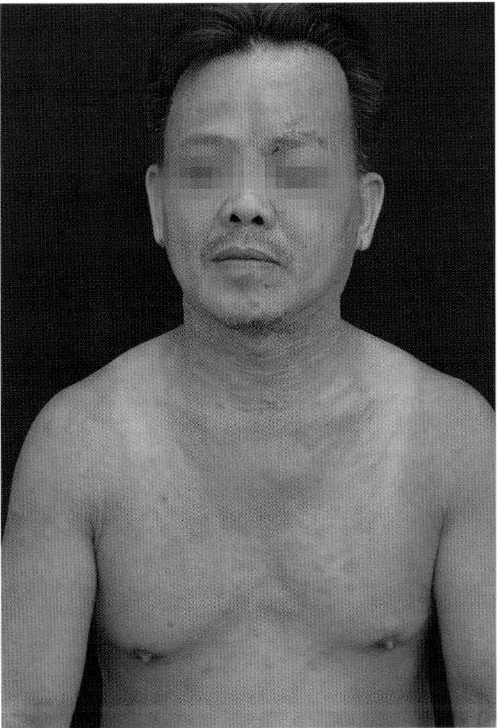

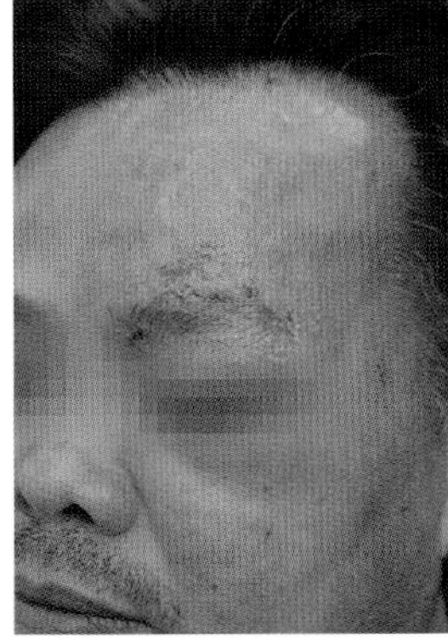

Severe ACD to PPD In hair dye can result in both facial swelling and secondary spread of dermatitis to other body areas.

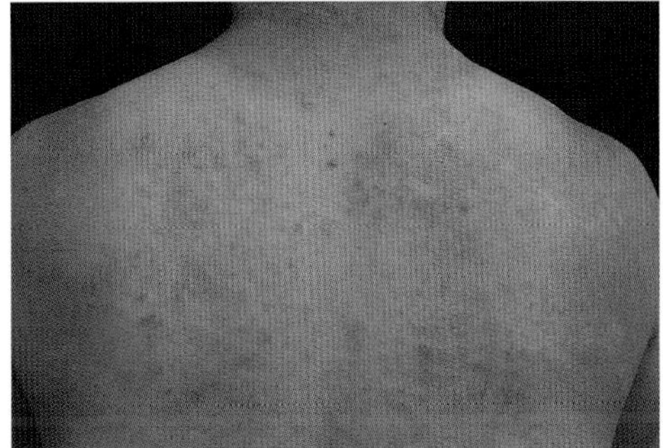

Figure 22.3 "Pseudoangioedema" from severe ACD to PPD.

- *Neutrophilic and eosinophilic dermatitis*

A 58-year-old woman presented with nummular erythematous excoriated plaques with crusts on her neck, upper chest and scalp. There were a few lesions on her arms and right ankle. The lesions then spread to the anogenital areas. She also had an episode of unexplained dyspnea. Skin biopsy revealed neutrophilic and eosinophilic infiltrates with marked dermal edema. Spongiosis was variable. Direct immunofluorescence microscopy showed negative results. Patch testing showed reactions to several allergens, including a +++ positive reaction to PPD and a positive reaction to Disperse Orange 3. The skin lesions recurred after she dyed her hair again [56]. Recently, the first pediatric case of eosinophilic cellulitis (Wells' syndrome) after having a temporary henna tattoo was reported. A 9-year-old boy presented with erythematous edematous papulonodules on the tattoo areas, and on his trunk and extremities. His absolute eosinophil count was 600/mm^3. Skin biopsy from the tattoo site revealed flame figures in the dermis. Patch testing indicated +++ positive reactions to PPD and black rubber mix at 48, 72, and 96 hours [57].

- *Chronic eczema: prurigo nodularis-like lesions and lichen simplex chronicus*

A 40-year-old man was initially diagnosed with perioral dermatitis. Three months later, he presented with symmetrical, discrete, eroded papulonodules with crusting and lichenification over his lower face. The only topical that he regularly used to this area was hair dye for his mustache. Patch testing revealed ++ positive reactions to PPD (at 72 hours and 7 days), as well as to his hair dye. The lesions resolved completely without any recurrence after he stopped using the dye [14].

A 62-year-old woman presented with lichen simplex chronicus that was aggravated by hair dyeing. Patch testing indicated weakly positive reactions to both PPD and her own hair dye. The lesions improved without recurrence after she stopped dyeing her hair [58].

A prospective and retrospective study to evaluate the association between lichen simplex chronicus and hair dye use demonstrated clinical relevance in 45.5% and 28.6%, respectively [58].

- *Hypertrophic scars and keloids.*

A 22-year-old man developed hypertrophic scars 2 weeks after beach "henna" tattooing. Patch testing showed a positive result to PPD [59]. Another case was a 16-year-old girl who presented with extensive keloids 5 days after getting tattoos. Patch tests were not performed in this patient [60].

- *Hair loss*

There have been a few case reports of PPD-allergic patients presenting with alopecia. A 41-year-old woman presented with severe alopecia after using PPD-containing hair dye. Hair loss began at day 6 after dyeing her hair and spread to 90% of the scalp within 4 months. Patch testing showed a ++ positive reaction to PPD at 48 and 72 hours [61]. A case of eyelash loss after using PPD-containing mascara was also reported [20].

- *Increased hair growth*

There was a case report of a woman whose hair growth increased after beach "henna" tattoo exposure. However, patch testing was not performed in this patient [62].

- *Xanthelasma palpebrarum*

A 38-year-old woman presented with an allergic reaction 1 day after she dyed her eyelashes. Xanthelasma appeared

6 weeks later. Patch testing revealed positive reactions to PPD and IPPD [21].

- *By proxy*
  Connubial contact dermatitis from PPD in hair dye in patients who did not use hair dye, but their partners did, has been reported. The patients may present with a unilateral rash [63] or tumid plaques [52]. The existence of by-proxy ACD to PPD demonstrates that in common hair dye practice polymerization of PPD is not 100% complete and that allergic, unpolymerized hair dye chemicals can remain on the hair after the process.
- *Patients who are allergic to PPD will often continue to dye their hair*
  Patients who are allergic to PPD will often continue to dye their hair, even against medical advice. Ho et al. observed that 73% of patients with a + patch test reaction to PPD continue to dye their hair, 49% with ++ reactions also continue but all patients with a +++ reaction had to stop dyeing their hair [64].

Adverse reactions (non-allergic)

- *Local toxic effects* of PPD include skin irritation and edema [65].
- PPD has been used as a *systemic poison* [65].

Occupational use

- In one UK study, 13/37 hairdressers with dermatitis referred for patch testing were allergic to PPD, making it more common than other specific hair dye allergens and only less common than nickel allergy [66]. Information Network of Departments of Dermatology data between 2003 and 2006 showed PPD to be the third most common allergen amongst hairdressers, with 18.1% positive patch test reactions [67].
- Skin lesions in professional hairdressers are almost always localized to the hands. Lesions on the face, forearms, or knees are less frequent [2]. A study from Bangkok showed that the most common causative allergen in hairdressers with hand contact dermatitis was PPD (45.45%) [68]. A much rarer form of presentation of occupational allergic reactions to PPD is contact urticaria. Over an 11 year period, the Finnish Institute of Occupational Health recorded 11 cases of type 1 allergic reactions to PPD, confirmed by open and prick tests, in hairdressers presenting with occupational asthma, rhinitis, and/or contact urticaria [69].

Exposure

- *Hair dyes.* In Japan, market research demonstrates that there are more people dyeing their hair and doing so at a younger age. In 1992, a survey of young people in Tokyo reported that 13% of girls in high school, 6% of women, and 2% of men in their 20s reported using hair colorants [70]. By 2001, the proportions had increased to 41%, 85%, and 33%, respectively.
  In Denmark, 75% of women and 18% of men used hair dye. The median age for first use of hair dye was during their teenage years in both men and women [55].
- *"Henna" tattoos.* The prevalence of PPD allergy is rising in children. "Henna" tattoos and hair dyes appear to be important sources of exposure as more younger people are dyeing their hair for fashion [4, 71, 72]. Temporary "henna" tattoos are also becoming very popular among travelers going to Southeast Asia [28].
  Concentrations of PPD in temporary henna tattoos were measured to be as high as 15.7%, much higher than the maximum limited concentration in hair dyes [53, 73]. Prolonged exposure to such high concentrations on non-hair bearing skin would be predicted to result in the production of large amounts of auto-oxidized products and severe allergic reactions [74]. In a review from St John's, 2.5% of PPD allergic patients had a history of temporary black henna tattoos, though there may be a higher prevalence now [64].
- *Other sources.* Other historical sources of PPD and PPD-like agents included fur dyes, textile dyes, printer ink, photographic work, X-ray film, and lacquers.

Patch testing

1% PPD in petrolatum is included in the baseline series of patch tests to screen for contact allergy to PPD and related aromatic amine dyes [75].

In children and adults with a clear history of allergy to hair dyes or exposure to henna tattoos, initial testing at a lower concentration is recommended [4, 76].

- *Complications from patch testing to PPD*
  - Severe positive patch test reactions
    Severe positive patch test reactions are particularly seen in either patients who have been sensitized with high doses of PPD contained in black henna tattoos or those with a history of severe reactions to hair dye and then tested with the standard 1% petroleum PPD concentration [76]. The reactions can be very uncomfortable and painful. +++ reactions may take several days or weeks to resolve.
  - Active sensitization
    There was a report of active sensitization to PPD with a late irrelevant reaction at 15 days [77]. It has been thought that patch testing to 1% PPD carries a high risk of active sensitization [78]. However, one study showed no significant increase in PPD-positive patch test reactions when individuals received repeat patch tests [79]. These findings indicate that active sensitization from PPD patch testing may be an uncommon phenomenon. This is confirmed by the results of the Bangkok hair dye study, which found that only 1 in 600 may have been actively sensitized by patch testing. Late patch test reactions (i.e. after 7 days) may often have clinical relevance and may not necessarily be due to active sensitization [5]. It has been claimed that late elicitation patch test

reactions to PPD are more common than active sensitization reactions [80]. PPD could be excluded in testing patients with no previous exposure to PPD (but be careful not to miss 'by proxy' dermatitis).

Co-sensitization/cross-reactivity

- "Caine" mix contains the potentially cross-reacting agent benzocaine. Reactions to "caine" mix were found in 10% of PPD-allergic patients and increased linearly with the strength of a positive PPD patch test reaction, suggesting cross-sensitivity [64].
- Only 3% of individuals with PPD allergy reacted to *N*-isopropyl-*N*-phenyl-PPD (black rubber) and *p*-aminobenzoic acid (PABA sunscreens). No relationship with the strength of PPD reactivity was observed, suggesting a more complex relationship than simple immunological cross-reactivity [64].
- We found that the most common azo dye coexisting allergen in PPD-allergic patients was Disperse Orange 3 (46%) [81]. Moreover, we observed that patients who had stronger PPD patch test reactions (++, +++) were more likely to display reactivity to azo dyes (80%). Co-sensitization to PPD was present in two-thirds of individuals sensitized to Disperse Orange 3 [82]. Most of them had a clear history of hair dye allergy. The authors suggested that this may represent cross-reactivity and hair dyes would usually be the source of primary sensitization in these patients. However, Disperse Orange can be degraded to PPD and nitroaniline within the skin [83]. As a result, a simultaneous patch test reaction to Disperse Orange 3 may represent local production of PPD within the test site [81]. In clinical practice, most PPD allergic patients do not suffer from clothing dye reactions.
- PPD can cross-sensitize with *N*-isopropyl-*N*-phenyl-4-phenylenediamine, which is the main sensitizer in black rubber. A 10-year-old non-atopic boy presented with severe pruritic erythematous vesicles on his palms and flexural sides of his fingers for 2 years. The lesions started after a few weeks of intensive use of a new bicycle and cleared completely with topical corticosteroids within 10 days. The dyshidrosiform eruption recurred within 1–2 days each time he rode his bicycle. Patch testing showed a ++ positive reaction to *N*-isopropyl-*N*-phenyl-4-phenylenediamine on days 2 to 4 and questionable papular reactions to pieces of his bicycle's handgrip. As the patient had never had contact with any PPD-containing products, his + positive reaction to PPD was considered to be cross-sensitization [84].
- PPD may theoretically cross-react with other chemically related compounds, including parabens, sulfonamides [85], sulfonylureas, benzoic acids [28], dapsone, thiazide diuretics, mesalazine, *p*-aminosalicylic acid, *p*-amino hair dyes, anthraquinone [86], toluene-2,5-diamine, and aminophenol [87].
- There were two cases of possible cross-sensitivity in PPD allergic subjects after ingestion of the anti-histamine polaronil, which contains dexamethasone and dexchlorpheniramine [88].
- *Cross-reactivity to other permanent hair dyes*
Nowadays, there are many alternative hair dyes marketed as PPD-free products. However, these hair dyes can contain other aromatic amines such as toluene-2,5-diamine (PTD), 2,4-diamino-anisole, *m*-aminophenol, *o*-aminophenol, and/or *p*-aminophenol. These agents can cross-react with PPD dyes [89]. An *in vitro* study showed wide cross-reactivity (64.7%) amongst aromatic amines, including PPD, *p*-toluenediamine, Bandrowski's base, and *p*-aminoazobenzene [90]. In clinical studies, 93% of PPD allergic patients had reactions to at least two hair dye-related chemicals [91]. A clinical study to assess the benefits of additional patch testing with non-PPD hair dye allergens appeared to be of limited value [92]. The best way to avoid potentially severe hair dye reactions is to advise PPD-allergic patients to avoid all permanent and semi-permanent hair dyes [89].
- In 2009, a retrospective analysis of patch test results with hair dye allergens was performed, focusing on the extent to which patients who were positive for allergic reactions to other hair dye allergens also had a concomitant reaction to PPD. Patients who were patch test positive to *p*-toluenediamine also reacted to PPD in five out of six cases (40/48 *p*-toluenediamine patch test + patients also reacted to PPD on patch testing). However, for the other aromatic amines reviewed, there was a high degree of concordance with positive patch tests to PPD: 2-nitro-PPD 14/14, 3- aminophenol 9/9, and 4-aminophenol 12/13. Patch testing to PPD is, therefore, a relatively effective screening test for ACD to hair dye [92].

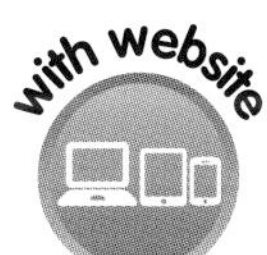

Go to www.wiley.com/go/mcfadden/common_contact_allergens to find the E-supplement for this chapter:
Para-Phenylenediamine: E-Supplement

References

1 Thyssen, J.P. and White, J.M. (2008). European Society of Contact D. Epidemiological data on consumer allergy to p-phenylenediamine. *Contact Dermatitis* 59 (6): 327–343.

2 Mqalvestio, A., Bovenzi, M., Hoteit, M. et al. (2010). p-Phenylenediamine sensitization and occupation. *Contact Dermatitis* 64: 37–42.

3 Almeida, P.J., Borrego, L., and Limiñana, J.M. (2011). Age-related sensitization to p-phenylenediamine. *Contact Dermatitis* 64 (3): 172–174.

4 Spornraft-Ragaller, P., Schnuch, A., and Uter, W. (2011). Extreme patch test reactivity to p-phenylenediamine but not to other allergens in children. *Contact Dermatitis* 65 (4): 220–226.

5 White, J.M., Gilmour, N.J., Jeffries, D. et al. (2007). A general population from Thailand: incidence of common allergens with emphasis on para-phenylenediamine. *Clinical and Experimental Allergy* 37 (12): 1848–1853.

6 Jenkins, D. and Chow, E.T. (2015). Allergic contact dermatitis to para-phenylenediamine. *Australasian Journal of Dermatology* 56 (1): 40–43.
7 Kiec-Swierczynska, M., Krecisz, B., and Swierczynska-Machura, D. (2007). Contact allergy to paraphenylenediamine; a 10-year observation held in the Nofer Institute of Occupational Medicine. *Lodz. Med Pr.* 58: 215–222.
8 Cheng, S., Cao, M., Zhang, Y. et al. (2011). Time trends of contact allergy to a modified European baseline series in Beijing between 2001 and 2006. *Contact Dermatitis* 65 (1): 22–27.
9 Hillen, U., Grabbe, S., and Uter, W. (2007). Patch test results in patients with scalp dermatitis: analysis of data of the Information Network of Departments of Dermatology. *Contact Dermatitis* 56 (2): 87–93.
10 Rastogi, M.K., Gupta, A., Soodan, P.S. et al. (2015). Evaluation of suspected cosmetic induced facial dermatoses with the use of Indian standard series and cosmetic series patch test. *Journal of Clinical and Diagnostic Research* 9 (3): WC07–WC10.
11 Uchida, S., Oiso, N., Matsunaga, K., and Kawada, A. (2013). Patch test reaction to p-phenylenediamine can persist for more than 1 month. *Contact Dermatitis* 69 (6): 382–383.
12 Ho, S.G., White, I.R., Rycroft, R.J., and McFadden, J.P. (2004). Allergic contact dermatitis from para-phenylenediamine in Bigen powder hair dye. *Contact Dermatitis* 51 (2): 93–94.
13 Hsu, T.S., Davis, M.D., El-Azhary, R. et al. (2001). Beard dermatitis due to para-phenylenediamine use in Arabic men. *Journal of the American Academy of Dermatology* 44 (5): 867–869.
14 Verma, P. and Yadav, P. (2014). Paraphenylenediamine dye allergic contact dermatitis of mustache region manifesting as prurigo nodularis-like lesions. *Dermatitis: Contact, Atopic, Occupational, Drug* 25 (2): 91–92.
15 Chan, H.P. and Maibach, H.I. (2008). Moustache p-phenylenediamine dye allergic contact dermatitis with distant site involvement – an atypical presentation. *Contact Dermatitis* 58 (3): 179–180.
16 Vogel, T.A., Coenraads, P.J., and Schuttelaar, M.L. (2014). Allergic contact dermatitis presenting as severe and persistent blepharoconjunctivitis and centrofacial oedema after dyeing of eyelashes. *Contact Dermatitis* 71 (5): 304–306.
17 Pas-Wyroślak, A., Wiszniewska, M., Kręcisz, B. et al. (2012). Contact blepharoconjunctivitis due to black henna – a case report. *International Journal of Occupational Medicine and Environmental Health* 25 (2): 196–199.
18 Kaiserman, I. (2003). Severe allergic blepharoconjunctivitis induced by a dye for eyelashes and eyebrows. *Ocular Immunology and Inflammation* 11 (2): 149–151.
19 Guchlerner, M. and Luchtenberg, M. (2014). A 16-year-old female patient with massive bilateral blepharedema. *Der Ophthalmologe : Zeitschrift der Deutschen Ophthalmologischen Gesellschaft* 111 (12): 1207–1209.
20 Wachsmuth, R. and Wilkinson, M. (2006). Loss of eyelashes after use of a tinting mascara containing PPD. *Contact Dermatitis* 54 (3): 169–170.
21 Bhat, J. and Smith, A.G. (2003). Xanthelasma palpebrarum following allergic contact dermatitis from para-phenylenediamine in a black eyelash-tinting product. *Contact Dermatitis* 49 (6): 311.
22 Teixeira, M., de Wachter, L., Ronsyn, E., and Goossens, A. (2006). Contact allergy to para-phenylenediamine in a permanent eyelash dye. *Contact Dermatitis* 55 (2): 92–94.
23 Hansson, C. and Thorneby-Andersson, K. (2001). Allergic contact dermatitis from 2-chloro-p-phenylenediamine in a cream dye for eyelashes and eyebrows. *Contact Dermatitis* 45 (4): 235–236.
24 Søsted, H., Rastogi, S.C., and Thomsen, J.S. (2007). Allergic contact dermatitis from toluene-2,5-diamine in a cream dye for eyelashes and eyebrows – quantitative exposure assessment. *Contact Dermatitis* 57 (3): 195–196.
25 Wong, G.A. and King, C.M. (2003). Immediate-type hypersensitivity and allergic contact dermatitis due to para-phenylenediamine in hair dye. *Contact Dermatitis* 48 (3): 166.
26 Kumaran, M.S., Narang, T., and Parsad, D. (2016). Contact Urticaria With Paraphenylene Diamine, Rare or Underreported? *Skinmed* 14 (5): 389–390.
27 Sahoo, B., Handa, S., Penchallaiah, K., and Kumar, B. (2000). Contact anaphylaxis due to hair dye. *Contact Dermatitis* 43 (4): 244.
28 Felix, B.Y. (2011). An itchy erythematous temporary holiday tattoo. *Tzu Chi Medical Journal* 23: 58–59.
29 Worsnop, F.S., Craythorne, E.E., and du Vivier, A.W. (2011). A blistering eruption after a holiday in India. *British Medical Journal* 343: d7474.
30 Najem, N. and Bagher, Z.V. (2011). Allergic contact dermatitis to black henna. *Acta Dermatovenerologica Alpina, Pannonica, et Adriatica.* 20 (2): 87–88.
31 Matulich, J. and Sullivan, J. (2005). A temporary henna tattoo causing hair and clothing dye allergy. *Contact Dermatitis* 53 (1): 33–36.
32 Di Landro, A., Valsecchi, R., and Marchesi, L. (2005). Allergic reaction with persistent hypopigmentation due to temporary tattoing with henna in a baby. *Contact Dermatitis* 52 (6): 338–339.
33 Neri, I., Guareschi, E., Savoia, F., and Patrizi, A. (2002). Childhood allergic contact dermatitis from henna tattoo. *Pediatric Dermatology* 19 (6): 503–505.
34 Schultz, E. and Mahler, V. (2002). Prolonged lichenoid reaction and cross-sensitivity to para-substituted amino-compounds due to temporary henna tattoo. *International Journal of Dermatology* 41 (5): 301–303.
35 Wohrl, S., Hemmer, W., Focke, M. et al. (2001). Hypopigmentation after non-permanent henna tattoo. *Journal of the European Academy of Dermatology and Venereology* 15 (5): 470–472.
36 Wakelin, S.H., Creamer, D., Rycroft, R.J. et al. (1998). Contact dermatitis from paraphenylenediamine used as a skin paint. *Contact Dermatitis* 39 (2): 92–93.
37 Farsani, T.T., Jalian, H.R., and Young, L.C. (2012). Chemical leukoderma from hair dye containing para-phenylenediamine. *Dermatitis: Contact, Atopic, Occupational, Drug* 23 (4): 181–182.
38 Korsaga-Some, N., Barro-Traoré, F., Andonaba, J.B. et al. (2012). Vitilgoid achromia after temporary tattooing. *International Journal of Dermatology* 51 (Suppl 1):54–6, 60–2.
39 Valsecchi, R., Leghissa, P., Di Landro, A. et al. (2007). Persistent leukoderma after henna tattoo. *Contact Dermatitis* 56 (2): 108–109.
40 Lee, J.H., Ahn, B.J., Noh, M., and Lee, A.Y. (2014). Patch test reactions in patients with the additional diagnosis of vitiligo. *International Journal of Dermatology* 53 (2): 187–191.
41 Wolf, R., Wolf, D., Matz, H., and Orion, E. (2003). Cutaneous reactions to temporary tattoos. *Dermatology Online Journal* 9 (1): 3.
42 Chung, W.H., Chang, Y.C., Yang, L.J. et al. (2002). Clinicopathologic features of skin reactions to temporary tattoos and analysis of possible causes. *Archives of Dermatology* 138 (1): 88–92.

43 Rubegni, P., Fimiani, M., de Aloe, G., and Andreassi, L. (2000). Lichenoid reaction to temporary tattoo. *Contact Dermatitis* 42 (2): 117–118.

44 Barrientos, N., Abajo, P., de Vega, M.M., and Dominguez, J. (2014). Erythema multiforme-like eruption following allergic contact dermatitis in response to para-phenylenediamine in a temporary henna tattoo. *International Journal of Dermatology* 53 (7): e348–e350.

45 Jappe, U., Hausen, B.M., and Petzoldt, D. (2001). Erythema-multiforme-like eruption and depigmentation following allergic contact dermatitis from a paint-on henna tattoo, due to para-phenylenediamine contact hypersensitivity. *Contact Dermatitis* 45 (4): 249–250.

46 Mikkelsen, C.S., Liljefred, F., and Mikkelsen, D.B. (2011). Erythema multiforme-like reaction to para-phenylenediamine. *Ugeskrift for Laeger* 173 (1): 51–52.

47 Sidwell, R.U., Francis, N.D., Basarab, T., and Morar, N. (2008). Vesicular erythema multiforme-like reaction to para-phenylenediamine in a henna tattoo. *Pediatric Dermatology* 25 (2): 201–204.

48 Spornraft-Ragaller, P., Kämmerer, E., Gillitzer, C., and Schmitt, J. (2012). Severe allergic reactions to para-phenylenediamine in children and adolescents: should the patch test concentration of PPD be changed? *Journal der Deutschen Dermatologischen Gesellschaft* 10 (4): 258–264.

49 Neri, I., Giacomini, F., Raone, B., and Patrizi, A. (2009). Generalized erythema multiforme after localized allergic dermatitis from dark henna tattoo. *Pediatric Dermatology* 26 (4): 496.

50 Allione, A., Dutto, L., Castagna, E. et al. (2011). Erythema multiforme caused by tattoo: a further case. *Internal and Emergency Medicine* 6 (3): 263–265.

51 Calzavara-Pinton, P., Capezzera, R., Zane, C. et al. (2002). Lymphomatoid allergic contact dermatitis from para-phenylenediamine. *Contact Dermatitis* 47 (3): 173–174.

52 Veysey, E.C., Burge, S., and Cooper, S. (2007). Consort contact dermatitis to paraphenylenediamine, with an unusual clinical presentation of tumid plaques. *Contact Dermatitis* 56 (6): 366–367.

53 Tukenmez Demirci, G., Kivanc Altunay, I., Atis, G., and Kucukunal, A. (2012). Allergic contact dermatitis mimicking angioedema due to paraphenylendiamine hypersensitivity: a case report. *Cutaneous and Ocular Toxicology* 31 (3): 250–252.

54 van Genderen, M.E., Carels, G., Lonnee, E.R., and Dees, A. (2014). Severe facial swelling in a pregnant woman after using hair dye. *BMJ Case Reports* 2014.

55 Søsted, H., Agner, T., Andersen, K.E., and Menné, T. (2002). 55 cases of allergic reactions to hair dye: a descriptive, consumer complaint-based study. *Contact Dermatitis* 47 (5): 299–303.

56 Lönngren, V., Young, E., Simanaitis, M., and Svedman, C. (2012). Neutrophilic and eosinophilic dermatitis caused by contact allergic reaction to paraphenylenediamine in hair dye. *Archives of Dermatology* 148 (11): 1299–1301.

57 Nacaroglu, H.T., Celegen, M., Karkiner, C.S. et al. (2014). Eosinophilic cellulitis (Wells' syndrome) caused by a temporary henna tattoo. *Postepy Dermatologii Alergologii* 31 (5): 322–324.

58 Chey, W.Y., Kim, K.L., Yoo, T.Y., and Lee, A.Y. (2004). Allergic contact dermatitis from hair dye and development of lichen simplex chronicus. *Contact Dermatitis* 51 (1): 5–8.

59 Gunasti, S. and Aksungur, V.L. (2010). Severe inflammatory and keloidal, allergic reaction due to para-phenylenediamine in temporary tattoos. *Indian Journal of Dermatology, Venereology and Leprology* 76 (2): 165–167.

60 Vasilakis, V., Knight, B., Lidder, S., and Frankton, S. (2010). Severe type IV hypersensitivity to 'black henna' tattoo. *BMJ Case Reports* 2010.

61 Ishida, W., Makino, T., and Shimizu, T. (2011). Severe hair loss of the scalp due to a hair dye containing para phenylenediamine. *ISRN Dermatology* 2011: 947284.

62 O'Brien, T.J. and McColl, D.M. (1999). Unusual reactions to paint-on tattoos. *Australasian Journal of Dermatology* 40 (2): 120.

63 Lopez, I.E., Turrentine, J.E., and Cruz, P.D. Jr. (2014). Clues to diagnosis of connubial contact dermatitis to paraphenylenediamine. *Dermatitis: Contact, Atopic, Occupational, Drug* 25 (1): 32–33.

64 Ho, S.G., Basketter, D.A., Jefferies, D. et al. (2005). Analysis of para-phenylenediamine allergic patients in relation to strength of patch test reaction. *British Journal of Dermatology* 153 (2): 364–367.

65 Namburi, R.P., Aparna, R.R.B., Suchitra, M.M. et al. (2011). A retrospective study on the biochemical profile of self poisoning with a popular Indian hair dye. *Journal of Clinical and Diagnostic Research: JCDR* 5 (7): 1343–1346.

66 Shah, M., Lewis, F.M., and Gawkrodger, D.J. (1996). Occupational dermatitis in hairdressers. *Contact Dermatitis* 35 (6): 364–365.

67 Uter, W., Lessmann, H., Geier, J., and Schnuch, A. (2007). Contact allergy to hairdressing allergens in female hairdressers and clients – current data from the IVDK, 2003–2006. *Journal der Deutschen Dermatologischen Gesellschaft* 5 (11): 993–1001.

68 Tresukosol, P. and Swasdivanich, C. (2012). Hand contact dermatitis in hairdressers: clinical and causative allergens, experience in Bangkok. *Asian Pacific Journal of Allergy and Immunology* 30 (4): 306–312.

69 Helaskoski, E., Suojalehto, H., Virtanen, H. et al. (2014). Occupational asthma, rhinitis, and contact urticaria caused by oxidative hair dyes in hairdressers. *Annals of Allergy, Asthma & Immunology* 112 (1): 46–52.

70 Japan Soap and Detergent Association (2002). The 44th Clean Survey on Hair Color and Hair Coloring Japan: Japan Soap and Detergent News; [cited 2002]. Available from: http://www.jsda.org/w/e_engls/e_news16.html#16-2.

71 McFadden, J.P., White, I.R., Frosch, P.J. et al. (2007). Allergy to hair dye. *British Medical Journal* 334 (7587): 220.

72 Jacob, S.E. and Brod, B.A. (2011). Paraphenylenediamine in black henna tattoos: sensitization of toddlers indicates a clear need for legislative action. *Journal of Clinical and Aesthetic Dermatology* 4 (12): 46–47.

73 Brancaccio, R.R., Brown, L.H., Chang, Y.T. et al. (2002). Identification and quantification of para-phenylenediamine in a temporary black henna tattoo. *American Journal of Contact Dermatitis* 13 (1): 15–18.

74 Aeby, P., Sieber, T., Beck, H. et al. (2009). Skin sensitization to p-phenylenediamine: the diverging roles of oxidation and N-acetylation for dendritic cell activation and the immune response. *Journal of Investigative Dermatology* 129 (1): 99–109.

75 Toholka, R., Wang, Y.S., Tate, B. et al. (2015). The First Australian Baseline Series: Recommendations for patch testing in suspected contact dermatitis. *Australasian Journal of Dermatology* 56 (2): 107–115.

76 Ho, S.G., White, I.R., Rycroft, R.J., and McFadden, J.P. (2004). A new approach to patch testing patients with para-phenylenediamine allergy secondary to temporary black henna tattoos. *Contact Dermatitis* 51 (4): 213–214.

77 Le Coz, C.J., El Bakali, A., Untereiner, F., and Grosshans, E. (1998). Active sensitization to budesonide and para-phenylenediamine from patch testing. *Contact Dermatitis* 39 (3): 153–155.

78 Devos, S.A. and Van Der Valk, P.G. (2001). The risk of active sensitization to PPD. *Contact Dermatitis* 44 (5): 273–275.

79 Dawe, S.A., White, I.R., Rycroft, R.J. et al. (2004). Active sensitization to para-phenylenediamine and its relevance: a 10-year review. *Contact Dermatitis* 51 (2): 96–97.

80 Gawkrodger, D.J. and Paul, L. (2008). Late patch test reactions: delayed immune response appears to be more common than active sensitization. *Contact Dermatitis* 59 (3): 185–187.

81 Goon, A.T., Gilmour, N.J., Basketter, D.A. et al. (2003). High frequency of simultaneous sensitivity to Disperse Orange 3 in patients with positive patch tests to para-phenylenediamine. *Contact Dermatitis* 48 (5): 248–250.

82 Seidenari, S., Mantovani, L., Manzini, B.M., and Pignatti, M. (1997). Cross-sensitizations between azo dyes and para-amino compound. A study of 236 azo-dye-sensitive subjects. *Contact Dermatitis* 36 (2): 91–96.

83 Le Coz, C.J. (2001). Clothing. In: *Contact Dermatitis*, 3e. Berlin: Springer.

84 Ozkaya, E. and Elinc-Aslan, M.S. (2011). Black rubber sensitization by bicycle handgrips in a child with palmar hyperhidrosis. *Dermatitis: Contact, Atopic, Occupational, Drug* 22 (4): E10–E12.

85 Thyssen, J.P., Menne, T., and Johansen, J.D. (2011). The increase in p-phenylenediamine allergy in Denmark is not explained by an increase in contact allergy to para group chemicals. *Contact Dermatitis* 64 (3): 176–179.

86 Hald, M., Menne, T., Johansen, J.D., and Zachariae, C. (2013). Severe occupational contact dermatitis caused by black rubber as a consequence of p-phenylenediamine allergy resulting from a temporary henna tattoo. *Contact Dermatitis* 68 (6): 377–379.

87 Lee, J.Y., Kim, C.W., and Kim, S.S. (2015). Analysis of the results from the patch test to para-phenylenediamine in the TRUE test in patients with a hair dye contact allergy. *Annals of Dermatology* 27 (2): 171–177.

88 Sornin de Leysat, C., Boone, M., Blondeel, A., and Song, M. (2003). Two cases of cross-sensitivity in subjects allergic to paraphenylenediamine following ingestion of Polaronil. *Dermatology* 206 (4): 379–380.

89 Ingram, J.R., Hughes, T.M., and Stone, N.M. (2014). Potential danger of hair dyes marketed as free from para-phenylenediamine. *International Journal of Dermatology* 53 (4): e257–e258.

90 Skazik, C., Grannemann, S., Wilbers, L. et al. (2008). Reactivity of in vitro activated human T lymphocytes to p-phenylenediamine and related substances. *Contact Dermatitis* 59 (4): 203–211.

91 Xie, Z., Hayakawa, R., Sugiura, M. et al. (2000). Experimental study on skin sensitization potencies and cross-reactivities of hair-dye-related chemicals in guinea pigs. *Contact Dermatitis* 42 (5): 270–275.

92 Basketter, D.A. and English, J. (2009). Cross-reactions among hair dye allergens. *Cutaneous and Ocular Toxicology* 28 (3): 104–106.

Exposure Color Code

- Clothing, jewelry, adornments
- Personal care products, cosmetics/cosmetic procedures
- Household products, domestic environment, including furniture and refurbishment
- Occupational dermatoses, work environment
- Medicines, surgical/dental procedures, herbal/alternative medicines
- Personal appliances/aids
- Leisure activities, sport, travel
- Other exposures (including dietary)
- Not relevant or multiple/general exposure

CHAPTER 23

Disperse Blue 106

CHAPTER CONTENTS

Allergen profile

Disperse Blue 106 is one of the more allergenic textile dyes found in clothing.

Aspects of daily life with potential exposure to textile dye allergens (regarding textile dyes in general):

- *Clothing*, all types, including shirts, trousers, stockings, brassieres, underclothing, and gloves.
- *Occupational*, e.g. work clothes, textile dye manufacturing, dress making factory.
- *Leisure and sports activities*, e.g. sports garments, shin pads, fishing – hand dermatitis from dyed maggot exposure (red, orange and black dyes) [1], red carpets, e.g. judo club [2].
- *Ornamentation*, e.g. textile necklace (azo dyes orange and yellow) [3], azo dye in red tattoo [4].
- *Medical, dental procedures/devices*, e.g. knee brace (disperse blue 85) [5].
- *Personal appliances*, e.g. spectacle frames.
- *Travel*, e.g. car seat belt.
- *Cosmetics*, e.g. from disperse dye use in temporary hair dye (not Disperse Blue 106)

Potential routes of exposure

- Direct contact
- Airborne (rare)

Potential clinical manifestations of contact allergy to textile dyes

Common

- Direct ACD
- Mimicking or exacerbation of endogenous or pre-existing eczema, including atopic and nummular eczema

Less common

- Multifactorial
- Airborne contact dermatitis (rare single case)
- Non-eczematous – pseudolymphomatoid, erythema multiforme-like, pigmented purpuric contact dermatitis, prurigo
- Contact urticaria
- Erythroderma

Key points

- Disperse Blue 106 is a potent sensitizer; its release will depend on the textile and degree of sweat and friction.
- It is found in synthetic fibers that are usually navy blue, black or dark green in color. Ingredients are not labeled in clothing, so allergic patients are at a disadvantage and it may be difficult to avoid the allergen.
- Can be present in all types of clothing.
- Clinical presentations vary:
  - *Classical eczematous*. Periaxillary, neck, perineum, buttocks, upper inner thighs, waistband, wrists.
  - *Non-classical eczematous 1*. Atopic dermatitis-like/flexural.
  - *Non-classical eczematous 2*. Widespread, patchy, nummular, erythroderma, linear.
  - *Non-eczematous*. Pseudolymphomatoid, erythema multiforme-like, pigmented/purpuric, pruritus/burning, prurigo, urticarial, lichenoid, papulosquamous.
- Occupational cases are usually from work-related clothing items or the textile industry.
- A late patch test reading may detect up to 20% more cases. False-positive patch tests are common.
- Practical advice includes wearing natural fibers, avoiding tight-fitting clothing, and washing new garments three times before wearing.
- The clinical relevance may not always be current and therefore some caution may be advised in avoiding all blue clothes.

Common Contact Allergens: A Practical Guide to Detecting Contact Dermatitis, First Edition. Edited by John McFadden, Pailin Puangpet, Korbkarn Pongpairoj, Supitchaya Thaiwat, and Lee Shan Xian.

© 2020 John Wiley & Sons Ltd. Published 2020 by John Wiley & Sons Ltd.

Companion website: www.wiley.com/go/mcfadden/common_contact_allergens

Introduction

- Disperse dyes are partially soluble in water and can be used as fabric coloring of synthetic textiles, especially polyester and acetate. They have also been identified as potential contact allergens causing textile dermatitis [6].
- Disperse Blue 106 is a thiazol-azoyl-*p*-phenylene diamine derivative which can produce a dark blue dye and can also be used in combination with other dyes to give brown, black, violet or green.
- Disperse Blue 106 has been used commercially since the 1980s and was also reported as an allergen causing textile ACD in the same year [7]. *In vitro* studies reveal Disperse Blue 106 to be an extremely potent sensitizer, comparable to 2,4 dinitrochlorobenzene [8].
- Disperse Blue 106 is in the standard series of the T.R.U.E.® test. It has been described as an important contact allergen that may be frequently missed [9, 10].

Molecular formula: $C_{14}H_{17}N_5O_3S$

Exposure

- Disperse Blue 106 was reported as a dark coloring in many synthetic fabrics such as navy blue or black color in 100% polyester, dark or blue green color in 100% wool synthetic, black/blue/dark green in 100% acetate or 100% polyester, mixed acetate/cotton, black velvet (70% acetate, 20% polyamide, and 10% elastane) and blue dye in cotton/polyester [7, 9, 11–15]. The synthetic materials were used in clothing such as brassieres, skirts, dresses, stockings, leggings, military uniforms, professional uniforms, undergarments, bed sheets, and certain parts of some shoes [15, 16].

Age

- Textile contact dermatitis (TCD) is more frequent in the fourth decade of life in males and in the fifth decade of life in females [6].

Children

- Disperse Blue 106 was the most common positive disperse dye contact allergy found in children, being more common in girls [17] and ranging in frequency from 0.4% to 8.8% [18, 19]. The most common locations of contact sensitization in children were the lower extremities and flexural areas (axilla and groin); there was an association with atopic children [18].

Sex

- TDD is more common in women, 56–100% of cases being female [14, 20]. One speculation was that tighter clothing is more common in female fashion [16].

Associated disease

- One study cites TDD as being more common in patients with atopic dermatitis [6]. Children with TDD were more likely to present with a flexural dermatitis [14].

Patch testing

The concentration of Disperse Blue 106 for patch testing is usually 1% but reactions have been recorded at 0.1% and 0.3% [21]. Screening tests with a 'dye mix' may miss some patients who are allergic to azo dye 106 [22].

- Disperse Blue 106 and 124 can elicit purpuric allergic reactions from patch testing, with correlating histopathological features [23].
- An irritant patch test reaction to Disperse Blue 106 can occur with a frequency of up to 5% [16].
- Disperse Blue 106 is also included in a textile dye mix (TDM) at a concentration of 0.3%. This TDM includes Disperse Blue 35, Disperse Yellow 3, Disperse Orange 1 and 3, Disperse Red 1 and 17, Disperse Blue 106, and Disperse Blue 124 at a concentration of 6.6% in petrolatum. The European Environmental and Contact Dermatitis Research Group (EECDRG) study identified 2.1–6.9% of dermatitis patients who had positive reactions to TDM and more than 30% of these also had positive relevance [24]. The International Contact Dermatitis Research Group (ICDRG) study showed that some patients who had TDM allergy also reacted to 1% and 0.3% Disperse Blue 106 (13.2% and 6.7%, respectively) [25].

Frequency of sensitization

Among the azo dyes, disperse dye is the most common textile allergen [6]. The prevalence of positive reactions to Disperse Blue 106 on routine patch testing ranged from 0.2 to 1.9%, being one of the most common positive azo dye allergens detected [14, 22].

Clinical relevance

- The relevance of positive reactions to disperse dyes was >70% in most studies [6, 14].

Cross-reactions

- Concomitant positive patch tests to disperse blue dyes and *p*-phenylenediamine (PPD) are uncommon [7, 10, 13].
- Co-reactions to Azo Blue 124 are common, occurring in over half of cases [20].

Clinical/case reports

- The clinical presentation of textile dermatitis is classically an eczematous eruption located on the skin in contact with the garment and/or areas of friction (Figures 23.1–23.2). The most common locations include the extremities, trunk, face, and buttocks [16, 20]. Axillary TDD classically affects the periphery but not the vault. Another classical presentation affects the perineum, buttocks, and upper inner thighs. The flexures were noted as a common location for atopic children [18]. The palms, soles, and eyelids are not commonly involved. Eyelid dermatitis can be caused by airborne allergy in an occupational setting in the dyeing process (Figures 23.1–23.2) [6].
- The other less common clinical presentations are erythemato-squamous, pustular, purpuric, hyperpigmented, nummular-like lesions, and lichenification [16, 26].
- A case of seat belt dermatitis on the exposed skin of the left shoulder from Disperse Blue dyes was reported [27].
- Disperse Blue textile dye dermatitis was reported as mimicking severe atopic dermatitis that had been resistant to treatment in an adult [28].
- A healthy 63-year-old woman presented with non-pruritic well-demarcated non-indurated macular erythema on both breasts. The differential diagnosis included metastatic intravascular breast cancer, panniculitis (reticular erythematous mucinosis), early morphoea, and erysipelas. After biopsy suggested dermatitis, patch testing revealed positive reactions to Disperse Blue 106 and 124. Changing her black bra to white led to resolution of the dermatitis [29].
- A 35-year-old woman had recurrent inflammation over the incision scar of her previous right total hip replacement surgery, which did not respond to treatment. Patch testing was positive to Disperse Blue 106/124 and the inflammation resolved when the patient stopped wearing dark underwear [30].
- Black velvet clothing has been described as a source of TDD from Disperse Blue 106 [15].
- A series of textile dye dermatitis to Azo Blue 106 in dark polyester blouses was described with axillary involvement in all and the neck, upper back, and elbow flexures being variously involved [7].
- A 33-year-old man presented with a severe reaction around the ears after having replacement plastic tips for his spectacle frames. He was patch test positive to multiple azo dyes, including Disperse Blue 106. The dermatitis improved when he covered the plastic tips, assumed to contain dyes, with tape [31].
- An 11-year-old presented with shin dermatitis coinciding with a change of shin pads to one with a colored cloth over protective foam. Patch testing showed multiple azo dye positivity including to Disperse Blue 106. The dermatitis improved with removal of the implicated shin pad [32].

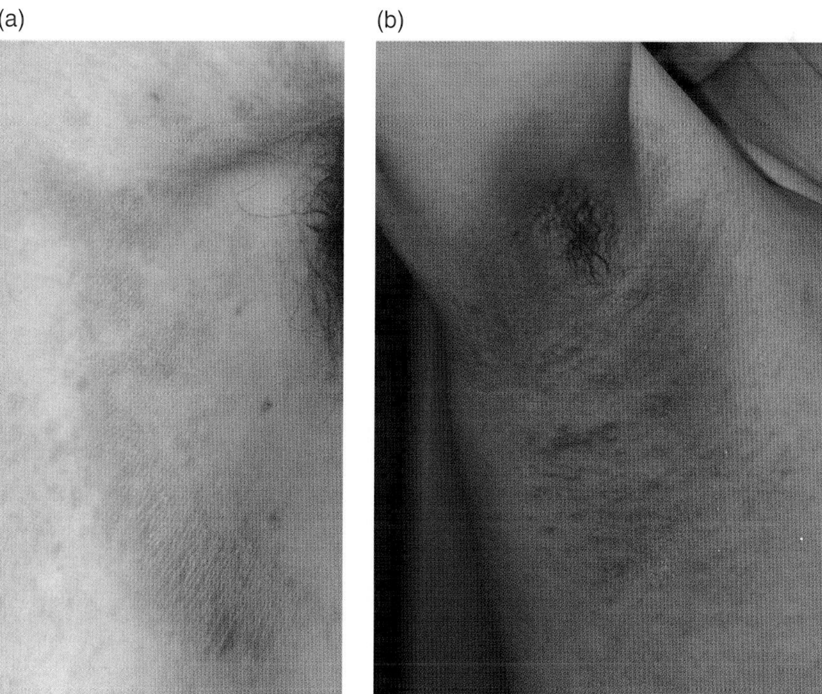

Figure 23.1 Axillary dermatitis. (a) ACD to disperse dyes with accentuation around the periphery and relative sparing of the vault. (b) ACD to fragrance with dermatitis involving the vault. Endogenous dermatitis such as seborrheic dermatitis may also affect the axillary area.

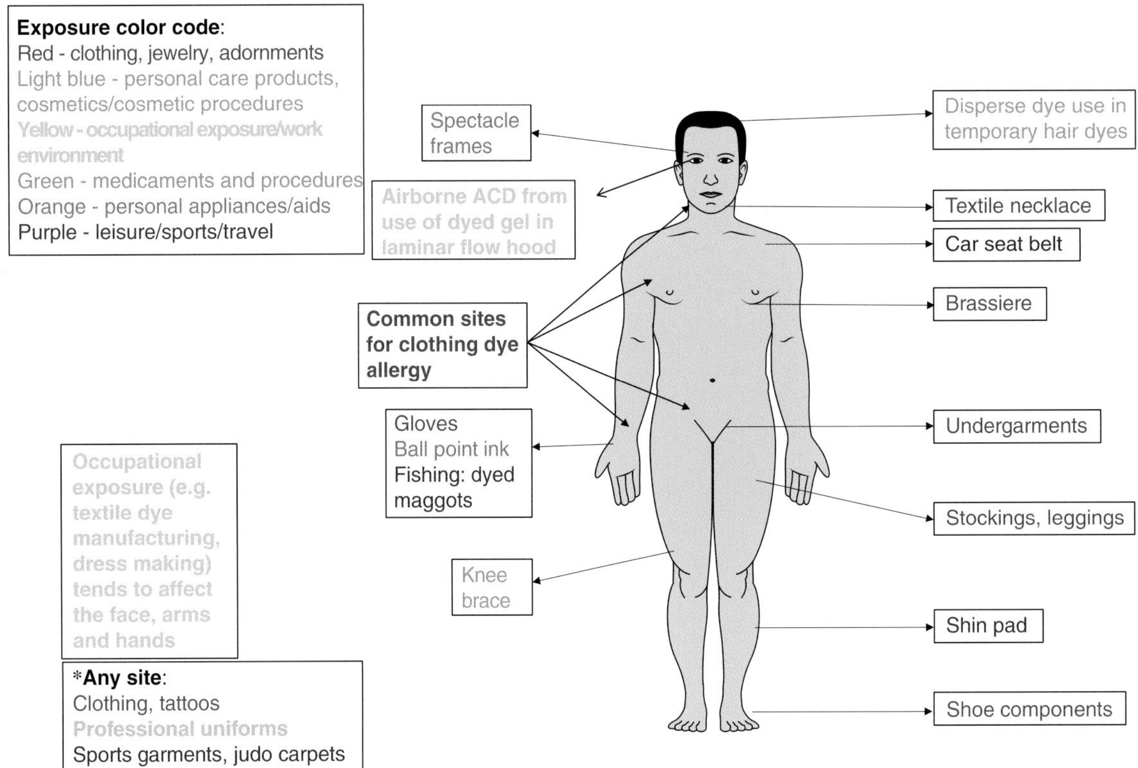

Figure 23.2 Reported exposure sources for ACD to disperse dyes.

- A competitive hockey player developed widespread dermatitis during the playing season. He wore a black lycra bodysuit under his hockey team clothes. Patch tests were positive to Disperse Blue 106, and on reverting to cotton as an underclothing his dermatitis resolved. Dark lycra may contain TDD [33].
- Linear dermatitis: A 43-year-old woman presented with dermatitis in a somewhat linear pattern under her breasts, across her back, and around her waist. This dermatitis occurred after wearing a new blue dress with a blue lining. Patch testing showed a strong reaction to Disperse Blue 106 and a weak reaction to the blue dress lining [10].
- Disperse Blue 106 was the most common dye allergen associated with hand dermatitis, including an atopic dermatitis patient who developed hand eczema after wearing a synthetic fiber garment. Black velvet gloves were also quoted as a potential source of dye exposure [34].
- Of 100 patients presenting with textile dye dermatitis, seven had transient wheals/urticaria and/or urticated dermatitis and four had pruritus [35].
- A Canadian series reviewed 40 patients allergic to textile dyes, the majority [33] of whom reacted to Disperse Blue 106. Fifteen of these patients had widespread dermatitis, 14 of whom required oral prednisolone and two required hospitalization. Some of these cases presented as erythroderma and others as widespread nummular dermatitis on the trunk and extremities. Four presented with genital pruritus and burning, developing into dermatitis of the vulva, perineum, buttocks, and upper inner thighs [9].
- Airborne ACD to Disperse Blue 106 from use of a dyed ultrasound gel used within a laminar flow hood has been reported [8]. A 28-year-old researcher presented with a 1-year history of intermittent swollen itchy eyelids. She was patch test positive to Disperse Blue 106. The ultrasound gel contained Disperse Blue 106 and the dermatitis resolved when she switched to colorless ultrasound gel [36].

Non-eczematous contact dermatitis

- ACD to clothing dyes can present as non-eczematous dermatitis, erythema multiforme, pseudolymphomatoid contact dermatitis and pigmented purpuric contact dermatistis.
- A 46-year-old woman developed pruritic pseudolymphoma-like and erythema multiforme-like lesions on the posteromedial thigh area after wearing dark tights or skirts. Skin biopsy revealed moderately superficial lymphocytic infiltration in the dermis. Patch testing showed positive reactions to cobalt, nickel, and Disperse Blue 106 and 124. The TDD resolved after the patient avoided wearing dark-colored garments [37].
- A 37-year-old male who wore a blue uniform developed a widespread erythematous rash, with sparing of the skin folds, for 10 months. Skin biopsy revealed an inflammatory atypical lymphocyte infiltration in the superficial dermis with the immunohistochemical phenotype of T helper cells (CD3+ CD4+,

polyclonality). Patch testing showed positive reactions to Disperse Yellow 3 +, Disperse Red 1 ++, Disperse Orange +++, Disperse Red 17 ++, aminophenol +++, aminobenzene +++ and Disperse Blue 106/124 +++. He was diagnosed with lymphomatoid contact dermatitis caused by textiles and the clinical presentation disappeared by avoiding colored clothes [38].

- A 48-year-old male patient had a 4-year history of a relapsing erythematous, pruritic, and mildly scaly plaque on his glans penis. Histology showed a lymphomatoid appearance, with epidermal lymphocytes showing hyperchromatic nuclei with cerebriform configurations. Patch testing revealed a ++ reaction to Disperse Blue 106. Treatment of the lymphomatoid dermatitis with topical steroids and reverting to white undergarments led to quick resolution of the lesion [39].
- Pigmented purpuric dermatitis was reported in a 52-year-old female, who presented with nummular erythematous plaques and purpuric macules on both legs. Histopathology revealed lymphohistiocytic lichenoid infiltration with extravasation of red blood cells, which was compatible with a diagnosis of lichenoid purpura of Gougerot and Blum. Patch testing showed positive reactions to nickel, thimerosal, Disperse Blue 106, 124, and 106/124 on day 3. They also patch tested with Disperse Blue 106/124 on an area with previous petechiae, which showed a positive reaction with both erythema and petechiae. The diagnosis was confirmed by an exacerbation on wearing a blue dress [40].

Occupational allergic contact dermatitis (ACD)

- An occupational component was reported in 14.8% of cases [20]. The hands are the main site for occupational contact dermatitis from textiles [6].
- There are two case reports of occupational contact dermatitis, mostly from uniforms, in airline personnel who had ++ positive patch tests to Disperse Blue 106 and 124. One of these also had a positive reaction to the fabric material of airline seats [12].
- A 33-year-old woman working in a dressmaking factory developed eczema on the face, eyelids, neck, forearms, and hands after she started ironing clothes with steam. The dermatitis was work-related. She also developed eczema on the thighs, where she rested the clothes [41]. Patch testing showed multiple positives to azo dyes including Disperse Blue 106 (+/++).

Patient education

- The avoidance of exposure to Disperse Blue 106 is advised by wearing pure natural-made fabrics such as cotton, linen, silk or wool, light-colored garments, and loose-fitting clothing. Washing of clothing three times before wearing is recommended [16].

References

1 Warren, L.J. and Marren, P. (1997). Textile dermatitis and dyed maggot exposure. *Contact Dermatitis* 36 (2): 106.

2 Foussereau, J. (1985). An allergen in a judo club? *Contact Dermatitis* 13 (4): 283.

3 Nygaard, U., Kralund, H.H., and Sommerlund, M. (2013). Allergic contact dermatitis induced by textile necklace. *Case Reports in Dermatology* 5 (3): 336–339.

4 Waldmann, I. and Vakilzadeh, F. (1997). [delayed type allergic reaction to red azo dye in tattooing]. Der Hautarzt. *Zeitschrift fur Dermatologie, Venerologie, und verwandte Gebiete* 48 (9): 666–670.

5 Lazarov, A. and Ingber, A. (1998). Textile dermatitis from disperse blue 85 in a knee brace. *Contact Dermatitis* 38 (6): 357.

6 Lisi, P., Stingeni, L., Cristaudo, A. et al. (2014). Clinical and epidemiological features of textile contact dermatitis: an Italian multicentre study. *Contact Dermatitis* 70 (6): 344–350.

7 Menezes Brandão, F., Altermatt, C., Pecegueiro, M. et al. (1985). Contact dermatitis to disperse blue 106. *Contact Dermatitis* 13 (2): 80–84.

8 Betts, C.J., Dearman, R.J., Kimber, I., and Maibach, H.I. (2005). Potency and risk assessment of a skin-sensitizing disperse dye using the local lymph node assay. *Contact Dermatitis* 52 (5): 268–272.

9 Pratt, M. and Taraska, V. (2000). Disperse blue dyes 106 and 124 are common causes of textile dermatitis and should serve as screening allergens for this condition. *American Journal of Contact Dermatitis* 11 (1): 30–41.

10 Dawes-Higgs, E. and Freeman, S. (2004). Allergic contact dermatitis caused by the clothing dye, disperse blue 106, an important contact allergen that may be frequently missed. *Australasian Journal of Dermatology* 45 (1): 64–66.

11 Lodi, A., Ambonati, M., Coassini, A. et al. (1998). Textile dye contact dermatitis in an allergic population. *Contact Dermatitis* 39 (6): 314–315.

12 Khanna, M. and Sasseville, D. (2001). Occupational contact dermatitis to textile dyes in airline personnel. *American Journal of Contact Dermatitis* 12 (4): 208–210.

13 Dejobert, Y., Martin, P., Thomas, P., and Bergoend, H. (1995). Multiple azo dye sensitization revealed by the wearing of a black "velvet" body. *Contact Dermatitis* 33 (4): 276–277.

14 Malinauskiene, L., Bruze, M., Ryberg, K. et al. (2013). Contact allergy from disperse dyes in textiles: a review. *Contact Dermatitis* 68 (2): 65–75.

15 Hausen, B.M. (1993). Contact allergy to disperse blue 106 and blue 124 in black "velvet" clothes. *Contact Dermatitis* 28 (3): 169–173.

16 Lazarov, A. (2004). Textile dermatitis in patients with contact sensitization in Israel: a 4-year prospective study. *Journal of the European Academy of Dermatology and Venereology* 18 (5): 531–537.

17 Seidenari, S., Giusti, F., Pepe, P., and Mantovani, L. (2005). Contact sensitization in 1094 children undergoing patch testing over a 7-year period. *Pediatric Dermatology* 22 (1): 1–5.

18 Giusti, F., Massone, F., Bertoni, L. et al. (2003). Contact sensitization to disperse dyes in children. *Pediatric Dermatology* 20 (5): 393–397.

19 Jacob, S.E., Brod, B., and Crawford, G.H. (2008). Clinically relevant patch test reactions in children – a United States based study. *Pediatric Dermatology* 25 (5): 520–527.

20 Uter, W., Geier, J., Lessmann, H., and Hausen, B.M. (2001). Contact allergy to disperse blue 106 and disperse blue 124 in German and Austrian patients, 1995 to 1999. *Contact Dermatitis* 44 (3): 173–177.

21 Hausen, B.M. and Menezes Brandão, F. (1986). Disperse blue 106, a strong sensitizer. *Contact Dermatitis* 15 (2): 102–103.

22 Ryberg, K., Goossens, A., Isaksson, M. et al. (2011). Patch testing with a textile dye mix in a baseline series in two countries. *Acta Dermato-Venereologica* 91 (4): 422–427.
23 Lazarov, A. and Cordoba, M. (2000). The purpuric patch test in patients with allergic contact dermatitis from azo dyes. *Contact Dermatitis* 42 (1): 23–26.
24 Isaksson, M., Ryberg, K., Goossens, A., and Bruze, M. (2015). Recommendation to include a textile dye mix in the European baseline series. *Contact Dermatitis* 73 (1): 15–20.
25 Isaksson, M., Ale, I., Andersen, K.E. et al. (2015). Patch testing to a textile dye mix by the International Contact Dermatitis Research Group. *Dermatitis* 26 (4): 170–176.
26 Lazarov, A., Trattner, A., David, M., and Ingber, A. (2000). Textile dermatitis in Israel: a retrospective study. *American Journal of Contact Dermatitis* 11 (1): 26–29.
27 Guin, J.D. (2001). Seat-belt dermatitis from disperse blue dyes. *Contact Dermatitis* 44 (4): 263.
28 Mohamoud, A.A. and Andersen, F. (2017). Allergic contact dermatitis caused by textile dyes mimicking atopic dermatitis. *Contact Dermatitis* 76 (2): 119–120.
29 Wong, A., Ball, N., and de Gannes, G. (2011). Nonpruritic contact dermatitis from disperse blue dyes. *Dermatitis* 22 (5): 278–280.
30 Caliskaner, Z., Kartal, O., Baysan, A. et al. (2012). A case of textile dermatitis due to disperse blue on the surgical wound. *Human & Experimental Toxicology* 31 (1): 101–103.
31 Batchelor, R.J. and Wilkinson, S.M. (2006). Contact allergy to disperse dyes in plastic spectacle frames. *Contact Dermatitis* 54 (1): 66–67.
32 Powell, D. and Ahmed, S. (2010). Soccer shin guard reactions: allergic and irritant reactions. *Dermatitis* 21 (3): 162–166.
33 Marzario, B., Burrows, D., and Skotnicki, S. (2016). Contact dermatitis to personal sporting equipment in youth. *Journal of Cutaneous Medicine and Surgery* 20 (4): 323–326.
34 Giusti, F., Mantovani, L., Martella, A., and Seidenari, S. (2002). Hand dermatitis as an unsuspected presentation of textile dye contact sensitivity. *Contact Dermatitis* 47 (2): 91–95.
35 Seidenari, S., Manzini, B.M., and Danese, P. (1991). Contact sensitization to textile dyes: description of 100 subjects. *Contact Dermatitis* 24 (4): 253–258.
36 Skalina, K.A. and Ramesh, M. (2018). A case of allergic contact dermatitis caused by disperse blue dye in ultrasound gel. *Contact Dermatitis* .
37 Pecquet, C., Assier-Bonnet, H., Artigou, C. et al. (1999). Atypical presentation of textile dye sensitization. *Contact Dermatitis* 40 (1): 51.
38 Narganes, L.M., Sambucety, P.S., Gonzalez, I.R. et al. (2013). Lymphomatoid dermatitis caused by contact with textile dyes. *Contact Dermatitis* 68 (1): 62–64.
39 Uzuncakmak, T.K., Akdeniz, N., Ozkanli, S. et al. (2015). Lymphomatoid contact dermatitis associated with textile dye at an unusual location. *Indian Dermatology Online Journal* 6 (Suppl 1): S24–S26.
40 Komericki, P., Aberer, W., Arbab, E. et al. (2001). Pigmented purpuric contact dermatitis from disperse blue 106 and 124 dyes. *Journal of the American Academy of Dermatology* 45 (3): 456–458.
41 Anibarro, P.C., Brenosa, B.G., Madoz, S.E. et al. (2000). Occupational airborne allergic contact dermatitis from disperse dyes. *Contact Dermatitis* 43 (1): 44.

Exposure Color Code

- Clothing, jewelry, adornments
- Personal care products, cosmetics/cosmetic procedures
- Household products, domestic environment, including furniture and refurbishment
- Occupational dermatoses, work environment
- Medicines, surgical/dental procedures, herbal/alternative medicines
- Personal appliances/aids
- Leisure activities, sport, travel
- Other exposures (including dietary)
- Not relevant or multiple/general exposure

CHAPTER 24

Rubber: Mercaptobenzothiazole, Mercapto Mix, Thiurams, Carbamates, Thioureas, *N*-Isopropyl-*N*′-Phenyl-*p*-phenylenediamine

CHAPTER CONTENTS

Allergen profiling

Aspects of daily life with potential for contact allergen exposure to rubber chemicals

- *Work environment*: work gloves, shoes, multiple others.
- *Home environment*: gloves, garden hoses, mattresses, pillows, hot water bottles, rubber bands, toys, bath mats.
- *Clothing*: footwear, gloves, elasticated clothing, headwear, boots.
- *Leisure/sports activities*: swim caps, goggles, squash and other balls, sports shoes and gloves, shin guards, racket and golf handles, rubber mats, sport equipment "grips".
- *Personal appliances*: earplugs/pieces, watchstraps/bands, bridge of spectacle frames.
- *Medical and dental procedures*: healthcare workers' gloves, catheters, blood pressure cuffs, dental dams, orthopedic braces, elasticated bandaging.
- *Ornamentation*: rubber bracelets, necklaces.
- *Personal care products*: rubber sponge applicators, eyelash curlers.
- *Cosmetic procedures*: hair nets, its use in temporary beach "henna tattoo" applications, gloves.
- *Travel*: bicycle handles, escalator handles, travel neck cushions.
- *Physical intimacy*: condoms, diaphragms.

Potential routes of contact to rubber chemical allergens

- *Direct contact*, e.g. gloves, footwear.
- *Hands to face, neck, and body*, e.g. gloves.
- *By-proxy*, e.g. gloves from healthcare workers causing allergic contact dermatitis (ACD) in patients, from condoms.
- *Airborne*, e.g. rubber chemicals borne on powder from gloves, pesticides (uncommon/rare).
- *Mucosal*, e.g. dentists' gloves/dams (uncommon).

Clinical manifestations of contact allergy to rubber chemicals

- Direct exposure contact dermatitis, e.g. gloves (common).
- Mimicking or exacerbation of pre-existing dermatitis.
- Multifactorial dermatitis, e.g. glove allergy in an occupational setting with irritant contact dermatitis (ICD) and/or atopic hand dermatitis (common).
- By-proxy dermatitis, e.g. gloves from health care workers, condoms.
- Airborne contact dermatitis, e.g. accelerator in glove powder particles (uncommon).
- Non-eczematous dermatitis, e.g. lichenoid, pseudolymphomatous, erythema multiforme.
- Contact urticaria, e.g. rubber accelerator contact urticaria is rare in comparison to latex allergy but isolated cases of contact urticaria to rubber chemicals have been reported.
- Mucosal symptoms, e.g. from dentists' gloves (uncommon).
- Erythroderma, e.g. from healthcare workers' gloves (isolated report).

Common Contact Allergens: A Practical Guide to Detecting Contact Dermatitis, First Edition. Edited by John McFadden, Pailin Puangpet, Korbkarn Pongpairoj, Supitchaya Thaiwat, and Lee Shan Xian.
© 2020 John Wiley & Sons Ltd. Published 2020 by John Wiley & Sons Ltd.
Companion website: www.wiley.com/go/mcfadden/common_contact_allergens

Key points

- Thiurams, carbamates, and mercaptobenzothiazoles are used as vulcanization accelerators in the manufacturing of both natural rubber and synthetic rubber products.
- Thioureas are used as accelerators and antioxidants in the manufacture of rubber, especially neoprene. They are also used as fixatives in photography and photocopy paper.
- IPPD is an antioxidant used in rubber production to reduce the effects of perishing by atmospheric oxygen. It classically presents as an occupational source of ACD.
- The frequencies of allergy amongst eczema patients from 12 European countries are 0.72% (mercapto mix), 0.58% (mercaptobenzathiazole, MBT), 1.98% (thiuram miz), and 0.67% (*N-i*sopropyl-*N'*-*p*henyl-*p*-phenylenediamine, IPPD) The frequency of contact allergy to carbamates is 0.9–3.4% and 1% for thioureas. There are multiple sources of exposure to rubber accelerators other than from gloves and shoes. These include household products, personal appliances, clothing, recreational/sports appliances and sportswear, cosmetic agents and appliances, occupational sources, medical appliances and non-rubber products. Therefore, a careful history of potential exposures covering all aspects of daily life is required in patients who have contact allergy to rubber accelerators.
- Thiuram is the most common cause of rubber glove contact allergy. Non-rubber gloves, especially nitrile, also contain rubber accelerators. Carbamates and thioureas may also be used in glove production.
- Mercaptos are the most common rubber accelerator to cause contact allergy to footwear. However, thiurams are occasionally the sole cause of contact allergy to footwear. Contact allergy to footwear has a good prognosis if the allergen is avoided, although this may prove difficult in practice.
- Thiurams and carbamates are closely related, both chemically and immunologically.
- Sweat promotes the leaching of rubber accelerators from gloves and shoes – contact allergy from footwear may be more prominent during the summer/hot months and with sporting activities.
- Healthcare staff who are allergic to rubber accelerators can usually wear vinyl or specialized rubber accelerator free gloves. It is necessary to advise which gloves to use based on the profile of rubber accelerators to which the individual is sensitized.
- Unusual forms of presentation include airborne (accelerators contained within airborne glove powder) and erythroderma (in a patient with creams applied by nurses wearing rubber gloves).
- Non-eczematous clinical presentations of rubber accelerator allergy include pseudolymphomatoid dermatitis, purpuric dermatitis, and pigmented dermatitis.
- Many cases of ACD to black rubber are occupationally related. There are individual case reports of contact allergy to IPPD/black rubber from tires, shoes, boots, video cameras and microscope eyepieces, stamping devices, swimming goggles, handlebars, the black rubber parts of spectacle chains, orthopedic bandages, fishing rods, and elastics.
- There is some immunological cross-reactivity between the hair dye chemical *p*-phenylenediamine (PPD) and black rubber IPPD.

Pitfalls

- Patients can become confused between latex allergy (type 1 hypersensitivity to latex proteins resulting in contact urticaria, rhinoconjunctivitis symptoms from airborne spread, and rarely anaphylaxis, diagnosed with prick testing/specific IgE testing) and ACD to rubber chemicals (type IV hypersensitivity to rubber accelerator/antioxidant chemicals resulting in dermatitis, diagnosed by patch testing). It is necessary to make sure that the patient understands which allergy he/she has. However, type 1 allergy to natural rubber latex and type 4 allergy to rubber accelerator chemicals may occasionally coexist in the same patient.
- Patch testing with a glove or shoe sample in addition to the standard series will increase the sensitivity of detecting contact allergy to gloves or shoes. The material may need to be steamed by a kettle to help leaching of the sensitizing chemical.
- Rubber chemicals may occasionally cause airborne or distant site (ectopic) dermatitis.
- Nitrile gloves may contain considerable amounts of accelerator chemicals such as carbamates or MBT.
- Vinyl gloves are usually free of rubber accelerator chemicals (although there is one report in 1993 of vinyl household gloves releasing carbamate chemicals).

Exposure and use

There are multiple sources of exposure to rubber accelerators other than from gloves and shoes. These include household products, personal appliances, clothing, recreational/sports appliances and sportswear, cosmetic and healthcare agents and appliances, occupational sources, exposure from travel/transport, medical appliances, and non-rubber products. A careful history covering all aspects of daily life is therefore required in patients who have contact allergy to rubber accelerators.

- Thiurams, carbamates, and mercaptobenzothiazole are used as rubber accelerators to speed up the manufacturing process of rubber vulcanization. They are used in the manufacturing of both natural rubber and synthetic rubber products [1].
- Thioureas are used as accelerators and antioxidants in the manufacture of rubber, especially neoprene (e.g. wetsuits).
- IPPD is an antioxidant used in rubber production to reduce the effects of perishing by atmospheric oxygen. It is therefore used in products where anti-corrosion is an important feature e.g. vehicle tires, fan belts, and industrial machine belts.

Patch testing

There are five rubber chemicals usually included in the baseline series:

1. Mercaptobenzothiazole 2% pet.
2. Mercapto mix 1% pet. consisting of 0.33% each of:
   N-cyclohexylbenzothiazyl-sulfenamide
   dibenzothiazyl disulfide
   morpholinylmercaptobenzothiazole
3. Thiuram mix 1% pet. consisting of 0.25% each of:
   tetramethylthiuram disulfide (TMTD)
   tetramethylthiuram monosulfide (TMTM)
   tetraethylthiuram disulfide (TETD)
   dipentamethylenethiuram disulfide (DPTD)

4. IPPD 0.1% pet.
5. Carba mix 3% pet.

Frequency of sensitization

The average frequencies of positive patch tests (in petroleum) to rubber chemicals from 12 European clinics were mercapto mix 0.72%, MBT 0.58%, thiuram mix 1.98%, and IPPD/black rubber 0.67% [2].

Age

- The mean age of patients with accelerator allergy is 39 years [3].
- There were no significant differences in MBT allergy rates between people older than 40 years and younger individuals, and between children and adults [4].

Sex

- The prevalence of rubber contact allergy is equivalent between males and females.
- Most studies found no significant difference in the prevalence of mercapto compound sensitivity between males and females. In Taiwan, the ratio of female to male was 1 : 1 for thiuram mix allergy and 3:2 for mercapto mix allergy [3]. Data from the NACDG between 1985 and 1989 showed that men were more likely to have contact dermatitis to MBT (3.2% vs 1.3%, $p<0.05$) and mercapto mix (2.8% vs 1.5%, $p<0.05$). This difference was thought to be due to variation in exposure rather than gender tendency itself [4].

Clinical disease

ACD to rubber can present in a multitude of ways (Figures 24.1–24.6).

Gloves

- Thiuram is the most common cause of ACD to rubber gloves. Non-rubber gloves, especially nitrile, often contain accelerators as well (Figure 24.2).
- The classical clinical presentation is that of dorsal hand and finger involvement with involvement of and cut-off at the wrist [5]. Sometimes, the changes can be unusual or subtle. The palmar thenar eminence and palmar digits can also be involved [6].
- Local secondary spread of the rubber glove ACD often conceals the typical pattern.
- Thiurams were the most important sensitizers in patients exposed to rubber gloves (2.8%). Zinc diethyldithiocarbamate (ZDC) was the most frequent sensitizer amongst the carbamates in rubber gloves (0.5%). ZDC patch test positivity was also found to be associated with the strength of patch test reactions to thiuram mix [7].
- Powdered gloves had higher rubber accelerator levels than powder-free gloves from the same company. Powder-free nitrile gloves were found to contain either carbamates or MBT or both [8]. There has been a changing trend of contact sensitization to rubber gloves from thiurams only to a combination of carbamates, thiurams, and diphenylguanidine (DPG) [9].
- Nitrile gloves may contain considerable amounts of rubber allergens, e.g. dithiocarbamate. Bergendorff et al. [10] analyzed 19 disposable medical gloves used in Sweden by high-perfomance liquid chromatography. In this study, ten gloves contained zinc diethyldithiocarbamate (ZDC), three contained zinc pentamethylenedithiocarbamate, four contained zinc dibutyldithiocarbamate (ZBC), and two contained 2-mercaptobenzothiazole. Two nitrile gloves contained the highest amounts of ZDC (3–3.5 mg/g).

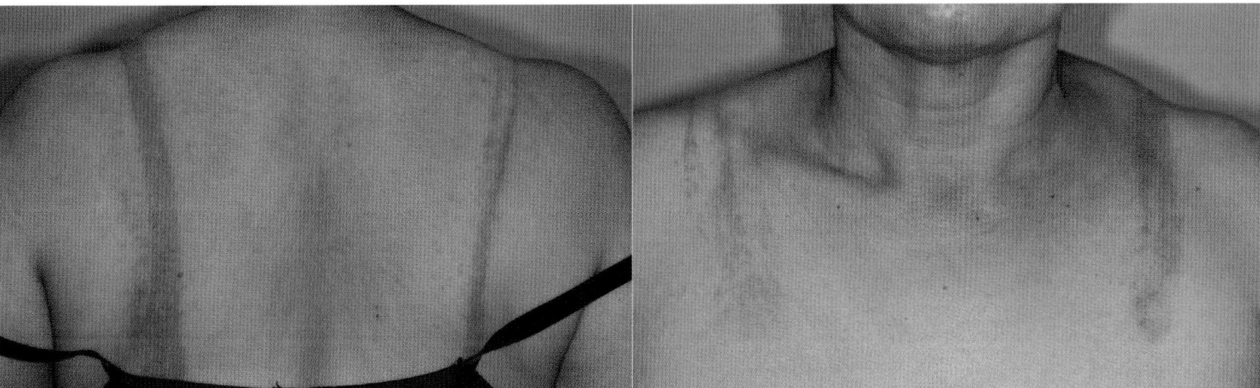

Elastane is now often used as a substitute for rubber/elastic in clothing.

Figure 24.1 Well-demarcated contact dermatitis from bra straps.

(a)

Wilson's original sketch of rubber glove pattern dermatitis (6)

Involvement of palmar thenar eminence and palmar digits

(b)

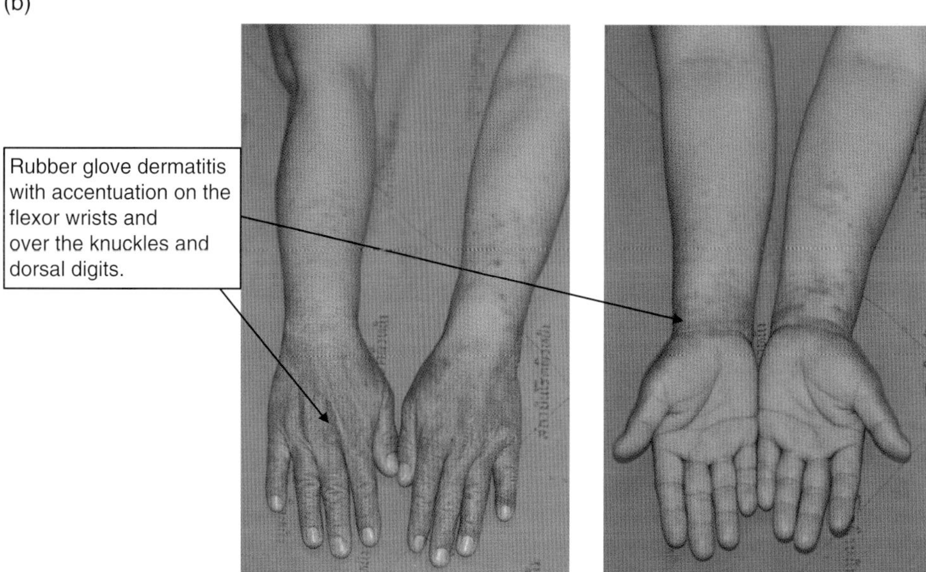

Rubber glove dermatitis with accentuation on the flexor wrists and over the knuckles and dorsal digits.

Figure 24.2 (a and b) Rubber glove allergy mainly affects the dorsal aspects of both hands and forearms but can affect the palmar areas.

Footwear

- Mercapto chemicals are the most common rubber accelerators (and overall) to cause ACD to footwear. However, thiuram allergy can also occasionally be the sole cause of contact allergy to footwear. Contact allergy to footwear has a good prognosis if the allergen is avoided (87.5% improvement/resolution after a mean follow-up period of 3 years) (Figure 24.3) [11].
- In one series of ACD to rubber in footwear, all areas of the feet could be involved except the interdigital spaces. The dorsal aspect of the foot was the most common site affected (40%), followed by the weight-bearing areas of the soles (27.3%). The sides of the heels (10.9%) were affected in those allergic to shoe adhesive [11].
- There is a high percentage of atopic dermatitis patients (46%) amongst patients with ACD to footwear [11].

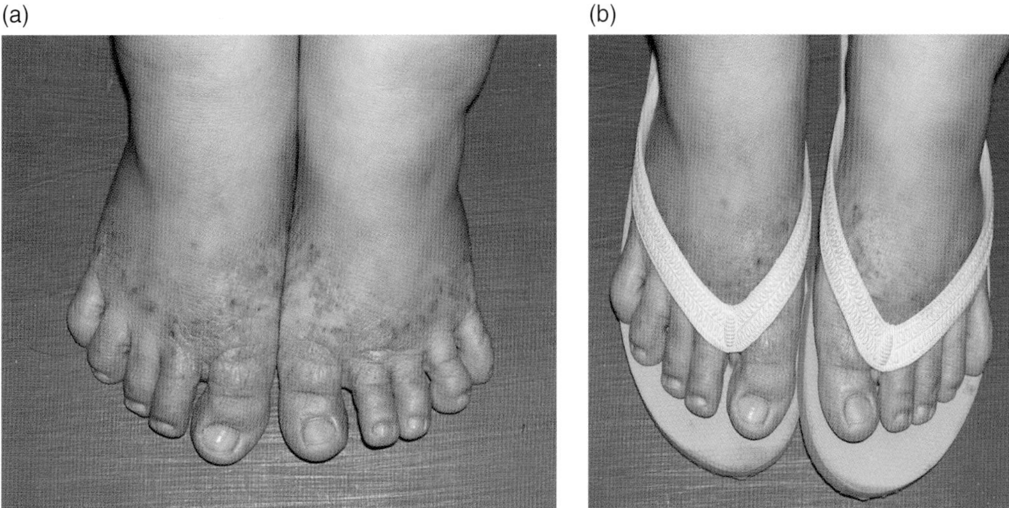

Figure 24.3 (a and b) Rubber sandal allergy frequently affects the dorsal aspects of the feet.

- 14.5% of patients with footwear ACD will not react to allergens in the baseline series but may react to a sample of the footwear [11].
- A study between 1997 and 2009 in 41 children aged <18 years old presenting with plantar dermatitis showed that 41% (17/41) had at least one relevant positive patch test reaction. The most common allergens were rubber chemicals and potassium dichromate [12].
- Hand involvement can also be found in up to 13.5% of cases with contact allergy to MBT in shoes. The cause can either be an id reaction or unidentified contact with rubber products [13].

Occupational disease (see also section "Gloves" and e-supplement chapter)

- Rubber allergy, including contact urticaria, is frequently associated with occupational contact dermatitis [14] from glove use, especially in dental practitioners, hospital workers, and allied healthcare professionals. The North American Contact Dermatitis Group (NACDG) tested 1097 patients for occupational contact dermatitis from 1998 to 2000 and thiuram allergy was found in 85 cases, mercaptobenzothiazole in 30 cases, and mercapto mix in 20 cases [15]. Thiuram was an important allergen amongst US healthcare workers comprising 24.5% of currently relevant occupational allergies compared with 6.9% in non-healthcare workers with dermatitis ($p < 0.001$) [16].
- IPPD/black rubber is an important occupational allergen. Of 56 cases of contact allergy to IPPD, 42 were occupational in origin. Seventeen cases were found in tire manufacturers, nine in car mechanics, nine in drivers and seven from other industrial branches [17].
- A case of occupational ACD to black rubber in the ocular pieces of an otomicroscope was reported. The patient was an otorhinolaryngologist who presented with recurrent symmetrical periorbital eczema [18].
- Occupational thiuram contact dermatitis of the ears was reported in a 56-year-old secretary. She had been transcribing letters for 30 years using a headset with rubber ear piece "olives" for 6 hours a day. Patch testing showed positive reactions to TMTD, TMTM, TETD, DPTD, cobalt, nickel, Fragrance Mix II, and the ear "olives" of the headset [19].
- A 27-year-old professional diver of 6 years developed an extensive dermatitis on the areas covered by his *wetsuit*. He was patch test positive to the wetsuit and then on subsequent testing to diethylthiourea. He was able to find an alternative wet suit without thioureas and the dermatitis resolved. The authors note that diethylthiourea is commonly used in the manufacture of rubber for wetsuits [20].
- A 52-year-old woman developed dermatitis beginning on her left index finger and spreading to the palm from handling *gas masks* during their production. She was allergic to DPG on patch testing [21].

Case reports

- *Different body regions can be affected*: In Taiwan, the sites of involvement in cases of mercapto mix allergy were the feet (36%), face/neck (18%), hands (18%), and arms (10%); in thiuram mix the sites were the hands (28%), face/neck (17%), arms (17%), and feet (9%) [3].
- *Dental by proxy*: Yilmaz et al. [22] reported three patients with ACD to thiuram from doctors"/dentists' gloves which was mistaken for local anesthetic intolerance, and Schwensen et al. reported two cases who presented with perioral ACD to rubber chemicals in rubber gloves used by dentists during dental procedures [23].
- *Hemodialysis*: Contact dermatitis sited near the shunt area in a hemodialysis patient was probably due to the hemodialysis equipment or nurses' gloves [24].

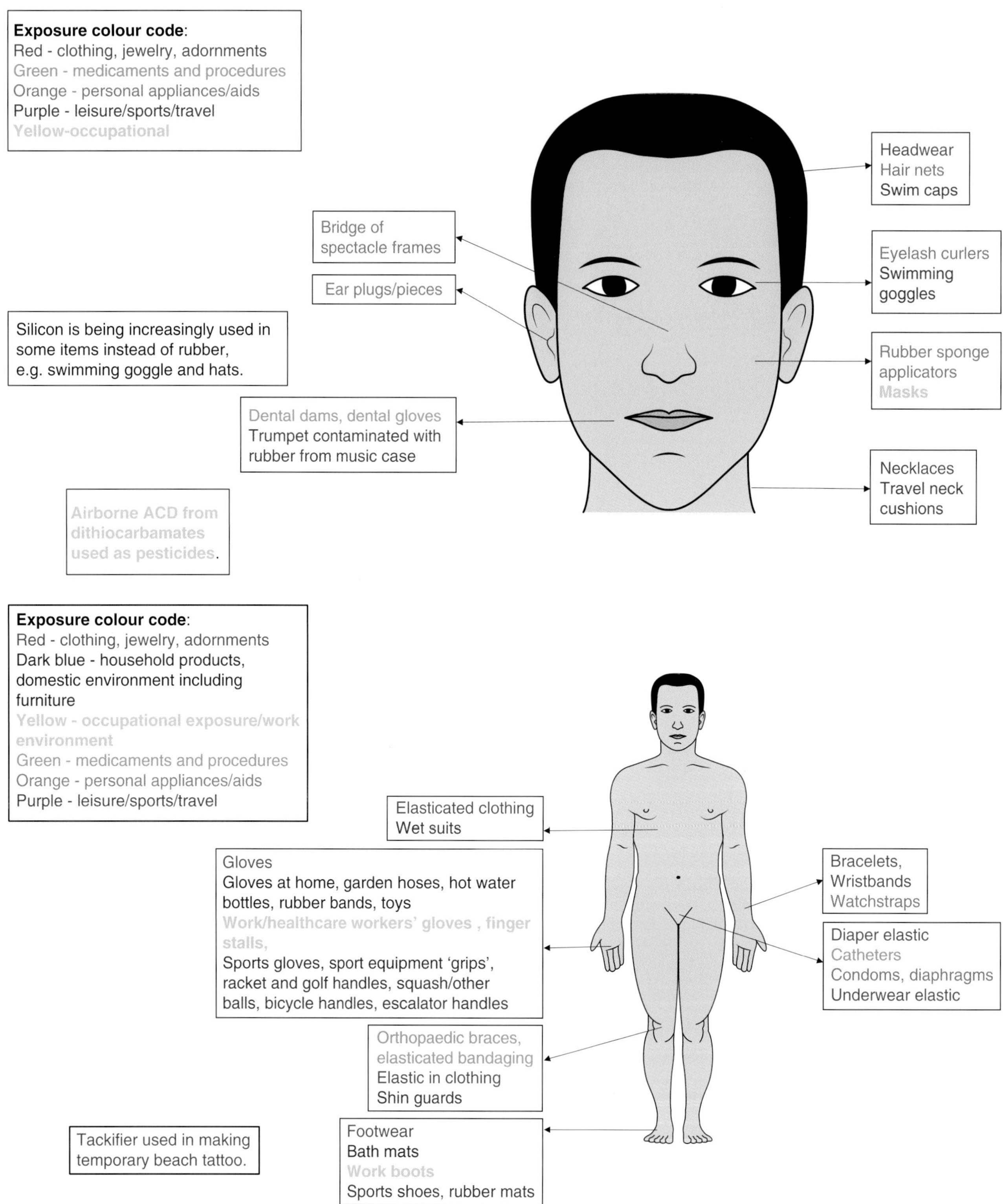

Figure 24.4 Reported exposure sources for ACD to non-black rubber.

- *Compression bandages*: ACD to rubber chemicals (e.g. in elastic compression bandages) occurs in 11–15.6% of patients with leg ulcers [25].
- *Pseudolymphomatoid CD*: Lymphomatoid-like contact dermatitis resembling cutaneous T-cell lymphoma has been reported.

The skin eruption began on the left anterior thigh, before spreading to the buttocks, lateral thighs, and genitals. This was associated with the wearing of panty hose. Histopathology revealed non-diagnostic superficial and deep perivascular lymphoid infiltration with palisading granulomas. However,

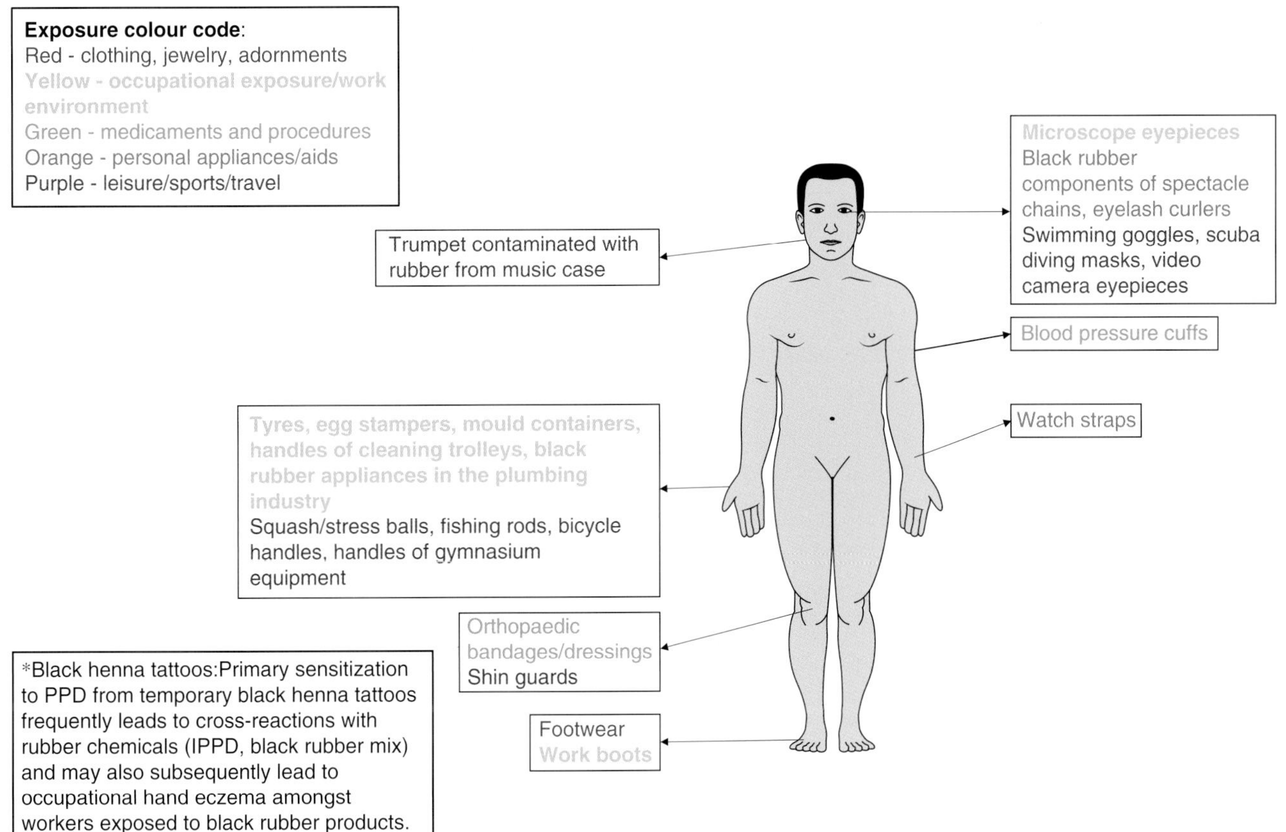

Figure 24.5 Reported exposure sources for ACD to black rubber.

no T-cell clone was detected. Patch tests showed positive reactions to multiple clothing azo dyes and to diphenylguanidine, which was assumed to be present in clothing elastic [26]. The rash resolved on wearing white non-elastic undergarments.

- *Erythema multiforme-like CD*: A 38-year-old woman, after using new rubber gloves for housework, developed erythematous plaques, 1 to 1.5 cm with some showing targetoid features on the dorsal and ventral aspects of the hand and lower third of the forearm, in keeping with a glove distribution [27]. There were strongly positive patch tests (++/+++) to both thiuram and carbamates. Secondary spread of rubber ACD with erythema multiforme-like lesions has been reported [28].
- *Diapers*: MBT was a component of the elastic border of a diaper causing ACD in an 18-month-old boy. He presented with oozing oval to linear erythematous plaques on his upper thighs, lower abdomen, and genital area. Patch test results at 72 hours showed positive reactions to MBT and mercapto mix [29].
- *Pesticide, Koebnerising of psoriasis*: A Koebnerizing psoriasis on the forearm spreading to the trunk from occupational contact dermatitis to thiuram contained in a seed protectant at a concentration of 32% was reported in a greenhouse worker [30]. The positive patch test to thiuram also koebnerised into psoriasis.
- *Possible Koebnerising of pemphigus*: It has been reported that ACD to thiuram may induce pemphigus. A 42-year-old woman developed vesiculopustular and crusted lesions due to ACD to thiurams in rubber gloves worn by her carer to apply emollients and topical corticosteroids. This patient also had mild superficial acantholysis, specific pemphigus autoantibodies as well as weak serum positivity to desmogleins 1 and 3 [31] *(Note: This may represent the koebnerisation of pemphigus [32].)*
- *Music case*: A 12-year-old boy presented with recurrent lip swelling after playing the cornet and trumpet. The instrument cases contained blue and black lined rubber foam. Patch testing showed +++ to PPD, ++ to thiuram mix, and + to IPPD. The original sensitization exposure may have derived from a previous henna beach tattoo, with PPD from the tattoo dye, IPPD as a cross-reaction, and thiuram from adhesive application as a tackifier immediately prior to the tattoo application [33].
- Use of stick-on rubber stencils, in order to apply designs more easily, is a technique of henna tattooing. Patients can therefore be not only sensitized to PPD, but also to thiuram, natural rubber latex, and colophonium [34, 35].
- *Disulfiram allergy (TETD) cross-reacting with trimethylthiuram disulfide (TMTD)*: Three alcoholic patients developed nonhealing wounds followed by dermatitis at the implant sites of *disulfiram*, which is used to treat alcoholism. They subsequently

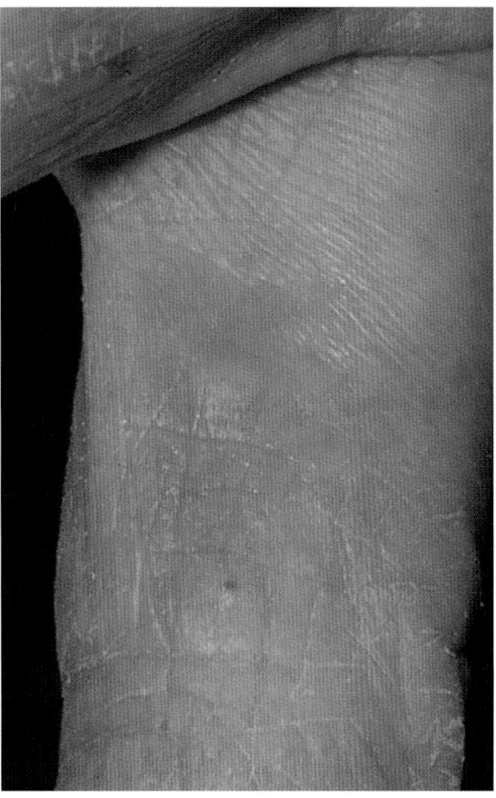

Figure 24.6 Allergic urticarial reaction to latex.

went on to develop ACD reactions to gloves and thiuram pesticide spray (airborne CD) [36].

- *Genital ACD from condoms*: A 32-year-old construction worker had a history of glove dermatitis. Use of condoms resulted in severe contact dermatitis of the penis within 24 hours which lasted for several days. He was patch test positive to thiuram. A 30-year-old female teacher was treated by her gynecologist for recurrent vulvovaginitis. An itchy dermatitis of the vulva and vagina with discharge usually started 24 hours after intercourse if a condom was used by her partner. With no condom, no symptoms occurred. She was patch test positive to thiuram [37].
- *Purpuric CD*: A presumed TMTD-induced Henoch–Schonlein purpura was reported in a 23-year-old Mexican male tree planter. The illness coincided with workplace exposure to tree seedlings treated with a solution of 42% TMTD, although patch testing was not performed [38].
- *Nodular CD*: A 57-year-old cleaner presenting with linear lichenified nodules on the back of the hands caused by ACD to thiuram in gloves was reported [39].
- *Erythroderma*: A 50-year-old acromegalic woman presented with recurrent erythrodermic psoriasis caused by ACD to thiuram in nurses' rubber gloves during the application of topical agents. The patient suffered from psoriasis for 18 years prior to two occasions of severe erythrodermic flare-ups during each admission. Patch testing showed +++ reactions to thiuram mix and to a piece of the nurses' rubber gloves, while prick tests and specific IgE tests to latex were negative [40].
- *Contact urticaria* from thiuram was suspected in a surgical assistant who developed hand swelling and itching 15–20 minutes after wearing rubber gloves. Patch testing revealed positive reactions to thiuram mix, TMTD, TMTM, and a piece of the glove. Open and closed immediate tests with the rubber series and latex were negative [41] (Figure 24.6).
- *Airborne and distal site dermatitis*: [42] A nurse presented with work-related periorbital and glabella dermatitis caused by the airborne spread of rubber accelerators transported by powder starch. Patch tests revealed ++ reactions to TMTM, TMTD, TETD, CBS, MBTS, MOR, and surgical gloves. A prick test to latex was negative [43]. Another case of airborne ACD to thiuram presenting with hand eczema and persistent periorbital dermatitis was reported in a dental technician [44].
- *Facial dermatitis*: A recent study found that rubber accelerator allergy was not only associated with hand involvement, an occupational setting and age over 40 years but also facial involvement. The authors speculate that indirect contact (i.e. manual transmission/hand to face) or even airborne contact may contribute [45].

ACD to thioureas

ACD to thioureas is uncommon. Contact allergy to thiourea was detected in 1% of patients when added to a baseline patch test screen [46]. Eczematous lesions localized to the contact sites or a generalized skin eruption are possible manifestations [47]. Photodermatitis has also been reported. Occupational airborne ACD from dibutylthiourea has been reported in a polyurethane machine operator and a laboratory technician [48]. One survey of thiourea ACD found that the most common sources of sensitization included various neoprene-containing orthopedic braces, sports equipment, and footwear [49].

- rubber latex, and colophonium [34, 35].

ACD to black rubber/IPPD: case reports

Many reported cases are occupational. There are individual case reports of ACD to IPPD/black rubber from tires, shoes, boots, video camera and microscope eyepieces, a stamping device, swimming goggles, handlebars, black rubber parts of a spectacle chain, orthopedic bandages, a fishing rod and elastics (Figure 24.5).

- *Tires*: Among 1798 rubber factory employees (tires and shoes), 50 workers were given compensation for skin problems, 21 for ACD. 14 of these were ACD to black rubber chemicals. The main causes of irritant/toxic dermatitis were solvents (16 cases) and handling bulk rubber (6 cases) [50].
- A 67-year-old retired railworker developed pigmentation and purpura on the volar aspects of the wrists spreading over the following months to both ring fingers. There was also

well-defined erythema over the back of both hands. Patch testing was ++ to IPPD and other rubber chemicals. The authors speculated that the sensitization to black rubber came from exposure to tires [51].

- *Boots*: Shortly after wearing boots, a patient developed an eczematous and purpuric eruption over the dorsa and soles of his feet. Patch testing was positive for both thioureas (synthetic rubber) and IPPD (++) [52].
- *Black rubber eyepieces*: A patient developed an edematous vesiculobullous dermatitis on the periocular region a few hours after using a video camera with a black rubber eyepiece. Patch testing was positive to IPPD [53]. A 24-year-old laboratory technician developed bilateral periorbital dermatitis 8 months after working with microscopes with black rubber eyepieces. Patch testing was ++ to IPPD, other black rubber chemicals, and the eye piece [54].
- *Plumbing*: A 22-year-old man started work in the plumbing business which involved handling, amongst other agents, black rubber appliances. After 3 months, he developed hand eczema which spread to his arms, hands, and feet. It transpired that he had previously had a severe inflammatory skin reaction to a temporary "henna" beach tattoo, through which he was presumably sensitized to PPD. This then cross-reacted with black rubber, which led to occupational dermatitis. Patch testing to IPPD and other black rubber chemicals showed positive results (++) [55].
- *Bicycle handles*: A 10-year-old non-atopic boy presented with a history of severe erythematous pruritic vesicular lesions on the flexural aspects of his fingers and on the palmar region of his hands. The lesions had started 2 years ago after 2–3 weeks' intensive use of a new bicycle with black rubber handles. When he stopped using the bicycle, his hand eczema would resolve with topical steroids. The patient also suffered from palmar hyperhidrosis. Patch testing was positive (++) to IPPD [56]. *(Note: ACD to black rubber in the rubber handles of gymnasium equipment has personally been observed; ACD to diethylthiourea from a rubber handle of a cleaning trolley has also been described [57].)*
- *Shin guards*: Of a series of eight patients with shin guard dermatitis, one was allergic to black rubber. Other rubber allergens in this series included mercapto mix, carbas, and thioureas [58].
- *Egg stamper*: A 66-year-old right-handed man developed bilateral hyperkeratotic and lichenoid dermatitis of both his hands and lower arms. The dermatitis started 2 years after working at an egg-stamper factory where he continually handled a stamper made of black rubber. Patch testing to IPPD was positive (++) [59].
- *Footwear*: An Indian study of 155 patients with footwear dermatitis found that 20% were positive to black rubber mix; however, a third were also patch test + to PPD so some of these cases could be due to cross-reactivity with PPD *(Note: Even with some cases of cross reactivity this level of black rubber allergy is much higher than in European studies, where ACD to black rubber in footwear is uncommon [60].)*
- *Mold container*: An 18-year-old technician developed hyperkeratotic dermatitis on the left palm, limited to an area in repeated contact with a container made of black rubber in which he prepared molds. Patch testing was ++ to IPPD and black rubber chemicals. Thin-layer chromatographic analysis of the mold confirmed the presence of black rubber chemicals, and the dermatitis cleared after avoidance of exposure to the container [61].
- *Swimming goggles*: A 64-year-old presented with severe dermatitis of the eyelids and periorbital areas related to the use of swimming goggles with black rubber. Patch testing to the material was strongly positive (+++) [62].
- *Scuba diving mask*: A series of patients were seen with ACD to the black rubber of their scuba diving masks. The dermatitis involved the peripheral parts of the face in contact with the mask, sparing the central part of the face including the eyes and nose [63].
- *Spectacle chain*: A 42-year-old woman presented with facial dermatitis corresponding to where she wore a black rubber part of a spectacle chain. Patch tests were positive to IPPD and other black rubber chemicals [64].
- *Underwear elastic*: Nine females developed purpuric dermatitis correlating with exposure to underwear elastic. All were positive to IPPD and the elastic material on patch testing [65]. *(Note: This may be of historical interest only as IPPD allergy from underwear exposure has not been reported recently.)*
- *Watch strap*: A 33-year-old woman presented with vesicular eczema on her left wrist, correlating with the areas of contact with a black rubber watch strap. This occurred 2–3 weeks after she started wearing the watch. The only positive reaction on patch testing was to IPPD (++). Chemical analysis of the watch revealed that it contained IPPD [66]. In an earlier report of four cases of ACD to black rubber watch straps, IPPD was positive in only two cases but all four had positive patch tests to black rubber mix [67].
- *Fishing rod*: A 28-year-old man complained of right palmar dermatitis on four occasions, each starting after prolonged (approximately 4 hours) handling of a carbon-fiber fishing rod. He was strongly positive (+++) to IPPD and was also positive (+) to aminoazobenzene [68].
- *Lymphomatoid-like CD*: Two cases of ACD to IPPD presenting as lymphomatoid contact dermatitis have been reported [69]. Both patients presented with bilateral plaques confined to the temples and the black rubber exposure was from the chain of their spectacles.
- *Orthopedic dressing*: A 51-year-old male underwent a knee operation, then wore a textile bandage padded with black neoprene-like rubber. He was patch test positive (++) to IPPD. Mass spectrometry confirmed that the material did indeed contain IPPD [70].
- *Blood pressure cuff*: A single documented case of ACD to a blood pressure cuff from black rubber, the dermatitis developing at site of direct contact [71].
- *Black henna tattoos*: Primary sensitization to PPD from temporary black henna tattoos frequently leads to cross-reactions

with rubber chemicals (IPPD, black rubber mix [72]) and may also subsequently lead to occupational hand eczema amongst workers exposed to black rubber products [55].

- *Squash ball*: ACD to black rubber in a squash ball can present with dermatitis of the central palm in the non-dominant hand [73].
- *Bullous patch test reaction*: A 59-year-old bee keeper was diagnosed with ACD to IPPD in rubber boots and a bench covered with a piece of old tire. Patch tests had to be removed after 12 hours because of a severe bullous reaction to IPPD [74].
- *Eyelash curler*: Although ACD to eyelash curlers is usually caused by nickel, allergic reactions to the rubber component, including the black rubber chemical, can occur, with a clinical presentation of eyelid dermatitis [75].
- *"Stress ball"*: A 55-year-old secretary working at a ceramics factory presented with right-handed dermatitis spreading to the palmar areas of both hands. Patch testing found a + reaction to IPPD only. Further questioning revealed that she had used a black rubber "kidney" pattern material as a "stress ball," squeezing the material between her fingers during coffee breaks. The "kidneys" were formally used by the production workers to smooth decorative designs onto ceramic products [2].

Advice for individuals sensitized to rubber chemicals

Gloves: accelerator free gloves, vinyl gloves, leather gloves.

Shoes

Moccasins that are made entirely of leather without an inner or outer sole.

100% leather shoes.

Allergens may be leached, in particular, from older worn parts of shoes or in patients with hyperhidrosis.

Other tips include wearing cork insoles and discarding contaminated hosiery which could otherwise perpetuate the dermatitis.

Accelerator-free.

Clothing

Spandex products, Lycra, Blue C, Vyrene, or Nurma.

Condom: "Avanti".

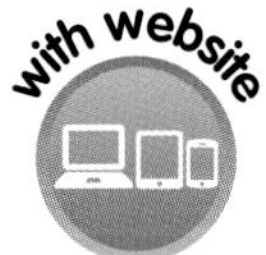

Go to www.wiley.com/go/mcfadden/common_contact_allergens to find the E-supplement for this chapter:

Rubber: E-Supplement

References

1 Adams, A.K. and Yiannias, J.A. (2008). Mercaptobenzothiazole and mercapto mix. *Dermatitis* 19 (5): E39–E41.

2 Lewis, V.J., Hughes, T.M., and Stone, N.M. (2006). Occupational allergic contact dermatitis to N-isopropyl-N-phenyl-p-phenylenediamine from a black rubber 'kidney' used in the ceramics industry. *Contact Dermatitis* 55 (4): 250–251.

3 Chen, H.H., Sun, C.C., and Tseng, M.P. (2004). Type IV hypersensitivity from rubber chemicals: a 15-year experience in Taiwan. *Dermatology* 208 (4): 319–325.

4 Adams, A.K. and Warshaw, E.M. (2006). Allergic contact dermatitis from mercapto compounds. *Dermatitis* 17 (2): 56–70.

5 Nedorost, S. (2009). Clinical patterns of hand and foot dermatitis: emphasis on rubber and chromate allergens. *Dermatologic Clinics* 27 (3): 281–287, vi.

6 Wilson, H.T. (1960). Rubber-glove dermatitis. *British Medical Journal* 2 (5191): 21–23.

7 Knudsen, B.B. and Menne, T. (1996). Contact allergy and exposure patterns to thiurams and carbamates in consecutive patients. *Contact Dermatitis* 35 (2): 97–99.

8 Depree, G.J., Bledsoe, T.A., and Siegel, P.D. (2005). Survey of sulfur-containing rubber accelerator levels in latex and nitrile exam gloves. *Contact Dermatitis* 53 (2): 107–113.

9 Cao, L.Y., Taylor, J.S., Sood, A. et al. (2010). Allergic contact dermatitis to synthetic rubber gloves: changing trends in patch test reactions to accelerators. *Archives of Dermatology* 146 (9): 1001–1007.

10 Bergendorff, O., Persson, C., and Hansson, C. (2006). High-performance liquid chromatography analysis of rubber allergens in protective gloves used in health care. *Contact Dermatitis* 55 (4): 210–215.

11 Freeman, S. (1997). Shoe dermatitis. *Contact Dermatitis* 36 (5): 247–251.

12 Darling, M.I., Horn, H.M., McCormack, S.K., and Schofield, O.M. (2012). Sole dermatitis in children: patch testing revisited. *Pediatric Dermatology* 29 (3): 254–257.

13 Lear, J.T. and English, J.S. (1996). Hand involvement in allergic contact dermatitis from mercaptobenzothiazole in shoes. *Contact Dermatitis* 34 (6): 432.

14 Bensefa-Colas, L., Telle-Lamberton, M., Faye, S. et al. (2015). Occupational contact urticaria: lessons from the French National Network for Occupational Disease Vigilance and Prevention (RNV3P). *British Journal of Dermatology* 173 (6): 1453–1461.

15 Rietschel, R.L., Mathias, C.G., Fowler, J.F. Jr. et al. (2002). Relationship of occupation to contact dermatitis: evaluation in patients tested from 1998 to 2000. *American Journal of Contact Dermatitis* 13 (4): 170–176.

16 Suneja, T. and Belsito, D.V. (2008). Occupational dermatoses in health care workers evaluated for suspected allergic contact dermatitis. *Contact Dermatitis* 58 (5): 285–290.

17 Foussereau, J. and Cavelier, C. (1977). Has N-isopropyl-N'-phenylparaphenylenediamine a place among standard allergens? Importance of this allergen in rubber intolerance. *Dermatologica* 155 (3): 164–167.

18 Bach, R.O., Thormann, H., and Christensen, L.P. (2016). Occupational periorbital allergic contact dermatitis caused by antioxidants in black rubber in an otorhinolaryngologist using an otomicroscope. *Contact Dermatitis* 74 (2): 117–119.

19 Pfohler, C., Korner, R., Muller, C.S., and Vogt, T. (2011). Occupational allergic contact dermatitis of the ears caused by thiurams in a headset. *Contact Dermatitis* 65 (4): 242–243.

20 Adams, R.M. (1982). Contact allergic dermatitis due to diethylthiourea in a wetsuit. *Contact Dermatitis* 8 (4): 277–278.

21 Bruze, M. and Kestrup, L. (1994). Occupational allergic contact dermatitis from diphenylguanidine in a gas mask. *Contact Dermatitis* 31 (2): 125–126.

22 Yilmaz, B., Courvoisier, S., and Bircher, A.J. (1999). Thiuram-elicited contact dermatitis mistaken for local anesthetic intolerance. *Contact Dermatitis* 41 (5): 301–302.

23 Schwensen, J.F., Menne, T., Hald, M. et al. (2016). Allergic perioral contact dermatitis caused by rubber chemicals during dental treatment. *Contact Dermatitis* 74 (2): 110–111.

24 Kruis-de Vries, M.H., Coenraads, P.J., and Nater, J.P. (1987). Allergic contact dermatitis due to rubber chemicals in haemodialysis equipment. *Contact Dermatitis* 17 (5): 303–305.

25 Cravo, M., Goncalo, M., and Figueiredo, A. (2008). Allergic contact dermatitis to rubber-containing bandages in patients with leg ulcers. *Contact Dermatitis* 58 (6): 371–372.

26 Hession, M.T. and Scheinman, P.L. (2010). Lymphomatoid allergic contact dermatitis mimicking cutaneous T cell lymphoma. *Dermatitis* 21 (4): 220.

27 Lu, C.Y. and Sun, C.C. (2001). Localized erythema-multiforme-like contact dermatitis from rubber gloves. *Contact Dermatitis* 45 (5): 311–312.

28 Bara, C., Milpied, B., Geraut, C., and Stalder, J.F. (2003). Erythema multiforme with occupational rubber contact sensitivity. *Contact Dermatitis* 49 (5): 269–270.

29 Onken, A.T., Baumstark, J., Belloni, B. et al. (2011). Atypical diaper dermatitis: contact allergy to mercapto compounds. *Pediatric Dermatology* 28 (6): 739–741.

30 Spiewak, R. (2004). Kobnerizing occupational contact allergy to thiuram in a farmer with psoriasis. *Contact Dermatitis* 51 (4): 214–215.

31 Gallo, R., Massone, C., Parodi, A., and Guarrera, M. (2002). Allergic contact dermatitis from thiurams with pemphigus-like autoantibodies. *Contact Dermatitis* 46 (6): 364–365.

32 Balighi, K., Daneshpazhooh, M., Azizpour, A. et al. (2016). Koebner phenomenon in pemphigus vulgaris patients. *JAAD Case Reports* 2 (5): 419–421.

33 Hallai, N., Meirion Hughes, T., and Stone, N. (2004). Contact allergy to thiuram in a musician. *Contact Dermatitis* 51 (3): 154.

34 Lim, S.P., Prais, L., and Foulds, I.S. (2004). Henna tattoos for children: a potential source of para-phenylenediamine and thiuram sensitization. *British Journal of Dermatology* 151 (6): 1271.

35 Martin, J.A., Hughes, T.M., and Stone, N.M. (2005). 'Black henna' tattoos: an occult source of natural rubber latex allergy? *Contact Dermatitis* 52 (3): 145–146.

36 Rebandel, P. and Rudzki, E. (1996). Secondary contact sensitivity to TMTD in patients primarily positive to TETD. *Contact Dermatitis* 35 (1): 48.

37 Bircher, A.J., Hirsbrunner, P., and Langauer, S. (1993). Allergic contact dermatitis of the genitals from rubber additives in condoms. *Contact Dermatitis* 28 (2): 125–126.

38 Duell, P.B. and Morton, W.E. (1987). Henoch–Schonlein purpura following thiram exposure. *Archives of Internal Medicine* 147 (4): 778–779.

39 Wedgeworth, E.K., Banerjee, P., and White, I.R. (2009). Linear lichenified nodules in a case of thiuram allergy. *Contact Dermatitis* 60 (3): 181–182.

40 Pagliaro, J.A. and Jones, S.K. (1999). Recurrent erythrodermic psoriasis in a thiuram-allergic patient due to contact with nurses' rubber gloves. *British Journal of Dermatology* 140 (3): 567–568.

41 Van Ketel, W.G. (1984). Contact urticaria from rubber gloves after dermatitis from thiurams. *Contact Dermatitis* 11 (5): 323–324.

42 Swinnen, I. and Goossens, A. (2013). An update on airborne contact dermatitis: 2007–2011. *Contact Dermatitis* 68 (4): 232–238.

43 Jensen, P., Menne, T., and Thyssen, J.P. (2011). Allergic contact dermatitis in a nurse caused by airborne rubber additives. *Contact Dermatitis* 65 (1): 54–55.

44 Schwensen, J.F., Menne, T., Johansen, J.D., and Thyssen, J.P. (2015). Persistent periorbital allergic contact dermatitis in a dental technician caused by airborne thiuram exposure. *Contact Dermatitis* 73 (5): 321–322.

45 Schwensen, J.F., Menne, T., Johansen, J.D., and Thyssen, J.P. (2016). Contact allergy to rubber accelerators remains prevalent: retrospective results from a tertiary clinic suggesting an association with facial dermatitis. *Journal of the European Academy of Dermatology and Venereology* 30 (10): 1768–1773.

46 Warshaw, E.M., Cook, J.W., Belsito, D.V. et al. (2008). Positive patch-test reactions to mixed dialkyl thioureas: cross-sectional data from the North American Contact Dermatitis Group, 1994 to 2004. *Dermatitis* 19 (4): 190–201.

47 Martinez-Gonzalez, M.C., Goday-Bujan, J.J., Almagro, M., and Fonseca, E. (2009). Allergic contact dermatitis to diethylthiourea in a neoprene wader. *Actas Dermo-Sifiliográficas* 100 (4): 317–320.

48 Kanerva, L., Estlander, T., Alanko, K., and Jolanki, R. (1998). Occupational airborne allergic contact dermatitis from dibutylthiourea. *Contact Dermatitis* 38 (6): 347–348.

49 Liippo, J., Ackermann, L., Hasan, T. et al. (2010). Sensitization to thiourea derivatives among Finnish patients with suspected contact dermatitis. *Contact Dermatitis* 63 (1): 37–41.

50 Kilpikari, I. (1982). Occupational contact dermatitis among rubber workers. *Contact Dermatitis* 8 (6): 359–362.

51 Roed-Petersen, J., Clemmensen, O.J., Menne, T., and Larsen, E. (1988). Purpuric contact dermatitis from black rubber chemicals. *Contact Dermatitis* 18 (3): 166–168.

52 Romaguera, C., Grimalt, F., and Vilaplana, J. (1989). Eczematous and purpuric allergic contact dermatitis from boots. *Contact Dermatitis* 21 (4): 269.

53 Soto, J., Vazquez, F.J., Yu, A. et al. (1989). Contact dermatitis by sensitization to amine-type antioxidants. *Allergologia et Immunopathologia* 17 (5): 263–265.

54 Kuijpers, D.I., Hillen, F., and Frank, J.A. (2006). Occupational periocular contact dermatitis due to sensitization against black rubber components of a microscope. *Contact Dermatitis* 55 (2): 77–80.

55 Hald, M., Menne, T., Johansen, J.D., and Zachariae, C. (2013). Severe occupational contact dermatitis caused by black rubber as a consequence of p-phenylenediamine allergy resulting from a temporary henna tattoo. *Contact Dermatitis* 68 (6): 377–379.

56 Ozkaya, E. and Elinc-Aslan, M.S. (2011). Black rubber sensitization by bicycle handgrips in a child with palmar hyperhidrosis. *Dermatitis* 22 (4): E10–E12.

57 Liippo, J., Ackermann, L., and Lammintausta, K. (2011). Occupational allergic contact dermatitis caused by diethylthiourea in a neoprene handle of a cleaning trolley. *Contact Dermatitis* 64 (6): 359–360.

58 Powell, D. and Ahmed, S. (2010). Soccer shin guard reactions: allergic and irritant reactions. *Dermatitis* 21 (3): 162–166.

59 Kroft, E.B. and van der Valk, P.G. (2008). Occupational contact dermatitis of both hands because of sensitization of black rubber. *Contact Dermatitis* 58 (2): 125–126.

60 Chowdhuri, S. and Ghosh, S. (2007). Epidemio-allergological study in 155 cases of footwear dermatitis. *Indian Journal of Dermatology, Venereology and Leprology* 73 (5): 319–322.

61 Conde-Salazar, L., Valks, R., Acebes, C.G., and Berto, J. (2004). Occupational allergic contact dermatitis from antioxidant amines in a dental technician. *Dermatitis* 15 (4): 197–200.

62 Vaswani, S.K., Collins, D.D., and Pass, C.J. (2003). Severe allergic contact eyelid dermatitis caused by swimming goggles. *Annals of Allergy, Asthma & Immunology* 90 (6): 672–673.

63 Maibach, H. (1975). Scuba diver facial dermatitis: allergic contact dermatitis to N-isopropyl-N-phenylpara-phenylenediamine. *Contact Dermatitis* 1 (5): 330.

64 Conde-Salazar, L., Guimaraens, D., Romero, L.V., and Gonzalez, M.A. (1987). Unusual allergic contact dermatitis to aromatic amines. *Contact Dermatitis* 17 (1): 42–44.

65 Batschvarov, B. and Minkov, D.M. (1968). Dermatitis and purpura from rubber in clothing. *Transactions of the St. John's Hospital Dermatological Society* 54 (2): 178–182.

66 Foussereau, J., Cavelier, C., and Protois, J.C. (1988). A case of allergic isopropyl-p-phenylenediamine (IPPD) dermatitis from a watch strap. *Contact Dermatitis* 18 (4): 253.

67 Romaguera, C., Aguirre, A., Diaz Perez, J.L., and Grimalt, F. (1986). Watch strap dermatitis. *Contact Dermatitis* 14 (4): 260–261.

68 Minciullo, P.L., Patafi, M., Ferlazzo, B., and Gangemi, S. (2004). Contact dermatitis from a fishing rod. *Contact Dermatitis* 50 (5): 322.

69 Marliere, V., Beylot-Barry, M., Doutre, M.S. et al. (1998). Lymphomatoid contact dermatitis caused by isopropyl-diphenylenediamine: two cases. *Journal of Allergy and Clinical Immunology* 102 (1): 152–153.

70 Carlsen, L., Andersen, K.E., and Egsgaard, H. (1987). IPPD contact allergy from an orthopedic bandage. *Contact Dermatitis* 17 (2): 119–121.

71 Milanesi, N., Francalanci, S., Gola, M. et al. (2013). Allergic contact dermatitis caused by a blood pressure cuff. *Journal of the American Academy of Dermatology* 69 (6): e301–e302.

72 de Groot, A.C. (2013). Side-effects of henna and semi-permanent 'black henna' tattoos: a full review. *Contact Dermatitis* 69 (1): 1–25.

73 Cronin E (1973). Squash ball dermatitis. *Contact Dermatitis* 13: 365–365.

74 Rudzki, E. and Rebandel, P. (2000). Sensitivity to IPPD diagnosed a posteriori. *Contact Dermatitis* 43 (6): 361.

75 Vestey, J.P., Buxton, P.K., and Savin, J.A. (1985). Eyelash curler dermatitis. *Contact Dermatitis* 13 (4): 274–275.

Exposure Color Code

- Clothing, jewelry, adornments
- Personal care products, cosmetics/cosmetic procedures
- Household products, domestic environment, including furniture and refurbishment
- Occupational dermatoses, work environment
- Medicines, surgical/dental procedures, herbal/alternative medicines
- Personal appliances/aids
- Leisure activities, sport, travel
- Other exposures (including dietary)
- Not relevant or multiple/general exposure

CHAPTER 25

Colophonium

CHAPTER CONTENTS

Key points

- Colophonium, a naturally occurring resin obtained from pine trees, is the base of many glues and adhesives.
- It is used in adhesives, cosmetics, plasticisers, fabric, finishers, varnishes, and waxes. It is also found in the protective coatings of glossy and photographic papers.
- A history of reacting to 'fabric plasters' usually indicates colophonium allergy.
- People at risk of colophonium allergy include wood workers, administrative workers, and users of cosmetics.
- There are three types: gum rosin, wood rosin, and tall oil rosin.
- Unmodified gum rosin is the material that is mainly used in the baseline series.
- Abitol is the most common modified colophonium used in cosmetics. Tall oil is used in some shampoos. Colophonium/modified colophonium is used in some lipsticks and eye cosmetics such as mascara.
- The relevance of positive reactions can sometimes be difficult to explain because of its widespread use.
- Recycled and mechanical pulp-manufactured paper as well as garden conifers may increase exposure to colophonium.
- Machinists are exposed to colophonium tall oil in cutting oils.
- Can be a marker of fragrance allergy.
- Allergic contact dermatitis (ACD) to colophonium can present as shoe dermatitis either from its use as a tackifier in shoe linings or as part of the leather finishing process.
- ACD to colophonium in violinists can present on the fingers, neck, chest, or jawline from either the application of or exposure to violin rosin.
- ACD to colophonium can occur in the context of leg ulcers due to exposure to hydrocolloid dressings containing the modified colophonium "pentaerythritol ester of rosin."
- Airborne ACD to colophonium can occur in woodworkers from exposure to pine wood dust, and in construction workers from exposure to soldering fumes.
- Some translucent soaps, polishes, and hair-removing waxes contain colophonium.
- Some sanitary pads contain colophonium and have been reported to cause ACD.
- Patients allergic to colophonium need to avoid its modified fractions including abitol (dihydroabietyl alcohol), abietic acid, dehydroabietic acid, tall oil, rosin, and glycerol ester of hydrogenated rosin/abietic acid.

Common Contact Allergens: A Practical Guide to Detecting Contact Dermatitis, First Edition. Edited by John McFadden, Pailin Puangpet, Korbkarn Pongpairoj, Supitchaya Thaiwat, and Lee Shan Xian.
© 2020 John Wiley & Sons Ltd. Published 2020 by John Wiley & Sons Ltd.
Companion website: www.wiley.com/go/mcfadden/common_contact_allergens

Exposure and use

Colophonium, a naturally occurring resin obtained from pine trees, is the natural base of many glues and adhesives [1]. It is used in a wide variety of agents, leading to diverse forms of ACD (Figures 25.1–25.4).

Uses of unmodified colophonium

Uses of unmodified colophonium include soldering fluxes, soaps, cutting fluids (these form a layer on the surface of the machining metal due to their polarity to reduce friction and cool the metal), insulation material to hold components in place in electronic equipment, adhesives, powder used by baseball pitchers to obtain a better grip on the ball (mixed with magnesium carbonate), drossing compounds (substances used to remove scum from molten metal), rosin oil-saturant for paper wrapped cables, depilatory powder, and to manufacture modified rosin [2].

Uses in cosmetic and household goods

- See Figure 25.3.
- Mascaras [3] were found to contain from <0.005% up to 0.7% resin acids [4], lipsticks [5], eyeshadows, concealer creams,

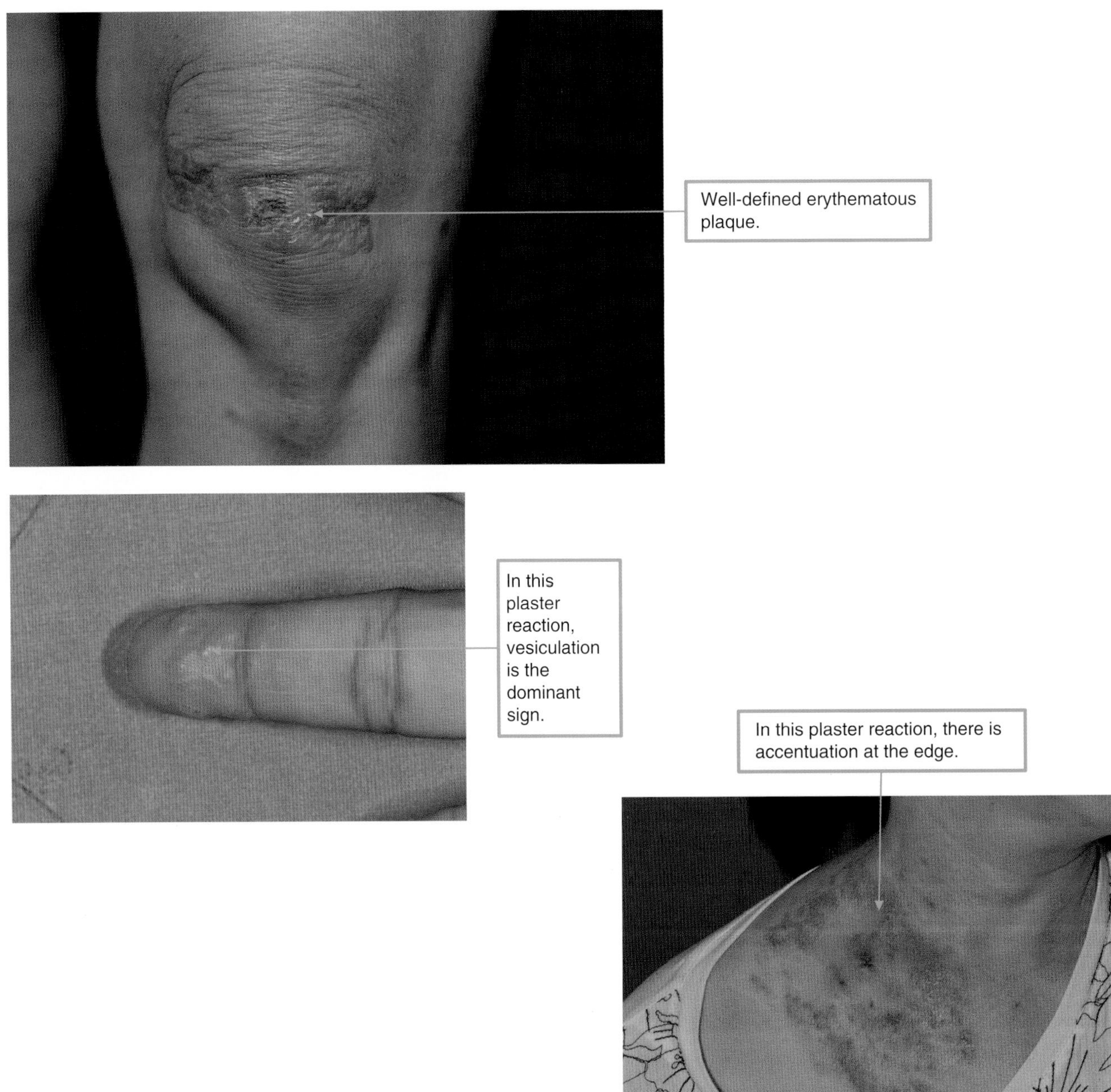

Well-defined erythematous plaque.
In this plaster reaction, vesiculation is the dominant sign.
In this plaster reaction, there is accentuation at the edge.

Figure 25.1 ACD to colophonium from fabric plasters.

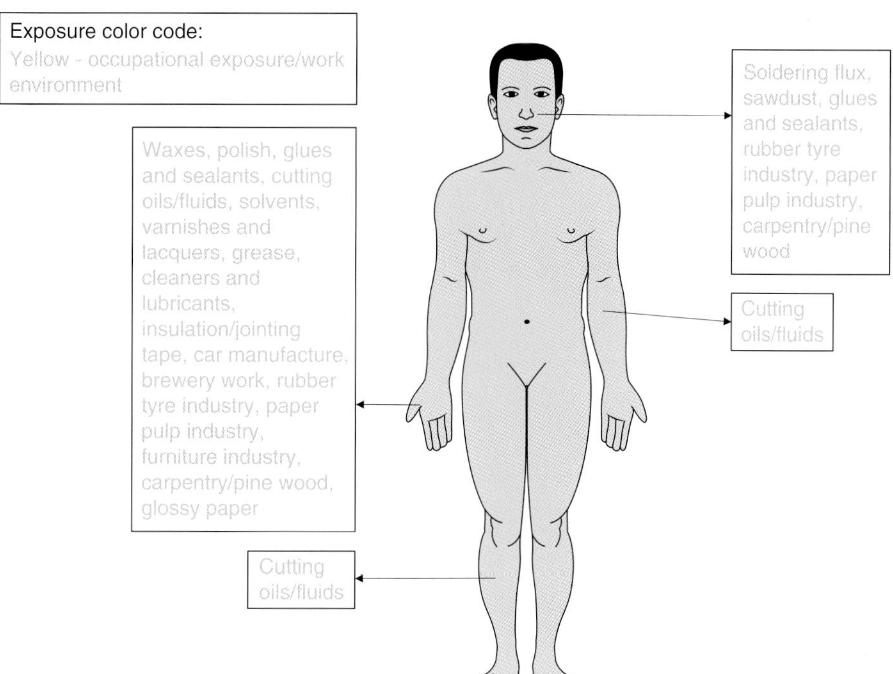

Figure 25.2 Sources of occupational colophonium exposure.

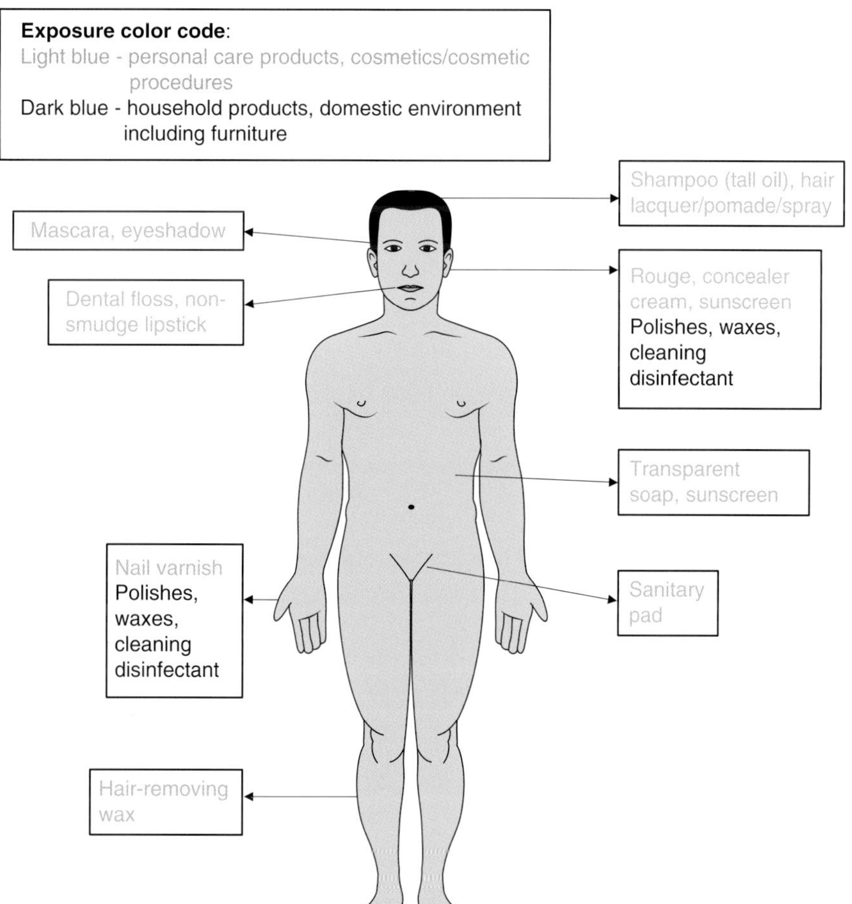

Figure 25.3 Sources of colophonium exposure from personal care products/cosmetics and the domestic environment.

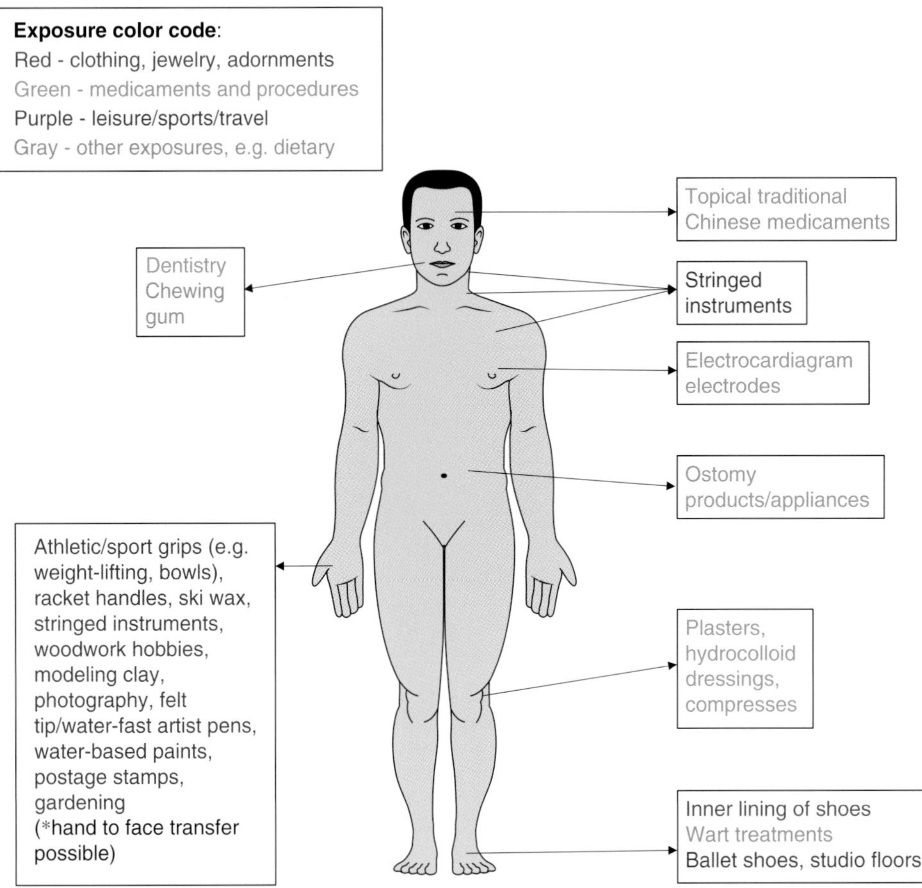

Figure 25.4 Other sources of colophonium exposure.

nail varnish, rouge, soap, shampoo, brilliantine, depilatory waxes [6], hair pomades and sprays, hair lacquer [7].

- Sanitary pads [8]: The highest content of resin acids was 0.056%, corresponding to 0.08% colophonium. Three products had >0.03% colophonium, whereas another four products contained very low levels of colophonium [9].
- Toiletries: transparent soaps, hair-removing wax, dental floss, sunscreens, blister creams and first-aid ointments.
- Household items: grease removers for clothes, shoe wax, polish for floors/cars/furniture, laundry soaps, fly strips.
- Dehydroabietyl alcohol/abitol) is the most common modified colophonium used in cosmetics [3]. There is no restriction on the use of colophonium in cosmetics.
- Colophonium must be declared in concentrations at or above 1% according to the EU legislation on dangerous substances – Annex 1 (Directive 67/548/EEC) and the product must be labeled with the risk phrase R 43 ("may cause sensitization by skin contact") [10].

Non-cosmetic exposure and use

- See Figures 25.2 and 25.4.
- Adhesive products, adhesive tapes, and plasters (salicylic acid plasters, Opsite®).
- Brewery pitch – a resinous compound especially used for coating the insides of beer casks.
- Cars: adhesives in the linings of the roof, doors, and the interior aspects of the dashboard caused airborne ACD [11].
- Caulking compounds (caulking means to fill cracks or crevices, such as windows or in tanks, to make them watertight).
- Lens coating, linoleum, shoe, thermoplastic tiles.
- Chewing gum.
- Christmas trees (the sticky sap).
- Cutting oil and soap water used as cutting fluid [12].
- Cleaners and lubricants (clothing, leather, office machines).
- Dentistry (antiseptics in root canal treatment, dental cements, impression pastes, liquids, and cavity varnishes).
- Dancing: athletic grips, floors of studios, anti-slipping cream for ballet shoes.
- Depilatory agents.
- Disposable diapers: infant, adult incontinence.
- Rosin components (mainly abietic acid and dehydroabietic acid) were detected in all six diapers analyzed using gas chromatography in Sweden. More rosin was found in the top layer than in the fluff. Occlusion and irritation enhance the risk of sensitization [13].
- Fabric finishes (historical) [14].
- Fillers (putty and wood).
- Fireworks – sometimes used as a binder in the fireworks.

- Flexible collodion – a syrupy liquid compound which dries to a transparent, tenacious film; used as a topical protectant, applied to the skin to close small wounds/abrasions/cuts, used to hold surgical dressings in place, and to keep medications in contact with the skin.
- Furniture, untreated pine wood [15].
- Glues, mastics, and sealants.
- Grease and lubricant thickeners, axle grease.
- Grippers for bowls, weight-lifting and sports.
- Insulation tape (electrical and thermal insulating tape).
- Inks (ceramic, marking pens, printing).
- Jointing tape.
- Linoleum (adhesive bedding and cements, floor covering [16], tiles).
- Lottery tickets [17].
- Machine belts (industrial).
- Match tips.
- Medical setting
  - Adhesives of tapes used to approximate the edges of incisions [18]. Tape skin closure (Steri-Strip®, 3M company) has previously contained Foral 85®, a glycerol ester of hydrogenated abietic acid [19]. However, the use of acrylates as an adhesive instead of colophonium is increasing.
  - Compresses [20].
  - ECG electrodes [21].
  - Dressings.
  - Granuflex E is a new formulation of Granuflex. This is a bilaminate, occlusive hydrocolloid dressing that contains pentaerythritol ester of hydrogenated rosin as a tackifying agent to make it adherent to skin. Granuflex E is also known as Duoderm E or Duoderm CGF (controlled gel formula) [22]. The pentaerythritol ester of hydrogenated colophonium, Pentalyn, was found to be a sensitizer in Granuflex E® hydrocolloid dressing, Duoderm CGF, and Duoderm Extrathin® [23] independent of unmodified colophony [24].
  - Sealant in dental prostheses: can cause oral lichen planus [25], impression materials, fluoride varnishes, Cavex® dental baseplate molding materials (an intermediate in making dental prostheses) [26].
  - Topical traditional Chinese medicaments: 5 out of 12 Chinese medicaments causing ACD contained colophonium [27]. Herbal medicated oil, vapor rubs [28].
  - Medicines (e.g. wart removers, cold sore creams, ostomy products, nappy creams, hemorrhoid creams, sprays).
- Modeling clay.
- Newspapers (controversial as to whether there is release).
- Oils (core oil, cutting oil, tall oil).
- Ostomy appliances.
- Water-based paints [29].
- Paper (glossy paper, photographic paper, plastics, price labels, stickers).
- In paper manufacturing, paper made from mechanical pulps that are considered to be environmentally friendly contains more rosin compounds than paper made from chemical pulps. Bleaching the pulp with hydrogen peroxide leads to more oxidized compounds. Recycled and mechanical pulp-manufactured paper may increase the prevalence of colophonium-related hand eczema in the future [30].
- Pens (felt tip, water-fast artist pens).
- Plastics (surface coating) (controversial as to whether there is release).
- Polishes (car, coffee beans, floor [16], furniture, metal, shoe, wood).
- Polyethylene.
- Postage stamps (adhesive).
- Traditional printing (ink, paper, photographs).
- Pruning *X Cupressocyparis leylandii* hedges [31].
- Rubber emulsifier, reclaiming agent in recycling of rubber, tire-compounding (mixing agents in rubber to improve performance).
- Sawdust (pine and spruce) in the furniture industry, woodwork hobbies, animal feeds.
- Sealants.
- Shoes: colophonium in leather tanning, finishing agent in Portuguese leather shoes can contaminate socks [32, 33].
- Clear soaps.
- Soldering flux in the electronics industry [34].
- Solvents.
- Stains (furniture, wood).
- Surface coatings (beer casks, rustproof coating, coatings on price labels, cans, paper).
- Tackifier (athletic/sport grips, sticky fly paper, stringed instruments, dancer's shoes, machine belts, postage stamps, etc.).
- Tapes (industrial, medical).
- Varnishes, lacquers, sealants.
- Veterinary products and medications.
- Waterproofing (cardboard, oil cloth, walls).
- Waxes (stringed musical instruments, car, grafting, floor, furniture, physiotherapy, sealing, shoemakers, ski).
- Recreational (e.g. sport racket handles, athletic grip aids, golf club grips, bows for stringed instruments, fireworks, ski wax).
- Firewood and pine trees in the garden.

Patch testing

Colophonium 20% in petrolatum is included in both the American and European baseline series. Unmodified gum rosin is the material that is mainly used in the baseline series [35]. The worldwide clinic prevalence of colophonium positive patch test reactions is 5.35%.

- The relevance of a positive reaction is sometimes difficult to explain because of its wide usage.
- The rosin mix for the European series has used American, Chinese, and Portuguese unmodified gum rosin [36].

Clinical disease

Case reports

- A 5-year-old girl presented with dermatitis on the heels and forefoot. Positive reactions were shown to unmodified rosin (colophonium 20% pet.) (++) and to the *shoe lining* (++). Linen, impregnated with a modified rosin tackifier, was glued under the leather. A sample of this modified rosin gave a ++ patch test reaction. Gas chromatographic analysis showed that the rosin components in this modified rosin included abietic acid, dehydroabietic acid, and maleopimaric acid (MPA). Patients with positive reactions to modified rosins such as MPA, but not to unmodified rosin in the standard series, have been reported [37].
- A case of *shoe dermatitis* due to colophonium used as *leather finishing* was reported. The patient developed acute vesicular dermatitis on the dorsa of his feet after wearing a new pair of shoes manufactured in Portugal. Patch testing was positive to the upper part of the shoe, colophonium, and ester gum rosin. The Portuguese manufacturer confirmed that gum rosins and tall oils could have been used in the leather-tanning process [33].
- Occupational contact dermatitis from colophonium in German *banknotes* was reported in a bank clerk. He developed squamous dermatitis on the tips of his right thumb and index finger 5 years after he started the job. Patch testing was + to colophonium on day 3 and ++ to formaldehyde and *p*-tert-butylcatechol [38].
- A professional *violinist* presented with a 6-month history of an eczematous eruption with vesiculation on the fingertips of his left hand. Positive patch test reactions were noted to nickel, cobalt, colophonium, his own rosin, neomycin, formaldehyde, and three releasers, as well as shavings from the finished ebony wood. Unfortunately, changing the rosin to a synthetic brand can adversely affect the tone and quality of the music and also affect adhesive friction [39].
- Another violinist had ACD from colophonium, turpentine (cross reaction), ebony, and the lacquer of the violin in the location of fiddler's neck. She presented with eczematous and erosive lesions where the violin touched her neck, jaw, and shoulder. Maleic resins (rosin and maleic anhydride) were used in the varnishes and lacquers. The differential diagnosis was fiddler's neck, an irritant contact dermatitis which is more common [40].
- Two *dental nurses* were diagnosed with occupational ACD of the fingertips and hands from colophonium in fluoride *tooth varnish*, containing 33% colophonium. Patch tests were ++ and +++ to colophonium. This fluoride-based agent was used for the prophylaxis of caries and the treatment of sensitive roots and shooting pains in teeth. Colophonium was added to make it stick but it was not listed in the material safety data sheet [41]. A colophonium-sensitive male patient developed contact stomatitis from a similar exposure [42].
- A *jeweler* involved in washing, dusting, oiling, grinding, *soldering*, and *polishing* precious metals was reported as having contact allergy to colophonium and silver nitrate. He has had a chronic dermatitis on his hands, forearms, and legs for 30 years [43].
- Two cases presented with recurrent painful oral ulcers and burning mouth with associated angioedema. They were diagnosed as ACD to colophonium in *chewing gum*. Patch tests were +++ and ++ to colophonium in each patient. The authors communicated with the company and found that colophony was a constituent of the base of chewing gums, particularly found in Juicy Fruit® and Hubba Bubba® gums [44].
- A 62-year-old female patient with a *venous leg ulcer* developed severe eczema during wound bed preparation with the *hydrocolloid dressing* Varihesive®. Patch tests were positive to the hydrocolloid dressing and colophonium. This dressing contained the pentaerythritol ester of hydrogenated rosin as a tackifying agent [45].
- ACD from a modified colophonium, glyceryl rosinate, in a hydrocolloid wound dressing was reported in a venous ulcer patient. The patient did not react to unmodified colophonium in the baseline series. Patch testing to modified colophonium should be performed when unmodified colophonium is negative [46].
- A 14-year-old Japanese male developed rectangular-shaped severe painful bullous and erythematous macular lesions on the left wrist 7 days after using a *compress*. The compress contained ketoprofen, menthol, and hydrogenated rosin glycerol ester. Patch tests were ++ to hydrogenated rosin glycerol ester and + to menthol. Ketoprofen was positive ++ only in the photopatch test [20].
- *Cross-reaction between colophonium and turpentine* was reported. Both colophonium and turpentine oil are isolated from the resin of pine trees by distillation [40].
- A 33-year-old male was suspected to have developed primary sensitization by accidental skin contact with a *permanent marker* containing colophonium. The patient had no previous history of contact allergy to sticking plaster or adhesives. After this episode, he developed a severe acute vesiculobullous dermatitis on the skin in contact with surgical adhesive tapes [47].
- A case of ACD caused by gum rosin and wood rosin in Tako-no-Sudashi ointment, an *old Japanese over-the-counter medicated ointment* used for pustular disease, was reported. The patient presented with pruritic well-demarcated crusted erythema of the left cheek 4 days after using this ointment. Patch testing showed ++ reactions to Tako-no-Sudashi ointment, gum rosin, and wood rosin on day 3 [48].
- A 13-year-old girl presented with recurrent vulval dermatitis after first using a *sanitary pad*. She had a +++ reaction to colophonium. A sample of the sanitary pad gave a + patch test reaction [49]. Another case report was a 36-year-old female patient who presented with acute facial dermatitis after applying a fragrance-containing moisturizer. She also had reactions to adhesive dressings and a history of intermittent vulval pain during her menstruation periods. Patch tests showed a ++ positive

reaction to colophonium and a + positive reaction to her sanitary pad, *Myroxylon pereirae*, fragrance mix 1, her fragranced moisturizer, lanolin, and neomycin [8].

- A 1-year-old girl presented with ACD at the site of *self-adhesive electrocardiography electrodes*. Patch testing showed ++ positive reactions to colophonium on both day 2 and day 4. In addition, a ++ positive reaction on day 2 and a +++ positive reaction on day 4 were demonstrated at the electrode patch test sites. Glyceryl rosinate and compositae mix also gave positive reactions (+ on day 2 and ++ on day 4) [50].
- ■■■■ ACD from multiple colophonium-related sources in one patient has been reported. The sources included adhesive tape, *depilating wax strips*, rosin for double bass playing, and shoes. The patient also gave positive reactions to instrument wax and garage door wax [51].

Hand to face/neck/trunk contact dermatitis

- An 84-year-old retired nurse presented with a 2-year history of severely pruritic eczematous patches on the face, neck, trunk, and extremities. Patch test was + to colophonium (10%), abietic acid (2%), benzophenone, and benzocaine. This patient bowled frequently and colophony in the form of 'rosin bags' or 'grip sacks' was used to enhance grip. Allergen was transferred from her hands to remote sites, especially the face [52]. *(Note: Colophonium fractions are also included in some nail varnishes.)*

Prognosis

- A 10-year follow-up of colophonium allergic patients showed that 19% had become anergic [53].
- A follow-up study of patients with hand eczema due to colophonium allergy showed that after 9–13 years, ≥ 30% still had hand eczema, 72% were still patch test positive to colophonium, and > 50% had new positive reactions to other allergens [54].

Occupational disease

- Colophonium was the fifth most common cause of occupational hand eczema in Sweden (3.2%). Women in administrative work were found to have a statistically significant increase in contact allergy to colophonium [55].
- Airborne contact dermatitis has been reported in the manufacturing of linoleum floor coverings and milk cartons [16]. An immediate phototoxic reaction was reported in a colophonium-sensitive electrician who presented with chronic facial dermatitis for 10 years. He was routinely exposed to vaporised colophonium from soldering tin threads. Patch testing showed a ++ reaction to colophonium. Photopatch testing showed a +++ reaction in the light-exposed patch of colophonium [56].

Metal workers

- Metal workers with occupational dermatitis and exposure to water-based metal-working fluids had an eightfold increased risk of sensitization to colophony compared to those with occupational dermatitis who were not exposed to metal-working fluids (OR 8.0; 95% CI 1.7–73.5). The content of resin acids in the water-based metal-working fluids was 0.06–0.12% [57].
- Colophonium in metal-working fluids originates mainly from distilled tall oil, which contains 10–30% colophonium. Resin acids of colophonium were detected in 7/15 samples of metal-working fluids, separated by gas chromatography and identified with mass spectrometric detection and ultraviolet detection. The concentrations ranged from 0.41% to 3.8% (median 1.7), whereas the content of resin acids was not declared in any of the safety data sheets [58].

Musicians

- Musicians may be exposed to colophonium in adhesive tapes, rosin, polish, cosmetics, and varnishes. Unmodified colophonium is commonly used by string players (violin, viola, and cello) to wax the strings. Colophony may cause dermatitis of the fingers and hands, face, and neck [59].

Healthcare workers

- An Information Network of Dermatological Clinics (IVDK) retrospective study on occupational contact allergy in nurses (2003–2012) showed a significant increase in colophonium sensitization rate of 3.4% [60].

Type 1 hypersensitivity

- A case of facial *allergic contact urticaria from colophonium in solder flux fume* has been reported by Rivers and Rycroft [61]. This patient was an inspector of printed circuit boards. She developed itching and swelling of the face, upper chest, and arms within 1–2 hours together with transient shortness of breath which subsided by the next day. A prick test with colophonium 20% pet. produced an immediate wheal and flare.
- *Contact urticaria to abietic acid in a sticking plaster* was reported. The lesions occurred within 10–30 minutes and improved within 30 minutes. Patch tests showed a + reaction to colophony at 30 minutes and a ++ reaction to abietic acid at 20 minutes [62].
- However, a retrospective study to evaluate the benefits of prick testing screening in the diagnosis of occupational contact urticaria and airway diseases caused by colophonium could not demonstrate relevant reactions [63].

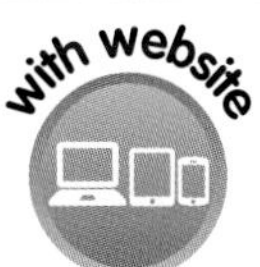

Go to www.wiley.com/go/mcfadden/common_contact_allergens to find the E-supplement for this chapter.

Colophonium: E-Supplement

References

1 Gebhardt, M. and Elsner, P. (2000). *Adhesives and Glues* (eds. L. Kanerva, P. Elsner, J. Wahlberg and H. Maibach). Berlin: Springer.

2 Sadhra, S., Foulds, I.S., Gray, C.N. et al. (1994). Colophony – uses, health effects, airborne measurement and analysis. *Annals of Occupational Hygiene* 38 (4): 385–396.

3 Dooms-Goossens, A., Degreef, H., and Luytens, E. (1979). Dihydroabietyl alcohol (Abitol): a sensitizer in mascara. *Contact Dermatitis* 5 (6): 350–353.

4 Sainio, E.L., Henriks-Eckerman, M.L., and Kanerva, L. (1996). Colophony, formaldehyde and mercury in mascaras. *Contact Dermatitis* 34 (5): 364–365.

5 Batta, K., Bourke, J.F., and Foulds, I.S. (1997). Allergic contact dermatitis from colophony in lipsticks. *Contact Dermatitis* 36 (3): 171–172.

6 de Argila, D., Ortiz-Frutos, J., and Iglesias, L. (1996). Occupational allergic contact dermatitis from colophony in depilatory wax. *Contact Dermatitis* 34 (5): 369.

7 Schwartz, L. (1943). An outbreak of dermatitis from hair lacquer. Public Health Reports (1896–1970) 58 (44): 1623–1625.

8 Wujanto, L. and Wakelin, S. (2012). Allergic contact dermatitis to colophonium in a sanitary pad – an overlooked allergen? *Contact Dermatitis* 66 (3): 161–162.

9 Kanerva, L., Rintala, H., Henriks-Eckerman, K., and Engström, K. (2001). Colophonium in sanitary pads. *Contact Dermatitis* 44 (1): 59–60.

10 Nilsson, U., Berglund, N., Lindahl, F. et al. (2008). SPE and HPLC/UV of resin acids in colophonium-containing products. *Journal of Separation Science* 31 (15): 2784–2790.

11 Danielsen, H. (1999). Airborne allergic contact dermatitis from colophony in a car. *Contact Dermatitis* 41 (1): 51.

12 Fregert, S. (1979). Colophony in cutting oil and in soap water used as cutting fluid. *Contact Dermatitis* 5 (1): 52.

13 Karlberg, A.T. and Magnusson, K. (1996). Rosin components identified in diapers. *Contact Dermatitis* 34 (3): 176–180.

14 Schwartz, L., Spolyar, L.W., and Gastineau, F.M. (1940). An outbreak of dermatitis from new resin fabric finishes. *Journal of the American Medical Association* 115: 906–911.

15 Booken, D., Velten, F.W., Utikal, J. et al. (2006). Allergic contact dermatitis from colophony and turpentine in resins of untreated pine wood. *Der Hautarzt* 57 (11): 1013–1015.

16 Karlberg, A.T., Gafvert, E., Meding, B., and Stenberg, B. (1996). Airborne contact dermatitis from unexpected exposure to rosin (colophony). Rosin sources revealed with chemical analyses. *Contact Dermatitis* 35 (5): 272–278.

17 Pereira, F., Manuel, R., Gäfvert, E., and Lacerda, M.H. (1997). Relapse of colophony dermatitis from lottery tickets. *Contact Dermatitis* 37 (1): 43.

18 James, W.D. (1984). Allergic contact dermatitis to a colophony derivative. *Contact Dermatitis* 10 (1): 6–10.

19 Sjöborg, S. and Fregert, S. (1984). Allergic contact dermatitis from a colophony derivative in a tape skin closure. *Contact Dermatitis* 10 (2): 114–115.

20 Ota, T., Oiso, N., Iba, Y. et al. (2007). Concomitant development of photoallergic contact dermatitis from ketoprofen and allergic contact dermatitis from menthol and rosin (colophony) in a compress. *Contact Dermatitis* 56 (1): 47–48.

21 Machovcova, A. (2011). Colophony, a hidden allergen on ECG electrodes in a boy after cardiovascular surgery. *Pediatric Dermatology* 28 (3): 345–347.

22 Mallon, E. and Powell, S.M. (1994). Allergic contact dermatitis from Granuflex hydrocolloid dressing. *Contact Dermatitis* 30 (2): 110–111.

23 Suhng, E.A., Byun, J.Y., Choi, Y.W. et al. (2011). A case of allergic contact dermatitis due to DuoDERM Extrathin(R). *Annals of Dermatology* 23 (Suppl 3): S387–S389.

24 Downs, A.M., Sharp, L.A., and Sansom, J.E. (1999). Pentaerythritol-esterified gum rosin as a sensitizer in Granuflex hydrocolloid dressing. *Contact Dermatitis* 41 (3): 162–163.

25 Garcia-Bravo, B., Pons, A., and Rodriguez-Pichardo, A. (1992). Oral lichen planus from colophony. *Contact Dermatitis* 26 (4): 279.

26 Cockayne, S.E., Murphy, R., and Gawkrodger, D.J. (2001). Occupational contact dermatitis from colophonium in a dental technician. *Contact Dermatitis* 44 (1): 42–43.

27 Li, L.F. and Wang, J. (2002). Patch testing in allergic contact dermatitis caused by topical Chinese herbal medicine. *Contact Dermatitis* 47 (3): 166–168.

28 Koh, D., Lee, B.L., Ong, H.Y., and Ong, C.N. (1997). Colophony in topical traditional Chinese medicaments. *Contact Dermatitis* 37 (5): 243.

29 Fischer, T., Bohlin, S., Edling, C. et al. (1995). Skin disease and contact sensitivity in house painters using water-based paints, glues and putties. *Contact Dermatitis* 32 (1): 39–45.

30 Karlberg, A.T., Gäfvert, E., and Lidén, C. (1995). Environmentally friendly paper may increase risk of hand eczema in rosin-sensitive persons. *Journal of the American Academy of Dermatology* 33 (3): 427–432.

31 Lovell, C.R., Dannaker, C.J., and White, I.R. (1985). Dermatitis from X *Cupressocyparis leylandii* and concomitant sensitivity to colophony. *Contact Dermatitis* 13 (5): 344–345.

32 Bugnet, L.D., Sanchez-Politta, S., Sorg, O., and Piletta, P. (2008). Allergic contact dermatitis to colophonium-contaminated socks. *Contact Dermatitis* 59 (2): 127 128.

33 Strauss, R.M. and Wilkinson, S.M. (2002). Shoe dermatitis due to colophonium used as leather tanning or finishing agent in Portuguese shoes. *Contact Dermatitis* 47 (1): 59.

34 Goh, C.L. and Ng, S.K. (1987). Airborne contact dermatitis to colophony in soldering flux. *Contact Dermatitis* 17 (2): 89–91.

35 Karlberg, A.T. (1988). Contact allergy to colophony. Chemical identifications of allergens, sensitization experiments and clinical experiences. *Acta Dermato-Venereologica* 139: 1–43.

36 Karlberg, A.T. and Gäfvert, E. (1996). Isolated colophony allergens as screening substances for contact allergy. *Contact Dermatitis* 35 (4): 201–207.

37 Lyon, C.C., Tucker, S.C., Gäfvert, E. et al. (1999). Contact dermatitis from modified rosin in footwear. *Contact Dermatitis* 41 (2): 102–103.

38 Koch, P. (1995). Occupational contact dermatitis from colophony and formaldehyde in banknote paper. *Contact Dermatitis* 32 (6): 371–372.

39 Alvarez, M.S. and Brancaccio, R.R. (2003). Multiple contact allergens in a violinist. *Contact Dermatitis* 49 (1): 43–44.

40 Kuner, N. and Jappe, U. (2004). Allergic contact dermatitis from colophonium, turpentine and ebony in a violinist presenting as fiddler's neck. *Contact Dermatitis* 50 (4): 258–259.

41 Kanerva, L. and Estlander, T. (1999). Occupational allergic contact dermatitis from colophony in 2 dental nurses. *Contact Dermatitis* 41 (6): 342–343.
42 Sharma, P.R. (2006). Allergic contact stomatitis from colophony. *Dental Update* 33 (7): 440–442.
43 Agarwal, S. and Gawkrodger, D.J. (2002). Occupational allergic contact dermatitis to silver and colophonium in a jeweler. *American Journal of Contact Dermatitis* 13 (2): 74.
44 Gupta, G. and Forsyth, A. (1999). Allergic contact reactions to colophony presenting as oral disease. *Contact Dermatitis* 40 (6): 332–333.
45 Körber, A., Kohaus, S., Geisheimer, M. et al. (2006). Allergic contact dermatitis from a hydrocolloid dressing due to colophony sensitization. *Der Hautarzt* 57 (3): 242–245.
46 Pereira, T.M., Flour, M., and Goossens, A. (2007). Allergic contact dermatitis from modified colophonium in wound dressings. *Contact Dermatitis* 56 (1): 5–9.
47 Fesquet, E., Guillot, B., and Raison-Peyron, N. (2006). Allergic contact dermatitis to rosin after a single accidental permanent marker skin contact. *Contact Dermatitis* 55 (1): 58–59.
48 Tsuruta, D., Sowa, J., Tsuruta, K. et al. (2011). Allergic contact dermatitis caused by gum rosin and wood rosin in Tako-no-Suidashi ointment. *The Journal of Dermatology* 38 (10): 993–995.
49 Rademaker, M. (2004). Allergic contact dermatitis to a sanitary pad. *Australasian Journal of Dermatology* 45 (4): 234–235.
50 Deswysen, A.C., Zimerson, E., Goossens, A. et al. (2013). Allergic contact dermatitis caused by self-adhesive electrocardiography electrodes in an infant. *Contact Dermatitis* 69 (6): 379–381.
51 Vandebuerie, L., Aerts, C., and Goossens, A. (2014). Allergic contact dermatitis resulting from multiple colophonium-related allergen sources. *Contact Dermatitis* 70 (2): 117–119.
52 Aboutalebi, A., Chan, C.S., and Katta, R. (2009). Transfer contact dermatitis caused by rosin use in bowling. *Dermatology Online Journal* 15 (12): 11.
53 Downs, A.M. and Sansom, J.E. (1999). Colophony allergy: a review. *Contact Dermatitis* 41 (6): 305–310.
54 Farm, G. (1996). Contact allergy to colophony and hand eczema. A follow-up study of patients with previously diagnosed contact allergy to colophony. *Contact Dermatitis* 34 (2): 93–100.
55 Meding, B. and Swanbeck, G. (1990). Occupational hand eczema in an industrial city. *Contact Dermatitis* 22 (1): 13–23.
56 Krutmann, J., Rzany, B., Schöpf, E., and Kapp, A. (1989). Airborne contact dermatitis from colophony: phototoxic reaction? *Contact Dermatitis* 21 (4): 275–276.
57 Geier, J., Lessmann, H., Schnuch, A., and Uter, W. (2004). Contact sensitizations in metalworkers with occupational dermatitis exposed to water-based metalworking fluids: results of the research project "FaSt". *International Archives of Occupational and Environmental Health* 77 (8): 543–551.
58 Henriks-Eckerman, M.L., Suuronen, K., and Jolanki, R. (2008). Analysis of allergens in metalworking fluids. *Contact Dermatitis* 59 (5): 261–267.
59 Gambichler, T., Boms, S., and Freitag, M. (2004). Contact dermatitis and other skin conditions in instrumental musicians. *BMC Dermatology* 4: 3.
60 Molin, S., Bauer, A., Schnuch, A., and Geier, J. (2015). Occupational contact allergy in nurses: results from the information network of departments of dermatology 2003-2012. *Contact Dermatitis* 72 (3): 164–171.
61 Rivers, J.K. and Rycroft, R.J. (1987). Occupational allergic contact urticaria from colophony. *Contact Dermatitis* 17 (3): 181.
62 el Sayed, F., Manzur, F., Bayle, P. et al. (1995). Contact urticaria from abietic acid. *Contact Dermatitis* 32 (6): 361–362.
63 Helaskoski, E., Suojalehto, H., Kuuliala, O., and Aalto-Korte, K. (2015). Prick testing with chemicals in the diagnosis of occupational contact urticaria and respiratory diseases. *Contact Dermatitis* 72 (1): 20–32.

Exposure Color Code

- Clothing, jewelry, adornments
- Personal care products, cosmetics/cosmetic procedures
- Household products, domestic environment, including furniture and refurbishment
- Occupational dermatoses, work environment
- Medicines, surgical/dental procedures, herbal/alternative medicines
- Personal appliances/aids
- Leisure activities, sport, travel
- Other exposures (including dietary)
- Not relevant or multiple/general exposure

CHAPTER 26

Epoxy Resin

CHAPTER CONTENTS

Key points

- Epoxy is a thermosetting polymer formed from the reaction of an epoxide "resin" with a polyamine "hardener."
- Allergic contact dermatitis (ACD) to epoxy resin systems is most likely to occur in the occupational setting.
- Epoxy is typically used in adhesives, surface coatings, electrical insulation, plasticizers, polymer stabilizers, laminates, surface coatings, paints and inks, product finishers, polyvinyl chloride (PVC) products, the building industry, electron microscopy, and sculptures.
- Clinical presentations can include hand, periorbital, or generalized dermatitis.
- ACD to epoxy resin in floor layers classically presents with dermatitis on the periorbital region, hands, flexor areas of the forearms, knees, and shins.
- Compounds containing epoxy groups causing ACD often but do not necessarily cross-react with the baseline series epoxy resin (diglycidyl ether of bisphenol A).
- Epoxy resin can be in a cured or uncured condition. "Cured" compounds may contain varying amounts of uncured residue.
- Cross-reactivity to fragrance chemicals, including isoeugenol, has been postulated.
- In some females, isolated epoxy resin contact allergy has been demonstrated without clinical relevance.
- Not all components of epoxy resin systems are available as a commercial patch test substance. Patch testing to patients' own epoxy products, at appropriate dilutions, may be important.
- Between less than 10% and 27% of epoxy resin allergy cases are due to the hardener or the diluent.
- Non-occupational sensitization sources from hobbies and leisure activities account for a third of epoxy resin sensitization cases.

Common "pitfalls"

- The baseline series epoxy resin is a useful screening agent to detect contact allergy. However, do not rely on epoxy resin in the standard series to fully exclude contact allergy to epoxy resin. When epoxy resin allergy is strongly suspected, add in an extensive epoxy series and dilute patients' own samples to appropriate levels.
- Testing with undiluted or inaccurately diluted epoxy resin samples can result in both false-positive patch test reactions and active sensitization.
- The relevance of ACD "by proxy" as with some construction workers, such that the patient is not directly handling epoxy resin but the resin is present in the workplace, can be easily missed. Workplace visits or photographic illustrations of the workplace and work practice can help in this situation.

Epoxy resin systems

Alternative name: diglycidyl ether of bisphenol A (DGEBA)

Epoxy resin systems [1] consist of:

- *Epoxy monomer*
- *Hardener*: Resin monomers are polymerized by cross-linking and become solid/hardened above a molecular weight of 900 daltons. Epoxy resins which harden at room temperature consist of two parts. The curing or hardening agents influence the properties and functions of the resin.

Common Contact Allergens: A Practical Guide to Detecting Contact Dermatitis, First Edition. Edited by John McFadden, Pailin Puangpet, Korbkarn Pongpairoj, Supitchaya Thaiwat, and Lee Shan Xian.

© 2020 John Wiley & Sons Ltd. Published 2020 by John Wiley & Sons Ltd.

Companion website: www.wiley.com/go/mcfadden/common_contact_allergens

- *Reactive diluent*: Diluents are added to the uncured resin to reduce its viscosity and facilitate its penetration into materials. Reactive diluents form chemical bonds with the epoxy compound during curing and become part of the final resin. They also accelerate and increase the efficiency of the curing process. Many of the reactive diluents are low-viscosity epoxy compounds [2], for example 1,4-butanediol diglycidyl ether. These compounds have greater allergenic potential than non-reactive diluents. Non-reactive diluents increase the pot life of the system by decreasing the activity of the curing agent, but the final resins have suboptimal performance. Examples include dibutyl phthalate and styrene [2].
- *Other additives* can include *fillers*, which are inert substances such as glass or minerals added to improve specific properties. *Resin modifiers*, such as polyurethane and plasticizers, can improve durability [2].

Exposure and use

Epoxy resins were first developed in the 1940s [3]. They are mainly used in [4] (Figure 26.1):

- *Adhesives and surface coatings* for cars, the electronics and aeronautics industries, home use (DIY), epoxy pipe relining [5], and parquet (type of wooden flooring) fitters [6].
- *Run-resins for models and molds*: foundry, prostheses, mounting for glasses, resin utensils, and capsules.
- *Composite material* used in aeronautical engineering [7], articles of sport and leisure (tennis rackets, skis, fishing rods, competitive boats, sailboards) [8].
- *Coating*: flooring [9], painting and varnish, electronic components (credit cards, printed circuits), coil insulation and wires, impermeable concrete for pipes or tanks, protection of the ground and walls against chemicals.
- *Tissue processing* in light, electron, and immunoelectron microscopy [10].
- Fluids such as cutting *oil* in machine operatives [11], neat oil in metal processing [12], and immersion oils for optical microscopy [10, 13].
- Epoxy resins are also used in plasticizers, polymer stabilizers, laminates, product finishers, PVC products (e.g. eyeglass frames, vinyl gloves, handbags, plastic necklaces), the building industry, sculptures [14], can and drum linings, flame retardants, marine varnishes, polymer stabilizers, automotive primers, model making, bridge coatings, steel pipe coatings, dental bonding agents, tools and die casting, joining of telephone cables, pacemakers [15], plumbing [16], hemodialysis needles [17], hemodialysis catheters [18], nasal cannulas [19], insulin pumps [20], and the restoration of window frames [21].

Frequency of sensitization

Most reports from clinics give a frequency of contact allergy to epoxy resin between 0.5%-1.5%.

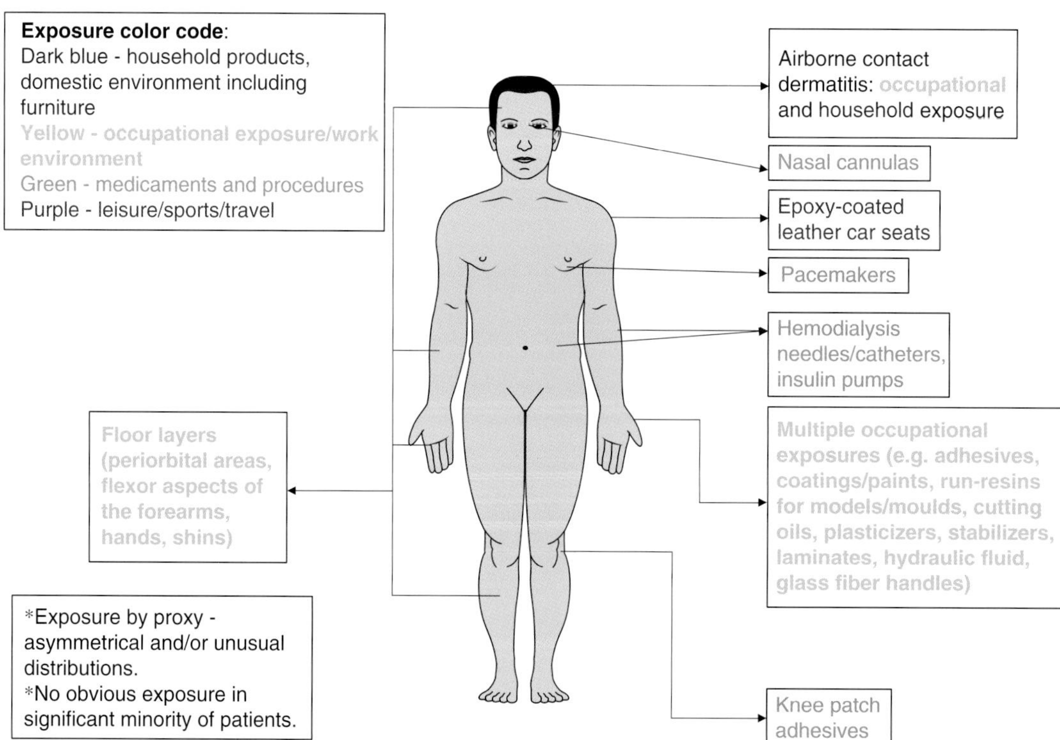

Figure 26.1 Reported exposure sources for ACD to epoxy resin.

Patch testing

1% epoxy resin in acetone or petrolatum/T.R.U.E.® test equivalent.

Epoxy products can generally be tested at 0.1-1% in petroleum or acetone (Figure 26.2). If the final concentration of the allergen exceeds the recommended concentration, this can induce active sensitization [22]. If there is no evidence of exposure, it may be excluded when patch testing children as there is a (very) low risk of active sensitization.

A commercially available 'epoxy series' is available to use when epoxy allergy is suspected.

An isolated allergy to non-DGEBA epoxy agents, reactive diluents, or hardeners without a positive patch test to epoxy resins may occasionally occur.

Clinical disease

- ■ 90% of patients present with dermatitis on the exposed areas of the hands and forearms and 50% have facial involvement. The mean exposure time to the time of development of dermatitis is 31 months [23]. Non-occupational sources were found in 21 of 59 (35%) patients with epoxy resin sensitization. The most common non-occupational sources were glues, paints, and coatings used in domestic renovation, construction projects, and boat repair [24]. *Poor prognostic factors* include older age, a history of atopy, longer duration of symptoms, and more severe disease at the time of diagnosis. Of 16 allergic patients who had stopped working with epoxy resin, nine reported complete healing and seven had ongoing dermatitis after 2 years [25].

Occupational disease

- Epoxy resins are a well-recognized and major source of *occupational ACD*, with reports relating to the construction industry, manufacturing, and their use in painting, laminates, electrical insulation, two-component bonding agents [26], electrical equipment, electronics, varnishes, immersion oil and plastics [26, 27]. Engineers, windscreen repairers, tile setters, aircraft industry workers [28], dentists and dental assistants, floor layers, carpenters, joiners, plastic products machine operators, bricklayers, stonemasons, precision workers in metal, wood treaters, cabinet-makers, plumbers, pipe-fitters, machinery mechanics, and fitters [29] can be at risk (Figures 26.1 and 26.3).
- Burrows et al. [8] describes dermatitis caused by allergy to epoxy resin systems in 14 out of 25 (56%) *aircraft manufacturing workers*. They gave positive patch test reactions to the composite material and/or DGEBA, tetraglycidyl-4,4′-methylene dianiline (TGMDA), and *o*-diglycidyl phthalate.
- Angelini et al. [30] describes another outbreak of epoxy resin allergy, this time amongst 10 out of 22 *marble workers* handling a resin based on epoxy resin and *o*-cresyl glycidyl ether, with exposure times of between 20 days and 2 months. They presented with hand dermatitis (nine cases) and eyelid dermatitis (six cases). All ten subjects were patch test positive

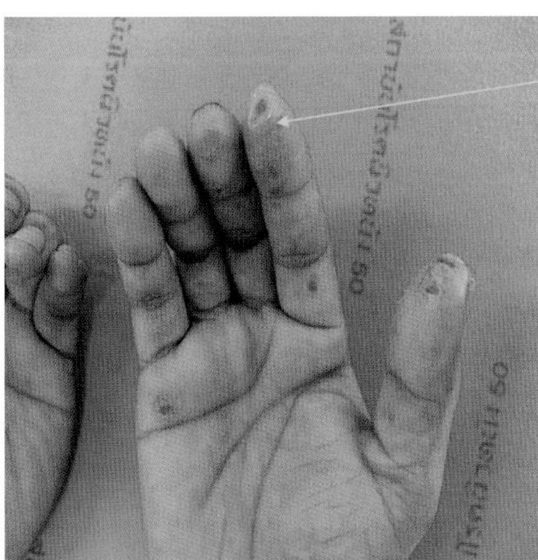

Chronic skin changes with fissuring from repeated occupational exposure. There is marked finger pulp involvement.

Multiple positive reactions to epoxy resin and diluted samples; multiple allergens can be involved from both cross-reaction and co-sensitisation.

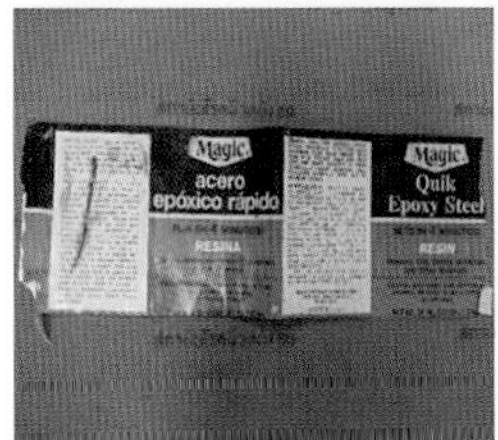

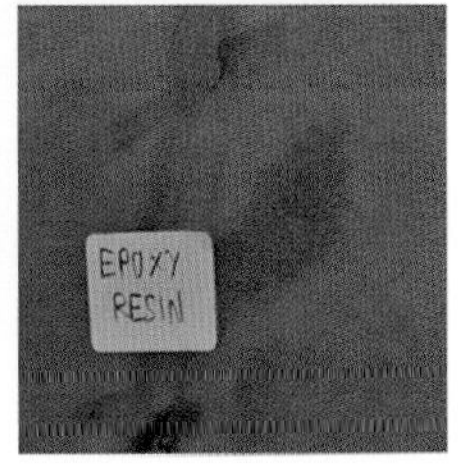

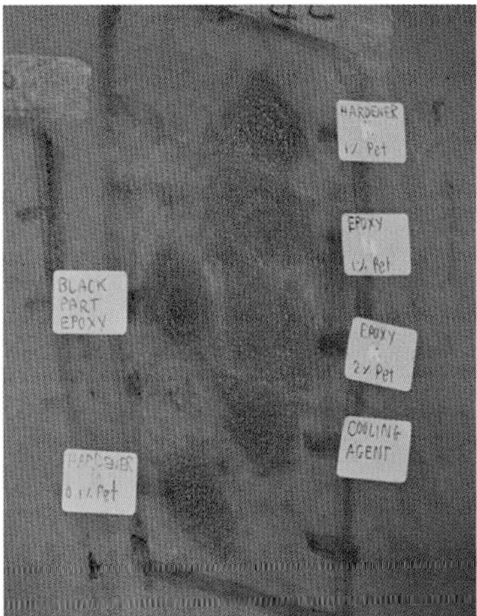

Figure 26.2 Multiple positive patch tests to chemicals used in epoxy resin systems.

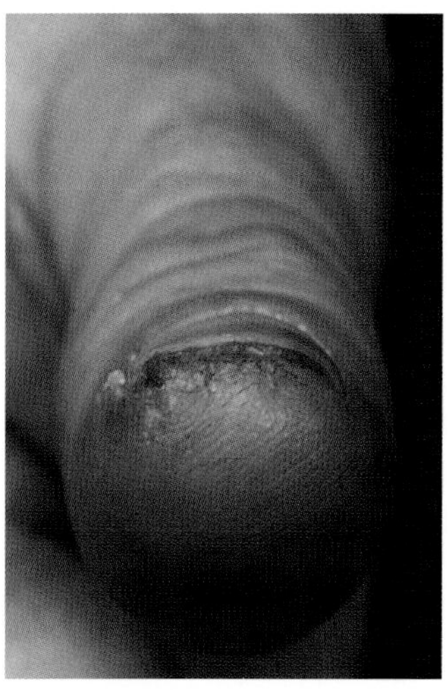
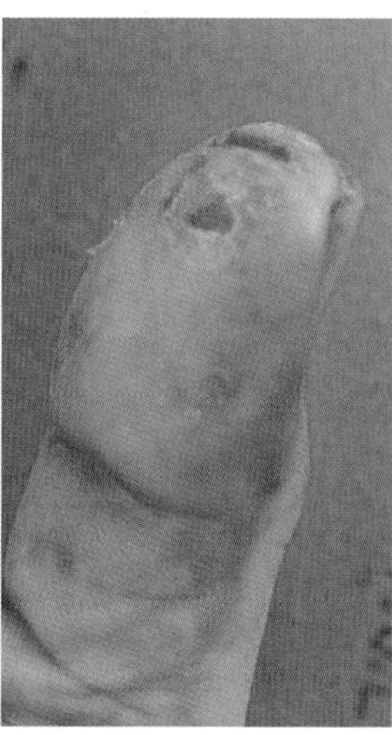

Figure 26.3 Occupational ACD to epoxy resin showing involvement of the finger pulp and hyponychium. "Ragged" nails may also be present.

to the reactive diluent *o*-cresyl glycidyl ether (0.25% pet.), but only four were reactive to the commercially available epoxy resin (1% pet.). Other outbreaks have been reported such as in factory workers manufacturing windmills, ski, paints, electronic circuit boards (case report), developmental chemists, making and assembling small electronic parts, as well as in grouters constructing the English Channel Tunnel [31–37].

- Contact allergy to special floor coverings containing epoxy resins and their derivatives was reported in 15 *special floor-laying workers* who had severe lesions on the face, i.e. eyelids (8/15), forearms (8/15), hands +/− feet (11/15), trunk (3/15), and legs (3/15). Clinical onset in these patients occurred less than 6 months after starting work. These floor coatings are mainly used in heavily frequented areas, such as hospitals, civic centers, laboratories, the chemical industry, the food sector, hypermarkets, computer centers, sports installations and the metallurgy industry because of high resistance to mechanical compression, water, chemicals, wear and tear, and other environmental and climatic factors [9]. Floor layers with ACD to epoxy resin typically have eczema involving the periorbital areas with edema and erythema, hands, flexor areas of the forearms, and shins.
- *Epoxy relining* is a method of repairing worn water pipes. Epoxy resin systems are involved in creating new pipes inside existing pipes, with large amounts of epoxy resin being handled at temporary worksites. Berglind et al. reported eight "relining" workers with suspected occupational dermatitis. Seven were positive to epoxy resin chemicals, six to the epoxy resin in the baseline series. Five were patch test positive to their own epoxy resins [5].

Further case reports

- ACD with eosinophilia secondary to the epoxy resin residing between the needle and silicone tubing in a blunt *hemodialysis cannula* was reported in two patients from Canada. After starting hemodialysis, they developed pruritic, erythematous, and papular eruptions at the arteriovenous fistula sites. Both patients reacted strongly to bisphenol A and bisphenol F [38].
- *Scleroderma-like lesions* have been described in workmen exposed to the vapors of epoxy resins. An epoxy amine [bis(4-amino-3-methylcyclohexyl) methane] was suspected [39].
- *Lichenoid dermatitis* with non-lichenoid allergic patch test reactions (days 2 and 7) has been reported from the USA. The patient was a floor layer who presented with well-defined violaceous lichenified plaques on the eyelids, volar wrists and elbows. Histopathological features were identical to that of lichen planus. The sealer and curing compound contained 4'-isopropylidenediphenol, epichlorohydrin, xylene, and propylene glycol monomethyl ether [40].
- Epoxy resins may produce *erythema multiforme-like* eruptions. A 46-year old man developed an eczematous erythematous papulovesicular and bullous eruption on the arms 10 days after repairing a swimming pool using a sealant that contained 55% epoxy resin (MW 380) and an epoxy hardener, isophorone diamine. Nine days later, a different, target-like eruption appeared on the arms and hands which healed in 2 weeks. Patch testing was positive to epoxy resin, fragrance mix, *Myroxylon pereirae*, and hardener in the sealant [41].
- *Some patients are highly sensitive and can react to minimal exposure*: Kanerva et al. [42] reported a patient with a previous subclinical allergy to DGEBA/epoxy resin who had ACD from very small amounts of DGEBA/epoxy resin (0.015%) in a mop handle made of glass fiber. Patch testing with DGEBA/epoxy resin was positive down to 0.00032% (3.2 ppm) and with bisphenol A-glycidyl methacrylate (Bis-GMA) down to 0.0001% (1 ppm).
- *Unexpected sources of exposure* can occur. These include knee patch adhesives [43] and coatings on leather car seats [44].

"Epoxy by proxy"

- Information about the occupations of other family members can be important when a positive patch test reaction to epoxy resin cannot be explained. A mother developed recurrent ACD on the face, eyelids, and neck 24 hours after hand washing her son's work-soiled clothes, wearing protective gloves. Her son worked at a paint factory preparing two-part epoxy paints. Two years previously, she presented with similar dermatitis. Patch testing showed a ++ reaction to epoxy resin [45].

Airborne contact dermatitis

- There is a predilection for airborne ACD to epoxy resin to affect the dorsal aspects of the hands as well as the forearms, face, and eyelids. Eyelid edema can be an isolated finding. Lesions may occur from just entering a room where epoxy is used [4]. A review of 40 cases of epoxy resin sensitivity found that 52.5% had involvement of the face [46]. In addition, airborne occupational contact dermatitis can present with conjunctivitis alone without eyelid and periorbital skin involvement [47].

Contact urticaria

- Contact urticaria from epoxy compounds is a well-recognized but rare occurrence. Acute urticarial reactions have been described from aliphatic polyamine hardeners more often than from reactive diluents. Contact urticaria with angioedema due to epoxy resin and its reactive diluents, phenylglycidyl ether and cresylglycidyl ether, has been reported in an aircraft factory worker [48].
- A patient developed an acute allergic type I reaction presenting as laryngeal swelling and respiratory distress followed by generalized urticaria with anaphylactic shock while having dental root canal treatment. Patch testing showed a strong urticarial reaction to the epoxy resin root canal filling material after 20 minutes and a positive delayed patch test reaction on day 3 [49].

Contact vitiligo

- Contact vitiligo secondary to an epoxy resin diluent was reported. This patient, who had worked in a marble factory for 5 years, had a 1-year history of vitiliginous lesions on the backs of his fingers. Patch testing was positive to phenylglycidyl ether, cresylglycidyl ether, hexanediol diglycidyl ether, and triphenyl phosphate. After a 2-year follow-up period, there were no further vitiligo-like lesions on the test area [50].

Isolated contact allergy to epoxy resin in females without exposure history

- Plausible explanations for this not uncommon observation include exposure to uncured epoxy resin in the coatings of furniture such as tables, cross-reactivity with unidentified fragrance agents, or by proxy exposure in the past (epoxy resin used at work or home easily contaminates surfaces).

Persistent photosensitivity

- Persistent photosensitivity following ACD to epoxy resin has been reported [51, 52]. In a series of five patients, symptoms of ACD to epoxy resin preceded photosensitivity by 5 months to 12 years in three cases and occurred simultaneously in two cases. Patch testing to epoxy resin was positive in all patients. Phototesting revealed a decreased minimal erythema dose to both ultraviolet A (UVA) and UVB in the three patients who were phototested [51].

Association with contact allergy to fragrance mix 1

- Andersen and colleagues found that of 145 epoxy resin allergic patients, 19 reacted to Fragrance Mix I (FMI) (13%, $p < 0.0001$). Of the individual ingredients in FMI, there were two significant associations: 8/31 epoxy resin allergic patients reacted to isoeugenol (26%, $p = 0.0045$) and 3/32 epoxy resin allergic patients reacted to amyl cinnamal ($p = 0.017$) [53].

Skin protection

- Protection for the skin and eyes with good ventilation can prevent epoxy resin dermatitis [26].
- Epoxy resin can penetrate rubber, leather, cotton, or PVC gloves. Long-sleeved heavy-duty vinyl gloves, neoprene, nitrile, or butyl rubber over thin cotton inner gloves to absorb moisture are recommended. Use of gloves only once and frequent changing of gloves is also recommended [54]. Double-layer PVC or latex gloves may provide protection in some occupational settings [26].
- A barrier cream was evaluated in a placebo-controlled double-blind study and found to be ineffective prevention for epoxy resin. Polyethylene laminate gloves (4-H glove; Safety 4 Company, Lyngby, Denmark) effectively protected two sensitized volunteers after 8 and 48 hours of exposure to epoxy resin [55].
- Epoxy resins can be removed with acetone, alcohol, or methyl ethyl ketone followed by acid-type cleansers [56].
- To reduce skin contact, workers should allow epoxy products on tools to cure first before scraping them off instead of cleaning with volatile solvents, use disposable tools where possible, and close used packages with epoxy resin or hardener immediately [54].

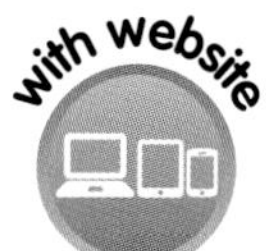

Go to www.wiley.com/go/mcfadden/common_contact_allergens to find the E-supplement for this chapter:

Epoxy Resin: E-Supplement

References

1 Amado, A. and Taylor, J.S. (2008). Contact allergy to epoxy resins. *Contact Dermatitis* 58 (3): 186–187.

2 Cronin, E. (1980). *Contact Dermatitis*. Chapter 12. Edinburgh: Churchill Livingstone.

3 Bray, P.G. (1999). Epoxy resins. *Occupational Medicine* 14 (4): 743–758.

4 Geraut, C., Tripodi, D., Brunet-Courtois, B. et al. (2009). Occupational dermatitis to epoxydic and phenolic resins. *European Journal of Dermatology* 19 (3): 205–213.

5 Anveden Berglind, I., Lind, M.L., and Lidén, C. (2012). Epoxy pipe relining – an emerging contact allergy risk for workers. *Contact Dermatitis* 67 (2): 59–65.

6 Geier, J., Krautheim, A., and Fuchs, T. (2012). Airborne allergic contact dermatitis in a parquet fitter. *Contact Dermatitis* 67 (2): 106–108.

7 Ayala, F., Lembo, G., Balato, N. et al. (1990). The use of laboratory methods in contact dermatitis induced by composite materials. *Contact Dermatitis* 22 (5): 262–266.

8 Burrows, D., Fregert, S., Campbell, H., and Trulsson, L. (1984). Contact dermatitis from the epoxy resins tetraglycidyl-4,4′-methylene dianiline and o-diglycidyl phthalate in composite material. *Contact Dermatitis* 11 (2): 80–82.

9 Condé-Salazar, L., Gonzalez de Domingo, M.A., and Guimaraens, D. (1994). Sensitization to epoxy resin systems in special flooring workers. *Contact Dermatitis* 31 (3): 157–160.

10 Geraut, C. and Tripodi, D. (1999). 'Airborne' contact dermatitis due to Leica immersion oil. *International Journal of Dermatology* 38 (9): 676–679.

11 English, J.S., Foulds, I., White, I.R., and Rycroft, R.J. (1986). Allergic contact sensitization to the glycidyl ester of hexahydrophthalic acid in a cutting oil. *Contact Dermatitis* 15 (2): 66–68.

12 Jensen, C.D. and Andersen, K.E. (2003). Two cases of occupational allergic contact dermatitis from a cycloaliphatic epoxy resin in a neat oil: case report. *Environmental Health* 2: 3.

13 Hughes, R. and Taylor, J.S. (2002). Surveillance of allergic contact dermatitis: epoxy resin and microscopic immersion oil. *Journal of the American Academy of Dermatology* 47 (6): 965–966.

14 Kanerva, L., Elsner, P., Wahlberg, J., and Maibach, H. (2000). Epoxy resins. In: *Handbook of Occupational Dermatology* (eds. R. Jolanki, T. Estlander, K. Alanko and L. Kanerva). Berlin Heidelberg New York: Springer Verlag.

15 Skoet, R., Tollund, C., and Bloch-Thomsen, P.E. (2003). Epoxy contact dermatitis due to pacemaker compounds. *Cardiology* 99 (2): 112.

16 Condé-Salazar, L., Gorospe, M., and Guimaraens, D. (1993). A new source of sensitivity to epoxy resin. *Contact Dermatitis* 28 (5): 292.

17 Brandao, F.M. and Pinto, J. (1980). Allergic contact dermatitis to epoxy resin in hemodialysis needles. *Contact Dermatitis* 6 (3): 218–219.

18 Hanson, J., Ward, K., Van Beck, J., and Warshaw, E. (2015). Allergic contact dermatitis to a hemodialysis catheter: epoxy is an occult allergen in medical devices. *Minnesota Medicine* 98 (4): 39–40.

19 Wright, R.C. and Fregert, S. (1983). Allergic contact dermatitis from epoxy resin in nasal canulae. *Contact Dermatitis* 9 (5): 387–389.

20 Boom, B.W. and van Driel, L.M. (1985). Allergic contact dermatitis to epoxy resin in infusion sets of an insulin pump. *Contact Dermatitis* 12 (5): 280.

21 Brooke, R.C. and Beck, M.H. (1999). Occupational allergic contact dermatitis from epoxy resin used to restore window frames. *Contact Dermatitis* 41 (4): 227–228.

22 Kanerva, L., Jolanki, R., and Estlander, T. (2001). Active sensitization by epoxy in Leica immersion oil. *Contact Dermatitis* 44 (3): 194–196.

23 Yung, A. and Wilkinson, S.M. (2003). Allergic contact dermatitis from the epoxy resin plasticizer diglycidyl ether of propylene glycol. *Contact Dermatitis* 49 (2): 109–110.

24 Majasuo, S., Liippo, J., and Lammintausta, K. (2012). Non-occupational contact sensitization to epoxy resin of bisphenol A among general dermatology patients. *Contact Dermatitis* 66 (3): 148–153.

25 Cahill, J., Keegel, T., Dharmage, S. et al. (2005). Prognosis of contact dermatitis in epoxy resin workers. *Contact Dermatitis* 52 (3): 147–153.

26 Lee, Y.C., Gordon, D.L., and Gordon, L.A. (1999). Epoxy resin allergy from microscopy immersion oil. *Australasian Journal of Dermatology* 40 (4): 228–229.

27 Rademaker, M. (2000). Occupational epoxy resin allergic contact dermatitis. *Australasian Journal of Dermatology* 41 (4): 222–224.

28 Aalto-Korte, K., Pesonen, M., and Suuronen, K. (2015). Occupational allergic contact dermatitis caused by epoxy chemicals: occupations, sensitizing products, and diagnosis. *Contact Dermatitis* 73 (6): 336–342.

29 Pesonen, M., Jolanki, R., Larese Filon, F. et al. (2015). Patch test results of the European baseline series among patients with occupational contact dermatitis across Europe – analyses of the European Surveillance System on Contact Allergy network, 2002–2010. *Contact Dermatitis* 72 (3): 154–163.

30 Angelini, G., Rigano, L., Foti, C. et al. (1996). Occupational sensitization to epoxy resin and reactive diluents in marble workers. *Contact Dermatitis* 35 (1): 11–16.

31 Irvine, C., Pugh, C.E., Hansen, E.J., and Rycroft, R.J. (1994). Cement dermatitis in underground workers during construction of the Channel Tunnel. *Occupational Medicine* 44 (1): 17–23.

32 Jolanki, R., Tarvainen, K., Tatar, T. et al. (1996). Occupational dermatoses from exposure to epoxy resin compounds in a ski factory. *Contact Dermatitis* 34 (6): 390–396.

33 Omer, S.A. and Al-Tawil, N.G. (1994). Contact sensitivity among workers in a paint factory. *Contact Dermatitis* 30 (1): 55–57.

34 Ponten, A., Carstensen, O., Rasmussen, K. et al. (2004). Epoxy-based production of wind turbine rotor blades: occupational contact allergies. *Dermatitis: Contact, Atopic, Occupational, Drug* 15 (1): 33–40.

35 Craven, N.M., Bhushan, M., and Beck, M.H. (1999). Sensitization to triglycidyl isocyanurate, epoxy resins and acrylates in a developmental chemist. *Contact Dermatitis* 40 (1): 54–55.

36 Schroder, C., Uter, W., and Schwanitz, H.J. (1999). Occupational allergic contact dermatitis, partly airborne, due to isocyanates and epoxy resin. *Contact Dermatitis* 41 (2): 117–118.

37 Fowler, J.F. (1990). Occupational dermatitis of the fingertips. *American Journal of Contact Dermatitis* 1: 210–211.

38 Haussmann, J., Pratt, M., Linett, L., and Zimmerman, D. (2005). Allergic contact dermatitis and eosinophilia in association with a hemodialysis cannula. *American Journal of Kidney Diseases* 45 (2): e23–e26.

39 Yamakage, A., Ishikawa, H., Saito, Y., and Hattori, A. (1980). Occupational scleroderma-like disorder occurring in men engaged in the polymerization of epoxy resins. *Dermatologica* 161 (1): 33–44.

40 Lichter, M., Drury, D., and Remlinger, K. (1992). Lichenoid dermatitis caused by epoxy resin. *Contact Dermatitis* 26 (4): 275.

41 Whitfeld, M.J. and Rivers, J.K. (1991). Erythema multiforme after contact dermatitis in response to an epoxy sealant. *Journal of the American Academy of Dermatology* 25 (2 Pt 2): 386–388.

42 Kanerva, L., Jolanki, R., Estlander, T., and Alanko, K. (2000). Latent (subclinical) contact dermatitis evolving into occupational allergic contact dermatitis from extremely small amounts of epoxy resin. *Contact Dermatitis* 43 (1): 47–49.

43 Taylor, J.S., Bergfeld, W.F., and Guin, J.D. (1983). Contact dermatitis to knee patch adhesive in boys' jeans: a nonoccupational cause of epoxy resin sensitivity. *Cleveland Clinic Quarterly* 50 (2): 123–127.

44 Wurpts, G. and Merk, H.F. (2010). Allergy to car seat. *Der Hautarzt* 61 (11): 933–934.

45 Lyon, C.C. and Beck, M.H. (2000). Epoxy-by-proxy dermatitis. *Contact Dermatitis* 42 (5): 306.
46 Jolanki, R., Kanerva, L., Estlander, T. et al. (1990). Occupational dermatoses from epoxy resin compounds. *Contact Dermatitis* 23 (3): 172–183.
47 Goodson, A. and Powell, D. (2014). Contact dermatitis to epoxy resins presenting as conjunctivitis. *Dermatitis* 25 (1): 34.
48 Sasseville, D. (1998). Contact urticaria from epoxy resin and reactive diluents. *Contact Dermatitis* 38 (1): 57–58.
49 Stutz, N., Hertl, M., and Loffler, H. (2008). Anaphylaxis caused by contact urticaria because of epoxy resins: an extraordinary emergency. *Contact Dermatitis* 58 (5): 307–309.
50 Silvestre, J.F., Albares, M.P., Escutia, B. et al. (2003). Contact vitiligo appearing after allergic contact dermatitis from aromatic reactive diluents in an epoxy resin system. *Contact Dermatitis* 49 (2): 113–114.
51 Kwok, T., Rosen, C.F., Storrs, F.J. et al. (2013). Persistent photosensitivity after allergic contact dermatitis to epoxy resin. *Dermatitis: Contact, Atopic, Occupational, Drug* 24 (3): 124–130.
52 Allen, H. and Kaidbey, K. (1979). Persistent photosensitivity following occupational exposure to epoxy resin. *Archives of Dermatology* 115 (11): 1307–1310.
53 Andersen, K.E., Christensen, L.P., Vølund, A. et al. (2009). Association between positive patch tests to epoxy resin and fragrance mix I ingredients. *Contact Dermatitis* 60 (3): 155–157.
54 Spee, T., Van Duivenbooden, C., and Terwoert, J. (2006). Epoxy resins in the construction industry. *Annals of the New York Academy of Sciences* 1076: 429–438.
55 McClain, C. and Storrs, F. (1992). Protective effect of both a barrier cream and a polyethylene laminate glove against epoxy resin, glyceryl monothioglycolate, Frullania, and Tansy. *American Journal of Contact Dermatitis* 3 (4): 201–205.
56 Rietschel, R. and Fowler, J. (2001). *Fisher's Contact Dermatitis*, 6e, 727. Philadelphia: Lippincott Williams & Wilkins.

Exposure Color Code

- Clothing, jewelry, adornments
- Personal care products, cosmetics/cosmetic procedures
- Household products, domestic environment, including furniture and refurbishment
- Occupational dermatoses, work environment
- Medicines, surgical/dental procedures, herbal/alternative medicines
- Personal appliances/aids
- Leisure activities, sport, travel
- Other exposures (including dietary)
- Not relevant or multiple/general exposure

CHAPTER 27

Tosylamide Formaldehyde Resin

CHAPTER CONTENTS

Key points

- A nail varnish allergen.
- Although the source of exposure is almost exclusively from nail varnish, there are multiple potential routes of exposure (direct contact, airborne, hand-to-face/neck/body, and by proxy).
- The classical form of presentation is eyelid dermatitis, possibly associated with multiple annular patches on the face, neck, and upper chest.
- There are, however, diverse presentations such as cheilitis, otitis externa, nail fold dermatitis, groin dermatitis, seborrheic dermatitis-like, and a photosensitive rash.
- Co-sensitization with formaldehyde is very uncommon, as the resin releases little formaldehyde, but this can occur.
- False-positive reactions on patch testing can occur if the varnish has not been allowed to dry on the test disc before application to the back.
- Allergic contact dermatitis (ACD) to alternative resins, such as phthalic anhydride/trimellitic anhydride/glycols copolymer, polyester resins, and acrylates, are also common and have similar clinical features as ACD to tosylamide formaldehyde resin (TSFR).

Introduction

- TSFR has been one of the commonest cosmetic contact allergens [1, 2].
- Physical properties: nearly colorless, weak formaldehyde odor.
- TSFR is a thermoplastic resin which hardens as it dries. It facilitates adhesion and improves shine, rigidity, and flow in the application of nail polish to nails. In addition, it helps nail varnish last on nails.
- Synonyms [1]: TSFR-80, 4-toluenesulfonamide formaldehyde resin, benzenesulfonamide. For cosmetic labeling 'tosylamide formaldehyde resin' is always used.
- Basic constituents: despite its name, there is a very small amount of free formaldehyde. The actual allergen is predominantly the resin [1].
- The classical nail varnish allergens are the water-soluble components (including monomers and dimers) of TSFR in dry polish [2].
- Sources: nail polish [3, 4], nail lacquers [5], nail cosmetic resins, nail polish enamel, and nail hardeners [2].

Routes of exposure

- Direct contact dermatitis.
- Airborne ACD.
- Manual transmission [3].

Frequency of sensitization (patch test clinic data available only)

- 1% is a good approximation.
- Brazil (high rates documented, possibly from more extensive use; see Table 27.1).

Common Contact Allergens: A Practical Guide to Detecting Contact Dermatitis, First Edition. Edited by John McFadden, Pailin Puangpet, Korbkarn Pongpairoj, Supitchaya Thaiwat, and Lee Shan Xian.

© 2020 John Wiley & Sons Ltd. Published 2020 by John Wiley & Sons Ltd.

Companion website: www.wiley.com/go/mcfadden/common_contact_allergens

Table 27.1 Frequency of sensitization from patch test clinics: Brazil (1–3) vs. North America (4).

1996–2001	Brazil, age 10–19 years old (n = 1027)	12%	[4]
2003–2010	Brazil, age 1–19 years old (n = 125)	6.8%, 100% clinical relevance	[3]
2003–2010	Brazil (n = 792)	10.4%	[6]
2007–2008	North America (n = 5078)	1%	[7]

Clinical presentations

- *Location*: In one study the three principal sites affected were [8]:
  1. the eyelids, especially the upper eyelids; usually bilateral but can be unilateral (Figure 27.1)
  2. the lower half of the face, especially the corners of the mouth and chin (the presentation often comprises a blotchy and ill-defined eczematous rash, with erythematous scaly patches)
  3. the sides of the neck and the upper chest, with similar morphology to the lower face (Figures 27.2 and 27.3).

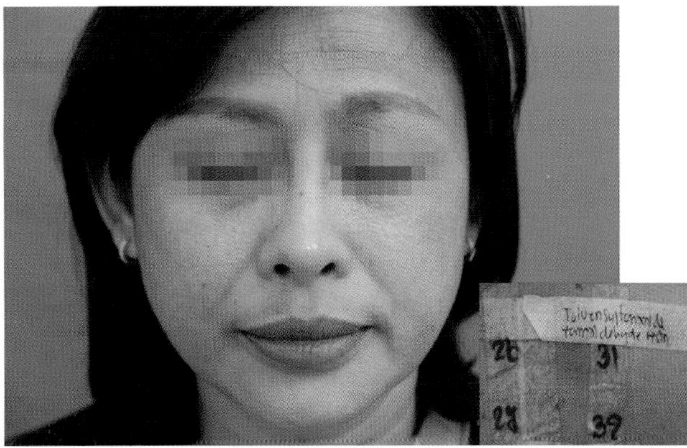

Figure 27.1 ACD to TSFR, demonstrating a classical airborne distribution with upper and lower eyelid, forehead and early malar cheek involvement.

- *Wide diversity of anatomical sites*: In another large study of patients with ACD to nail varnish, the involved anatomical locations documented were as shown in Table 27.2 [9]. *(Note: Some patients had more than one location involved.)*
- In another series, ACD to TSFR involved areas other than the head and neck in 23% (20/88) of patients [10]. This included the upper chest (n = 9), shoulders and arms (n = 6), antecubital fossa (n = 4), knee or popliteal fossa (n = 4), patches on the trunk (n = 4), thighs (n = 2), groin (n = 1), and vulva (n = 1).
- The diagnosis is often not suspected before the patch test consultation. In one survey, only 2/18 cases of nail varnish allergy had been suspected [11]. Mistaken pre-patch test diagnoses included atopic eczema, otitis externa, rosacea, urticaria, and "VDU (visual display unit) sickness" [11].
- The sides of the neck and the lower face may be involved from "hand-touching."
- The first description of ACD to nail varnish occurred in 1925. Two female patients presented with erythematous dermatitis on the sides of the neck [12].
- *Periungual lesions* [13]: In one series, 11/18 patients with ACD to TSFR had periungual skin involvement [11].
- *Worsening of atopic dermatitis* and periorbital dermatitis in a 4-year-old child with varnished nails has been reported as a clinical presentation of ACD to TSFR. The authors speculated that the itch–scratch–itch cycle had contributed to both sensitization to nail varnish and the worsening atopic dermatitis [14].
- Similarly, any itchy dermatitis may be aggravated by ACD to TSFR, as a result of exposure to nail varnish from scratching [15, 16].
- *Cheilitis*: 8/88 cases of ACD to TSFR had involvement of the lips or angles of the mouth. Cheilitis was pronounced in one patient with a habit of pressing her nails against the lips [10]. In 2/19 cases of allergic contact cheilitis, TSFR was implicated [17].
- *Desquamative gingivitis*: There is a single case report of ACD to TSFR with gingival inflammation adjacent to the incisors in a patient who was a habitual "nail biter" [18].

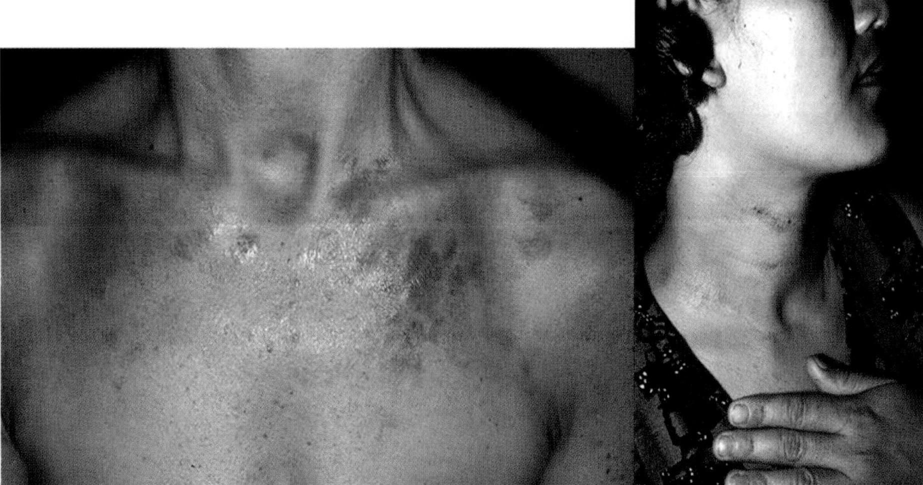

Figure 27.2 ACD to TSFR with patchy involvement of the neck and upper chest from "hand-to-neck/chest" exposure.

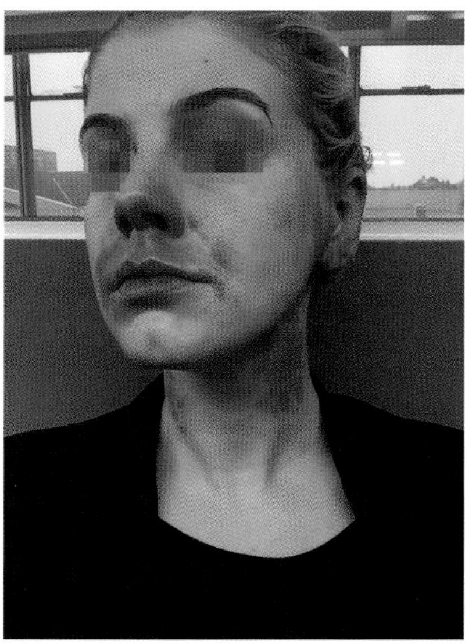
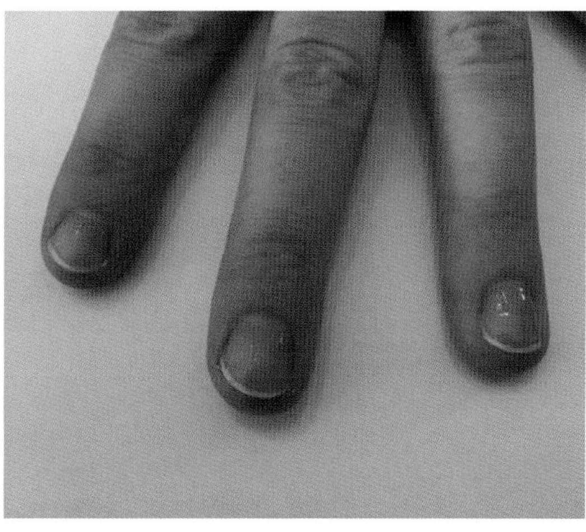

Figure 27.3 ACD to TSFR demonstrating extensive head and neck involvement from both airborne and "hand-to-face/neck" exposure. There is also nailfold involvement from direct contact exposure.

Table 27.2 The wide diversity of anatomical sites that can be involved in ACD to TSFR.

Face and sublocations of face affected were:	*n* = 135 (87%)
of which Periorbital	*n* = 86 (71% of facial lesions)
Perioral	*n* = 40 (30% of facial lesions)
Mentum	*n* = 35 (23% of facial lesions)
Frontal	*n* = 25 (19% of facial lesions)
Auricular	*n* = 25 (19% of facial lesions)
Nasolabial sulcus	*n* = 22 (16% of facial lesions)
Zygomatic region	*n* = 17 (13% of facial lesions)
Maxillary region	*n* = 13 (10% of facial lesions)
Lips	*n* = 10 (7% of facial lesions)
Temporal region	*n* = 6 (4% of facial lesions)
Neck	*n* = 86 (55%)
Trunk and abdomen	*n* = 45 (29%)
Upper limbs	*n* = 31 (20%)
Periungual region of the fingernails	*n* = 33 (21%)
Palms	*n* = 19 (12%)
Lower limbs	*n* = 10 (6%)
Toenails	*n* = 9 (6%)
Sole	*n* = 4 (3%)
Scalp	*n* = 3 (2%)
Gluteal/perianal, genitalia	*n* = 2 each (1% each)

- *Otitis externa*: Of 88 patients with ACD to TSFR, the pinnae was involved in four, the retroauricular areas in six, and five had otitis externa [10]. The dermatitis may spread to involve the face, neck, and chest and may easily be misdiagnosed as seborrheic dermatitis [10].
- *Seborrheic dermatitis-like lesions*: ACD to TSFR has been reported with facial dermatitis mimicking seborrheic dermatitis but without scalp involvement [19].
- *Photosensitivity* (isolated case report) [20].
- *Onycholysis* (mimicking onychomycosis) [21].
- *On sites of nickel exposure*: Nail varnish is frequently used by nickel-allergic subjects to coat nickel to prevent allergic reactions. This may, however, lead to ACD to TSFR at the same sites [22].

Patch testing

- 10% in pet.
- Test the patients' own samples of nail varnish. It is important that the varnish is dry before applying the patch, as false-positive irritant reactions to wet nail varnish can occur (likewise clinical irritant [non-allergic] contact reactions from the transfer of wet nail varnish to skin are also theoretically possible).

Other nail varnish allergens

- The increasing use of *phthalic anhydride/trimellitic anhydride/glycols copolymer* as an alternative resin system in nail varnishes has led to this agent becoming another common nail varnish allergen, presenting in a similar way as ACD to TSFR [23].
- Similarly, *acrylates* are now another major nail varnish allergen and 2-hydroxyethyl-methacrylate (HEMA) 2% in pet. is a useful screen for acrylic nail varnish allergy [24].
- Solvents, plasticizers, dyes, pigments, couplers, and film-building materials have been implicated but only in single case reports (i.e. uncommon) [12].

- Nail varnish can contain low amounts of *formaldehyde*
- *Sunscreen chemicals*
- *Colophonium*
- *Metal* in "glitter" allergens
- Adipic acid.

References

1 Stechschulte, S.A., Avashia, N., and Jacob, S.E. (2008). Tosylamide formaldehyde resin. *Dermatitis* 19 (3): E18–E19.

2 Orton, D.I. and Wilkinson, J.D. (2004). Cosmetic allergy: incidence, diagnosis, and management. *American Journal of Clinical Dermatology* 5 (5): 327–337.

3 Rodrigues, D.F. and Goulart, E.M. (2015). Patch test results in children and adolescents. Study from the Santa casa de Belo Horizonte dermatology clinic, Brazil, from 2003 to 2010. *Anais Brasileiros de Dermatologia* 90 (5): 671–683.

4 Duarte, I., Lazzarini, R., and Kobata, C.M. (2003). Contact dermatitis in adolescents. *American Journal of Contact Dermatitis* 14 (4): 200–202.

5 Amin, K.A. and Belsito, D.V. (2006). The aetiology of eyelid dermatitis: a 10-year retrospective analysis. *Contact Dermatitis* 55 (5): 280–285.

6 Rodrigues, D.F., Neves, D.R., Pinto, J.M. et al. (2012). Results of patch-tests from Santa Casa de Belo Horizonte Dermatology Clinic, Belo Horizonte, Brazil, from 2003 to 2010. *Anais Brasileiros de Dermatologia* 87 (5): 800–803.

7 Fransway, A.F., Zug, K.A., Belsito, D.V. et al. (2013). North American Contact Dermatitis Group patch test results for 2007–2008. *Dermatitis* 24 (1): 10–21.

8 Calnan, C.D. and Sarkany, I. (1958). Studies in contact dermatitis iii nail varnish. *Transactions of the St John's Hospital Dermatological Society* 40: 1–10.

9 Lazzarini, R., Duarte, I., de Farias, D.C. et al. (2008). Frequency and main sites of allergic contact dermatitis caused by nail varnish. *Dermatitis* 19 (6): 319–322.

10 Cronin E (1980). *Contact Dermatitis*. Chapter 4 Cosmetics, 93–171. Edinburgh: Churchill Livingstone.

11 Lidén, C., Berg, M., Färm, G., and Wrangsjö, K. (1993). Nail varnish allergy with far-reaching consequences. *British Journal of Dermatology* 128 (1): 57–62.

12 Hausen, B.M., Milbrodt, M., and Koenig, W.A. (1995). The allergens of nail polish. (I). Allergenic constituents of common nail polish and toluenesulfonamide-formaldehyde resin (TS-F-R). *Contact Dermatitis* 33 (3): 157–164.

13 Ozkaya, E. and Mirzoyeva, L. (2009). Tosylamide/formaldehyde resin allergy in a young boy: exposure from bitter nail varnish used against nail biting. *Contact Dermatitis* 60 (3): 171–172.

14 Jacob, S.E. and Stechschulte, S.A. (2008). Tosylamide/formaldehyde resin allergy – a consideration in the atopic toddler. *Contact Dermatitis* 58 (5): 312–313.

15 Nardelli, A., Degreef, H., and Goossens, A. (2004). Contact allergic reactions of the vulva: a 14-year review. *Dermatitis* 15 (3): 131–136.

16 Lazarov, A. (1999). Perianal contact dermatitis caused by nail lacquer allergy. *American Journal of Contact Dermatitis* 10 (1): 43–44.

17 Freeman, S. and Stephens, R. (1999). Cheilitis: analysis of 75 cases referred to a contact dermatitis clinic. *American Journal of Contact Dermatitis: Official Journal of the American Contact Dermatitis Society* 10 (4): 198–200.

18 Staines, K.S., Felix, D.H., and Forsyth, A. (1998). Desquamative gingivitis, sole manifestation of tosylamide/formaldehyde resin allergy. *Contact Dermatitis* 39 (2): 90.

19 Pongpairoj, K., Morar, N., and McFadden, J.P. (2016). 'Seborrheic dermatitis' of the head and neck without scalp involvement – remember nail varnish allergy. *Contact Dermatitis* 74 (5): 306–307.

20 Vilaplana, J. and Romaguera, C. (2000). Contact dermatitis from tosylamide/formaldehyde resin with photosensitivity. *Contact Dermatitis* 42 (5): 311–312.

21 Paltzik, R.L. and Enscoe, I. (1980). Onycholysis secondary to toluene sulfonamide formaldehyde resin used in a nail hardener mimicking onychomycosis. *Cutis* 25 (6): 647–648.

22 Shergill, B. and Goldsmith, P. (2004). Nail varnish is a potential allergen in nickel allergic subjects. *Clinical and Experimental Dermatology* 29 (5): 545–546.

23 Gach, J.E., Stone, N.M., and Finch, T.M. (2005). A series of four cases of allergic contact dermatitis to phthalic anhydride/trimellitic anhydride/glycols copolymer in nail varnish. *Contact Dermatitis* 53 (1): 63–64.

24 Montgomery, R., Stocks, S.J., and Wilkinson, S.M. (2016). Contact allergy resulting from the use of acrylate nails is increasing in both users and those who are occupationally exposed. *Contact Dermatitis* 74 (2): 120–122.

Exposure Color Code

- Clothing, jewelry, adornments
- Personal care products, cosmetics/cosmetic procedures
- Household products, domestic environment, including furniture and refurbishment
- Occupational dermatoses, work environment
- Medicines, surgical/dental procedures, herbal/alternative medicines
- Personal appliances/aids
- Leisure activities, sport, travel
- Other exposures (including dietary)
- Not relevant or multiple/general exposure

CHAPTER 28

para-Tertiary-Butylphenol Formaldehyde Resin

CHAPTER CONTENTS

Key points

- PTBP formaldehyde resin is an alkylphenol resin made from PTBP and formaldehyde that is in widespread everyday use.
- It is used in glued leather goods such as shoes, handbags, belts, and watchstraps.
- It is used occupationally in conjunction with materials such as plywood and fiberglass.
- PTBP allergy has been one of the most common causes of dermatitis reactions to shoes and watchstraps.
- Allergic contact dermatitis (ACD) to PTBP in shoes is commonly found on the soles of the feet.
- Potential occupational exposures include shoemakers, adhesive workers, box makers, leather finishers, and dentists. ACD to PTBP is the most common occupational allergen in cobblers.
- PTBP may occasionally be present in cosmetics such as deodorants, lip liners, and plastic nail adhesives (mostly of historical interest).
- There are case reports of ACD from exposure to athletic tape, knee braces, knee supports, padded bras, temporary henna tattoos, and neoprene components in a face mask.
- Depigmentation has been reported with and without preceding inflammation.
- Diagnostic patch testing is with PTBP resin 1% pet. The reported frequency of positive reactions in contact clinics in Europe, America, and Asia is usually between 0.3 and 2.0%.

Common pitfalls

- Sensitivity to formaldehyde does not imply allergy to formaldehyde resins.
- Patch testing with PTBP formaldehyde resin in most baseline series may not be sufficient to detect patients with contact allergy to all phenol-formaldehyde resins (PFRs).
- Other resins may now be used in the manufacturing of shoes.

Exposure and use

PTBP resin is used as an adhesive because it sticks rapidly, is durable and pliable, and maintains good bond strength at raised temperatures (Figure 28.1). PTBP is also found in certain neoprene adhesives [1, 2]. PTBP resins have also been used as adhesives with paper and wood [2].

Cosmetics

PTBP may have occasionally been included in cosmetics such as deodorants, lip liners, and plastic nail adhesives, though current exposure would be unlikely. Angelini et al. [3] described the use of gas chromatography combined with mass spectrometry

Common Contact Allergens: A Practical Guide to Detecting Contact Dermatitis, First Edition. Edited by John McFadden, Pailin Puangpet, Korbkarn Pongpairoj, Supitchaya Thaiwat, and Lee Shan Xian.
© 2020 John Wiley & Sons Ltd. Published 2020 by John Wiley & Sons Ltd.
Companion website: www.wiley.com/go/mcfadden/common_contact_allergens

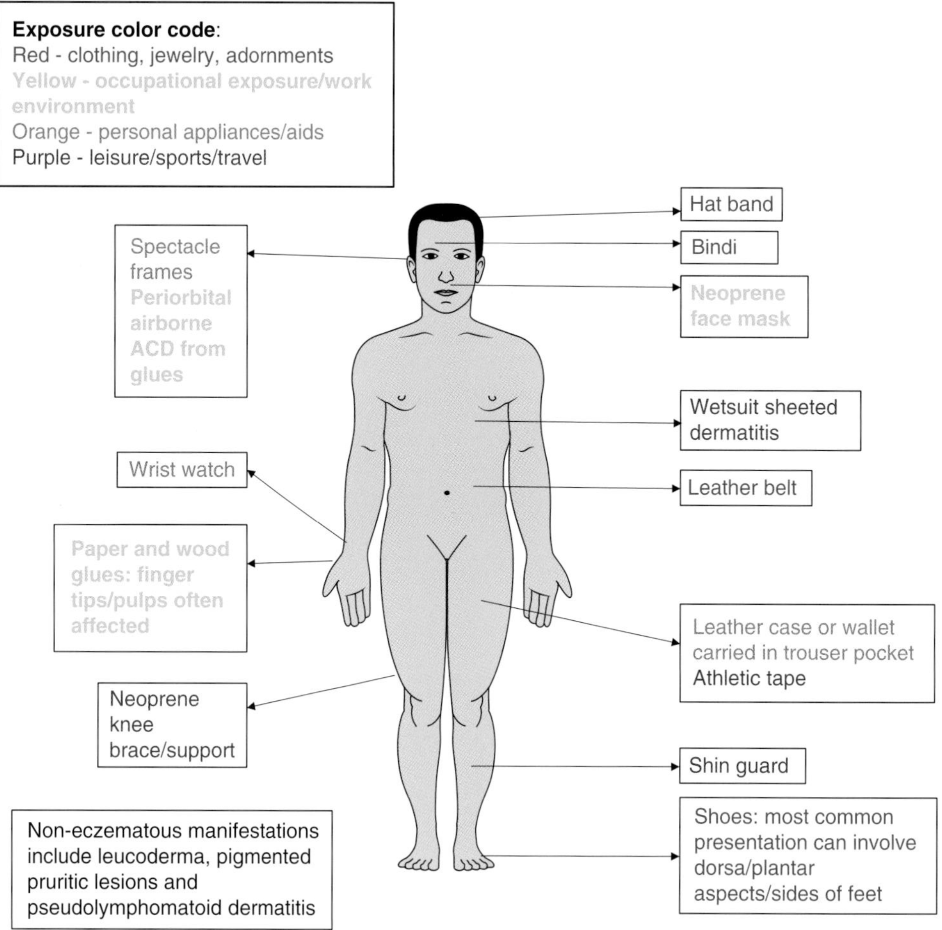

Figure 28.1 Reported exposure sources for ACD to PTBP resin.

(GC-MS) in the investigation of a case of ACD of the lip margins caused by a PTBP-containing lip liner.

Non-cosmetic exposure and use

PTBP is an adhesive commonly used to bond leather, rubber-to-rubber, or rubber-to-metal surfaces. It is principally found in shoes, handbags, belts, and watchstraps. When shoes get wet, the allergen in these glues dissolves and comes into contact with the skin.

Products that may contain para-tertiary-butylphenol (PTBP) formaldehyde resin

- Domestic wood adhesives.
- Adhesive tape.
- Adhesive labels.
- Automobile components: motor oils, upholstery, brake lining.
- Bindi.
- Boxes.
- Deodorants (historical).
- Diapers.
- Disinfectant (historical).
- Duplicating paper.
- Fabric labels, glued and glossy fabrics.
- Film developers.
- Furniture.
- Glues (DIY glues).
- Hat bands.
- Insecticides.
- Leather and rubber products: handbags, shoes, belts, hats, watchbands.
- Masonry sealant.
- Paints.
- Playing cards, glossy paper.
- Polychloroprene adhesives.
- Surface coatings, varnishes, printing inks.
- Medical items: hearing aids, prostheses [4], adhesive dressings [5], electrocardiograph monitoring electrodes [6], athletic tape, braces (knee), dental bonding materials.
- Building industry: plywood manufacturing, insulation materials (rock wool), casting molds, fiberglass products.

Patch testing

- 1% PTBP in petrolatum is included in the International Contact Dermatitis Research Group (ICDRG) standard patch test series.
- The worldwide patch test clinic prevalence of positive patch test reactions to PTBP approximates to 1.3%.
- Irritant reactions are not uncommon.

Clinical disease

- Rashes are commonly found on the feet, hands, and wrists. In most cases involving the feet the source of exposure is the *adhesive in shoes* (Figure 28.2). Leather gloves and watch-straps are also commonly implicated in cases involving the hands and wrists.
- *Watchstrap* (Figure 28.3) dermatitis is clinically less severe than that of metals and dyes in the straps. It is often more intense at the margins of the strap, where the allergen reaches the skin [7].

Case reports

- ACD to PTBP resin was reported in a retired man who took up painting and decorating as a hobby for 2 months prior to developing eczematous and desquamative lesions. He handled glue, metal, wood, and plastic and had lesions on the palms and backs of the fingers, as well as fissures on the fingertips [8].
- Downs and Sansom [9] described seven patients with palmoplantar dermatitis from PTBP with clinical similarities to mercaptobenzothiazole allergy. The plantar areas (especially pressure) and/or dorsal aspects of the feet can be involved.
- A 32-year-old Japanese man experienced adhesive dermatitis after having a knee operation. He had worn a *knee brace* for 2 months prior to developing an erythemato-vesicular eruption at the site of contact with the brace. Patch tests were positive to the pads of the brace, raincoat fabric, PTBP, and tetramethylthiuram disulfide (TMTD), but negative to non-formaldehyde PTBP, phenol formaldehyde resin, and formaldehyde. The pads and raincoat fabric were analyzed. PTBP formaldehyde resin was detected by high-performance liquid chromatography and PTBP by flame ionization detection-gas chromatography

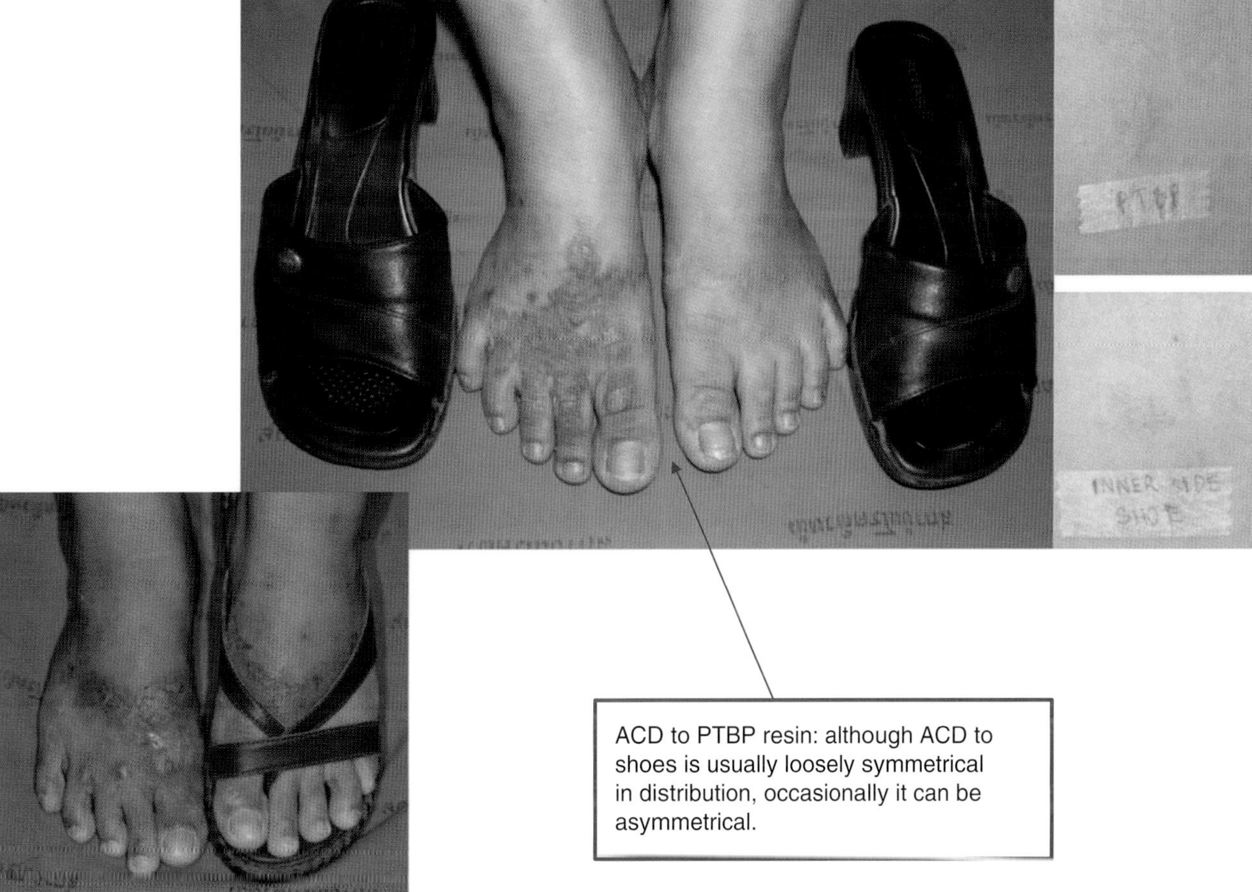

PTBP
INNER SIDE
SHOE
ACD to PTBP resin: although ACD to shoes is usually loosely symmetrical in distribution, occasionally it can be asymmetrical.

Figure 28.2 ACD to PTBP resin from shoes – note that the dermatitis is usually but not necessarily symmetrical.

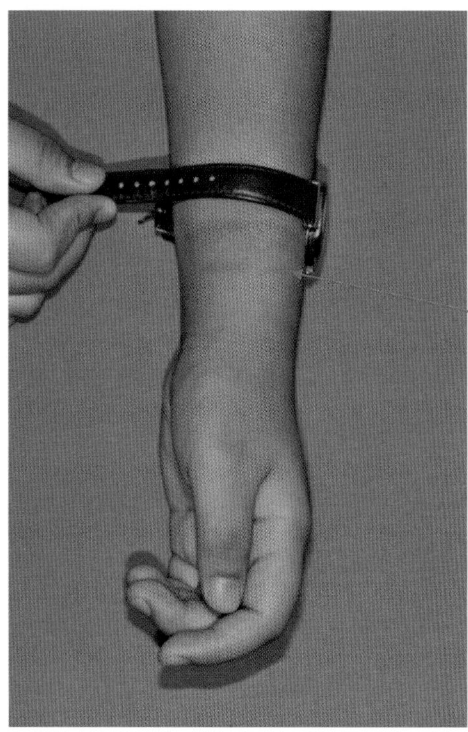
Accentuation of inflammation at the edge of the dermatitis.

Figure 28.3 ACD to PTBP resin from a watchstrap. In the "PTBP watchstrap sign," as opposed to metal and leather ACD, the intensity of inflammation is often less and there is accentuation at the edge of the dermatitis.

and gas chromatography mass spectrometry, but TMTD was not detected [10] (Figure 28.4).

- Four teenage girls diagnosed with ACD from *athletic tape* were reported. One of them had foot dermatitis from new *sneakers*. They presented with severe vesicular ankle dermatitis. All four patients reacted positively to alkyl phenol resin and PTBP formaldehyde resin, but negatively to PTBP, form aldehyde, and phenol formaldehyde resin. PTBP formaldehyde resin was detected in the extract of the adhesive from both the athletic tape and sneakers [11].
- Ozkaya et al. [12] reported a case with severe eczema caused by PTBP and colophonium in a novel product, *neoprene thermal sauna shorts*. A pruritic, erythematous, and vesicular eruption developed on the upper thighs, abdomen, and buttocks, sparing areas of contact with the seams. Neoprene products may contain numerous sensitizing additives such as antioxidants, accelerators (thioureas, carbamates), or adhesives (PTBP).
- A 58-year-old Japanese woman experienced itchy erythema on the neck and thighs, sparing the areas covered by a new *wetsuit*, 12 hours after wearing it. She reacted positively to PTBP, mercuric chloride, potassium dichromate, urushiol, and a piece of her wetsuit. The adhesive made of rubber material in the wetsuit, namely polychloroprene rubber, was the most likely cause. The polychloroprene rubber adhesives contain PTBP as a tackifier [13].
- In a UK series of patients with suspected shoe ACD, only 1/230 (0.5%) had a positive reaction to PTBP [14]. This is in contrast to a previous study from Italy, where patch test results to a shoe battery in patients with contact dermatitis of the feet showed PTBP reactions in 5.5% (9/165) [15].
- ACD to a *temporary henna tattoo* from the presumed inclusion of PTBP resin as an adhesive agent, with subsequent *leucoderma*, has been reported [16].
- A 28-year-old non-atopic woman who played soccer as a hobby complained of a relapsing itching linear dermatitis of the right popliteal area after using a neoprene knee brace. Patch tests showed ++/+++ reactions to both PTBP 1% pet and the seamed part of the brace. Spectroscopy confirmed the presence of PTBP in the seamed area of the brace [17].
- A 73-year-old man presented with pruritic scaly plaques localized to the posterior scalp, forehead, bilateral cheeks, and angle of his mandible. The areas of dermatitis correlated with the areas of contact with the neoprene strap of his mask used for continuous positive airway pressure (CPAP). Patch test was positive (+) to PTBP as well as to a sample of the neoprene strap. Covering the strap with cotton led to resolution of the dermatitis [18].
- A 14-year-old girl presented with a 7-month history of severe, recurrent breast dermatitis. She was noted to have bilateral hyperpigmented, erythematous, lichenified, and crusted plaques with effacement of the nipple and areola areas. Patch testing showed + reactions to PTBP and the padded area of her bra. Avoidance of the padded bra led to resolution of the dermatitis [19].

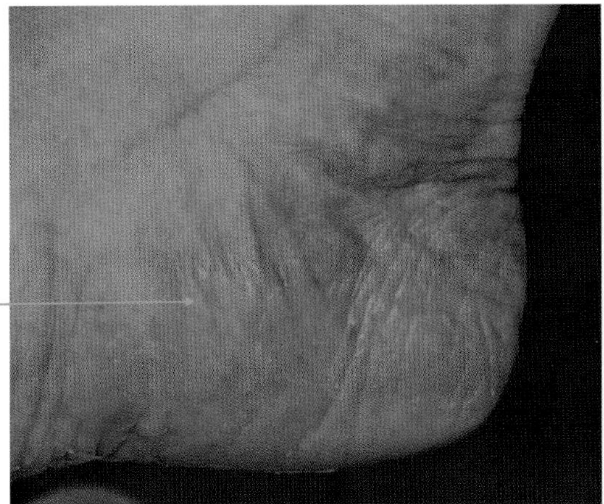

Clinical changes of ACD from a prosthesis are often chronic and the dermatitis can be very pruritic.

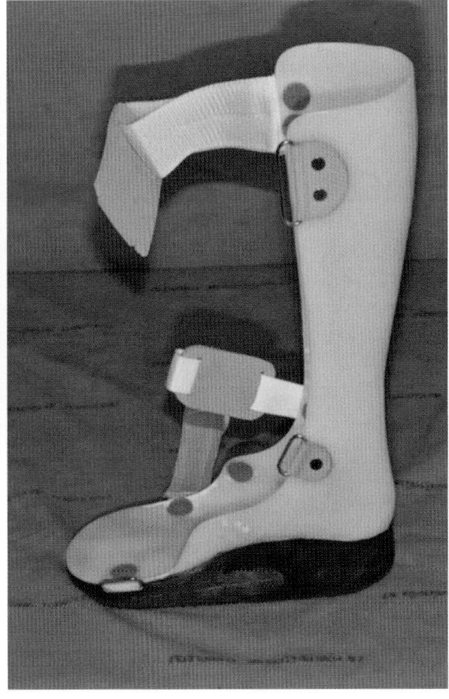

Figure 28.4 ACD to PTBP resin from a prosthesis.

Contact leucoderma

- ACD to PTBP resin can cause leucoderma. ACD to PTBP in watchstraps, lip liners, and bindi causing leucoderma have all been recorded [20, 21]. There may not always be preceding inflammation. Multiple cases in an occupational setting have been recorded [3, 22].

Non-eczematous dermatoses

- A 51-year-old woman was reported with a 1.5 year history of well-defined pigmented pruritic lesions which were initially mildly erythematous on the left wrist. Patch tests showed ++ reactions to both PTBP (1% pet) and a piece of her leather watchstrap. Histopathology from the wrist and positive patch test site showed interface dermatitis [23].
- A case of lymphomatoid contact dermatitis to PTBP has been reported. This patient carried a leather spectacle case in the pocket of his trousers a few days prior to developing a persistent pruritic plaque on his thigh. Histopathology was consistent with a lichenoid variant of cutaneous T-cell lymphoma. Patch testing showed a + reaction to the spectacle case and a ++ reaction to PTBP resin [24].

Occupational disease

- PTBP formaldehyde resin was one of the most common occupational allergens in *shoemakers*. In Italian shoemakers, 6% (15/246) suffered hyperkeratosis of the fingertips and 3.2% had pruritus sine materia (generalized pruritus without skin lesions) [25].
- In 1958, Malten described ten cobblers sensitized by an adhesive in the soles of shoes in the Netherlands [26]. The fingertips of the left hand that held the sole were often involved. In 1959, Calnan and Harman also described three sensitized shoemakers and one worker from *handbag manufacturing* [27]. Among 106 PTBP allergic patients reported between 1958 and 1976, occupational allergies accounted for 71% (75 cases). The shoe-making industry was the main cause (42 cases), followed by the *automobile industry* (33 cases) [1]. Other potential occupational exposures are *adhesive workers, box makers* and *leather finishers.*
- *Adhesive labels* are another source of PTBP. When increased adhesion is required, esters of maleic or phthalic acids, terpenes or phenolic resins are added to the adhesive. These compounds can migrate to the surface and cause dermatitis. A worker in a supply depot, putting metal objects in cardboard boxes using tapes and adhesive labels, presented with vesicular dermatitis on the fingertips and hypothenar eminence. Patch tests showed positive reactions to PTBP and to the sticky side of used labels [28].

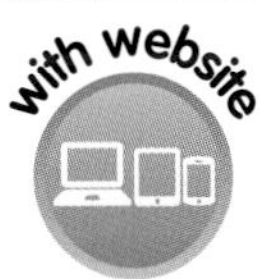

Go to www.wiley.com/go/mcfadden/common_contact_allergens to find the E-supplement for this chapter:
Para-tertiary-Butylphenol Formaldehyde Resin: E-Supplement

References

1 Foussereau, J., Cavelier, C., and Selig, D. (1976). Occupational eczema from para-tertiary-butylphenol formaldehyde resins: a review of the sensitizing resins. *Contact Dermatitis* 2 (5): 254–258.
2 Cronin, E. (1980). *Contact Dermatitis Chapter 3. Clothing Textiles*. Edinburgh: Churchill Livingstone.
3 Angelini, E., Marinaro, C., Carrozzo, A.M. et al. (1993). Allergic contact dermatitis of the lip margins from para-tertiary-butylphenol in a lip liner. *Contact Dermatitis* 28 (3): 146–148.
4 Romaguera, C., Grimalt, F., and Vilaplana, J. (1985). Paratertiary butylphenol formaldehyde resin in prosthesis. *Contact Dermatitis* 12 (3): 174.
5 Burden, A.D., Lever, R.S., and Morley, W.N. (1994). Contact hypersensitivity induced by p-tert-butylphenol-formaldehyde resin in an adhesive dressing. *Contact Dermatitis* 31 (4): 276–277.
6 Avenel-Audran, M., Goossens, A., Zimerson, E., and Bruze, M. (2003). Contact dermatitis from electrocardiograph-monitoring electrodes: role of p-tert-butylphenol-formaldehyde resin. *Contact Dermatitis* 48 (2): 108–111.
7 Mobacken, H. and Hersle, K. (1976). Allergic contact dermatitis by para-tertiary butylphenol-formaldehyde resin in watch straps. *Contact Dermatitis* 2 (1): 59.
8 Moran, M. and Pascual, A.M. (1978). Contact dermatitis to para-tertiary-butylphenol formaldehyde. *Contact Dermatitis* 4 (6): 372–373.
9 Downs, A.M. and Sansom, J.E. (1998). Palmoplantar dermatitis may be due to phenol-formaldehyde resin contact dermatitis. *Contact Dermatitis* 39 (3): 147–148.
10 Hayakawa, R., Ogino, Y., Suzuki, M., and Kaniwa, M. (1994). Allergic contact dermatitis from para-tertiary-butylphenol-formaldehyde resin (PTBP-F-R). *Contact Dermatitis* 30 (3): 187–188.
11 Shono, M., Ezoe, K., Kaniwa, M.A. et al. (1991). Allergic contact dermatitis from para-tertiary-butylphenol-formaldehyde resin (PTBP-FR) in athletic tape and leather adhesive. *Contact Dermatitis* 24 (4): 281–288.
12 Ozkaya, E., Elinc-Aslan, M.S., and Mirzoyeva, L. (2010). Allergic contact dermatitis caused by p-tert-butylphenol formaldehyde resin and colophonium in neoprene thermal sauna shorts. *Contact Dermatitis* 63 (4): 230–232.
13 Nagashima, C., Tomitaka-Yagami, A., and Matsunaga, K. (2003). Contact dermatitis due to para-tertiary-butylphenol-formaldehyde resin in a wetsuit. *Contact Dermatitis* 49 (5): 267–268.
14 Holden, C.R. and Gawkrodger, D.J. (2005). 10 years' experience of patch testing with a shoe series in 230 patients: which allergens are important? *Contact Dermatitis* 53 (1): 37–39.
15 Angelini, G., Vena, G.A., and Meneghini, C.L. (1980). Shoe contact dermatitis. *Contact Dermatitis* 6 (4): 279–283.
16 Rodrigo-Nicolas, B., de la Cuadra, J., Sierra, C., and Miquel, J. (2014). Contact dermatitis from a temporary tattoo in a boy with contact allergy to p-tert butyl phenol formaldehyde resin. *Dermatitis* 25 (1): 37–38.
17 Corazza, M., Zauli, S., Bernardi, T. et al. (2012). A linear allergic contact dermatitis to p-tert-butylphenol formaldehyde resin sectorially present in a neoprene orthopedic brace: role of spectroscopy. *Dermatitis* 23 (6): 292–293.
18 Herro, E.M. and Jacob, S.E. (2012). Allergic contact dermatitis to p-tert butylphenol formaldehyde resin in a continuous positive airway pressure strap. *Dermatitis* 23 (3): 125–126.
19 Herro, E.M., Friedlander, S.F., and Jacob, S.E. (2012). Bra-associated allergic contact dermatitis: p-tert-butylphenol formaldehyde resin as the culprit. *Pediatric Dermatology* 29 (4): 540–541.
20 Malten, K.E. (1975). Paratertiary butylphenol depigmentation in a "consumer". *Contact Dermatitis* 1 (3): 181–182.
21 Bajaj, A.K., Gupta, S.C., and Chatterjee, A.K. (1990). Contact depigmentation from free para-tertiary-butylphenol in bindi adhesive. *Contact Dermatitis* 22 (2): 99–102.
22 Romaguera, C. and Grimalt, F. (1981). Occupational leukoderma and contact dermatitis from paratertiary-butylphenol. *Contact Dermatitis* 7 (3): 159–160.
23 Ozkaya-Bayazit, E. and Buyukbabani, N. (2001). Non-eczematous pigmented interface dermatitis from para-tertiary-butylphenol-formaldehyde resin in a watchstrap adhesive. *Contact Dermatitis* 44 (1): 45–46.
24 Evans, A.V., Banerjee, P., McFadden, J.P., and Calonje, E. (2003). Lymphomatoid contact dermatitis to para-tertyl-butyl phenol resin. *Clinical and Experimental Dermatology* 28 (3): 272–273.
25 Mancuso, G., Reggiani, M., and Berdondini, R.M. (1996). Occupational dermatitis in shoemakers. *Contact Dermatitis* 34 (1): 17–22.
26 Malten, K.E. (1958). Occupational eczema due to para-tertiary-butylphenol in a shoe adhesive. *Dermatologica* 117: 103–109.
27 Calnan, C.D. and Harman, M.K. (1959). Sensitivity to para-tertiary-butylphenol. *Transantions of the St John's Hospital Dermatological Society* 43: 27–32.
28 Dahlquist, I. (1984). Contact allergy to paratertiary butylphenol formaldehyde resin in an adhesive label. *Contact Dermatitis* 10 (1): 54.

Exposure Color Code

- Clothing, jewelry, adornments
- Personal care products, cosmetics/cosmetic procedures
- Household products, domestic environment, including furniture and refurbishment
- Occupational dermatoses, work environment
- Medicines, surgical/dental procedures, herbal/alternative medicines
- Personal appliances/aids
- Leisure activities, sport, travel
- Other exposures (including dietary)
- Not relevant or multiple/general exposure

CHAPTER 29

Sesquiterpene Lactone Mix and Compositae Mix

CHAPTER CONTENTS

Key points

- Sesquiterpene lactone mix is a mixture of substances used as a screening test for allergy to members of the daisy family (Compositae or Asteraceae).
- Compositae is an alternative name for the official term Asteraceae. They comprise one of the largest groups of flowered plants (about 10%) and are present throughout the world.
- Members of this family include decorative and wild flowering plants, plants used for medicinal purposes, weeds, and edible plants.
- Trichomes/hairs on the plant surface are the primary sites of sesquiterpene lactone accumulation.
- Modes of sensitization include airborne, direct/indirect contact, inhalation, or ingestion of allergens. Direct contact is the most common cause.
- The most common sites affected in allergic contact dermatitis (ACD) to sesquiterpene lactones are the hands and/or the face.
- Classic Compositae contact allergy presents in older men as an airborne pattern of chronic lichenified and intensely pruritic eczema. Seasonal variations, with recurrences in summer months and remissions in winter, are typical.
- Systemic contact dermatitis and an eruption resembling erythema multiforme are uncommon forms of presentation of Compositae allergy.
- Patch testing is with 0.1% pet. preparation of a mix of three sesquiterpene lactones/T.R.U.E.® test equivalent.
- In Europe, most clinics report a frequency of 0.5–2.2% of positive patch tests to sesquiterpene lactone mix; a large multicenter study reports a mean frequency of 0.9%.
- Compositae mix patch tests usually include common yarrow, mountain arnica, German chamomile, feverfew, and common tansy.
- Sesquiterpene lactone mix screening alone may detect only about 60% of sensitized patients and in patients with a high index of suspicion additional testing with additional Compositae mix and extra single Compositae agents has been recommended by some authors. However, there have also been concerns regarding the theoretical potential for active sensitization with some Compositae mix patch test preparations.
- Sesquiterpene lactone mix may be an inadequate screen for sensitivity to a single individual Compositae plant.
- Cross-reactivity of sesquiterpene lactones with terpenes may occur and may be associated with fragrance allergy.
- Sesquiterpene lactone allergy is associated with chronic actinic (photosensitive) dermatitis.
- *Parthenium* dermatitis in the Indian subcontinent is a particularly severe form of Compositae ACD.
- Compositae allergy can result from occupational exposure in gardeners, forestry and outdoor workers, farmers, and florists.
- Reported ACD cases to Compositae from herbal remedies/creams are varied and numerous, and include exposure to yarrow, great burdock, arnica, mugwort, marigold, chamomile, echinacea, feverfew, and dandelion.
- Sesquiterpene lactone allergy has been noted in atopics of all ages, and if available testing with dandelion has also been recommended in atopic patients.

Common Contact Allergens: A Practical Guide to Detecting Contact Dermatitis, First Edition. Edited by John McFadden, Pailin Puangpet, Korbkarn Pongpairoj, Supitchaya Thaiwat, and Lee Shan Xian.

© 2020 John Wiley & Sons Ltd. Published 2020 by John Wiley & Sons Ltd.

Companion website: www.wiley.com/go/mcfadden/common_contact_allergens

Routes of compositae exposure for sensitization and allergic reactions

- Routes include airborne, direct contact, 'by proxy', manual transmission and less commonly, mucosal, inhalation or ingestion of allergens [1].

Exposure and use

- Compositae can be found in gardens, by the roadside, and in the wilderness.
- Sesquiterpene lactones are also present in several wood species [2]. These include tulip trees (*Liriodendron*), poplar, maple trees (possibly), the *Magnolia* species and bay trees (*Laurus nobilis*). *Frullania*, a genus of leafy liverworts that grows on tree bark and rocks worldwide, has caused occupational contact dermatitis due to the presence of sesquiterpene lactones.

Common plants containing sesquiterpene lactones

Patients allergic to sesquiterpene lactone should be given the following list of plants to avoid:

arnica, artichoke, bitterweed, boneset, broomweed, burdock, capeweed, chamomile, chicory, chrysanthemum, cineraria, cocklebur, cosmos, costus root, cotton thistle, dahlia, daisy, dandelion, elecampane, endive, feverfew, *Gaillardia*, golden rod, *Helenium*, ironweed, laurel bay or sweet bay (*Laurus nobilis*), laurel oil, leafcup, lettuce, marguerite, liatris, liverworts, magnolias, marigold, marsh elder, mugwort, *Parthenium*, poverty weed, *Pyrethrum*, ragweed, rudbeckia, sagebrush, sneezeweed, spinach, sunflower, tansy, tulip tree, whitewood of commerce, wild feverfew, wormwood, yarrow, yellow star thistle (Figure 29.1).

- Multiple exposures to Compositae have been associated with some reports of ACD.
- Apart from direct contact with the plants, other sources include creams, lotions, perfumes, cosmetics and toiletries, ointments, topical medications, aromatherapy oils (e.g. tagetes), herbal remedies, dried flowers (e.g. sunflowers, everlastings), teas, and herbal supplements.
- *Herbal remedies*: Many Compositae extracts have been used as herbal/medicinal agents. These include milfoil, yarrow, great burdock, arnica, mugwort, marigold, chamomile, echinacea, feverfew, and dandelion. They can be used in the form of creams, oral drugs, teas, and compresses.

Cosmetic regulation

- There is no effective regulatory control of Compositae use in cosmetics.

Patch testing

- There is a (very) low risk of active sensitization from Compositae mix patch testing.
- In contrast to Compositae plant extract, sesquiterpene lactone mix rarely elicits false-positive patch test reactions.
- 73.1% (19/26) of sesquiterpene lactone mix allergic patients also reacted to Compositae mix and 63.3% (19/30) of those with Compositae mix sensitivity reacted to sesquiterpene lactone mix. 0.4% (12/2818) of all patients in the whole tested population with Compositae mix sensitivity would have been missed by not testing with Compositae mix. The stronger the patch test reaction to Compositae mix, the more likely an allergic reaction to the sesquiterpene lactone mix [3].
- In a population from Austria, sensitization to arnica (*Arnica montana* L.) (n = 5) and marigold (*Calendula officinalis* L.) (n = 9) was accompanied by a reaction to Compositae mix in half of the cases and to sesquiterpene lactone mix in one case only. Patch testing with additional plant extracts was therefore recommended [4].
- Patients can react to plants or chemicals they have never been exposed to. These positive reactions are due to immunological cross-reactivity. A clinical and geographical history of relevant exposure is important [5].

Frequency of sensitization

- In Europe, most clinics report a frequency of 0.5–2.2% amongst all dermatitis patients patch tested. There is a mean frequency of 0.9%.
- North America has a mean frequency of 0.5% amongst all patch-tested patients.
- A healthy adult European population has a frequency of 0.1%.

Age and sex

- Any age can be affected, e.g. elderly gardeners, working age in floristry/farming/forestation occupations.
- In early studies, sesquiterpene lactone allergy was 20 times more common in men than women, especially those aged >40 years and working in the farming and forestry industries. However, more recent studies show a higher frequency in women who work in plant nurseries and florists' shops, or women who use certain cosmetics. Young women tend to have hand and/or face dermatoses, whereas older individuals have more generalized dermatitis and/or an airborne distribution [1].
- In children, a history of atopy appears to be a risk factor for developing contact allergy to Compositae. Compositae sensitization should also be suspected if their atopic dermatitis is exacerbated during the summer and there is a history of plant exposure. Screening with sesquiterpene lactone mix has shown prevalence rates of 0.5% and 1.8%, while screening with two Compositae plants could detect 4.2% and 2.6% among children

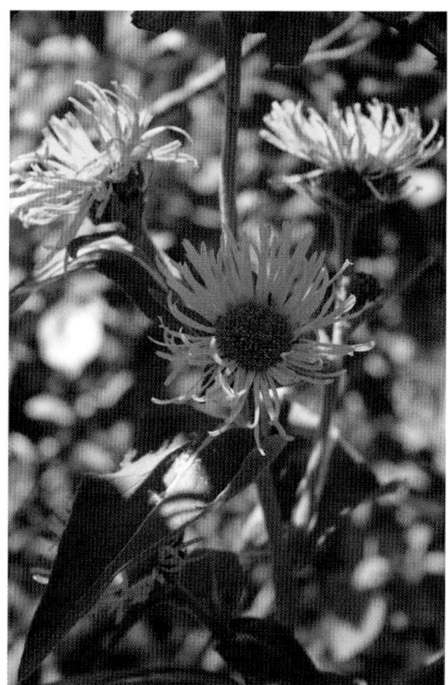

Inula helenium (horse-heal, elfdock)

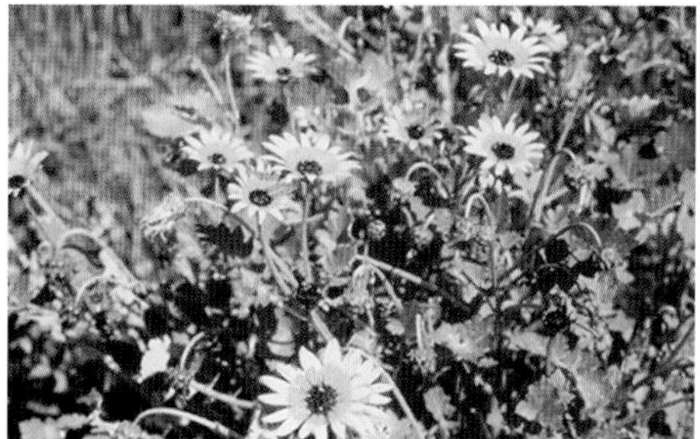

Arctotheca sp. (capeweed), a South African native growing as a weed in Australia

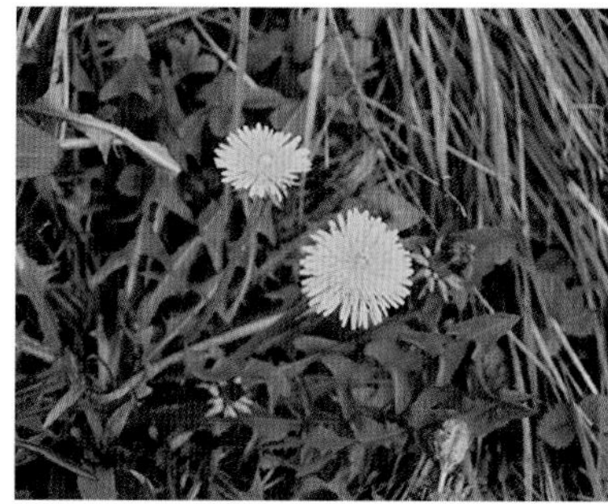

Taraxacum officinale (dandelion)

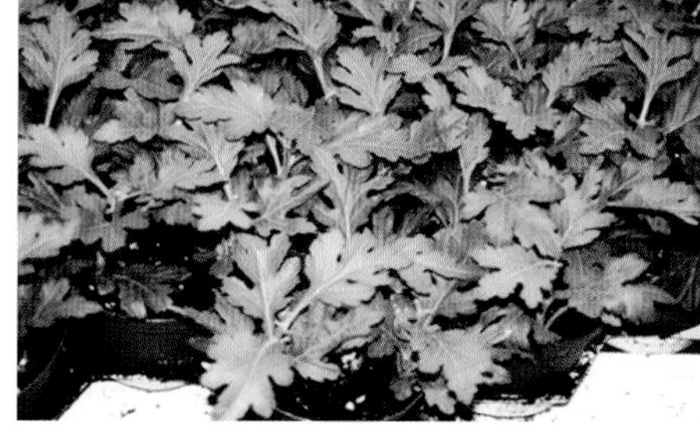

Disbudded X *Dendranthema* (florists' chrysanthemum) cultivar plants in a Danish nursery

Figure 29.1 Examples of Compositae plants.

and adolescent patients respectively [6]. Compositae weeds, especially dandelions, are important sensitizers in children [6] (can affect the feet) and can be patch tested in young patients [7].

- *Geographical variations*: An American study by Menz and Winkelmann [8] of 74 patients with Compositae sensitivity found a male/female ratio of 1.4:1, whereas in Singapore the ratio was 1:3.5 [9].

Clinical disease

- Clinical disease can present in the context of the domestic, occupational or leisure environments and exposure can be through various routes such as direct contact, airborne, systemic, mucosal, and by proxy (Figures 29.2–29.5).
- Chrysanthemum allergy was first reported by Howe in 1887. Ragweed dermatitis was reported in 1919. The North American feverfew (*Parthenium hysterophorus*) was brought from America to India in 1956 and has subsequently caused thousands of cases of *parthenium* dermatitis [10].
- In its classical form, Compositae contact allergy presents as a diffuse chronic lichenified eczematous and intensely pruritic eruption on areas exposed to flowers or pollen. It mainly occurs in middle-aged and elderly adults. Recurrences in summer months and remissions in winter are typical. When untreated, the eczema can progress and become more persistent [1, 11] (Figure 29.3).
- In rare cases, patients can develop generalized erythroderma. The widespread chronic eczema may imitate atopic dermatitis, seborrheic dermatitis, actinic reticuloid syndrome, and photodermatitis. However, involvement of the photoprotected upper eyelids [2], submental area, and retroauricular areas is usual. Contact urticaria is a possible presentation, usually in lettuce allergy [11].
- In one single series, 65% of patients had *vesicular hand eczema* [10]. *(Note: This is a high figure with respect to other reported series.)*
- *Recurrent facial edema*, accompanied by erythema and a burning sensation, was caused by allergy to a herbal oral medicine [12].
- *Systemic contact dermatitis* has been reported. Patients presented with exacerbations of previous eczema or mucosal and anogenital pruritus. The implicated foods were chamomile, chicory, lettuce, and echinacea. Dietary avoidance led to complete clearance in two patients [13].
- Most patients presented with *hand and/or face dermatitis* [14]. The rash may spread to unexposed sites. At St John's Institute of Dermatology, generalized eczema was found in 20%, hand and face involvement in 24%, hands alone in 36%, and face alone in 11% [15].

Airborne allergic contact dermatitis

- Information Network of Departments of Dermatology (IVDK) data showed a high sensitization prevalence rate of 13.4% (47/350 patch tested patients) to sesquiterpene lactone among patients presenting with airborne contact dermatitis (Figure 29.3) [16].
- Airborne contact dermatitis affects the face, upper eyelids, neck, hands, and arms or antecubital fossae, sometimes similar to photodermatitis [1].
- Common global sources for the classic airborne Compositae dermatitis are ragweed and *parthenium* [10].

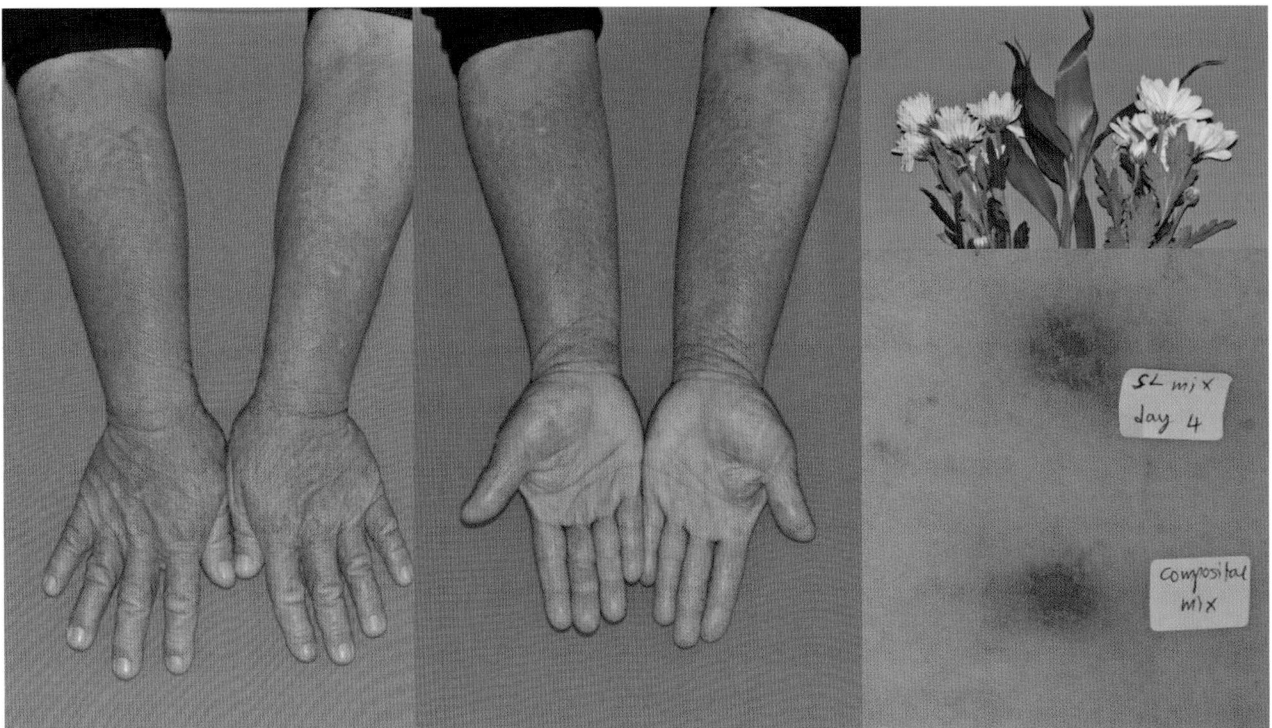

Figure 29.2 Occupational ACD in a florist from direct contact with Compositae plants. The dermatitis is affecting both the palmar and dorsal aspects of the hands, with spread to the forearms.

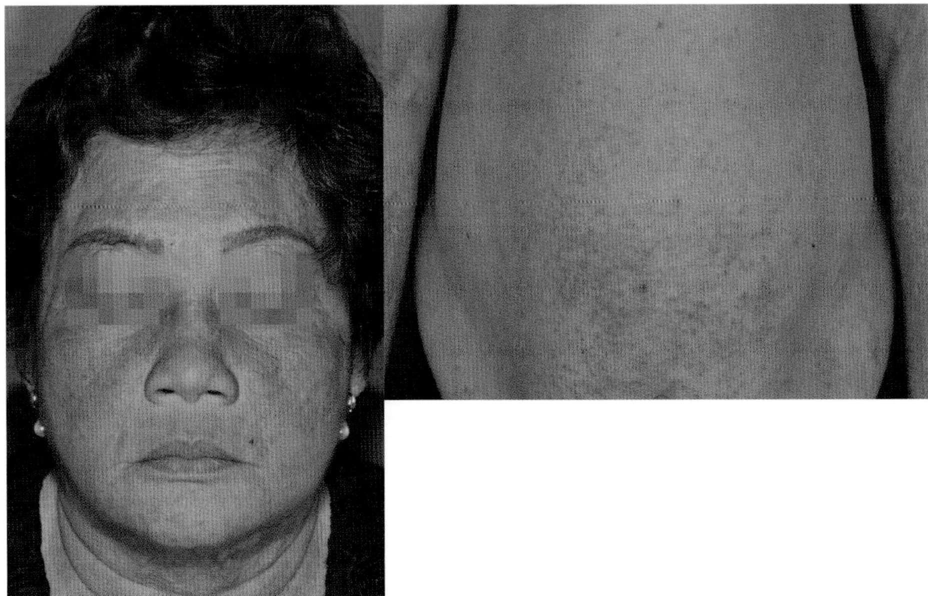

Figure 29.3 Airborne ACD to sesquiterpene lactones. In its classical form, this presents as a diffuse lichenified eczematous and intensely pruritic eruption on the exposed areas of skin. The dermatitis can then spread to the covered areas.

- Three cases of airborne contact dermatitis due to *Ambrosia deltoidea* (triangle-leaf bursage) were reported from the USA. Ivy Block® lotion may be useful in preventing exacerbations if applied prior to exposure, but may be irritating for eczematous skin [17].
- Seven patients were reported from Spain as having recurrent scaly erythematous dermatitis on sun-exposed areas, simulating a photodermatitis. All of them had dermatitis after walking in forests or parks during the summer. All patients had positive patch test responses to *Frullania dilatata*

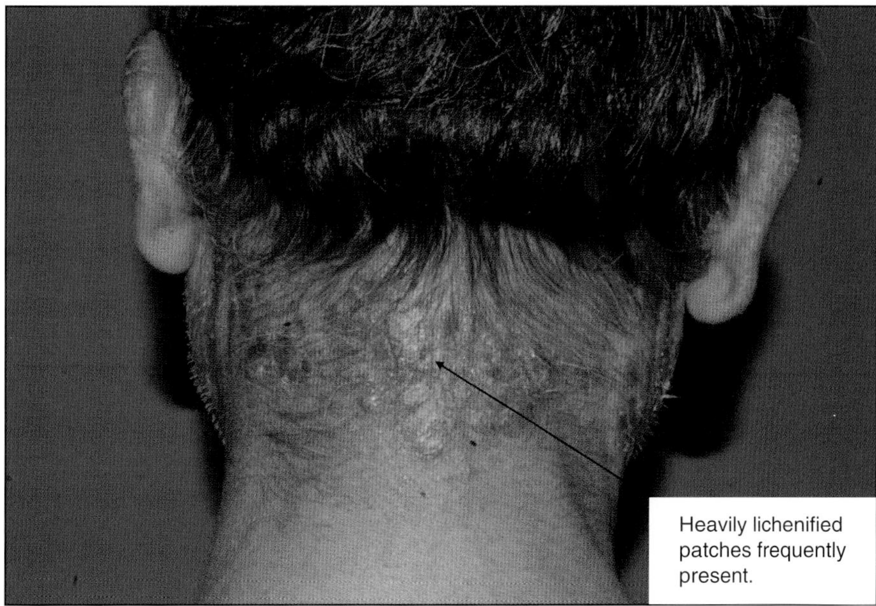

Figure 29.4 Chronic actinic dermatitis can be associated with contact allergy to sesquiterpene lactones. In this case, the photoprotected areas are spared, such as the submental and retroauricular areas.

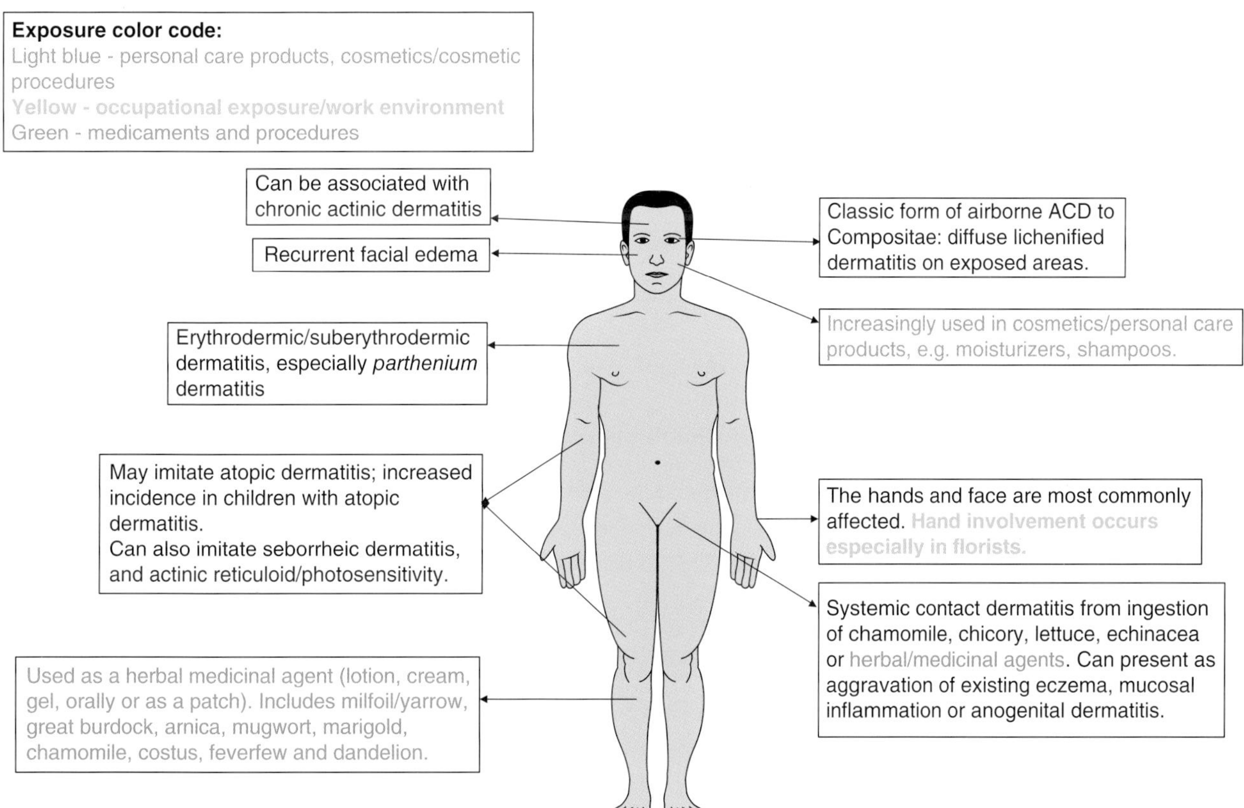

Exposure color code:
Light blue - personal care products, cosmetics/cosmetic procedures
Yellow - occupational exposure/work environment
Green - medicaments and procedures
Can be associated with chronic actinic dermatitis
Recurrent facial edema
Erythrodermic/suberythrodermic dermatitis, especially *parthenium* dermatitis
May imitate atopic dermatitis; increased incidence in children with atopic dermatitis.
Can also imitate seborrheic dermatitis, and actinic reticuloid/photosensitivity.
Used as a herbal medicinal agent (lotion, cream, gel, orally or as a patch). Includes milfoil/yarrow, great burdock, arnica, mugwort, marigold, chamomile, costus, feverfew and dandelion.
Classic form of airborne ACD to Compositae: diffuse lichenified dermatitis on exposed areas.
Increasingly used in cosmetics/personal care products, e.g. moisturizers, shampoos.
The hands and face are most commonly affected. Hand involvement occurs especially in florists.
Systemic contact dermatitis from ingestion of chamomile, chicory, lettuce, echinacea or herbal/medicinal agents. Can present as aggravation of existing eczema, mucosal inflammation or anogenital dermatitis.

Figure 29.5 Clinical manifestations of contact allergy to sesquiterpene lactones.

(a species of liverwort), and six of the seven cases reacted to sesquiterpene lactone mix [18].

Occupational disease: gardeners, chefs, forestry workers, and florists

- One of the most common causes of occupational contact dermatitis in florists is chrysanthemum (Figure 29.2). Hausen et al. [19] described three patients with sesquiterpene lactone ACD after prolonged cultivation contact with *Arnica* species.
- Menz and Winkelmann found that the most common sources of weed exposure causing ACD are from the garden (40%), outdoor work or recreational exposure (17%), and farming (15%) [8].
- Occupational ACD caused by decorative plants was reported from Finland. The mean exposure time before presentation was 13 years. Compositae allergy accounted for 5 out of 12 cases. Five of the 12 were not able to continue working because of severe relapses of skin symptoms [20].
- A supermarket worker handling fruit and vegetables developed chronic hand eczema from repeated exposure to lettuce for 6 months. She had positive skin prick tests and histamine release tests, as well as specific IgE antibodies to lettuce milky sap. Closed patch tests were negative. Occupational protein contact dermatitis was diagnosed [21].

Case reports: uncommon presentations

- ACD to a medicinal herb *Tanacetum balsamita* (bible leaf) was reported. The patient had used the leaf to treat a small wound on the fingertip and presented with acute eczema of the index finger and eyelid edema. He had strong patch test reactions to the leaf, Compositae mix, sesquiterpene lactone mix, and fragrance mix. This plant was used as a place marker in bibles. It has also been used for its astringent and antiseptic properties, to treat common colds or intestine problems, and as flavoring in salads, fatty meat, poultry, lamb, fish, potatoes, soups, sauces, beverages, cakes, and beer [22].
- A case of contact dermatitis from the Compositae plant *Dittrichia graveolens* (stinkwort) presented with hand dermatitis with marked erythema and hyperkeratosis on the dorsal aspects of the hands for 5 years. Patch tests with extracts diluted to 0.5% or 1% in pet. or patch testing with the leaf is recommended. Stinkwort is an invasive weed found in Mediterranean countries, Australia, and California. It adheres to clothing, machinery, and soil and can be airborne [23].
- An *erythema multiforme-like* eruption following ACD from exposure to *Inula helenium*-containing "herbal bags" was reported from Spain. Histology was consistent with erythema multiforme. Patch tests to sesquiterpene lactone mix and alantolactone were positive (+++) [24].
- A patient presented with contact dermatitis on the face and hands from exposure to both pesticides and Compositae plants. He had positive patch test reactions to sesquiterpene lactone mix, arnica tincture, pyrethrum, and captafol [25].
- Lettuce allergy can be urticarial, dermatitic, or combined. Although most cases have been reported in an occupational setting, it is probably more prevalent in a non-occupational setting. Patch testing should be supplemented with a patch of fresh cut lettuce. Persons at risk of occupational exposure, atopics, and patients with lettuce-eating pets should be alerted to the possibility of lettuce ACD [26].

Association with chronic actinic dermatitis

- Sesquiterpene lactone sensitivity has been associated with the development of chronic actinic dermatitis. These cases tend to be elderly men with dermatitis affecting the face, neck, and hands (Figure 29.4).
- Ross et al. [15] reported 135 (68 male, 67 female) patients with sesquiterpene lactone allergy. 29 of 48 tested by monochromator light tests were found to be photosensitive; 21 of these were men, with a mean age of 69 years.
- At St John's Institute of Dermatology, between 1987 and 1992, 36% (29 of 80) of patients with chronic actinic dermatitis were found to have contact allergy to sesquiterpene lactone mix on patch testing [27]. This decreased to 20% (10 of 50) in the years 2000–2005 [28].

Cross-reactivity with other plants

- Cross-reactions between Compositae and diterpenes, such as colophony, and monoterpenes, such as turpentine, may occur. They have common biosynthetic precursors such as farnesol. The tulip allergen does not cross-react with sesquiterpene lactones [1].

Co-reactions with other contact allergens

- Multiple simultaneous positive reactions to sesquiterpene lactones and different contact allergens have been reported [23]. The most common concurrent positive patch test reactions are to colophonium, *Myroxylon pereirae*, fragrance mix 1, turpentine, wood tar, metal, chromate, and *p*-phenylenediamine [1, 3].
- Compositae mix may co-react with fragrance chemicals [29].
- Among Compositae allergic patients, contact allergy to carvone was also found. The significance of these reactions remains unknown. L-carvone and D-carvone are found in *Tanaceta balsamita* and mugwort (*Artemisia vulgaris* L.), respectively. Carvone is found in many volatile oils such as spearmint, dill, and caraway seed oils and is widely used as a flavoring agent in toothpaste, chewing gum, and candy [30]. Carvone is chemically related to limonene.

Parthenium dermatitis

- *Parthenium* dermatitis is caused by the leaves, flowers, and hair-like structures (trichomes) of *Parthenium hysterophorus*. The most important allergens are the sesquiterpene lactones. Other common allergens are parthenin, coronopilin, tetraneurin A, hymenin, hysterin, ambrosin, and dihidroisoparthenin.
- The reported clinical manifestations (mostly from Southern Asia) include classical airborne contact dermatitis, chronic actinic dermatitis, exfoliative dermatitis, widespread, extensive, and chronic lichenified dermatitis [31], photo contact dermatitis, and adult-onset atopic dermatitis [32]. The "deck-chair sign" (sparing of the natural skin folds, resembling the slats of a deck chair) [33], lesions mimicking seborrheic dermatitis [34], and actinic prurigo-like dermatitis [35] have also been reported. The dermatitis can be of a severe and unremitting nature.

Systemic treatment

- Although primary treatment usually consists of topical corticosteroids [10], systemic corticosteroids and azathioprine are sometimes needed for severe persistent dermatitis [36]. Roed-Petersen and Thomsen [37] reported treatment of recalcitrant airborne contact dermatitis from Compositae oleoresins with azathioprine, which improved skin lesions and prevented seasonal recurrence.
- Burke et al. [38] developed a prednisone-assisted psoralens-ultraviolet A light (PUVA) regimen to treat Compositae photosensitivity in which the prednisone dose decreased weekly, and the thrice weekly PUVA dose increased during the same time interval. Two patients with recalcitrant eruptions who were enrolled in this study showed dramatic improvement.

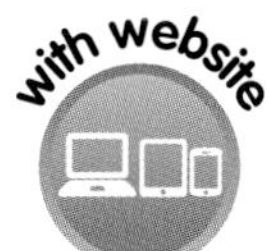

Go to www.wiley.com/go/mcfadden/common_contact_allergens to find the E-supplement for this chapter:

Sesquiterpene Lactone Mix and Compositae Mix: E-Supplement

References

1 Warshaw, E.M. and Zug, K.A. (1996). Sesquiterpene lactone allergy. *American Journal of Contact Dermatitis* 7 (1): 1–23.

2 Wenk, K.S., Tehrani, M., and Ehrlich, A. (2012). Sesquiterpene lactone-related allergic contact dermatitis after exposure to tulip poplar wood and bark. *Dermatitis: Contact, Atopic, Occupational, Drug* 23 (2): 89–90.

3 Isaksson, M., Hansson, C., Inerot, A. et al. (2011). Multicentre patch testing with compositae mix by the Swedish Contact Dermatitis Research Group. *Acta Dermato-Venereologica* 91 (3): 295–298.

4 Reider, N., Komericki, P., Hausen, B.M. et al. (2001). The seamy side of natural medicines: contact sensitization to arnica (*Arnica montana* L.) and marigold (*Calendula officinalis* L.). *Contact Dermatitis* 45 (5): 269–272.

5 Rodríguez, E., Epstein, W.L., and Mitchell, J.C. (1977). The role of sesquiterpene lactones in contact hypersensitivity to some North and South American species of feverfew (Parthenium-Compositae). *Contact Dermatitis* 3 (3): 155–162.

6 Paulsen, E., Otkjaer, A., and Andersen, K.E. (2008). Sesquiterpene lactone dermatitis in the young: is atopy a risk factor? *Contact Dermatitis* 59 (1): 1–6.

7 Paulsen, E. and Andersen, K.E. (2013). Sensitization patterns in *Compositae*-allergic patients with current or past atopic dermatitis. *Contact Dermatitis* 68 (5): 277–285.

8 Menz, J. and Winkelmann, R.K. (1987). Sensitivity to wild vegetation. *Contact Dermatitis* 16 (3): 169–173.

9 Tan, E., Leow, Y.H., Ng, S.K., and Goh, C.L. (1999). A study of the sensitization rate to sesquiterpene lactone mix in Singapore. *Contact Dermatitis* 41 (2): 80–83.

10 Jovanović, M. and Poljacki, M. (2003). *Compositae* dermatitis. *Medicinski Pregled* 56 (1–2): 43–49.

11 Paulsen, E. (1992). *Compositae* dermatitis: a survey. *Contact Dermatitis* 26 (2): 76–86.

12 Engebretsen, K.A., Johansen, J.D., and Thyssen, J.P. (2015). Herbal medicine as a cause of recurrent facial oedema. *Contact Dermatitis* 72 (5): 342–344.

13 Fabbro, S.K. and Zirwas, M.J. (2014). Systemic contact dermatitis to foods: nickel, BOP, and more. *Current Allergy and Asthma Reports* 14 (10): 463.

14 Ducombs, G., Benezra, C., Talaga, P. et al. (1990). Patch testing with the "sesquiterpene lactone mix": a marker for contact allergy to *Compositae* and other sesquiterpene-lactone-containing plants. A multicentre study of the EECDRG. *Contact Dermatitis* 22 (5): 249–252.

15 Ross, J.S., du, Menagé Peloux, H., Hawk, J.L., and White, I.R. (1993). Sesquiterpene lactone contact sensitivity: clinical patterns of *Compositae* dermatitis and relationship to chronic actinic dermatitis. *Contact Dermatitis* 29 (2): 84–87.

16 Breuer, K., Uter, W., and Geier, J. (2015). Epidemiological data on airborne contact dermatitis – results of the IVDK. *Contact Dermatitis* 73 (4): 239–247.

17 Schumacher, M.J. and Silvis, N.G. (2003). Airborne contact dermatitis from *Ambrosia deltoidea* (triangle-leaf bursage). *Contact Dermatitis* 48 (4): 212–216.

18 Quirce, S., Tabar, A.I., Muro, M.D., and Olaguibel, J.M. (1994). Airborne contact dermatitis from *Frullania*. *Contact Dermatitis* 30 (2): 73–76.

19 Hausen, B.M., Herrmann, H.D., and Willuhn, G. (1978). The sensitizing capacity of *Compositae* plants. I. Occupational contact dermatitis from *Arnica longifolia* Eaton. *Contact Dermatitis* 4 (1): 3–10.

20 L.A., Estlander, T., Jolanki, R., and Kanerva, L. (1996). Occupational allergic contact dermatitis caused by decorative plants. *Contact Dermatitis* 34 (5): 330–335.

21 Alonso, M.D., Martin, J.A., Cuevas, M. et al. (1993). Occupational protein contact dermatitis from lettuce. *Contact Dermatitis* 29 (2): 109–110.

22 Lucidarme, N., Cattaert, N., De Haes, P., and Goossens, A. (2008). Contact allergy to 'bible leaf' used in folk medicine. *Contact Dermatitis* 59 (1): 57–59.

23 Thong, H.Y., Yokota, M., Kardassakis, D., and Maibach, H.I. (2008). Allergic contact dermatitis from *Dittrichia graveolens* (L.) Greuter (stinkwort). *Contact Dermatitis* 58 (1): 51–53.

24 Mateo, M.P., Velasco, M., Miquel, F.J., and de la Cuadra, J. (1995). Erythema-multiforme-like eruption following allergic contact dermatitis from sesquiterpene lactones in herbal medicine. *Contact Dermatitis* 33 (6): 449–450.
25 Spettoli, E., Silvani, S., Lucente, P. et al. (1998). Contact dermatitis caused by sesquiterpene lactones. *American Journal of Contact Dermatitis* 9 (1): 49–50.
26 Paulsen, E. and Andersen, K.E. (2016). Lettuce contact allergy. *Contact Dermatitis* 74 (2): 67–75.
27 Menagé, H., Ross, J.S., Norris, P.G. et al. (1995). Contact and photocontact sensitization in chronic actinic dermatitis: sesquiterpene lactone mix is an important allergen. *British Journal of Dermatology* 132 (4): 543–547.
28 Chew, A.L., Bashir, S.J., Hawk, J.L. et al. (2010). Contact and photocontact sensitization in chronic actinic dermatitis: a changing picture. *Contact Dermatitis* 62 (1): 42–46.
29 Paulsen, E. and Andersen, K.E. (2005). Colophonium and *Compositae* mix as markers of fragrance allergy: cross-reactivity between fragrance terpenes, colophonium and compositae plant extracts. *Contact Dermatitis* 53 (5): 285–291.
30 Paulsen, E., Andersen, K.E., Carlsen, L., and Egsgaard, H. (1993). Carvone: an overlooked contact allergen cross-reacting with sesquiterpene lactones? *Contact Dermatitis* 29 (3): 138–143.
31 Sharma, V.K., Verma, P., and Maharaja, K. (2013). Parthenium dermatitis. *Photochemical & Photobiological Sciences* 12 (1): 85–94.
32 Zahra, S., Ahmad, W., and Jamil, S. (2012). Clinical spectrum of disease in patients of parthenium dermatitis. *Pakistan Journal of Medical and Health Sciences* 6 (2): 397–399.
33 Pai, S., Shetty, S., and Rao, R. (2015). Parthenium dermatitis with deck-chair sign. *JAMA Dermatology* 151 (8): 906–907.
34 Sethuraman, G., Bansal, A., Sharma, V.K., and Verma, K.K. (2008). Seborrheic pattern of parthenium dermatitis. *Contact Dermatitis* 58 (6): 372–374.
35 Singh, S., Khandpur, S., and Sharma, V.K. (2015). Allergic contact dermatitis to *Parthenium hysterophorus* mimicking actinic prurigo. *Indian Journal of Dermatology, Venereology and Leprology* 81 (1): 82–84.
36 Sharma, V.K. and Sethuraman, G. (2007). Parthenium dermatitis. *Dermatitis: Contact, Atopic, Occupational, Drug* 18 (4): 183–190.
37 Roed-Petersen, J. and Thomsen, K. (1980). Azathioprin in the treatment of airborne contact dermatitis from *Compositae* oleoresins and sensitivity to UVA. *Acta Dermato-Venereologica* 60 (3): 275–277.
38 Burke, D.A., Corey, G., and Storrs, F.J. (1996). Psoralen plus UVA protocol for *Compositae* photosensitivity. *American Journal of Contact Dermatitis* 7 (3): 171–176.

Exposure Color Code

- Clothing, jewelry, adornments
- Personal care products, cosmetics/cosmetic procedures
- Household products, domestic environment, including furniture and refurbishment
- Occupational dermatoses, work environment
- Medicines, surgical/dental procedures, herbal/alternative medicines
- Personal appliances/aids
- Leisure activities, sport, travel
- Other exposures (including dietary)
- Not relevant or multiple/general exposure

CHAPTER 30

Primin

CHAPTER CONTENTS

Allergen profile

Potential exposure from aspects of daily life
- Household environment (potted plants, furnishings contaminated by primin)
- Occupational (gardeners, florists)
- Leisure (gardening)
- Clothing (contaminated by primin)

Potential routes of exposure
- Direct contact
- Airborne
- By proxy (partner, contaminated clothing/furnishings)
- Mucosal (conjunctival airborne, rare)

Clinical manifestations of contact allergy to primin
- Direct contact dermatitis
- Airborne contact dermatitis
- By proxy contact dermatitis
- Non-eczematous contact dermatitis
  - Erythema multiforme
  - Vitiligo-like
  - Lichenoid dermatitis
- Oral/mucosal contact dermatitis (rare)

Known cross-reactions (uncommon)
- Epoxy hardener diaminodiphenylmethane
- Hardwoods (rosewood, jacaranda and teak) and orchids

Key points

- Primin is found in the house plant *Primula obconica*.
- The main allergens are: primin (2-methoxy-6-pentyl-1,4-benzoquinone), primetin, miconidin (2-methoxy-6-pentyl-1,4-dihydroxybenzene), and quinones.
- The allergens are most concentrated in the glandular hairs on the calyx (the bract surrounding the flower head).
- Contact allergy to primin is now uncommon.
- Allergy may occur through either directly touching the plant or indirect contact (by proxy). Indirect contact, such as handshakes or door handles, can elicit an allergic reaction.
- Direct emission of primin from intact *Primula obconica* plants is a possible cause of airborne contact dermatitis.
- The main sites of dermatitis are the hands, face, neck, and forearms.
- Some people who are allergic to *Primula* will also be allergic to certain orchids and tropical hardwoods such as rosewood (dalbergione), jacaranda, and teak.
- Active sensitization is rare but patch testing with fresh plants may marginally increase the risk.
- Patch test positivity has been reported to be between 0.12% and 2% and is highest in Europe.
- Allergic contact dermatitis (ACD) to primin presenting as vitiligo or erythema multiforme-like lesions has been reported.
- Common clinical features include a streaky rash or dermatitis of the face, eyelids, neck, arms, and hands.
- The interdigital spaces and back of the non-dominant hand may be involved due to the frequent pulling of dead flowers and leaves of the plant to improve tidiness.

Common Contact Allergens: A Practical Guide to Detecting Contact Dermatitis, First Edition. Edited by John McFadden, Pailin Puangpet, Korbkarn Pongpairoj, Supitchaya Thaiwat, and Lee Shan Xian.

© 2020 John Wiley & Sons Ltd. Published 2020 by John Wiley & Sons Ltd.

Companion website: www.wiley.com/go/mcfadden/common_contact_allergens

Patch testing

- 0.1% pet. synthetic primin or T.R.U.E.® test equivalent.

Patch test highlights

- Optimal reading times are 48 hours and 7 days, and the reading is most likely to be positive at 7 days [1].
- False-negative reactions to primin can occur. Dooms-Goossens et al. reported two patients who gave ++ reactions to plant material, while primin in the standard series remained completely negative. The possible reasons were primin retained in the patch test unit, higher concentrations in the plant, and the presence of more than one allergen. They suggested testing with pieces of the plant itself as testing with primin alone may give false-negative reactions [2].

Immunological cross-reactions

- Primin has the structure of a *p*-benzoquinone derivative. Cross-reactions may occur between primin and *para*-(amino) compounds, since *p*-benzoquinone is a common oxidation product of these compounds. Highly statistically significant concomitant positive patch test reactions were found for *diaminodiphenylmethane* (DDM) and primin (8% in 132 patients with positive patch tests to DDM; $p < 0.001$). DDM is an aromatic diamine used as a hardener for epoxy resins, to prevent oxidation and ozone damage in rubber products, and in synthetic textile fibers (Spandex) and polyurethanes [3].
- ■ ■ Similarly, patients with contact allergy to primula may cross-react to quinone-containing hardwoods such as *jacaranda* and *teak* [4].

Frequency of sensitization

- Currently in most clinics less than 1%. Most common in northern Europe.
- Declining trend in allergy due to decreased use and introduction of hypoallergenic primulas.

Age

- More common in the older age group (median age 62 years) [1].

Sex

- In many reports over 90% female [1].

Clinical disease

Primula dermatitis was first described by White in 1888. It has variable clinical manifestations that can be misdiagnosed (Figures 30.1–30.4). Only 50% of cases had typical features [5].

Morphology

- Typical rashes are linear streaks that can vary from erythematous papules to vesicles and bullae [6, 7] (Figure 30.2).
- Mitchell (1980) noted that the clinical presentation can be influenced by season, route of exposure and degree of hypersensitivity [7].
- Seasonal variations are determined by the varying allergen content of the plant. Symptoms may be least pronounced during spring. In summer more severe and frequent attacks of dermatitis occur with the severity waning during winter [7].
- The degree of hypersensitivity varies between individuals; removing dead leaves may cause severe dermatitis in some individuals but trivial attacks in others [7].
- Exposure to the allergen is usually from direct contact but indirect contact can occur through handshakes, furniture, or doorknobs [7, 8].
- Unusual presentations include erythema multiforme-like lesions with histology showing hyperkeratotic orthokeratosis, mild spongiosis, exocytosis, and a few necrotic keratinocytes [9, 10], herpes simplex-like facial eruptions [11], lichen planus-like eruptions [12], and possible photoallergic contact dermatitis [13].

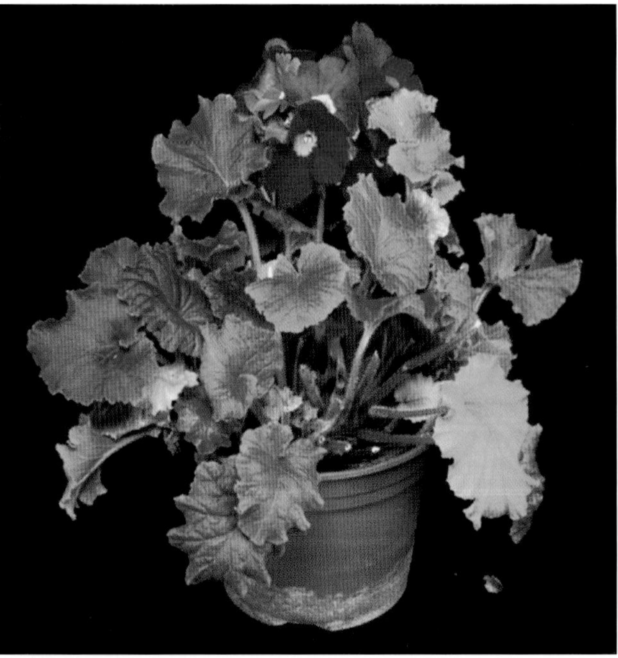

Figure 30.1 Primulas bloom in spring. The flowers appear in spherical shapes on thick stems with rosettes of leaves. The flowers colors can be purple, yellow, red, pink, blue, or white. ACD is often from direct contact with *Primula obconica*. Other routes of exposure include airborne, by proxy and hand-to-face/body.

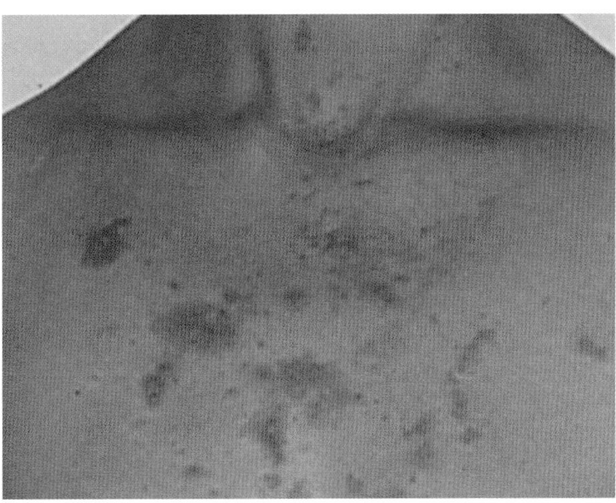

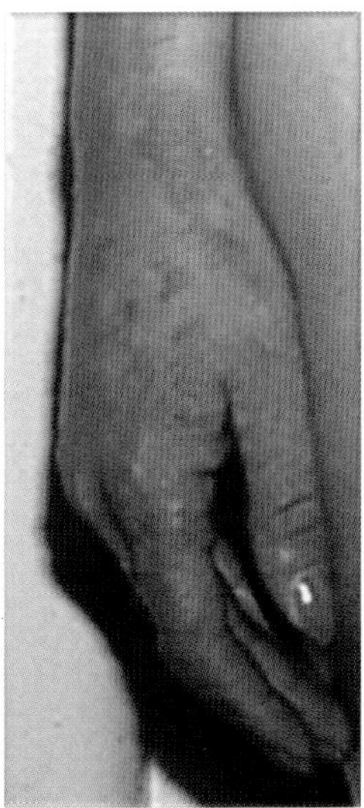

Figure 30.2 ACD to primula showing a classical "streaky" pattern. Erythematous papular streaky lesions can be observed.

- *Primula* sensitivity presenting as vitiligo has been reported. The irreversible pigmentary loss at the sites of previous eczema and patch test sites may be an isomorphic phenomenon of autoimmune vitiligo. Another mechanism may be the destruction of melanocytes by primin, resulting in leukoderma [14].

Sites

- Involvement of the neck, arm, and face (i.e. perioral, periorbital [15]) with redness and swelling of the eyelids, as well as vesicular hand eczema (left hand especially), are common clinical features.
- Hand eczema was the most common presentation in 151 patients having positive reactions to primin [16].
- The interdigital spaces or sides of the fingers of the left hand are often involved because of the frequent pulling of dead flowers and leaves off the plant to make it look tidy and prevent rotting. Large blisters can form at times. Mucosal lesions are rare; itching and burning sensations of the lips and tongue have been reported [17].
- Rarely, the ears, thighs, buttocks, or ankles can be affected. In severe cases, extensive rash, facial edema, and systemic symptoms such as pyrexia, coryza, and conjunctivitis can occur [18].

Duration

The mean duration of symptoms before diagnosis was 17 months [18].

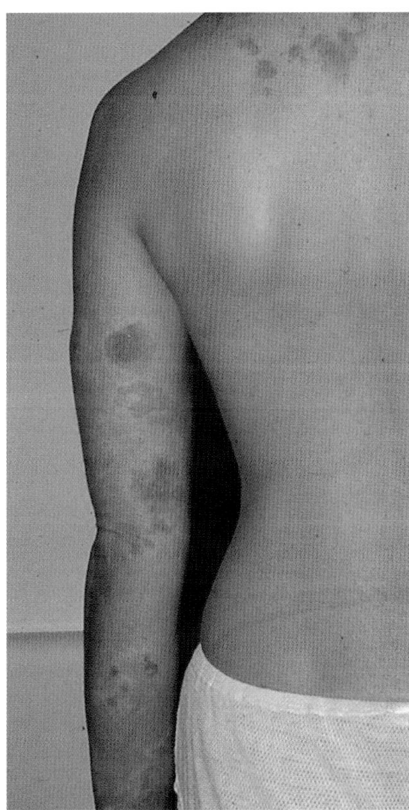

Figure 30.3 ACD to primula with extensive involvement. Some of the lesions are beginning to take on a targetoid/erythema multiforme-like appearance.

Erythema multiforme-like eruptions

Erythema multiforme-like lesions can be an unusual manifestation of contact allergy to primin with consistent histological findings and the positive patch test reaction can also be erythema multiforme-like (Figure 30.3).

A 30-year-old horticulturist with a previous history of hand eczema worked for the first time in a greenhouse where primulas were grown. Within a few hours of handling the plants, a pruriginous erythema appeared on the backs of his hands.

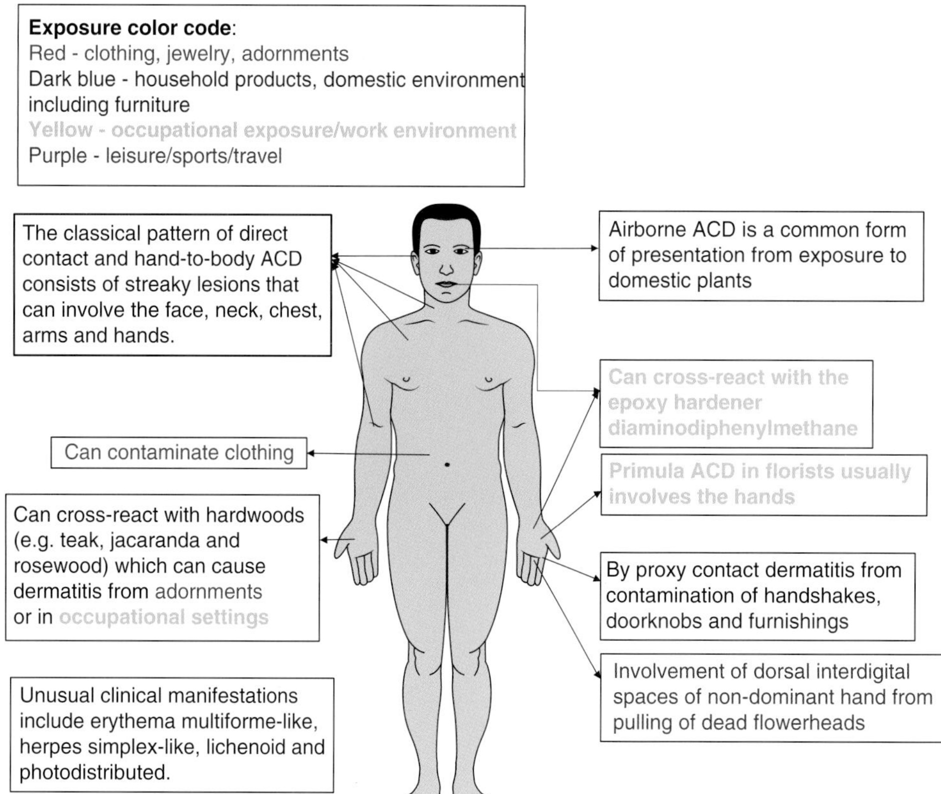

Exposure color code:
Red - clothing, jewelry, adornments
Dark blue - household products, domestic environment including furniture
Yellow - occupational exposure/work environment
Purple - leisure/sports/travel
The classical pattern of direct contact and hand-to-body ACD consists of streaky lesions that can involve the face, neck, chest, arms and hands.
Can contaminate clothing
Can cross-react with hardwoods (e.g. teak, jacaranda and rosewood) which can cause dermatitis from adornments or in occupational settings
Unusual clinical manifestations include erythema multiforme-like, herpes simplex-like, lichenoid and photodistributed.
Airborne ACD is a common form of presentation from exposure to domestic plants
Can cross-react with the epoxy hardener diaminodiphenylmethane
Primula ACD in florists usually involves the hands
By proxy contact dermatitis from contamination of handshakes, doorknobs and furnishings
Involvement of dorsal interdigital spaces of non-dominant hand from pulling of dead flowerheads

Figure 30.4 Clinical manifestations of contact allergy to primula/primin.

The next day, erythematous urticarial papules were disseminated over the backs of his hands and forearms. Some lesions had a targetoid appearance, resembling erythema multiforme morphologically. The lesions became purpuric on the back of the hands. Two days later, the eruption spread to the face with erythematous urticarial papules and plaques, sharply delineated on the cheeks and chin. Pustulation of his perioral lesions with lip edema, but no mucosal involvement, was observed. Patch tests showed ++ reactions to primin 0.01% pet., the leaf and the flower and +++ (bullous) reactions to the stem [10].

- A 68-year-old woman presented with pruritic, purplish papules coalescing into linear streaks and small plaques on the dorsa of her hands, fingers, and wrists. This started shortly after she handled primula plants. Patch testing was + for primin 0.01% pet. A biopsy showed interface dermatitis with basal layer vacuolization, subepidermal edema, and some necrotic keratinocytes in the epidermis, a picture strikingly consistent with the pathology of erythema multiforme [7].
- A 35-year-old female working in a plant nursery developed itchy eczematous lesions on her hands followed by an erythematouspapules polymorphous rash with confluence on her forearms and face. She was patch tested to primin 0.01%, the leaves, and the flower and was ++ to all. The patch test reaction to primin extended beyond the site of the test and had an erythema multiforme-like appearance. Biopsy of the original rash was consistent with erythema multiforme [9].

Occupational disease

- Primin allergy was work-related in seven of 149 patients (4.7%) from a study in Denmark (five women, two men). Most of them worked as florists. Hand eczema was present in six patients [16].
- In a study population of specialized *Primula* growers, cutaneous reactions to *Primula* species were found in 26% (male: female 2.4:1). *Primula auricula* was the most common, followed by *Primula obconica* and *Primula vulgaris*. A facial flare was noted in a 77-year-old male grower who entered a room containing *P. obconica*, suggestive of airborne contact dermatitis [13].
- Primin sensitization was significantly associated with household workers, retired people, woodworkers, chemical industry workers [19], and plant nursery workers [6].

Other areas of interest

Active sensitization

Historical patch testing with ether extract of fresh plant material often led to active sensitization. However patch testing with synthetic primin reduced this risk.

Primin-free *P. obconica*

- *P. obconica* cultivars, which contain less primin, have been developed since 1995 to reduce contact allergy. A seed producer in the USA has bred this allergen-free strain, which is available for purchase [20].
- Microscopy showed a higher density of trichomes in allergenic *P. obconica* than primin-free genotypes. Only the trichomes of the former contained allergenic resinous secretions. Primin was not present in the primin-free plants.
- A telephone survey showed that 50% of suppliers were selling the primin-free variant [21].

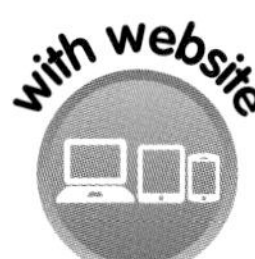

Go to www.wiley.com/go/mcfadden/common_contact_allergens to find the E-supplement for this chapter:

Primin: E-Supplement

References

1 Ingber, A. and Menné, T. (1990). Primin standard patch testing: 5 years experience. *Contact Dermatitis* 23 (1): 15–19.

2 Dooms-Goossens, A., Biesemans, G., Vandaele, M., and Degreef, H. (1989). Primula dermatitis: more than one allergen? *Contact Dermatitis* 21 (2): 122–124.

3 Fortina, A.B., Piaserico, S., Larese, F. et al. (2001). Diaminodiphenylmethane (DDM): frequency of sensitization, clinical relevance and concomitant positive reactions. *Contact Dermatitis* 44 (5): 283–288.

4 Hjorth, N., Fregert, S., and Schildknecht, H. (1969). Cross-sensitization between synthetic primin and related quinones. *Acta Dermato-Venereologica* 49 (6): 552–555.

5 Hjorth, N. (1966). Primula dermatitis. Sources of errors in patch testing and patch test sensitization. *Transactions of the St John's Hospital Dermatological Society* 52 (2): 207–219.

6 Lee, J., Warshaw, E., and Zirwas, M.J. (2011). Allergens in the American Contact Dermatitis Society Core Series. *Clinics in Dermatology* 29 (3): 266–272.

7 Mitchell, J.N.S. (1980). Plants. Chapter 10. In: *Contact Dermatitis* (ed. E. Cronin), 461–547. Edinburgh: Churchill Livingstone.

8 Hjorth, N. (1970). Primula dermatitis. *Current Problems in Dermatology* 3: 31.

9 Bonamonte, D., Filotico, R., Mastrandrea, V. et al. (2008). Erythema multiforme-like contact dermatitis from primin. *Contact Dermatitis* 59 (3): 174–176.

10 Lengrand, F., Tellart, A.S., Segard, M. et al. (2001). Erythema multiforme-like eruption: an unusual presentation of primula contact allergy. *Contact Dermatitis* 44 (1): 35.

11 Thomson, K.F., Charles-Holmes, R., and Beck, M.H. (1997). Primula dermatitis mimicking herpes simplex. *Contact Dermatitis* 37 (4): 185–186.

12 Lapière, K., Matthieu, L., Meuleman, L., and Lambert, J. (2001). Primula dermatitis mimicking lichen planus. *Contact Dermatitis* 44 (3): 199.

13 Aplin, C.G. and Lovell, C.R. (2001). Contact dermatitis due to hardy *Primula* species and their cultivars. *Contact Dermatitis* 44 (1): 23–29.

14 Bhushan, M. and Beck, M.H. (1999). Allergic contact dermatitis from primula presenting as vitiligo. *Contact Dermatitis* 41 (5): 292–293.

15 Gündüz, O. (2012). Occupational allergic contact dermatitis due to primula sensitivity: case report. *Turkiye Klinikleri Journal of Dermatol* 22 (2): 125–128.

16 Zachariae, C., Engkilde, K., Johansen, J.D., and Menné, T. (2007). Primin in the European standard patch test series for 20 years. *Contact Dermatitis* 56 (6): 344–346.

17 de Fernández, Corres, L., Leanizbarrutia, I., and Muñoz, D. (1987). Contact dermatitis from *Primula obconica* Hance. *Contact Dermatitis* 16 (4): 195–197.

18 Rook, A. and Wilson, H.T. (1965). Primula dermatitis. *British Medical Journal* 1 (5429): 220–222.

19 Bongiorni, L., Prodi, A., Rui, F. et al. (2015). Primin sensitization in north-eastern Italy: a temporal trend from 1996 to 2012. *Contact Dermatitis* 73 (2): 108–112.

20 Engasser, P.G. (1995). Primin-free *Primula obconica* seeds are available. *American Journal of Contact Dermatitis* 6: 252.

21 Connolly, M., Mc Cune, J., Dauncey, E., and Lovell, C.R. (2004). *Primula obconica* – is contact allergy on the decline? *Contact Dermatitis* 51 (4): 167–171.

Exposure Color Code

- Clothing, jewelry, adornments
- Personal care products, cosmetics/cosmetic procedures
- Household products, domestic environment, including furniture and refurbishment
- Occupational dermatoses, work environment
- Medicines, surgical/dental procedures, herbal/alternative medicines
- Personal appliances/aids
- Leisure activities, sport, travel
- Other exposures (including dietary)
- Not relevant or multiple/general exposure

CHAPTER 31
Neomycin

CHAPTER CONTENTS

Key points

- Neomycin is an aminoglycoside antibiotic commonly used in topical medications such as creams, ointments, and eyedrops. It is usually combined with corticosteroids and other antimicrobial agents.
- Neomycin contact dermatitis is common in patients with lower leg dermatitis, atopic dermatitis, groin dermatitis, and both chronic ear and eye inflammation.
- As with other medicaments, contact dermatitis to neomycin should be suspected when the skin disease fails to respond or there is worsening of the skin condition.
- The incidence of neomycin allergy is around 3.6% in patch test populations and 1% in healthy subjects.
- The risk of sensitization correlates with the frequency of use and chronicity of treatment.
- Kanamycin, gentamicin, paromomycin, spectinomycin, tobramycin and, to a lesser extent, streptomycin are known neomycin cross-reactors. Patients allergic to neomycin should avoid all aminoglycosides.
- Late patch test readings (>3 days) may be necessary to detect allergic patch test reactions to neomycin.

Exposure and use

Neomycin is an aminoglycoside antibiotic commonly used in topical medications such as creams and ointments, as well as eye and eardrops. It is usually combined with corticosteroids and other antimicrobial agents. An oral drug has been used to prevent infections in gastrointestinal surgery [1].

Sources of neomycin

- First-aid medicines.
- Topical antibiotic creams, lotions, and ointments used to treat skin, eye, and ear infections.
- Pet care and veterinary products – medications for the skin, eyes, and ears.
- Preservative in vaccines.

Common Contact Allergens: A Practical Guide to Detecting Contact Dermatitis, First Edition. Edited by John McFadden, Pailin Puangpet, Korbkarn Pongpairoj, Supitchaya Thaiwat, and Lee Shan Xian.
© 2020 John Wiley & Sons Ltd. Published 2020 by John Wiley & Sons Ltd.
Companion website: www.wiley.com/go/mcfadden/common_contact_allergens

Patch testing

- Neomycin 20% in petrolatum is the usual patch test concentration. There is a T.R.U.E.® test equivalent.
- *False-negative patch tests* to 0.5% neomycin suspension and 20% neomycin in pet. were demonstrated (read at 3, 6, and 13 days) in an otitis externa patient by Epstein [2]. The diagnosis was eventually made by an intradermal test with 1% neomycin that showed a 7 mm reaction at 3 days and a 9 mm reaction at 6 days. A usage test with 0.5% neomycin in pet. also showed dermatitis at 1 week.
- *Positive patch test reactions have high specificity*: The relationship between positive patch tests and a positive repeated open application test (ROAT) was examined using a neomycin cream and ointment (although the concentrations of neomycin in these agents is not stated). The ROAT was positive in 7/8 subjects with a strong positive patch test reaction to neomycin and in 2/4 subjects with a weakly positive patch test reaction [3]. However, neomycin is a weak allergen and probably gives very weak "danger" signaling. It is conceivable that these ROAT-negative patients could still react when neomycin is applied to inflamed skin.
- *Delayed patch test reactions*: A retrospective study that investigated the incidence of positive patch tests at days 6 or 7 (results were negative at day 3) showed that among 77 late positive reactions, neomycin was the second most common allergen (7 reactions) after nickel (20 reactions) [4].

Frequency of sensitization

Europe

St John's UK (1998, n = 1119)	3.6% [5]
European Surveillance System on Contact Allergies (ESSCA)	1.3% [6]

America

USA (*n* = 127)	6.3% [7]
North American Contact Dermatitis Group (NACDG) (2001–2002)	11.6% [8]
Mayo Clinic (2006–2010)	10.3% [9]

Asia

Singapore (1984–1985)	5.7% [10]

General population

USA (*n* = 1158)	1.1% [7]

Age

USA (2002–2008; age 3–36 months)	5% [11]
(Note: Topical aminoglycosides should be used with caution in children due to the risk of ototoxicity.)	

- The NACDG reported an overall clinic incidence of positive reactions to neomycin of about 10.64% between 1994 and 2008, being statistically more common in the older age group [12].

Elderly	≥ 65 years	13%, relevant 5.1%
Adult	19–64 years	10.3%, relevant 3.6%
Children	≤ 18 years	7.6%, relevant 2.3%

Sex

The majority of reports found that neomycin sensitivity was more common in females.

Clinical disease

- The clinical presentation is often an existing inflammatory dermatosis which flares or does not improve [13]. These chronic inflammatory dermatoses include lower leg dermatitis, chronic atopic dermatitis, and groin dermatitis, as well as chronic ear and eye inflammation (Figures 31.1 and 31.2).
- In 12 American patients who had positive reactions to neomycin, ten (seven female, three male) gave a history of applying neomycin for at least 1 week on an inflammatory dermatosis [7].
- The risk of neomycin sensitivity correlates with the number of additional positive reactions to other standard series allergens (polysensitisation) [14].
- Among 40 neomycin sensitive cases at St. John's, 42.5% of patients had dermatitis of more than 5 years' duration. The main sites of involvement were the face/neck in 15 cases, "generalized" in 12 cases, hands in 4 cases, and legs/feet in 3 cases [5].

Otitis externa

- Neomycin was the most common sensitizer in a series of 179 patients with chronic inflammatory ear disorders (76%), followed by framycetin (62%), gentamicin (31%), quinoline mix (18%), and caine mix (11%). The ear disorders comprised otitis externa, seborrheic dermatitis, atopic dermatitis, contact dermatitis, and psoriasis [15].
- Among patients with chronic otitis externa in the UK, neomycin sensitivity rate was 32% [16].

Hailey-Hailey disease

- Medicament allergic contact dermatitis (ACD) is common in Hailey-Hailey disease. In one study, neomycin was the most common contact allergy found in this group, with 3/15 patch

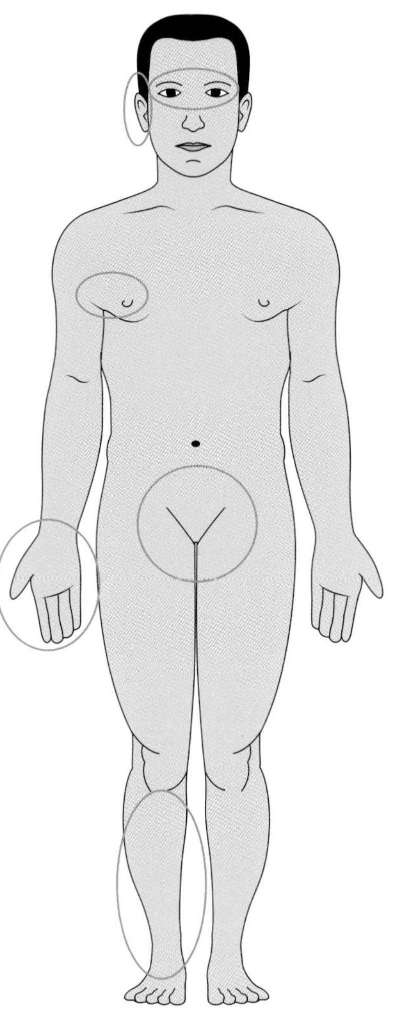

Figure 31.1 Skin areas which are prone to developing medicament contact dermatitis.

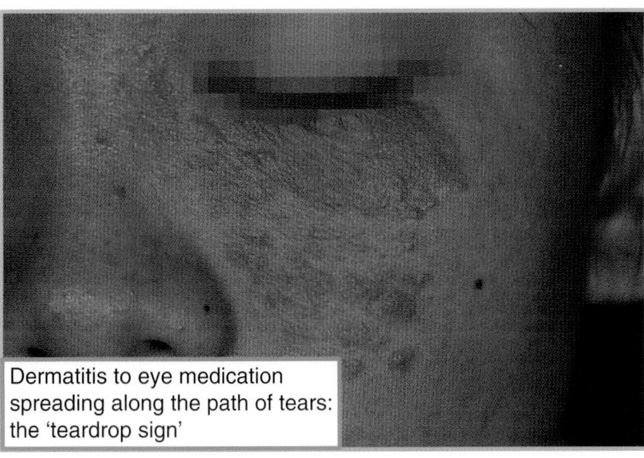

Dermatitis to eye medication
spreading along the path of tears:
the 'teardrop sign'

Figure 31.2 Medicament allergy to aminoglycosides in eyedrops, detected by a positive patch test to neomycin. There is a high degree of immunological cross-reactivity between the aminoglycosides. A patient with a positive patch test to neomycin should avoid all aminoglycosides.

testing positive for neomycin [17]. *(Note: Care should be taken when patch testing patients with Hailey-Hailey disease – to reduce the risk of koebnerisation and induction of the dermatosis at the site of tape application, patches should be removed the morning after application.)*

Ophthalmic and eyelid contact dermatitis

- 7 of 90 patients (8%) suspected of having an allergic reaction to eye medications had neomycin sensitivity [18].
- A study of 79 patients with eyelid dermatitis revealed that neomycin was the fourth most common contact allergen identified in this group, 11.8% of whom had neomycin-positive patch tests compared to 3.5% in a large control population. Although causation was not verified, one plausible contributing factor could have been the current/past use of aminoglycoside eye medications [19].

Leg ulcers and stasis dermatitis

- Neomycin is consistently reported as one of the most common agents in patients with leg ulcers, who as a group have a high incidence of medicament sensitivity. Three more recent reports give patch test positivity rates of 5%, 10.7%, and 13% [20–22].

Ano-genital dermatitis

- A retrospective study of 37 patients diagnosed with genital contact dermatitis showed that neomycin was the fifth most common allergen in the baseline series (5.4%) [23].

Case reports: atypical presentations

Systemic contact dermatitis

- Systemic contact dermatitis was reported in a neomycin-sensitive patient who was accidentally given oral neomycin with a resulting "baboon"-type rash, including eczema on the axillae, genitals, and neck, and later pompholyx on the hands and feet [24].

Diffuse cutaneous reactions

- Baldinger and Weiter reported a diffuse cutaneous hypersensitivity reaction in a 72-year-old woman 5 days after using dexamethasone/polymyxin B/neomycin combination eyedrops, with a positive patch test to neomycin [25].

Erythroderma

- A severe exfoliative erythroderma was reported after intravenous gentamicin administration to a neomycin-sensitive patient [26]. The authors state that approximately half of patients with contact allergy to neomycin will also react to gentamicin.

Recall dermatitis

- Recall dermatitis was reported in a 61-year-old man who developed flare-up reactions to neomycin at previous neomycin-treated biopsy sites following a positive patch test reaction to neomycin [27].

Erythema multiforme

- Severe allergic keratoconjunctivitis and erythema multiforme after a routine eye examination occurred as a consequence of neomycin ACD from a topical eye medicament [28].

Lichenoid reaction

- A 12-year-old boy presented with a chronic lichenoid rash on his hands, feet, and buttocks, not responding to long term use of corticosteroid/aminoglycoside creams [29]. Patch testing showed positive patch tests to several aminoglycosides including neomycin, with the reactions showing a lichenoid morphology. The dermatitis cleared on withdrawal of the aminoglycoside creams without relapse.

Follicular contact dermatitis

- Follicular contact dermatitis can be caused by both allergens as well as irritants. These allergens include antibiotics, in particular neomycin, and metals. It presents with multiple papules with hair at the core of the papules. Atopic patients may be more at risk and there may be multiple sensitivities. The differential diagnosis includes bacterial infection, systemic drug eruptions, infundibulofolliculitis, Kyrle's disease, Darier's disease, keratosis pilaris, and viral exanthemata [30].

Immediate allergic reactions

- A 33-year-old woman with previous contact hypersensitivity to neomycin, benzocaine, and *p*-aminodiphenylamine had anaphylactic shock following the application of Leukase®-Kegel (contains framycetin, trypsin, and lignocaine) liquid dressing on her incisional wound. A scratch test was performed with neomycin and within a few minutes she reproduced generalized itching, erythema, a feeling of heat, and again anaphylactic shock [31]. She had both immediate and delayed allergy to neomycin and this case suggests that cross-reactivity to other aminoglycosides can occur not only with delayed but also immediate hypersensitivity.
- A 52-year-old man developed acute facial swelling, widespread urticaria, rhinoconjunctivitis, and pruritus of the ears and throat within 3 minutes after using a neomycin-containing nasal ointment (Rinobanedif®) to treat recurrent nasal scabs. Skin prick tests produced a 12 mm wheal to the ointment and an 18 mm wheal to neomycin. There were no delayed skin reactions [1].

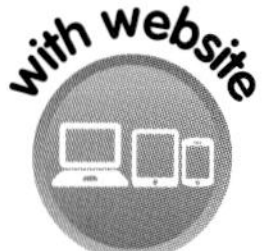

Go to www.wiley.com/go/mcfadden/common_contact_allergens to find the E-supplement for this chapter:

Neomycin: E-Supplement

References

1 Añíbarro, B. and Seoane, F.J. (2009). Immediate allergic reaction due to neomycin. *Journal of Investigational Allergology & Clinical Immunology* 19: 64–65.

2 Epstein, E. (1980). Contact dermatitis to neomycin with false negative patch tests: allergy established by intradermal and usage tests. *Contact Dermatitis* 6: 219–220.

3 Prystowsky, S.D., Nonomura, J.H., Smith, R.W., and Allen, A.M. (1979). Allergic hypersensitivity to neomycin. Relationship between patch test reactions and 'use' tests. *Archives of Dermatology* 115: 713–715.

4 Jonker, M.J. and Bruynzeel, D.P. (2000). The outcome of an additional patch-test reading on days 6 or 7. *Contact Dermatitis* 42: 330–335.

5 Morris, S.D., Rycroft, R.J., White, I.R. et al. (2002). Comparative frequency of patch test reactions to topical antibiotics. *British Journal of Dermatology* 146: 1047–1051.

6 Uter, W., Spiewak, R., Cooper, S.M. et al. (2016). Contact allergy to ingredients of topical medications: results of the European Surveillance System on Contact Allergies (ESSCA), 2009–2012. *Pharmacoepidemiology and Drug Safety* 25: 1305–1312.

7 Prystowsky, S.D., Allen, A.M., Smith, R.W. et al. (1979). Allergic contact hypersensitivity to nickel, neomycin, ethylenediamine, and benzocaine. Relationships between age, sex, history of exposure, and reactivity to standard patch tests and use tests in a general population. *Archives of Dermatology* 115: 959–962.

8 Pratt, M.D., Belsito, D.V., DeLeo, V.A. et al. (2004). North American Contact Dermatitis Group patch-test results, 2001–2002 study period. *Dermatitis* 15: 176–183.

9 Wentworth, A.B., Yiannias, J.A., Keeling, J.H. et al. (2014). Trends in patch-test results and allergen changes in the standard series: a Mayo Clinic 5-year retrospective review (January 1, 2006, to December 31, 2010). *Journal of the American Academy of Dermatology* 70:269–275.

10 Goh, C.L. (1988). Epidemiology of contact allergy in Singapore. *International Journal of Dermatology* 27: 308–311.

11 Belloni Fortina, A., Romano, I., Peserico, A., and Eichenfield, L.F. (2011). Contact sensitization in very young children. *Journal of the American Academy of Dermatology* 65: 772–779.

12 Warshaw, E.M., Raju, S.I., Fowler, J.F. Jr. et al. (2012). Positive patch test reactions in older individuals: retrospective analysis from the North American Contact Dermatitis Group, 1994–2008. *Journal of the American Academy of Dermatology* 66: 229–240.

13 Uter, W., Geier, J., Pfahlberg, A., and Effendy, I. (2002). The spectrum of contact allergy in elderly patients with and without lower leg dermatitis. *Dermatology* 204: 266–272.

14 Menezes de Pádua, C.A., Schnuch, A., Lessmann, H. et al. (2005). Contact allergy to neomycin sulfate: results of a multifactorial analysis. *Pharmacoepidemiology and Drug Safety* 14: 725–733.

15 Millard, T.P. and Orton, D.I. (2004). Changing patterns of contact allergy in chronic inflammatory ear disease. *Contact Dermatitis* 50: 83–86.

16 Smith, I.M., Keay, D.G., and Buxton, P.K. (1990). Contact hypersensitivity in patients with chronic otitis externa. *Clinical Otolaryngology and Allied Sciences* 15: 155–158.

17 Reitamo, S., Remitz, A., Lauerma, A.I., and Forstrom, L. (1989). Contact allergies in patients with familial benign chronic pemphigus (Hailey-Hailey disease). *Journal of the American Academy of Dermatology* 21: 506–510.

18 Wijnmaalen, A.L., van Zuuren, E.J., de Keizer, R.J., and Jager, M.J. (2009). Cutaneous allergy testing in patients suspected of an allergic reaction to eye medication. *Ophthalmic Research* 41: 225–229.

19 Nethercott, J.R., Nield, G., and Holness, D.L. (1989). A review of 79 cases of eyelid dermatitis. *Journal of the American Academy of Dermatology* 21: 223–230.

20 Erfurt-Berge, C., Geier, J., and Mahler, V. (2017). The current spectrum of contact sensitization in patients with chronic leg ulcers or stasis dermatitis – new data from the Information Network of Departments of Dermatology (IVDK). *Contact Dermatitis* 77: 151–158.

21 Jankićević, J., Vesić, S., Vukićević, J. et al. (2008). Contact sensitivity in patients with venous leg ulcers in Serbia: comparison with contact dermatitis patients and relationship to ulcer duration. *Contact Dermatitis* 58: 32–36.

22 Saap, L., Fahim, S., Arsenault, E. et al. (2004). Contact sensitivity in patients with leg ulcerations: a North American study. *Archives of Dermatology* 140: 1241–1246.

23 Bhate, K., Landeck, L., Gonzalez, E. et al. (2010). Genital contact dermatitis: a retrospective analysis. *Dermatitis* 21: 317–320.

24 Menné, T. and Weismann, K. (1984). Hematogenous contact eczema following oral administration of neomycin. *Hautarzt* 35: 319–320.

25 Baldinger, J. and Weiter, J.J. (1986). Diffuse cutaneous hypersensitivity reaction after dexamethasone/polymyxin B/neomycin combination eyedrops. *Annals of Ophthalmology* 18: 95–96.

26 Guin, J.D. and Phillips, D. (1989). Erythroderma from systemic contact dermatitis: a complication of systemic gentamicin in a patient with contact allergy to neomycin. *Cutis* 43: 564–567.

27 Jacob, S.E., Barland, C., and ElSaie, M.L. (2008). Patch-test-induced "flare-up" reactions to neomycin at prior biopsy sites. *Dermatitis* 19: E46–E48.

28 Sherertz, E.F., Reed, J.W., Zanolli, M.D., and Goldsmith, S.M. (1991). Severe allergic keratoconjunctivitis and erythema multiforme after a routine eye examination: discerning the cause. *Annals of Ophthalmology* 23: 173–176.

29 Lembo, G., Balato, N., Patruno, C. et al. (1987). Lichenoid contact dermatitis due to aminoglycoside antibiotics. *Contact Dermatitis* 17: 122–123.

30 Cohen, P.R. (2014). Follicular contact dermatitis revisited: a review emphasizing neomycin-associated follicular contact dermatitis. *World Journal of Clinical Cases* 2: 815–821.

31 Agathos, M. (1980). Anaphylactic reaction to framycetin (neomycin B) and lignocaine. *Contact Dermatitis* 6: 236–237.

Exposure Color Code

- Clothing, jewelry, adornments
- Personal care products, cosmetics/cosmetic procedures
- Household products, domestic environment, including furniture and refurbishment
- Occupational dermatoses, work environment
- Medicines, surgical/dental procedures, herbal/alternative medicines
- Personal appliances/aids
- Leisure activities, sport, travel
- Other exposures (including dietary)
- Not relevant or multiple/general exposure

CHAPTER 32

Clioquinol

CHAPTER CONTENTS

Key points

- As with other medicament allergens, allergic contact dermatitis (ACD) to clioquinol can present as a reaction to a medicated cream, worsening of dermatitis or non-response to treatment of a dermatitis.
- Clioquinol is used as an antiseptic preservative and antibacterial topical drug.
- The halogenated hydroxyquinolines are iodochlorhydroxyquin, iodoquinol, broxyquinoline, chlorquinaldol, clioquinol, and chlorhydroxyquinoline.
- Clioquinol is tested at 5% pet. or the T.R.U.E.® test equivalent. The alternative quinoline mix patch test preparation comprises clioquinol and chlorquinaldol.
- Two-thirds of patients sensitized to quinoline mix have positive reactions to clioquinol.
- In the UK, clioquinol-containing corticosteroid creams are indicated by a "C" in the name such as "Betnovate C."

Exposure and use

- Vioform (clioquinol) was first used as a topical preparation at the Manchester Skin Hospital in 1949 and was combined with hydrocortisone as vioform-hydrocortisone ointment in the 1950s [1]. Since quinolines are only weak allergens and are often in corticosteroid formulations that suppress inflammation, sensitivity to quinolines may be overlooked if the allergen is not included in a standard series of patch tests [2]. The usual concentrations are 1% and 3% in creams and ointment bases. Clioquinol is also used as antibacterial agent in ear drops [3].
- The halogenated hydroxyquinolines are widely used not only as topical antiseptic agents, but also as systemic treatment for intestinal or urinary infections. Clioquinol has been a more frequent sensitizer than other quinolines due to its cutaneous and more common use [4]. In the UK, clioquinol-containing corticosteroid creams are indicated by a "C" in the name.
- *Ethoxyquin* (6-ethoxy-1,2-dihydro-2,2,4-trimethylquinoline) is used as an antioxidant in animal feed to inhibit vitamin degradation. It is sprayed on stored apples and pears to prevent scalding and is used to preserve the color of chili powder and paprika (cayenne pepper, capsicum). It is also used as a stabilizer in the rubber industry [5]. Ethoxyquin may cause occupational ACD in apple packers, farmers handling chicken feed [6], and processors and handlers of pig and cattle feeds [5].
- *Polymerized 1,2-dihydro-2,2,4-trimethylquinoline* (TDQ-polymer) is used as an antioxidant in greases, *hydraulic fluids* and *rubber products* [7].

Patch testing

- Clioquinol 5% pet. has been included in the European standard series, extended international series, British Society of Cutaneous Allergy Series (BCDS), and Swedish series. However, it is not included in the American Contact Dermatitis Society (ACDS) and North American Contact Dermatitis Group (NACDG) Core Allergen Series (CAS) because it is uncommonly used and has low rates of positive patch test reactions

Common Contact Allergens: A Practical Guide to Detecting Contact Dermatitis, First Edition. Edited by John McFadden, Pailin Puangpet, Korbkarn Pongpairoj, Supitchaya Thaiwat, and Lee Shan Xian.
© 2020 John Wiley & Sons Ltd. Published 2020 by John Wiley & Sons Ltd.
Companion website: www.wiley.com/go/mcfadden/common_contact_allergens

(0.1–0.7%) in the US [8]. Quinoline mix (6% pet.) is an alternative patch test screen and comprises of clioquinol 3% and chlorquinaldol 3% (T.R.U.E.® test equivalent 160 μg/cm²).

Patch test highlights

- Sensitization to clioquinol persisted in ten patients who were retested. Although nine of those had completely avoided contact with clioquinol and related compounds during the interval, all were positive to clioquinol on re-patch testing [9]. Cross-reactions to other halogenated hydroxyquinolines were common; 4/10 were positive to quinolones used for malaria prohylaxis and 2/10 reacted to iodine.
- In a Danish population, 21 of 32 patients (66%) sensitized to quinoline mix also had positive reactions to clioquinol, seven (22%) to chlorquinaldol, ten (31%) to neither and one case reacted to chlorquinaldol only. Therefore, testing with clioquinol alone would miss 34% of patients who reacted to quinoline mix [2]. However, chlorquinaldol is now used less commonly.
- In the 664 patients evaluated for immediate contact reactions, clioquinol elicited immediate patch test reactions in 13 out of the 327 reactions in total. However it is not clear that any had clinical relevance [10].

Frequency of sensitization

Europe		0–2%, median 0.3%	[11–17]
America		0.1–0.7%	[8]
Asia			
Singapore			
1984–1985	$n = 2471$	2.6%	[18]
1985–1986	$n = 1685$	4.3%	[19]
1985–1987	$n = 3145$	2.7%	[20]

Age

The mean age of patients with clioquinol sensitivity was 48.5 years. Clioquinol mix positive reactions were slightly more common in the elderly in Singapore [21].

Sex

Out of 4000 consecutive eczema patients in a European five-center study, clioquinol sensitivity was found in 1.9% of female and 1.4% of male patients [22]. In contrast, studies from Singapore showed that clioquinol dermatitis was more common in men than in women (2.7% vs 2.4% [18], 5.1% vs 3.6% [19], and 3% vs 2.4% [20]). A recent UK study also found it to be more common in men, accounting for seven of eight patients [15].

Clinical disease

- Clioquinol ACD usually presents as a reaction to a topical medicament cream or poor response/relapse of dermatitis.
- As with other topical antibiotic and/or cortisone sensitivity, contact allergy to clioquinol is more frequent in patients with otitis externa.
- In the UK, clioquinol was the third most common sensitizer in patients with chronic inflammatory ear disease, accounting for 5 out of 40 patients (12%), after neomycin (15%) and framycetin (15%) [3].
- In a retrospective study of eight patients the primary sites of clioquinol dermatitis were the hands, legs/feet, and face/neck. Two cases (25%) had dermatitis for more than 5 years [15].
- In Singapore, clioquinol was the third most common allergen among topical medicaments after neomycin and proflavine. Most patients who had topical medicament sensitivity had dermatitis on their arms (44.3%) and legs (43%) [19].
- Clioquinol sensitivity was found to be statistically more common in 145 patients diagnosed with polymorphic light eruption type eczema than in the comparison series of 1714 patients (7% vs 1.8%; $p < 0.001$) [23].

Case reports

- *Fixed drug eruption* due to hydroquinoline is rare. It was reported in two patients from France [24]. The first case was an 84-year-old man who took tiliquinol and tilbroquinol (halogenated derivatives of 8-hydroxyquinolines) for colitis. He developed recurrent episodes of a typical non-bullous fixed drug eruption on the trunk and genitalia. The second case was a 64-year-old man who developed a bullous fixed drug eruption on the glans penis a few days after taking clioquinol for diarrhea.
- *Contact urticaria* and an *anaphylactoid* reactions from topical clioquinol and bacitracin powder have been reported. The patient reacted positively with a wheal and flare response to both compounds in the skin prick test [25].

Occupational disease

- A hydraulics mechanic developed contact dermatitis to polymeric quinoline (TDQ-polymer) present in *hydraulic fluid*. The patient had dermatitis on the lateral trunk, arms, back of the hands, face, neck, upper chest, and anterior thighs. Patch testing showed a ++ positive reaction to his hydraulic fluid (as is), diaminodiphenylmethane, cinnamic alcohol and TDQ polymer. There was no cross-reactivity between TDQ-polymer and TDQ-monomer, nor to other quinoline compounds (iodochlorhydroxyquin, ethoxyquin, 8-hydroxyquinoline) [7].

Irritant contact dermatitis *(Note: uncommon)*

- Primary irritant dermatitis from topical clioquinol preparations was found in seven out of 1756 patients assessed in a dermatitis clinic in Finland. All were male. The scrotum was affected in five cases and the other two cases had dermatitis only on the inguinal folds. During the same period of study, delayed contact hypersensitivity from clioquinol was found in 35 patients, five times more frequent than irritant dermatitis cases [26].
- A distinctive morphology of irritant contact dermatitis from clioquinol-containing ointment was reported. The clinical presentation was scaly red to purple fine reticular eruption mainly affecting the flexural areas, especially the neck and axillae. The reticular pattern was due to the weave of tubegauze dressings. Symptoms included mild burning and itching. Patch testing with 3% vioform was negative. The rash settled down within 48–72 hours after discontinuing treatment [1].

Systemic contact dermatitis

- Two patients were diagnosed with systemic eczematous contact-type dermatitis induced by clioquinol and chloroquine phosphate. The first case was a 40-year-old woman who developed widespread severe pruritic edematous plaques and papulovesicular dermatitis on the breast, abdomen, back, and hands 2 days after taking Entero-Vioform (clioquinol) tablets as prophylactic treatment for traveler's diarrhea. Patch testing showed ++ positive reactions to clioquinol (vioform) and chlorquinaldol (sterosan). The second patient was a 56-year-old woman who had taken oral chloroquine for malaria prophylaxis. After 2 weeks she developed widespread dermatitis and pyrexia and was patch test +++ to chloroquine [27].
- A 70-year-old male patient presented with systemic contact dermatitis from *norfloxacin* to treat a urinary tract infection. The clinical appearance, described as "toxicoderma," started 3 days after treatment with pruritus in the genital area, abdomen, lumbosacral area, and thighs which later evolved into a papulopustular rash on an erythematous edematous base. Patch testing to quinoline mix was positive and associated with a flare of papulopustular lesions on the genitalia and inner thighs [28].
- A 31-year-old woman presented with vaginal erythema, itching, edema, and eczema on the abdomen and chest 24 hours after using a Colposeptine (promestriene and chlorquinaldol) vaginal ovule. She had previously been diagnosed with contact dermatitis to clioquinol in an antiseptic ointment to treat otitis externa. Patch testing was positive to clioquinol and chlorquinaldol [4].

Cross-reactivity

- Clioquinol often cross-reacts with other halogenated hydroxyquinolines such as chlorquinaldol and 5,7-dibromo-8-hydroxy quinoline [29], in addition to oral quinoline-based antimalarial drugs, e.g. resorquine [30]. Because of the possibility of cross-reactivity, systemic contact dermatitis to antimalarial drugs has the potential to occur in quinoline allergic patients, but in practice is not commonly observed [4].
- Although most patients with chlorquinaldol hypersensitivity are also allergic to clioquinol, isolated allergy to chlorquinaldol has been reported in two patients by Myatt and Beck [31].

The chelating effect on nickel

- Clioquinol was found to be a potent *inhibitor of nickel dermatitis*. 3% clioquinol-containing barrier ointment coated on nickel containing-coins inhibited the nickel-induced hypersensitivity reactions in all 29 nickel-sensitive subjects [32].

Cutaneous pigmentation side effects (not related to allergy)

- Oral form: green hairy tongue, green discoloration of urine and feces.
- Creams: yellow discoloration of nails, red discoloration of white hair [33].

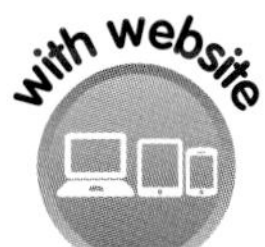

Go to www.wiley.com/go/mcfadden/common_contact_allergens to find the E-supplement for this chapter:
Clioquinol: E-Supplement

References

1 Beck, M.H. and Wilkinson, S.M. (1994). A distinctive irritant contact reaction to Vioform (clioquinol). *Contact Dermatitis* 31 (1): 54–55.

2 Agner, T. and Menné, T. (1993). Sensitivity to clioquinol and chlorquinaldol in the quinoline mix. *Contact Dermatitis* 29 (3): 163.

3 Holmes, R.C., Johns, A.N., Wilkinson, J.D. et al. (1982). Medicament contact dermatitis in patients with chronic inflammatory ear disease. *Journal of the Royal Society of Medicine* 75 (1): 27–30.

4 Rodríguez, A., Cabrerizo, S., Barranco, R. et al. (2001). Contact cross-sensitization among quinolines. *Allergy* 56 (8): 795.

5 Alanko, K., Jolanki, R., Estlander, T., and Kanerva, L. (1998). Occupational 'multivitamin allergy' caused by the antioxidant ethoxyquin. *Contact Dermatitis* 39 (5): 263–264.

6 Rubel, D.M. and Freeman, S. (1998). Allergic contact dermatitis to ethoxyquin in a farmer handling chicken feeds. *Australasian Journal of Dermatology* 39 (2): 89–91.

7 Morello, J., Fellman, J.H., and Storrs, F.J. (1992). Polymeric quinoline (polymerized 1,2-dihydro-2,2,4-trimethylquinoline); hydraulic fluid contact dermatitis. *American Journal of Contact Dermatitis* 3: 70–73.

8 Lee, J., Warshaw, E., and Zirwas, M.J. (2011). Allergens in the American Contact Dermatitis Society Core Series. *Clinics in Dermatology* 29 (3): 266–272.

9 Soesman-van Waadenoijen Kernekamp, A. and van Ketel, W.G. (1980). Persistence of patch test reactions to clioquinol (Vioform) and cross-sensitization. *Contact Dermatitis* 6 (7): 455–460.

10 Katsarou, A., Armenaka, M., Ale, I. et al. (1999). Frequency of immediate reactions to the European standard series. *Contact Dermatitis* 41 (5): 276–279.

11 Uter, W., Aberer, W., Armario-Hita, J.C. et al. (2012). Current patch test results with the European baseline series and extensions to it from the 'European Surveillance System on Contact Allergy' network, 2007–2008. *Contact Dermatitis* 67 (1): 9–19.

12 Wantke, F., Götz M, and Jarisch, R. (1995). Contact dermatitis from cloxyquin. *Contact Dermatitis* 32 (2): 112–113.

13 Thyssen, J.P., Johansen, J.D., Linneberg, A. et al. (2012). The association between contact sensitization and atopic disease by linkage of a clinical database and a nationwide patient registry. *Allergy* 67 (9): 1157–1164.

14 García-Gavín, J., Armario-Hita, J.C., Fernández-Redondo, V. (2011). Epidemiology of contact dermatitis in Spain. Results of the Spanish Surveillance System on Contact Allergies for the year 2008. *Actas Dermo-Sifiliográficas* 102 (2): 98–105.

15 Morris, S.D., Rycroft, R.J., White, I.R. et al. (2002). Comparative frequency of patch test reactions to topical antibiotics. *British Journal of Dermatology* 146 (6): 1047–1051.

16 Schoeffler, A., Waton, J., Latarche, C. et al. (2013). Changes in the European baseline series from 1981 to 2011 in a French dermatology-allergology centre. *Annales de Dermatologie et de Vénéréologie* 140 (8–9): 499–509.

17 Simonsen, A.B., Deleuran, M., Mortz, C.G. et al. (2014). Allergic contact dermatitis in Danish children referred for patch testing – a nationwide multicentre study. *Contact Dermatitis* 70 (2): 104–111.

18 Goh, C.L. (1988). Epidemiology of contact allergy in Singapore. *International Journal of Dermatology* 27 (5): 308–311.

19 Goh, C.L. (1989). Contact sensitivity to topical medicaments. *International Journal of Dermatology* 28 (1): 25–28.

20 Goh, C.L. (1989). Contact sensitivity to topical antimicrobials (I). Epidemiology in Singapore. *Contact Dermatitis* 21 (1): 46–48.

21 Goh, C.L. and Ling, R. (1998). A retrospective epidemiology study of contact eczema among the elderly attending a tertiary dermatology referral centre in Singapore. *Singapore Medical Journal* 39 (10): 442–446.

22 Bandmann, H.J., Calnan, C.D., Cronin, E. et al. (1972). Dermatitis from applied medicaments. *Archives of Dermatology* 106 (3): 335–337.

23 Hannuksela, M., Suhonen, R., and Förström, L. (1981). Delayed contact allergies in patients with photosensitivity dermatitis. *Acta Dermato-Venereologica* 61 (4): 303–306.

24 Janier, M. and Vignon, M.D. (1995). Recurrent fixed drug eruption due to clioquinol. *British Journal of Dermatology* 133 (6): 1013–1014.

25 Palungwachira, P. (1991). Contact urticaria syndrome and anaphylactoid reaction from topical clioquinol and bacitracin (Banocin): a case report. *Journal of the Medical Association of Thailand* 74 (1): 43–46.

26 Kero, M., Hannuksela, M., and Sothman, A. (1979). Primary irritant dermatitis from topical clioquinol. *Contact Dermatitis* 5 (2): 115–117.

27 Skog, E. (1975). Systemic eczematous contact-type dermatitis induced by iodochlorhydroxyquin and chloroquine phosphate. *Contact Dermatitis* 1 (3): 187.

28 Silvestre, J.F., Alfonso, R., Moragón, M. et al. (1998). Systemic contact dermatitis due to norfloxacin with a positive patch test to quinoline mix. *Contact Dermatitis* 39 (2): 83.

29 van Ketel, W.G. (1975). Cross-sensitization to 5,7-dibromo-8-hydroxy quinoline (D.B.O.) [a compound of Synalar + D.B.O. cream]. *Contact Dermatitis* 1 (6): 385.

30 Bielický, T. and Novák, M. (1969). Group sensitization to quinoline derivatives. *Dermatologica* 138 (1): 45–58.

31 Myatt, A.E. and Beck, M.H. (1983). Contact sensitivity to chlorquinaldol. *Contact Dermatitis* 9 (6): 523.

32 Memon, A.A., Molokhia, M.M., and Friedmann, P.S. (1994). The inhibitory effects of topical chelating agents and antioxidants on nickel-induced hypersensitivity reactions. *Journal of the American Academy of Dermatology* 30 (4): 560–565.

33 Bandmann, H.J. and Speer, U. (1984). Red hair after application of chinoform. *Contact Dermatitis* 10 (2): 113.

Exposure Color Code

- Clothing, jewelry, adornments
- Personal care products, cosmetics/cosmetic procedures
- Household products, domestic environment, including furniture and refurbishment
- Occupational dermatoses, work environment
- Medicines, surgical/dental procedures, herbal/alternative medicines
- Personal appliances/aids
- Leisure activities, sport, travel
- Other exposures (including dietary)
- Not relevant or multiple/general exposure

CHAPTER 33
Benzocaine

CHAPTER CONTENTS

Key points

- A medicament allergen.
- A moderate experimental sensitizer.
- Exposure includes application for hemorrhoids, anogenital pruritus, and painful skin conditions.
- Patch testing is with benzocaine 5% pet., T.R.U.E.® test, and as part of a caine mix.
- Benzocaine is used in anesthetic dental gels and creams to treat burns, bites, and hemorrhoids.
- Benzocaine is an ester caine/local anesthetic. Other ester caines include procaine, tetracaine, and cocaine. There is little or no cross-reactivity with amide caines such as lignocaine/lidocaine, articaine, bupivacaine, mepivacaine, and cinchocaine.
- Benzocaine is a poor screen for general caine sensitivity and should optimally be patch tested in conjunction with an amide local anesthetic (e.g. lidocaine) or as part of a caine mix.
- Benzocaine may cross-react with *para*-amino compounds such as *p*-phenylenediamine, other aromatic amine hair dye chemicals, parabens, and epoxy hardener.
- Allergic contact dermatitis (ACD) to benzocaine has also been described in the context of oral gel and condom use, and in the treatment of herpes zoster.

Exposure

- Benzocaine is commonly used as a topical anesthetic within cream/ointment preparations. It is used topically in painful conditions such as herpes zoster, insect bites, lumbago, and perniosis. It is also used for hemorrhoids, burns, and anogenital pruritus. It has been used to relieve symptoms of poison ivy dermatitis [1]. In addition, benzocaine is also commonly used as an oral mucosal anesthetic.

Patch testing

- Brinca et al. [2] suggested that almost 70% of allergic reactions to local anesthetics would have been missed if benzocaine had been used instead of caine mix as a screening allergen. They reviewed 2736 patch tests, identifying patients with positive reactions to caine mix or to one of seven local anesthetics. 112 patients (4.1%) had at least one reaction to a local anesthetic. Amongst the reactions to individual local anesthetic agents, cinchocaine gave the most reactions (50.7%), of which 97% were relevant. Benzocaine represented 22.5% of individual reactions, of which only 56% were relevant. Tetracaine was the next most common agent used. The authors remarked that cinchocaine and tetracaine were being increasingly used in hemorrhoid creams.
- Sidhu et al. [3] reviewed 10 years of patch testing to caine mix III constituents. Benzocaine (0.4% of patients patch tested) was the least common allergen of the mix causing reactions, with more positive reactions observed for tetracaine and dibucaine. Cross-reactivity between benzocaine and other caines occurred only infrequently.

Common Contact Allergens: A Practical Guide to Detecting Contact Dermatitis, First Edition. Edited by John McFadden, Pailin Puangpet, Korbkarn Pongpairoj, Supitchaya Thaiwat, and Lee Shan Xian.

© 2020 John Wiley & Sons Ltd. Published 2020 by John Wiley & Sons Ltd.

Companion website: www.wiley.com/go/mcfadden/common_contact_allergens

- A Danish group (Thyssen et al.) [4] noted that both lidocaine and benzocaine are available as over-the-counter preparations. They investigated temporal trends (1985–2010) of benzocaine and lidocaine allergy in dermatitis patients who underwent patch testing. The overall prevalence of benzocaine allergy was 0.5% and for lidocaine 0.3%. No temporal changes in the prevalence of allergy were seen over the study period other than a slight decrease in lidocaine allergy in more recent years. There were 103 positive reactions to benzocaine, but only 22 (21.3%) were thought to have past or current clinical relevance. 34 (33%) patients who were allergic to benzocaine had concomitant/cross-reactions to the hair dye chemical *p*-phenylenediamine (PPD), paraben mix or *N*-isopropyl-*N*'-phenyl-*p*-phenylenediamine (IPPD)/black rubber.

Frequency of sensitization

Europe

Europe	Clinics	Benzocaine	Range 0.36–5.9%, median 1.3%
		Caine mix	Range 0.1–4.6%, median 1.5%
	General population	Benzocaine	Range 0.1–1.0%, median 0.17%
		Caine mix	Range 0–1.0%, median 0.2%

North America

Clinics	Benzocaine	Range 1.5–7.7%, median 2.1%

Asia

Clinics	Benzocaine	Range 0–6.5%, median 1.5%
	Caine mix	Range 0.9–4.5%, median 1.8%

Australia

General population	Benzocaine	0.9%

For individual clinic rates see e-supplement

Patch testing – concomitant and cross-reactions

p-Phenylenediamine and other aromatic amines

- The North American Contact Dermatitis Group (NACDG) [5] looked for statistically significant concomitant patch test results in 4055 individuals patch tested between 1985 and 1989. With benzocaine allergy, there were statistically significant concomitant positive patch test reactions to both PPD and diaminodiphenylmethane (DDM) (used as a hardener in some epoxy resin systems and in the production of polyurethane foam). The authors attributed this to cross-reactions.
- Of 22 volunteers allergic to PPD, two were patch test positive to benzocaine [6].
- 134 patients with positive patch tests to PPD were analyzed by the Ottawa group for concomitant reactions [7]. 7.5% also reacted to benzocaine, whereas 24.6% reacted to azo clothing dyes.

Parabens

- A series of 4368 patients were patch tested to a standard series containing paraben mix, benzocaine, and PPD. None of the benzocaine+/PPD– patients reacted to parabens; however, 2 (8.6%) of the 23 patients who reacted positively to both benzocaine and PPD also reacted to parabens. The authors note that cross-reactivity among various *para*-amino compounds such as PPD, benzocaine, *p*-amino benzoic acid (PABA), and sulfonamides has been noted previously [8].

Cross-reactions with epoxy hardener

- DDM is an aromatic diamine used as a hardener in epoxy glue systems, to prevent ozone damage in rubber products, and in the production of synthetic textile fibers (Spandex) and polyurethanes. Exposure to DDM may occur in the manufacture of rubber, plastics, diisocyanates, dyes, and adhesives. Workers in the boat, automobile, electronic, and electrical industries are at risk of sensitization to this agent. Fortina et al. [9] reported on 132 DDM allergic patients. Twelve also reacted to benzocaine, with a highly significant association ($p < 0.0001$). A similar value was also reported by Holness [5].

Amide and ester local anesthetic allergy

- Local anesthetic agents can be divided into amides, such as lidocaine/lignocaine, bupivacaine, mepivacaine, prilocaine and articaine, and esters, such as benzocaine, procaine, and tetracaine.
- Several reports show a lack of cross-reactivity between these different groups, but some cross-reactivity within the groups. Amado et al. [10] reported on 16 patients with lidocaine allergy. Only one was also positive to benzocaine on patch testing, indicating little or no cross-reactivity.
- Handfield-Jones and Cronin [11] reported a case of lignocaine ACD from the use of a lignocaine-containing preparation for pruritus ani. They commented that lignocaine allergy is much less common than benzocaine allergy.
- Bircher et al. [12] described a 43-year-old woman with recurrent localized swelling and an eczematous dermatitis starting 1 day after an injection of lidocaine. Intradermal, patch, and

lymphocyte transformation tests revealed sensitization to lidocaine and cross-reactivity to the amide local anesthetics bupivacaine, mepivacaine, and prilocaine but not to articaine. Patch tests to the ester local anesthetics benzocaine, procaine, and tetracaine were all negative.

- A UK study of 3000 consecutive patients who were patch tested with a mix of benzocaine (ester), amethocaine (amide), and cinchocaine (amide) showed that 84 (2.8%) were allergic to this mix [13]. Forty of these were additionally tested to the constituents of the mix and 21 (52.5%) were sensitive to amethocaine and/or cinchocaine but not to benzocaine. They concluded that benzocaine as a solitary screening agent is unsatisfactory for general caine screening [13].

Vulval and anogenital dermatitis

- O'Gorman and Torgerson from the Mayo Clinic (2013) [14] reviewed patch test results from patients with vulval dermatitis. Benzocaine was the third most common contact allergy detected (7/59, 12%), after fragrance markers and quaternium-15. 0/89 reacted to lidocaine.
- The NACDG [15] reviewed the patch test positivity rate amongst 537 patients with anogenital dermatitis. Both benzocaine (13/342, 3.8%) and cinchocaine (6/146, 4.1%) had significantly higher clinically relevant rates amongst patients with anogenital disease only compared to the patch test population in general (benzocaine 121/20 796 or 0.58%, cinchocaine 7/9763 or 0.07%). The authors note that local anesthetic agents can be present in hemorrhoid and vaginal preparations.
- Brenan [16] found that 6% of patients with chronic vulvar symptoms had positive patch tests to caine mix.
- Bauer et al. [17] found that positive reactions to both methylchloroisothiazolinone and benzocaine were observed more frequently among patients with anogenital complaints as compared to the total clinic population (3.7% vs 2.5% and 2.7% vs 1.5%, respectively). They concluded that active agents of topical medications and popular remedies, preservatives and ointment bases appeared to frequently cause allergic reactions in this group.
- Goldsmith et al. [18] found that 17/201 (8.5%) patients with anogenital dermatitis had positive reactions to caine mix. However, they found that the allergy was more commonly detected when the dermatitis involved the perianal area alone (21%) compared to when the vulva alone was involved (3%).

Leg ulceration

- Artüz et al. (Ankara, Turkey, 2015) demonstrated an association between contact sensitization to benzocaine and chronic leg ulceration (12/40 or 20%) [19].
- Beliauskienė et al. [20] reviewed contact sensitization to the allergens of the European baseline series in patients with chronic leg ulcers. Benzocaine was the most common allergen found in leg ulcer patients, with 12/35 (32%) with classic leg ulcers and surrounding dermatitis having positive patch tests to benzocaine compared to 1/59 (1.7%) with lower leg or foot dermatitis without ulceration. This report from Lithuania exceeds the benzocaine allergy rate reported elsewhere and suggests a possible high rate of benzocaine use with leg ulcer pain. Generally, local anesthetic use is not recommended for leg ulcer management [21] and if local anesthetics are required urgently, amide anesthetics are preferred to benzocaine.
- Angelini et al. [22] reported on patch test results from 306 patients with stasis dermatitis, the majority of whom had leg ulcers. Benzocaine was positive in 31 cases (10.1%). They postulate, however, that many positive responses reflect a cross-reaction response (to PPD and other members of the *para*-amino group).

Foot dermatitis

- Angelini et al. [23] studied a series of 165 patients with foot dermatitis. Allergy to benzocaine was found in nine cases (5.5%) and was the most common medicament allergen; however, a high number of patients were positive to PPD as well, so at least some of the cases may have been cross-reactions.

Benzocaine-induced photosensitivity

- Two patients developed severe dermatitis after using a PABA-containing sunscreen whilst sunbathing and applying benzocaine-containing lotion afterwards [24]. One patient had photocontact allergy (i.e. irradiated site patch test positive, non-irradiated site patch test negative) to both PABA and benzocaine, and one to benzocaine alone. Benzocaine failed to produce phototoxic reactions in normal volunteers. Efforts to induce photocontact allergy in guinea pigs were unsuccessful. However, it was noted that benzocaine strongly absorbed ultraviolet energy and was chemically related to PABA.

Case reports

- *Dental gel*: González-Rodríguez et al. [25] reported a 53-year-old woman who had an episode of left-sided facial edema followed by dyspnea after dental surgery. During the procedure, 20% benzocaine gel was applied to the oral mucosa before an injection of mepivacaine. On patch testing, the patient had a ++ patch test reaction to benzocaine. The authors remark that as many as 5% of patients who use benzocaine may develop an allergy.

- Carazo et al. [26] report a patient who developed a generalized itchy dermatitis after the application of a medical aerosol containing ethyl chloride, as well as facial angioedema and tongue swelling after the local application of benzocaine. Patch tests were ++ for ethyl chloride (as is), ++ for benzocaine and +++ for caine mix at 96 hours. The authors concluded that this was a case of concomitant sensitivity as benzocaine and ethyl chloride are not chemically related.
- Ryan et al. [27] reported a 39-year-old man who developed edema and vesiculation of the oral mucosa following the application of benzocaine gel. An open test demonstrated an immediate urticarial reaction. A passive transfer test was negative, indicating a non-immunological etiology. Patch testing was positive after 48 hours and a diagnosis of ACD and non-immunological contact urticaria to benzocaine gel was made.
- A 65-year-old woman presented with painful mouth lesions 8 days after repair of a dental bridge [28]. She had been instructed to apply a local anesthetic gel containing 20% benzocaine to the painful gingivae. On the fifth day of gel application, painful blisters developed on the right side of the mouth. Patch testing was positive to benzocaine (++) and to the commercial gel (+++). The authors note the marked inflammation and blisters of the mucosa as characteristic manifestations of mucosal ACD to benzocaine.
- *Condom use*: Muratore et al. [29] reported a 22-year-old non-atopic man who presented with a recurrent erythematous-edematous dermatitis on the shaft of the penis with balanoposthitis. His female partner noticed the onset of his symptoms after intercourse, when he always wore condoms. On patch testing, there were reactions to thiuram (+ at day 2) and benzocaine (++ at day 2 and +++ at day 4). The thiuram allergy related to the patient's use of condoms, while the benzocaine allergy was related to the patient's use of a 5% benzocaine gel to improve his sexual performance.
- *ACD to benzocaine ointment during the treatment of herpes zoster*: During the treatment of thoracic herpes zoster with oral acyclovir and topical 20% benzocaine ointment, a 72-year-old woman developed a painful pruritic eruption on the involved area, spreading to the right arm. Patch tests showed +++ reactions to both the benzocaine ointment and benzocaine in the standard series. The authors highlighted the difficulties faced in diagnosing medicament allergy as the areas of skin affected were already inflamed [30].

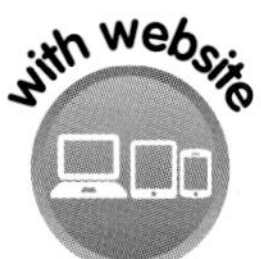

Go to www.wiley.com/go/mcfadden/common_contact_allergens to find the E-supplement for this chapter:

Benzocaine: E-Supplement

References

1 Fisher, A.A. (1972). Treatment of Rhus dermatitis with non-prescription products. *Journal of the American Medical Women's Association* 27 (9): 482–485.
2 Brinca, A., Cabral, R., and Gonçalo, M. (2013). Contact allergy to local anaesthetics-value of patch testing with a caine mix in the baseline series. *Contact Dermatitis* 68 (3): 156–162.
3 Sidhu, S.K., Shaw, S., and Wilkinson, J.D. (1999). A 10-year retrospective study on benzocaine allergy in the United Kingdom. *American Journal of Contact Dermatitis* 10 (2): 57–61.
4 Thyssen, J.P., Engkilde, K., Menné, T., and Johansen, J.D. (2011). Prevalence of benzocaine and lidocaine patch test sensitivity in Denmark: temporal trends and relevance. *Contact Dermatitis* 65 (2): 76–80.
5 Holness, D.L., Nethercott, J.R., Adams, R.M. et al. (1995). Concomitant positive patch test results with standard screening tray in North America 1985-1989. *Contact Dermatitis* 32 (5): 289–292.
6 Lisi, P. and Hansel, K. (1998). Is benzoquinone the prohapten in cross-sensitivity among aminobenzene compounds? *Contact Dermatitis* 39 (6): 304–306.
7 LaBerge, L., Pratt, M., Fong, B., and Gavigan, G. (2011). A 10-year review of p-phenylenediamine allergy and related para-amino compounds at the Ottawa Patch Test Clinic. *Dermatitis: Contact, Atopic, Occupational, Drug* 22 (6): 332–334.
8 Turchin, I., Moreau, L., Warshaw, E., and Sasseville, D. (2006). Cross-reactions among parabens, para-phenylenediamine, and benzocaine: a retrospective analysis of patch testing. *Dermatitis* 17 (4): 192–195.
9 Fortina, A.B., Piaserico, S., Larese, F. et al. (2001). Diaminodiphenylmethane (DDM): frequency of sensitization, clinical relevance and concomitant positive reactions. *Contact Dermatitis* 44 (5): 283–288.
10 Amado, A., Sood, A., and Taylor, J.S. (2007). Contact allergy to lidocaine: a report of sixteen cases. *Dermatitis: Contact, Atopic, Occupational, Drug* 18 (4): 215–220.
11 Handfield-Jones, S.E. and Cronin, E. (1993). Contact sensitivity to lignocaine. *Clinical and Experimental Dermatology* 18 (4): 342–343.
12 Bircher, A.J., Messmer, S.L., Surber, C., and Rufli, T. (1996). Delayed-type hypersensitivity to subcutaneous lidocaine with tolerance to articaine: confirmation by in vivo and in vitro tests. *Contact Dermatitis* 34 (6): 387–389.
13 Beck, M.H. and Holden, A. (1988). Benzocaine – an unsatisfactory indicator of topical local anaesthetic sensitization for the UK. *British Journal of Dermatology* 118 (1): 91–94.
14 O'Gorman, S.M. and Torgerson, R.R. (2013). Allergic contact dermatitis of the vulva. *Dermatitis: Contact, Atopic, Occupational, Drug* 24 (2): 64–72.
15 Warshaw, E.M., Furda, L.M., Maibach, H.I. et al. (2008). Anogenital dermatitis in patients referred for patch testing: retrospective analysis of cross-sectional data from the North American Contact Dermatitis Group, 1994–2004. *Archives of Dermatology* 144 (6): 749–755.
16 Brenan, J.A., Dennerstein, G.J., Sfameni, S.F. et al. (1996). Evaluation of patch testing in patients with chronic vulvar symptoms. *Australasian Journal of Dermatology* 37 (1): 40–43.
17 Bauer, A., Geier, J., and Elsner, P. (2000). Allergic contact dermatitis in patients with anogenital complaints. *Journal of Reproductive Medicine* 45 (8): 649–654.

18 Goldsmith, P.C., Rycroft, R.J., White, I.R. et al. (1997). Contact sensitivity in women with anogenital dermatoses. *Contact Dermatitis* 36 (3): 174–175.

19 Artüz, F., Yilmaz, E., Külcü Çakmak, S., and Polat Düzgün, A. (2016). Contact sensitisation in patients with chronic leg ulcers. *International Wound Journal* 13: 1190–1192.

20 Beliauskienė, A., Valiukevičienė, S., Sitkauskienė, B. et al. (2011). Contact sensitization to the allergens of European baseline series in patients with chronic leg ulcers. *Medicina* 47 (9): 480–485.

21 Brandão, F.M., Goossens, A., and Tosti, A. (2006). *Topical Drugs. Contact Dermatitis*, 4e, 623–652. Berlin, Heidelberg: Springer Verlag.

22 Angelini, G., Rantuccio, F., and Meneghini, C.L. (1975). Contact dermatitis in patients with leg ulcers. *Contact Dermatitis* 1 (2): 81–87.

23 Angelini, G., Vena, G.A., and Meneghini, C.L. (1980). Shoe contact dermatitis. *Contact Dermatitis* 6 (4): 279–283.

24 Kaidbey, K.H. and Allen, H. (1981). Photocontact allergy to benzocaine. *Arch Dermatol* 117 (2): 77–79.

25 González-Rodríguez, A.J., Gutiérrez-Paredes, E.M., Revert Fernández, Á., and Jordá-Cuevas, E. (2013). Allergic contact dermatitis to benzocaine: the importance of concomitant positive patch test results. *Actas Dermo-Sifiliográficas* 104 (2): 156–158.

26 Carazo, J.L., Morera, B.S., Colom, L.P., and Gálvez Lozano, J.M. (2009). Allergic contact dermatitis from ethyl chloride and benzocaine. *Dermatitis: Contact, Atopic, Occupational, Drug* 20 (6): E13–E15.

27 Ryan, M.E., Davis, B.M., and Marks, J.G. Jr. (1980). Contact urticaria and allergic contact dermatitis to benzocaine gel. *Journal of the American Academy of Dermatology* 2 (3): 221–223.

28 Akhavan, A., Alghaithi, K., Rabach, M. et al. (2006). Allergic contact stomatitis. *Dermatitis: Contact, Atopic, Occupational, Drug* 17 (2): 88–90.

29 Muratore, L., Calogiuri, G., Foti, C. et al. (2008). Contact allergy to benzocaine in a condom. *Contact Dermatitis* 59 (3): 173–174.

30 Roos, T.C. and Merk, H.F. (2001). Allergic contact dermatitis from benzocaine ointment during treatment of herpes zoster. *Contact Dermatitis*. 44 (2): 104.

Exposure Color Code

- Clothing, jewelry, adornments
- Personal care products, cosmetics/cosmetic procedures
- Household products, domestic environment, including furniture and refurbishment
- Occupational dermatoses, work environment
- Medicines, surgical/dental procedures, herbal/alternative medicines
- Personal appliances/aids
- Leisure activities, sport, travel
- Other exposures (including dietary)
- Not relevant or multiple/general exposure

CHAPTER 34

Tixocortol-21-pivalate, Budesonide, and Hydrocortisone 17-butyrate

CHAPTER CONTENTS

Allergen profiling

Corticosteroids are a group of pharmacological agents used in different preparations such as ointments, tablets, inhalers, and intravenous applications.

Exposure from daily activities

- *Medications/medical procedures*: ointments, creams, tablets, lozenges, suppositories, pessaries, inhalers, eyedrops, eardrops, intravenous preparations, shampoos, and mousses.
- *Occupational*: healthcare workers.
- *Use of herbal or lightening agents*: The steroid may be added covertly.

Routes of exposure

Common
- *Direct contact*: ointments, creams

Less common
- *Mucosal*: inhalers, eyedrops, eardrops, lozenges
- *Airborne*: inhalers
- *Systemic*: tablets, intravenous preparations
- *By proxy*: e.g. application of creams, administration of inhalers to children
- *Hand to face/neck/body*

Clinical manifestations

Common
- Direct contact dermatitis
- Exacerbation of pre-existing dermatitis/non-response of pre-existing dermatitis to treatment

Less common
- Airborne contact dermatitis
- Mucosal contact dermatitis
- Non-eczematous contact dermatitis: erythema multiforme, anaphylaxis, angioedema, contact urticaria
- By proxy contact dermatitis
- Respiratory symptoms
- Systemic contact dermatitis

Common Contact Allergens: A Practical Guide to Detecting Contact Dermatitis, First Edition. Edited by John McFadden, Pailin Puangpet, Korbkarn Pongpairoj, Supitchaya Thaiwat, and Lee Shan Xian.

© 2020 John Wiley & Sons Ltd. Published 2020 by John Wiley & Sons Ltd.

Companion website: www.wiley.com/go/mcfadden/common_contact_allergens

Key points

- Tixocortol-21-pivalate has been used as a topical corticosteroid in the treatment of rhinitis (as nasal suspensions or aerosols), pharyngitis (as lozenges), ulcerative colitis (as an enema or rectal solution), and oral inflammatory conditions (as a suspension or powder).
- Tixocortol pivalate is an effective patch test marker for hydrocortisone allergy and a principal screening agent for corticosteroid allergy. Budesonide is a supplementary marker for corticosteroid allergy. However, they are not good markers for the less commonly occurring allergy to fluorinated steroids. Adding a fluorinated steroid to the patch test series (e.g. betamethasone valerate and clobetasol propionate) may therefore be of value in routine patch test screening.
- Both tixocortol pivalate and budesonide should be added to the baseline series, as they can detect the majority of corticosteroid allergic cases.
- In patients with prolonged, recalcitrant eczematous skin disease, corticosteroid and medicament contact allergy should be excluded.
- A false-negative patch test reaction can occur because of the anti-inflammatory action of the corticosteroid.
- As the anti-inflammatory action may suppress an allergic reaction at an early reading, final patch test readings are ideally performed on a late occasion i.e. day 7.
- A positive patch test to corticosteroids may show an "edge" effect due to relative central suppression of the reaction by the steroid's anti-inflammatory effect.
- Once a patient has reacted to a corticosteroid, then further patch testing with a specialized corticosteroid series is optimal.
- As there is a high rate of false-negative reactions to steroid patch tests and rules of cross-reactivity are not assured, the patients' own topical steroid products should also be tested, ideally by patch testing and, if patch test negative, by repeat open application test (ROAT).
- If patch testing to a certain corticosteroid is negative in a tixocortol and/or budesonide positive patient, a ROAT with the patient's own steroid can be performed by the patient before the agent is used in a widespread manner.
- Corticosteroids can be divided into four groups, A–D, depending on the cross-reactivity pattern. A patient allergic to a corticosteroid from one group could therefore be given a corticosteroid from another group that does not cross-react. However, the potential for cross reaction between the groups is still possible. An alternative approach is to substitute fluorinated for non-fluorinated steroids.
- Budesonide is a good marker for triamcinolone sensitivity.
- Mometasone and betamethasone valerate are relatively uncommon steroid sensitizers and cross-reactors. Thus, they are possible alternative agents to use in steroid allergic patients.
- Hydrocortisone-17 butyrate 1% ethanol is an effective supplementary patch test screen for steroid sensitivity.

Classification

Corticosteroids were classified into four groups in a literature review by Coopman et al. [1]: A–D, depending on the cross-reactivity pattern and differences in structure in terms of the D ring and its side chains. A subdivision of group D into D1 and D2 has been proposed [2] (see Table 34.1).

Group A: hydrocortisone type.
Group B: triamcinolone acetonide type.
Group C: betamethasone type – non esterified.
Group D: esters, hydrocortisone-17-butyrate type.
Group D1: halogenated and with C16 substitution.
Group D2: the labile prodrug esters without the latter characteristics.

Tixocortol-21-pivalate (Group A)

An alternative classification is into fluorinated and non-fluorinated steroids.

Cross-reactivity amongst different steroids

Cross-reactivity rules are complex (see notes below) and cross reactions do not always occur. An alternative approach is to see whether the steroid molecule is fluorinated or not.

- Within each group, there is potential for cross-reaction. A patient allergic to a corticosteroid from one group should, therefore, be given a corticosteroid from another group that is less likely to cross-react [3].
- Tixocortol pivalate is the most sensitive and specific marker for hypersensitivity to hydrocortisone and for screening for other corticosteroid allergies [4]. One-third of patients who are patch test positive to tixocortol will also be allergic to hydrocortisone-17-butyrate [5]. Cross-reactivity was found between tixocortol pivalate and hydrocortisone by guinea pig maximization tests, whereas cross-reactivity between tixocortol and both amcinonide and budesonide was much lower and not statistically significant [6].
- Budesonide is a better marker than triamcinolone for group B corticosteroids [7].
- Clinical observations and a conformational analysis of the electronic shapes of corticosteroids showed similar molecular structures within each group (A, B, and D). In addition, this also indicated statistically significant correlations between budesonide and amcinonide (both in group C), and between budesonide and some steroids in group D, such as hydrocortisone-17-butyrate and alclometasone dipropionate [8]. There is still controversy over the significance of budesonide-positive patch tests but cross-reactions with hydrocortisone-17-butyrate and probably triamcinolone are thought likeliest [9]. Cross-reactions to mometasone furoate and budesonide were not observed in guinea pig studies [10].
- Cross-reactions were proposed in patients who were allergic to tixocortol pivalate and other corticosteroids to which the patients had not previously been exposed [11]. The most common cross-reactions were between group A and group D2 corticosteroids [12].
- Mometasone furoate (Elocon®) is a synthetic non-fluorinated corticosteroid that is structurally related to prednisolone. It can usually be used as an alternative topical treatment in corticosteroid sensitive patients because cross-sensitization to mometasone is relatively uncommon [13].
- A recent variation on the cross-reactivities between corticosteroids clusters group A, D2 (including hydrocortisone-17 butyrate), and budesonide as a first group, group B as a second, and group C and D1 as a third [14].

Patch testing

Patch testing studies give highly different rates of sensitivity for steroid markers in the baseline series.

- Corticosteroids were introduced into routine patch testing in the late 1980s [15]. An earlier study by Lauerma [16] suggested using tixocortol pivalate and hydrocortisone-17-butyrate to screen for corticosteroid contact allergy. A combination of tixocortol pivalate and budesonide was later found to be able to detect 91.3% of corticosteroid allergic cases. It was suggested that both be included in the baseline series [17].
- Tixocortol and budesonide may be poor screening agents for betamethasone valerate (Betnovate®) and clobetasol propionate (Dermovate®). The mean prevalence of allergy to either betamethasone valerate or clobetasol propionate was 1% (16/1562 patients) in a multicenter UK study. Of these, 81% would have been missed if they had been routinely tested with tixocortol pivalate and budesonide only. The authors suggested adding betamethasone valerate and clobetasol propionate to the baseline series [18].
- One major difficulty is the possibility of false-negative patch test reactions due to the anti-inflammatory effects of corticosteroids.
- The overall reproducibility of patch test reactions to corticosteroids was assessed in 15 patients who were retested. The strength of reproducible reactions was related to the relevance: 100% for +/++ reactions versus 18.2% for doubtful reactions [19].

Low versus high patch test concentrations

- Testing with different concentrations and bases of suspicious corticosteroids may be useful as false-negative reactions can occur with both higher and lower concentrations. If testing with 0.1% tixocortol pivalate is negative and the clinical history is strongly suspected, additional testing with 1% can be performed. Some patients only react to very low concentrations of budesonide. If 0.01% testing is negative, a lower concentration of 0.001% budesonide can be tested [20].

Late reactions

- Due to the anti-inflammatory effects of corticosteroids, allergic reactions may be suppressed at an early reading. Therefore, patch test readings should ideally be performed at a relatively late time, e.g. day 7 [15]. Up to 19–30% of corticosteroid reactions will be missed if an additional reading on days 6/7 is not performed [21, 22]. Readings performed after day 3 in 2980 patients detected eight additional positive reactions to budesonide and six to tixocortol pivalate. 10 out of 29 cases who had positive reactions to the corticosteroid series had negative reactions on day 3 [23].

Edge effect

The edge effect is a ring-like eczematous reaction at the edge of the patch test site which can mistakenly result in false-negative patch test readings being made. This is due to inflammatory suppression in the middle of the site where the corticosteroid concentration is higher than at the edge. This phenomenon is more apparent on the first reading day [19].

Active sensitization

- The risk of patch test sensitization to tixocortol pivalate is very low. The first case of possible active sensitization to tixocortol pivalate was reported from St. John's Institute of Dermatology in 1995. The patient was diagnosed with irritant facial dermatitis. The negative initial patch test reaction to tixocortol pivalate became positive on day 16 [24].
- Another case described was a patient who had a positive reaction to budesonide on day 17. Retesting showed a positive reaction on day 2 [25]. However, two cases who had budesonide reactions on day 10 and day 13 were considered to be late corticosteroid reactions since positive reactions to corticosteroid mixes were seen on days 6/7 [26].

Frequency of sensitization

- Estimated at 0.9–4.4% in contact dermatitis clinics [21].

European patch test clinics [5, 27–30] (see E-Supplement for individual clinic figures)

- Tixocortol pivalate: median 1.6%. range 0.1–9.4%.
- Budesonide: median 1.43%. range 0.37–12.7%.
- Hydrocortisone 17-butyrate: median 4.5%. range 1–7.9%.

American clinics [7, 31, 32]

- Tixocortol pivalate: median 2.9%, range 2.3–5.03%.
- Budesonide: 3.7%.

Asian clinics [33–35]

- Tixocortol pivalate: median 2.27%. range 0.47–8.6%
- Budesonide: 1.9%
- Hydrocortisone 17-butyrate: 4.7%

Age

- Corticosteroid sensitivity has been reported in children as young as 18 months of age [36]. Among 641 children under the age of 16 with atopic dermatitis, one case (0.2%) had tixocortol pivalate allergy, and 41 patients had positive patch tests to any topical medicament agent [37].
- A large European study revealed that 0.5% of 5400 pediatric patients had a positive patch test to tixocortol pivalate [38].

Sex

- There is a female preponderance, with 13 women out of 15 steroid allergic cases in Foussereau and Jelen's study (1986) [39]. In Vancouver, female cases accounted for 15 out of 20 tixocortol pivalate sensitive patients [32].

Clinical disease

- The clinical manifestation is classically that of a *chronic, recalcitrant* eczematous skin disease or a worsening dermatosis that does not respond to topical corticosteroid treatment [41].
- Patients with *stasis eczema* and *leg ulceration* are more likely to be allergic to corticosteroids; other predisposed groups include hand, anogenital, atopic, foot, and facial eczemas [9].
- Patients allergic to corticosteroids were more likely to have *multiple contact sensitivities* [42].
- Lutz et al. [31] found that 14/45 patients with tixocortol pivalate allergy had dermatitis *involving the face*. 89% of these 45 patients had reactions to other allergens in the standard series.
- *Atopic dermatitis* and *leg dermatitis* were identified as particular risk factors for tixocortol pivalate allergy, whereas the duration of disease was associated with hydrocortisone-17-butyrate allergy [43].
- In a cohort study, four of 44 patients (9%) with *inflammatory bowel disease* had contact allergy to steroid enemas: two cases from budesonide and one from tixocortol pivalate. They presented with worsening diarrhea or local irritation. One case who had a positive patch test to tixocortol pivalate (Colifoam®) also developed two episodes of rashes after intravenous hydrocortisone administration [44].
- In patients with leg ulcers, tixocortol pivalate was the second most common medicament sensitizer, accounting for 5 of 38 cases (13.3%), equal to neomycin and parabens. Only lanolin/wool alcohol was more common (eight cases) [45].
- *Allergic contact stomatitis* from tixocortol pivalate-containing chewing tablets (Oropivalone, Bacitracine®, Jouveinal) was reported in a 71-year-old woman. The symptoms occurred 8 days after therapy. She developed pruritus, edema, and pain on the face without any overlying eczema, excessive salivation and laryngeal edema. Patch testing was positive to tixocortol pivalate 10% and Pivalone® nasal suspension [46].
- *Erythema multiforme-like* contact dermatitis from budesonide was reported in two patients [47].

Other areas of interest

Allergic reactions from inhaled/nasal/oral corticosteroids

- Allergic reactions to inhaled corticosteroids have been uncommonly reported. Amongst other causes of treatment failure, allergy should be suspected in patients with refractory disease. In one series, budesonide was the major allergen involving 11 of 12 cases. Patients who are allergic to budesonide can usually still be treated with beclomethasone, fluticasone, or mometasone containing aerosols (class D1) since they tend not to cross react with budesonide [48].
- Bircher [49] described a case of contact allergy to tixocortol who had been sensitized through mucosal surfaces from the use of a tixocortol nasal spray, with a short induction phase (11 days). The patient presented with symptoms of rhinitis followed by the appearance of a pruritic papulo-vesicular rash on the perinasal area, upper lips and both ear lobes. Mucosal erythema was also observed.
- Bircher also described a case of contact allergy to tixocortol from a nasal spray masquerading as infectious sinusitis [50].
- In addition, Bircher described another case of steroid contact allergy to a nasal spray with periorbital eczema and a further case of acute stomatitis from contact allergy to tixocortol lozenges associated with facial swelling and respiratory difficulty [51].
- Primary sensitization and airborne allergic contact dermatitis (ACD) can result from exposure to inhalation corticosteroids e.g. budesonide. However, patients who used the inhalation corticosteroids were found to be less sensitized than the carers applying the steroid inhalers i.e. exposed "by proxy." Oral tolerance was proposed to be the reason in this situation [52].

Reported adverse effects to inhaled steroids include [3, 48]:

- nasal: nasal congestion, exacerbation of rhinitis, pruritic burning vesicles, burning sensations
- oral: erythema and edema of mucosa
- pulmonary: worsening airway obstruction
- skin: eczematous lesions, particularly around the orifices, cheeks, neck, trunk, and flexures; periorbital edema, and eczema
- systemic: urticaria, generalized eczematous or maculopapular eruptions.

Allergic contact dermatitis from ocular corticosteroids

- The Leuven group analyzed their cohort for ACD to ocular corticosteroids [53].
  - 18/315 cases of ACD to corticosteroids were from ocular exposure.
  - All 18 tested positive to group A steroids (particularly tixocortol).
  - The patients had used hydrocortisone, prednisolone, dexamethasone, fluorometholone, and/or triamcinolone.
  - Areas of clinical involvement were the periocular region ($n = 13$), eyelids ($n = 3$), eyes/mucosa ($n = 3$), face ($n = 1$), and neck ($n = 1$).
  - 10/18 also reacted to additional agents in eye drops, e.g. antibiotics.

Systemic allergic contact dermatitis to corticosteroids

- The Leuven group analyzed their cohort for systemic ACD to corticosteroids [54]. 16/315 (5%) of their corticosteroid allergic cohort presented with systemic contact dermatitis – 11 had a maculopapular rash whilst the others had a generalized eczematous rash.

  Most had been exposed to methylprednisolone through the oral, intravenous, or intra-articular routes. There were more extensive cross reactions in comparison to patients presenting with ACD from cutaneous exposure, with 11/16 reacting to all groups. They speculate that these patients may be recognizing the corticosteroid skeleton common to all corticosteroids.
- Systemic contact dermatitis from oral prednisolone presented as worsening facial eczema in a 61-year-old female patient who was allergic to hydrocortisone cream. Patch testing with

tixocortol pivalate showed a + reaction on day 7. The rash cleared when the fluorinated steroid betamethasone was applied [55].

Immediate hypersensitivity to corticosteroids

- Immediate hypersensitivity reactions to corticosteroids including anaphylaxis, urticaria and/or angioedema can occur [56, 57]. A systematic review of the literature found 120 reported cases of immediate hypersensitivity to corticosteroids.
  - The most common manifestations were anaphylaxis (60.8%) and urticaria/angioedema (26.7%).
  - Exposure was through any route but intravenous was the most common (44.2%), followed by oral (25.8%).
  - The most common steroids implicated were methylprednisolone (40.8%), followed by prednisolone (20%).
  - The majority of patients tolerated at least one alternative.
  - Skin testing was positive in 74.1% of patients.

Systemic use of oral corticosteroids in patch test positive patients

- Systemic reactions to oral corticosteroids in patients who are patch test positive to corticosteroids have been infrequently reported. Little practical advice is available from the literature. Isaksson and Persson (1998) reported a patient who was allergic to hydrocortisone/tixocortol pivalate topically (group A) and had systemic reactions when given oral prednisolone (worsening of facial eczema and secondary spread). However, he was patch test negative to betamethasone (group C) and oral administration of betamethasone led to resolution of his eczema.
- A tixocortol pivalate sensitive patient had an outbreak of generalized dermatitis after being given an adrenocorticotropic hormone (ACTH) depot injection (McFadden, unpublished observation). The endogenous cortisol produced by the synthetic ACTH injection can cross-react with tixocortol pivalate (group A).

Proposed modification of the allergenic classification of corticosteroids

In 2012, the Leuven group proposed a modification of the allergenic classification of corticosteroids (Table 34.1).

Table 34.1 A proposed modification of the original classification of corticosteroids [58].

	Group 1	Group 2	Group 3
Characteristics	No C16-methyl substitution No halogenation (in most cases)	C16/C17 cis-ketal/diol structure Halogenation	C16-methyl substitution Halogenation (except *)
Typical members	Budesonide Cloprednol Cortisone acetate Dichlorisone acetate Difluprednate Fludrocortisone acetate Fluorometholone Fluprednisolone acetate Hydrocortisone Hydrocortisone aceponate Hydrocortisone acetate Hydrocortisone-17-butyrate Hydrocortisone-21-butyrate Hydrocortisone hemisuccinate Isofluprednone acetate Mazipredone Medrysone Methylprednisolone aceponate Methylprednisolone acetate Methylprednisolone hemisuccinate Prednicarbate Prednisolone Prednisolone caproate Prednisolone pivalate Prednisolone sodium metasulphobenzoate Prednisolone succinate Prednisone Tixocortol pivalate Triamcinolone	Amcinonide Budesonide (*R*-isomer) Desonide* Fluchloronide Flumoxonide Flunisolide Fluocinolone acetonide Fluocinonide Halcinonide* Triamcinolone acetonide Triamcinolone benetonide Triamcinolone diacetate Triamcinolone hexacetonide ^May exceptionally only cross-react with the acetonides	Alclomethasone dipropionate Beclomethasone dipropionate Betamethasone Betamethasone 17-valerate Betamethasone dipropionate Betamethasone sodium phosphate Clobetasol propionate Clobetasone butyrate Cortivazol* Desoxymethasone Dexamethasone Dexamethasone acetate Dexamethasone sodium phosphate Diflucortolone valerate Diflorasone diacetate Flumethasone pivalate Fluocortin butyl Fluocortolone Fluocortolone caprylate Fluocortolone pivalate Fluprednidene acetate Halomethasone Meprednisone* Fluticasone propionate Mometasone furoate
Relation to original classification	Class A, D2, and budesonide	Class B	Class C and D2

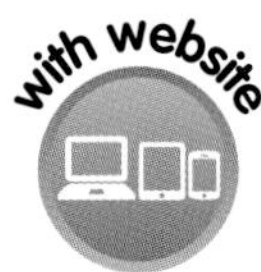

Go to www.wiley.com/go/mcfadden/common_contact_allergens to find the E-supplement for this chapter:

Tixocortol-21-pivalate, Budesonide, and Hydrocortisone 17-butyrate: E-Supplement

References

1 Coopman, S., Degreef, H., and Dooms-Goossens, A. (1989). Identification of cross-reaction patterns in allergic contact dermatitis from topical corticosteroids. *British Journal of Dermatology* 121 (1): 27–34.

2 Goossens, A., Matura, M., and Degreef, H. (2000). Reactions to corticosteroids: some new aspects regarding cross-sensitivity. *Cutis* 65 (1): 43–45.

3 Isaksson, M. (2001). Skin reactions to inhaled corticosteroids. *Drug Safety* 24 (5): 369–373.

4 Dooms-Goossens, A., Andersen, K.E., Burrows, D. et al. (1989). A survey of the results of patch tests with tixocortol pivalate. *Contact Dermatitis* 20 (2): 158.

5 Dooms-Goossens, A., Andersen, K.E., Brandao, F.M. et al. (1996). Corticosteroid contact allergy: an EECDRG multicentre study. *Contact Dermatitis* 35 (1): 40–44.

6 Frankild, S., Lepoittevin, J.P., Kreilgaard, B., and Andersen, K.E. (2001). Tixocortol pivalate contact allergy in the GPMT: frequency and cross-reactivity. *Contact Dermatitis* 44 (1): 18–22.

7 Davis, M.D., el-Azhary, R.A., and Farmer, S.A. (2007). Results of patch testing to a corticosteroid series: a retrospective review of 1188 patients during 6 years at Mayo Clinic. *Journal of the American Academy of Dermatology* 56 (6): 921–927.

8 Lepoittevin, J.P., Drieghe, J., and Dooms-Goossens, A. (1995). Studies in patients with corticosteroid contact allergy. Understanding cross-reactivity among different steroids. *Archives of Dermatology* 131 (1): 31–37.

9 English, J.S. (2000). Corticosteroid-induced contact dermatitis: a pragmatic approach. *Clinical and Experimental Dermatology* 25 (4): 261–264.

10 Bruze, M., Bjorkner, B., and Dooms-Goossens, A. (1996). Sensitization studies with mometasone furoate, tixocortol pivalate, and budesonide in the guinea pig. *Contact Dermatitis* 34 (3): 161–164.

11 Coopman, S. and Dooms-Goossens, A. (1988). Cross-reactions in topical corticosteroid contact dermatitis. *Contact Dermatitis* 19 (2): 145–146.

12 Mimesh, S. and Pratt, M. (2006). Allergic contact dermatitis from corticosteroids: reproducibility of patch testing and correlation with intradermal testing. *Dermatitis* 17 (3): 137–142.

13 Rasanen, L. and Tuomi, M.L. (1992). Cross-sensitization to mometasone furoate in patients with corticosteroid contact allergy. *Contact Dermatitis* 27 (5): 323–325.

14 Baeck, M., Chemelle, J.A., Goossens, A. et al. (2011). Corticosteroid cross-reactivity: clinical and molecular modelling tools. *Allergy* 66 (10): 1367–1374.

15 Isaksson, M. (2004). Corticosteroids. *Dermatologic Therapy* 17 (4): 314–320.

16 Lauerma, A.I. (1991). Screening for corticosteroid contact sensitivity. Comparison of tixocortol pivalate, hydrocortisone-17-butyrate and hydrocortisone. *Contact Dermatitis* 24 (2): 123–130.

17 Boffa, M.J., Wilkinson, S.M., and Beck, M.H. (1995). Screening for corticosteroid contact hypersensitivity. *Contact Dermatitis* 33 (3): 149–151.

18 Sommer, S., Wilkinson, S.M., English, J.S. et al. (2002). Type-IV hypersensitivity to betamethasone valerate and clobetasol propionate: results of a multicentre study. *British Journal of Dermatology* 147 (2): 266–269.

19 Devos, S.A. and Van Der Valk, P.G. (2001). Relevance and reproducibility of patch-test reactions to corticosteroids. *Contact Dermatitis* 44 (6): 362–365.

20 Isaksson, M., Brandao, F.M., Bruze, M., and Goossens, A. (2000). Recommendation to include budesonide and tixocortol pivalate in the European standard series. ESCD and EECDRG. European Society of Contact Dermatitis. *Contact Dermatitis* 43 (1): 41–42.

21 Kalavala, M., Statham, B.N., Green, C.M. et al. (2007). Tixocortol pivalate: what is the right concentration? *Contact Dermatitis* 57 (1): 44–46.

22 Isaksson, M., Andersen, K.E., Brandao, F.M. et al. (2000). Patch testing with corticosteroid mixes in Europe. A multicentre study of the EECDRG. *Contact Dermatitis* 42 (1): 27–35.

23 Uter, W., Geier, J., Richter, G., and Schnuch, A. (2001). Patch test results with tixocortol pivalate and budesonide in Germany and Austria. *Contact Dermatitis* 44 (5): 313–314.

24 Goldsmith, P.C., White, I.R., Rycroft, R.J., and McFadden, J.P. (1995). Probable active sensitization to tixocortol pivalate. *Contact Dermatitis* 33 (6): 429.

25 Le Coz, C.J., El Bakali, A., Untereiner, F., and Grosshans, E. (1998). Active sensitization to budesonide and para-phenylenediamine from patch testing. *Contact Dermatitis* 39 (3): 153–155.

26 Isaksson, M. and Bruze, M. (2003). Late patch-test reactions to budesonide need not be a sign of sensitization induced by the test procedure. *American Journal of Contact Dermatitis* 14 (3): 154–156.

27 Dooms-Goossens, A.E., Degreef, H.J., Marien, K.J., and Coopman, S.A. (1989). Contact allergy to corticosteroids: a frequently missed diagnosis? *Journal of the American Academy of Dermatology* 21 (3 Pt 1): 538–543.

28 Vestergaard, L. and Andersen, K.E. (1997). Contact allergy to local steroids. Contact allergy to corticosteroids among consecutively tested patients with eczema. *Ugeskrift for Laeger* 159 (38): 5662–5666.

29. Dooms-Goossens, A., Meinardi, M.M., Bos, J.D., and Degreef, H. (1994). Contact allergy to corticosteroids: the results of a two-centre study. *British Journal of Dermatology* 130 (1): 42–47.

30 Kot, M., Bogaczewicz, J., Kręcisz, B., and Woźniacka, A. (2016). Contact hypersensitivity to European baseline series and corticosteroid series haptens in a population of adult patients with contact eczema. *Acta Dermatovenerologica Croatica* 24 (1): 29–36.

31 Lutz, M.E., el-Azhary, R.A., Gibson, L.E., and Fransway, A.F. (1998). Contact hypersensitivity to tixocortol pivalate. *Journal of the American Academy of Dermatology* 38 (5 Pt 1): 691–695.

32 Morton, C.E. and Dohil, M.A. (1995). A survey of patch test results with tixocortol pivalate in Vancouver. *American Journal of Contact Dermatitis* 6 (1): 17–18.

33 Wattanakrai, P., Temnithikul, B., and Pootongkam, S. (2010). Pattern of corticosteroid allergy in Thailand. *Dermatitis: Contact, Atopic, Occupational, Drug* 21 (4): 203–206.
34 Khoo, B.P., Leow, Y.H., Ng, S.K., and Goh, C.L. (1998). Corticosteroid contact hypersensitivity screening in Singapore. *American Journal of Contact Dermatitis* 9 (2): 87–91.
35 Sarwar, U., Asad, F., Rani, Z. et al. (2016). Frequency of allergic contact dermatitis in hand eczema patients with European standard and corticosteroid series. *Journal of Pakistan Association of Dermatology.* 23 (3): 289–294.
36 Dooms-Goossens, A. and Morren, M. (1992). Results of routine patch testing with corticosteroid series in 2073 patients. *Contact Dermatitis* 26 (3): 182–191.
37 Mailhol, C., Lauwers-Cances, V., Rance, F. et al. (2009). Prevalence and risk factors for allergic contact dermatitis to topical treatment in atopic dermatitis: a study in 641 children. *Allergy* 64 (5): 801–806.
38 Belloni Fortina, A., Cooper, S.M., Spiewak, R. et al. (2015). Patch test results in children and adolescents across Europe. Analysis of the ESSCA Network 2002-2010. *Pediatric Allergy and Immunology* 26 (5): 446–455.
39 Foussereau, J. and Jelen, G. (1986). Tixocortol pivalate – an allergen closely related to hydrocortisone. *Contact Dermatitis* 15 (1): 37–38.
40 Ljubojevic, S., Lipozencic, J., Basta-Juzbasic, A., and Milavec-Puretic, V. (2005). What should we know about contact hypersensitivity to local glucocorticoids? *Liječnički Vjesnik* 127 (9–10): 237–240.
41 Wilkinson, S.M. and English, J.S. (1992). Hydrocortisone sensitivity: clinical features of fifty-nine cases. *Journal of the American Academy of Dermatology* 27 (5 Pt 1): 683–687.
42 Vind-Kezunovic, D., Johansen, J.D., and Carlsen, B.C. (2011). Prevalence of and factors influencing sensitization to corticosteroids in a Danish patch test population. *Contact Dermatitis* 64 (6): 325–329.
43 Malik, M., Tobin, A.M., Shanahan, F. et al. (2007). Steroid allergy in patients with inflammatory bowel disease. *British Journal of Dermatology* 157 (5): 967–969.
44 Wilkinson, M., Cartwright, P., and English, J.S. (1990). The significance of tixocortol-pivalate-positive patch tests in leg ulcer patients. *Contact Dermatitis* 23 (2): 120–121.
45 Callens, A., Vaillant, L., Machet, L. et al. (1993). Contact stomatitis from tixocortol pivalate. *Contact Dermatitis* 29 (3): 161.
46 Stingeni, L., Caraffini, S., Assalve, D. et al. (1996). Erythema-multiforme-like contact dermatitis from budesonide. *Contact Dermatitis* 34 (2): 154–155.
47 Baeck, M., Pilette, C., Drieghe, J., and Goossens, A. (2010). Allergic contact dermatitis to inhalation corticosteroids. *European Journal of Dermatology* 20 (1): 102–108.
48 Bircher, A.J. (1990). Short induction phase of contact allergy to tixocortol pivalate in a nasal spray. *Contact Dermatitis* 22 (4): 237–238.
49 Bircher, A.J., Hirsbrunner, P., Tschopp, K., and Wildermuth, V. (1995). Allergic contact dermatitis from tixocortol pivalate in a nasal spray masquerading as infectious complication of sinusitis. *ORL* 57 (1): 54–56.
50 Bircher, A.J., Pelloni, F., Langauer Messmer, S., and Muller, D. (1996). Delayed hypersensitivity reactions to corticosteroids applied to mucous membranes. *British Journal of Dermatology* 135 (2): 310–313.
51 Baeck, M. and Goossens, A. (2009). Patients with airborne sensitization/contact dermatitis from budesonide-containing aerosols 'by proxy'. *Contact Dermatitis* 61 (1): 1–8.
52 Baeck, M., De Potter, P., and Goossens, A. (2011). Allergic contact dermatitis following ocular use of corticosteroids. *Journal of Ocular Pharmacology and Therapeutics* 27 (1): 83–92.
53 Baeck, M. and Goossens, A. (2012). Systemic contact dermatitis to corticosteroids. *Allergy* 67 (12): 1580–1585.
54 Isaksson, M. and Persson, L.M. (1998). Contact allergy to hydrocortisone and systemic contact dermatitis from prednisolone with tolerance of betamethasone. *American Journal of Contact Dermatitis* 9 (2): 136–138.
55 Patel, A. and Bahna, S.L. (2015). Immediate hypersensitivity reactions to corticosteroids. *Annals of Allergy, Asthma & Immunology* 115 (3): 178–82.e3.
56 Vatti, R.R., Ali, F., Teuber, S. et al. (2014). Hypersensitivity reactions to corticosteroids. *Clinical Reviews in Allergy & Immunology* 47 (1): 26–37.
57 Baeck, M. and Goossens, A. (2012). Immediate and delayed allergic hypersensitivity to corticosteroids: practical guidelines. *Contact Dermatitis* 66 (1): 38–45.

Exposure Color Code

- Clothing, jewelry, adornments
- Personal care products, cosmetics/cosmetic procedures
- Household products, domestic environment, including furniture and refurbishment
- Occupational dermatoses, work environment
- Medicines, surgical/dental procedures, herbal/alternative medicines
- Personal appliances/aids
- Leisure activities, sport, travel
- Other exposures (including dietary)
- Not relevant or multiple/general exposure

CHAPTER 35 Lanolin

CHAPTER CONTENTS

Allergen profiling

Source

- Extracted from sheep wool (sheep sebum).
- Used in both topical medicaments and toiletries.
- Known as wool fat/alcohol in medicaments.

Potential exposure from aspects of daily life

- Personal care products.
- Medicaments.
- Sports – emollients.
- Occupational – healthcare workers, beauticians.
- Clothing – waxed wool garments *(Note: Rare case reports; for practical purposes lanolin allergic patients can wear wool garments.)*

Potential routes of exposure

- Direct contact (cosmetics, medicaments).
- Hand to face/trunk.
- By proxy (e.g. from someone else applying ointments).
- Mucosal (eye ointments).

Clinical presentations of contact allergy to lanolin

- Direct contact allergic contact dermatitis (ACD).
- Mimicking or exacerbation of pre-existing endogenous dermatitis, especially atopic dermatitis, groin or stasis dermatitis, and seborrheic dermatitis.
- Non-healing leg ulcers.
- Contact urticaria (rare – single report) [1].

Common Contact Allergens: A Practical Guide to Detecting Contact Dermatitis, First Edition. Edited by John McFadden, Pailin Puangpet, Korbkarn Pongpairoj, Supitchaya Thaiwat, and Lee Shan Xian.
© 2020 John Wiley & Sons Ltd. Published 2020 by John Wiley & Sons Ltd.
Companion website: www.wiley.com/go/mcfadden/common_contact_allergens

Tips

- Lanolin is produced from sheeps' sebum. It is used to retain skin moisture and is contained in many skin care products.
- Lanolin has been prescribed for the treatment of many skin conditions, including xerosis and eczema.
- Leg ulcer and leg dermatitis patients have high rates of lanolin allergy but this has diminished in recent years, probably due to the use of less allergenic lanolin in products.
- Lanolin is found in a variety of both cosmetics and topical medicaments.
- Patch testing with only one standard lanolin allergen may not detect all cases of lanolin allergy. If lanolin allergy is suspected, extra fractions (e.g. amerchol, crude lanolin) can be added to the screening patch test series.
- Some authors suggest that a later reading (e.g. at day 7) may increase the sensitivity of lanolin patch testing.
- The "lanolin paradox" has the same characteristics as the "paraben paradox" i.e. in patients with weak lanolin allergy, reactions may only occur on already inflamed skin.
- Sites commonly affected include the legs, ear canals, anogenital, flexural, and axillary areas.
- Lanolin is one of the more common contact allergies found amongst patients with facial dermatitis.
- Lanolin allergy is more common in females and older patients.
- ACD to lanolin from lipsticks and lip salves can cause lip and perioral dermatitis.
- Lanolin allergy can be one component of multiple allergies from medicaments, cosmetics, or both.
- Occupational relevance is most common amongst healthcare workers.
- Oleyl alcohol is derived from lanolin, and thus may have to be avoided in lanolin alcohol allergic patients.
- The frequency of sensitization is estimated to be 0.5% in the normal population and 2.5% in patch test populations.

Introduction

Lanolin is a waxy ingredient produced by sheeps' sebaceous glands. It has waterproofing properties and is used in many skincare products such as moisturizers, barrier creams, baby lotions, lip balms and glosses, hair conditioners, and eczema creams.

Synonyms

- Other names or subfractions include lanolin anhydrous, wool grease, wool wax, wool alcohol, amerchol, and wool fat.

Basic constituents

- Lanolin is a yellow waxy substance that can be extracted from sheeps' sebaceous glands. Its waterproofing properties help sheep to protect their wool and skin.
- The composition of lanolin is a mixture of long chain esters, fatty acids, and lanolin alcohols.
- Lanolin alcohols are a rich source of cholesterol, which is important for their skin emollient properties.

Structure

- Lanolin alcohol, wool wax alcohol.
- $C_{48}H_{69}NO_6$

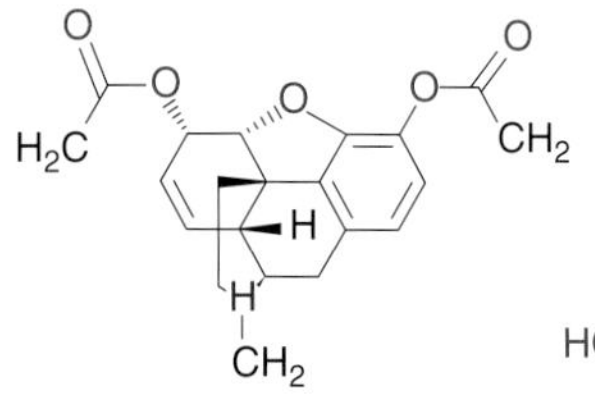

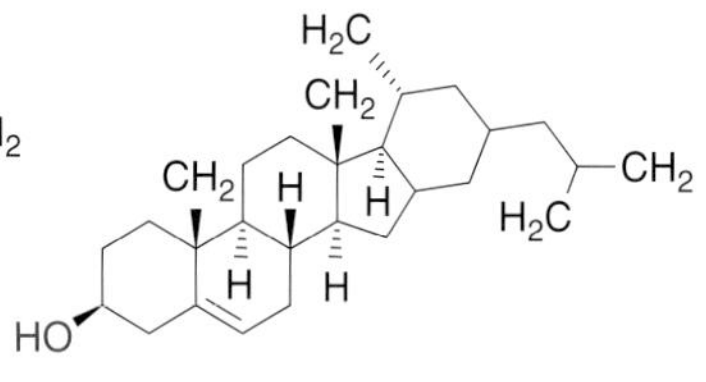

O O H$_2$C CH$_2$ H H CH$_2$ H$_2$C CH$_2$ CH$_2$ H H$_2$C CH$_2$ H H H HO

Uses

- Due to its ability to penetrate the epidermis to the depth of the stratum granulosum, lanolin has been used in the treatment of many skin conditions, including xerosis, eczema, and open wounds [2].
- Its occlusive properties help to store water in the stratum corneum. Combined with its soothing and hydrating properties, this makes lanolin valuable as an emollient and moisturizer [3].
- Lanolin is proven to help restore the barrier functions of skin. Within 1–2 weeks respectively of lanolin treatment, there was less cracking, peeling and bleeding in hand/heel dermatitis and healing of lip dermatitis [4].
- Lanolin is also found in a variety of skincare products such as lipsticks, cosmetic creams, powders, shampoos, liquid soaps, and topical medicament ointments.

Age

Lanolin sensitivity is most common in older adults and children.

Elderly

- An Italian review reported a high prevalence of contact allergy in elderly patients ranging from 33% to 64%. The authors postulated that the high rates of lanolin noted in this group were partly due to the common occurrence of lanolin allergy found in the leg ulcer patients being patch tested, who were mostly elderly people. Moreover, they noted that there may be a delay in patch test reactions to lanolin, and suggested a final patch test reading between day 5 and day 7 [5].
- A study from the UK reported 24 449 contact dermatitis patients who were patch tested to a standard series. The mean ages of both genders in lanolin allergic patients were significantly higher than those who did not have allergy to

lanolin: 48.4/49.2 years vs 41.4/35.9 years (male/female, respectively; $p < 0.0005$) [6].

Children

- In a study from Singapore, 2340 patients aged below 21 years were patch tested to a standard series and other additional series. 1063 of these (583 girls, 480 boys) had positive reactions to one or more allergens. The most common allergens identified were nickel 430/1063 (40%), thimerosal 120/1063 (15%), colophonium 96/1063 (9%), lanolin 86/1063 (8%), cobalt 83/1063 (8%), fragrance mix 49/1063 (5%), and neomycin 41/1063 (4%). Lanolin had significantly higher rates of positive reactions in the younger age groups compared to the older age groups. The peak rates found were in the 11–15 year age group in 27/375 (15%), in the 0–10 year age group in 9/176 (13%), and in the 16–20 year age group in 50/1789 (6%) (relative risk = 0.42, 95% confidence interval 0.27–0.64, $p < 0.01$) [7].
- 82 children with atopic dermatitis were patch tested with a baseline series and steroid series. 22 (26.8%) had positive reactions and the three most common allergens were amerchol L-101 (11.0%), potassium dichromate (7.3%), and nickel sulfate (4.9%). The patients with hand and/or foot eczema had statistically significant higher rates of allergic reactions than those without hand and/or foot eczema (14/32 or 43.8% and 8/50 or 16%, respectively). The authors noted that amerchol L-101 is a lanolin derivative, and lanolin is contained in emollients used by atopic dermatitis patients. They also noted that the 5% pet. composition of amerchol L-101 in patch tests could induce irritant/false positive reactions [8].

Sex

Lanolin sensitivity is reported as being more common in females in many but not all studies.

- In a study from the North American Contact Dermatitis Group (NACDG), 634 out of 25 811 patients (2.5%) patch tested to lanolin alcohol 30% in pet. had positive reactions. Amongst the lanolin sensitized patients, females had a higher rate of positive reactions than males (59.1% vs 40.9%). [9].

Frequency of sensitization

Derived from individual results reported in the Lanolin: E-Supplement chapter.

General population	Median 0.5%, range 0.2–4%
Patch test clinics	
Europe	Median 2.6%, range 0.3–7.4%
America	Median 2.5%, range 1.05–5.5%
Asia	Median 3.2%, range 0.4–5%

Clinical

- Over a 15-year period, 24 449 patients were patch tested with a baseline series which included lanolin 30% pet. The annual mean positive reaction rate to lanolin was 1.7%. The highest rates of lanolin allergy were found amongst patients with *leg dermatitis* (6.0%), followed by *anogenital dermatitis* (3.23%), *flexural dermatitis* (2.56%), *ear canal dermatitis* (2.45%), and *axillary dermatitis* (2.38%) [6]. The authors noted that lanolin allergy was more common in women and older age groups.
- In an American study, 634/25 811 (2.5%) patients had a positive patch test to lanolin alcohol. 529/634 (83.4%) were of current relevance and 81/634 (12.8%) had *leg dermatitis* [9].
- 18 572 patients with *facial dermatitis* were patch tested to a baseline and cosmetic series. A higher rate of reactions to cosmetic allergens was found in women. The most common allergens detected were fragrance mix (female versus male, 10.8% vs 8.3%), *p*-phenylenediamine (4.0% vs 2.8%) and lanolin alcohols (3.0% vs 2.2%) [10].
- A 27-year-old female presented with recurrent *severe lip and perioral dermatitis*. She had multiple positive patch test reactions including to lanolin (+++). Lanolin was found in three of her lip salves. This was a case of ACD to lanolin complicated by co-sensitization to the colophonium fraction abitol (also found in lip salves) and medicament allergy (tixocortol pivalate, bacitracin, and neomycin). The patient was a polysensitizer, with old allergies to nickel and acrylate as well [11].
- There is a higher rate of lanolin allergy reported in patients with *stasis dermatitis/leg ulcer* (Figure 35.1), even when compared to lanolin allergy rates in other chronic skin inflammatory dermatoses, such as a reported rate of 1% in

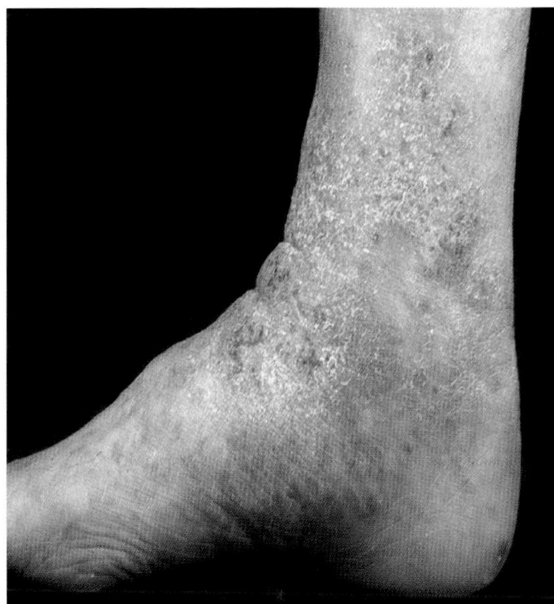

Figure 35.1 Lanolin is one of the most common contact allergens detected amongst reports of series of patients with stasis dermatitis or leg ulcers.

atopic dermatitis patients [12]. In a study from France of 106 leg ulcer patients who were patch tested, 75% had one or more positive reactions and 57% had two or more positive reactions. The most common allergens were balsam of Peru (40%), lanolin (21%), fragrance mix (18%), triclocarban (an antibacterial agent used in soaps) (13%), and colophony (11%) [13].

- A 13-year-old girl presented with chronic foot and ankle dermatitis. She used Bunga Pads™ inside her skates (gel pads used by athletes to protect their skin from friction). Physical examination revealed well-demarcated erythematous lichenified plaques on both ankles. Patch testing showed positive reactions to lanolin, amerchol L-101, and cocamidopropyl betaine. Bunga Pads contained lanolin. The rash improved after discontinuing the use of the pads [14].
- A 61-year-old man developed acute eczema on his thigh with secondary spread to the trunk after application of a fabric *plaster* bandage post-sclerotherapy. He was patch tested to a standard series and the plaster (both fabric and sticky sides), and had positive reactions to lanolin (+), neomycin (+), parabens (++), and the sticky side of the plaster (+). Lanolin was the only positive allergen which was contained within the plaster [15].
- A 19-year-old female had eczematous rashes on her hands and interphalangeal joints, spreading to both cheeks. The rash developed after self-treatment with propolis cream for a drug eruption from clindamycin that she took before dental treatment. She had previously been using propolis for dry lips. Patch testing showed positive reactions to *Myroxylon pereirae, c*olophonium, Fragrance Mix 1, Fragrance Mix 2, lanolin alcohol, and the propolis cream. The propolis cream that the patient had used contained lanolin [16].
- A 29-year-old-female presented with sore, cracked lips, followed 2 days later by vesicular facial eczema. She was patch tested with a standard, facial, and cosmetic series and the positive allergens were lanolin, amerchol L-101, castor oil, oleyl alcohol, ricinoleic acid, and her own *lipstick*. She was diagnosed with ACD to her *lipstick*. The authors noted that the positive reactions to oleyl alcohol and ricinoleic acid were possible cross-reactions from the same double bond and hydroxyl group, and that oleyl alcohol is derived from lanolin [17].

Occupational

Lanolin sensitivity is most common amongst healthcare workers.

- In the NACDG study on lanolin allergy, occupational relevance was infrequent but the most common occupation related to lanolin allergy was 'healthcare workers', such as registered nurses, nursing aides, and social workers. The sources of occupational related reactions were cosmetics, topical medicaments, and hand soaps [9].

Exposure

- Lanolin is found in a variety of products such as cosmetics and medicaments. Cosmetic products including lipsticks, powders, shampoos, lotions and soaps, and medicaments with ointment bases are common sources of lanolin exposure.

Cosmetic products

- In 2008, in a study from America, 276 moisturizers were examined for potentially allergenic ingredients. Lanolin was detected in 10% of these products [18].

Medical products

- In the USA, the vehicle allergens of 46 branded and 120 generic *topical steroids* were analyzed (including creams, ointments, liquids, and gels). 127 of 166 (76.5%) products contained at least one allergen. Lanolin was found in 10/166 or 6% of the topical steroids. [19]
- 4384 dermatitis patients were patch tested with a standard and medicament series. 901 (20.6%) had a positive reaction to one or more medicament allergens. Lanolin alcohol/amerchol L-101 (17.3%) was the second most common medicament allergy – this increased significantly with age. The authors recommended awareness of this when prescribing topical medicaments to elderly patients with dermatitis, especially those that contain perfumes and lanolin [20].
- Lanolin has been used as a treatment for postpartum *nipple soreness* [21].
- A case series from America reported three patients who had dermatitis after the use of Aquaphor™ (a post-surgical emollient to cover clean surgical wounds) – patch testing was positive to lanolin (wool) alcohol, one of Aquaphor's ingredients [22].

Patch testing

- Patch testing with only one standard lanolin allergen may not be adequately sensitive for testing in patients who have suspected lanolin allergy. If lanolin allergy is suspected, the patient's own products should also be patch tested and, if available, further subfractions of lanolin. Other subfractions of lanolin which have been used for patch testing include hydrogenated lanolin, amerchol L-101 (50% pet), crude lanolin, lanolin wax glyceride, lanolin acid, lanolin oil, cetyl acetate, and acetylated lanolin alcohol. However, many of these fractions may be difficult to obtain. A few reports suggest that lanolin patch test positivity may not always be repeatable or reproducible [23–27].

Co-sensitivity

- *Lanolin is a frequent co-sensitiser*. In a study from the NACDG, 25811 contact dermatitis patients were patch tested to a standard series. They divided patients into two groups, lanolin-positive patients (group A) and allergic but lanolin-negative patients (group B). The rates of positive reactions to one or more standard allergens in group A and group B were 89.9% and 68.4%, respectively ($p < 0.0001$). Lanolin allergic patients were 1.3 times more likely to react to at least one allergen when compared with non-lanolin allergic patients. The most common co-sensitized allergens included balsam of Peru, bacitracin, carba mix, and thiuram mix. Colophony, benzocaine, and cocamidopropyl betaine had significantly more than twice the rate of positive reactions in group A compared to group B (9.5%/3.4%, relative risk (RR) 2.78, 6.3%/2.6%, RR 2.44, and 4.3%/1.7%, RR 2.54, respectively, $p < 0.0001$). The authors note that lanolin is a common co-sensitizer [9].

The lanolin paradox

Wolf [28] noted the following: "Lanolin in topical therapeutic agents sensitizes a high proportion of patients, whereas the same lanolin is 'safe' in cosmetics so widely used by millions of individuals. Patients with an ACD to lanolin in a medication applied to a stasis ulcer can nevertheless use lanolin-containing cosmetics and not experience a reaction". The author noted that this lanolin paradox was similar to the paraben paradox.

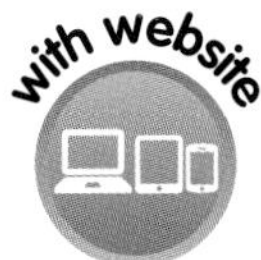

Go to www.wiley.com/go/mcfadden/common_contact_allergens to find the E-supplement for this chapter:

Lanolin: E-Supplement

References

1 von Liebe, V., Karge, H.J., and Burg, G. (1979). Contact urticaria. *Der Hautarzt; Zeitschrift fur Dermatologie, Venerologie, und verwandte Gebiete.* 30 (10): 544–546.

2 Suleyman, F. (2000). Role of lanolin in managing eczema and dry skin conditions. *Community Nurse* 6 (11): 30–31.

3 Stone, L. (2000). Medilan: a hypoallergenic lanolin for emollient therapy. *British Journal of Nursing* 9 (1): 54–57.

4 Joseph, L.B., Langley, N., Christiansen, M., and Kligman, A.M. (2007). Medical grade lanolin USP accelerates repair of hands, heels, and lips. *Journal of the American Academy of Dermatology* 56 (2): AB94.

5 Balato, A., Balato, N., Di Costanzo, L., and Ayala, F. (2011). Contact sensitization in the elderly. *Clinics in Dermatology* 29 (1): 24–30.

6 Wakelin, S.H., Smith, H., White, I.R. et al. (2001). A retrospective analysis of contact allergy to lanolin. *British Journal of Dermatology* 145 (1): 28–31.

7 Goon, A.T. and Goh, C.L. (2006). Patch testing of Singapore children and adolescents: our experience over 18 years. *Pediatric Dermatology* 23 (2): 117–120.

8 Isaksson, M., Olhardt, S., Rådehed, J., and Svensson, Å. (2015). Children with atopic dermatitis should always be patch-tested if they have hand or foot dermatitis. *Acta Dermato-Venereologica* 95(5): 583–586.

9 Warshaw, E.M., Nelsen, D.D., Maibach, H.I. et al. (2009). Positive patch test reactions to lanolin: cross-sectional data from the North American Contact Dermatitis Group, 1994 to 2006. *Dermatitis* 20 (2): 79–88.

10 Schnuch, A., Szliska, C., and Uter, W. (2009). Facial allergic contact dermatitis. Data from the IVDK and review of literature. *Der Hautarzt; Zeitschrift fur Dermatologie, Venerologie, und verwandte Gebiete* 60 (1): 13–21.

11 Fraser, K. and Pratt, M. (2015). Polysensitization in recurrent lip dermatitis. *Journal of Cutaneous Medicine and Surgery* 19 (1): 77–80.

12 Cronin, E., Bandmann, H.J., Calnan, C.D. et al. (1970). Contact dermatitis in the atopic. *Acta Dermato-Venereologica* 50 (3): 183–187.

13 Machet, L., Couhé, C., Perrinaud, A. et al. (2004). A high prevalence of sensitization still persists in leg ulcer patients: a retrospective series of 106 patients tested between 2001 and 2002 and a meta-analysis of 1975-2003 data. *British Journal of Dermatology* 150 (5): 929–935.

14 Mandell, J.A., Tlougan, B.E., and Cohen, D.E. (2011). Bunga Pad-induced ankle dermatitis in a figure skater. *Dermatitis* 22 (1): 58–59.

15 O'Donnell, B.F. and Hodgson, C. (1993). Allergic contact dermatitis due to lanolin in an adhesive plaster. *Contact Dermatitis* 28 (3): 191–192.

16 Fellinger, C., Hemmer, W., Wantke, F. et al. (2013). Severe allergic dermatitis caused by lanolin alcohol as part of an ointment base in propolis cream. *Contact Dermatitis* 68 (1): 59–61.

17 Tan, B.B., Noble, A.L., Roberts, M.E. et al. (1997). Allergic contact dermatitis from oleyl alcohol in lipstick cross-reacting with ricinoleic acid in castor oil and lanolin. *Contact Dermatitis* 37 (1): 41–42.

18 Zirwas, M.J. and Stechschulte, S.A. (2008). Moisturizer allergy: diagnosis and management. *Journal of Clinical and Aesthetic Dermatology* 1 (4): 38–44.

19 Coloe, J. and Zirwas, M.J. (2008). Allergens in corticosteroid vehicles. *Dermatitis* 19 (1): 38–42.

20 Green, C.M., Holden, C.R., and Gawkrodger, D.J. (2007). Contact allergy to topical medicaments becomes more common with advancing age: an age-stratified study. *Contact Dermatitis* 56 (4): 229–231.

21 Dodd, V. and Chalmers, C. (2003). Comparing the use of hydrogel dressings to lanolin ointment with lactating mothers. *Journal of Obstetric, Gynecologic & Neonatal Nursing* 32 (4): 486–494.

22 Nguyen, J.C., Chesnut, G., James, W.D., and Saruk, M. (2010). Allergic contact dermatitis caused by lanolin (wool) alcohol contained in an emollient in three postsurgical patients. *Journal of the American Academy of Dermatology* 62 (6): 1064–1065.

23 Miest, R.Y., Yiannias, J.A., Chang, Y.H., and Singh, N. (2013). Diagnosis and prevalence of lanolin allergy. *Dermatitis* 24 (3): 119–123.

24 Mortensen, T. (1979). Allergy to lanolin. *Contact Dermatitis* 5 (3): 137–139.

25 Edman, B. and Möller, H. (1989). Testing a purified lanolin preparation by a randomized procedure. *Contact Dermatitis* 20 (4): 287–290.

26 Brasch, J., Henseler, T., Aberer, W. et al. (1994). Reproducibility of patch tests. A multicenter study of synchronous left-versus right-sided patch tests by the German Contact Dermatitis Research Group. *Journal of the American Academy of Dermatology* 31 (4): 584–591.

27 Carmichael, A.J., Foulds, I.S., and Bransbury, D.S. (1991). Loss of lanolin patch-test positivity. *British Journal of Dermatology* 125 (6): 573–576.

28 Wolf, R. (1996). The lanolin paradox. *Dermatology* 192 (3): 198–202.

CHAPTER 36

Cetearyl Alcohol

CHAPTER CONTENTS

Key points

- Cetyl alcohol/cetearyl alcohol is a component of most topical medicament creams and cosmetic creams. Many topical medicament ointments *do not* contain it.
- Although most reports from patch test clinics show a prevalence rate of below 1%, cetyl/cetearyl alcohol is still included in most baseline patch test series because of its widespread use in cosmetic and topical medicament creams.
- Cetyl alcohol, and/or impurities in the commercial grade cetearyl preparation, are considered to be the active allergen(s), though this is still unclear.
- The prevalence of cetearyl alcohol allergy is higher in leg ulcer patients, as one might expect from a potential topical medicament allergen.
- The risk of allergic contact dermatitis (ACD) to cetearyl alcohol increases with the use of multiple topical medicaments (topical polypharmacy).
- Cetearyl alcohol may occasionally co-react with lanolin.
- There have been isolated reports of ACD to cetearyl alcohol presenting as contact urticaria and dermal reactions.

Molecular formula and chemical structure

Cetearyl alcohol is a mixture of two solid long-chain aliphatic fatty alcohols which are cetyl alcohol (C16) and stearyl alcohol (C18) [1–3].

Cetyl alcohol is used as an emollient in cosmetics. Stearyl alcohol is used as an antifoam and lubricant [4].

Cetostearyl alcohol is a synonym of cetearyl alcohol.

Immunology

- Many *in vitro* studies have shown that both are limited in their ability to penetrate intact skin. Cetyl alcohol can penetrate inflamed skin more readily than the longer-chained stearyl alcohol [5]. Cetyl alcohol is considered to be an allergen, especially in damaged skin, whereas it is doubtful if purified stearyl alcohol has sensitizing properties [1] or may be only a weak sensitizer [6]. As the number of carbon atoms in the molecules determines the properties of fatty alcohols, topical preparations often use mixtures of alcohols to adjust the viscosity and stability of different formulations [3]. Cetyl alcohol and stearyl alcohol are often combined [7]. According to the requirements of the US and European Pharmacopeia, cetearyl alcohol must contain at least 40% of stearyl alcohol and 90% or more of both alcohols combined [2]. A combination of these two aliphatic alcohols has long been identified as a possible sensitizer [1].
- Furthermore, it is unclear if contact allergy to cetyl and stearyl alcohols could actually be due to their impurities [3].

Common Contact Allergens: A Practical Guide to Detecting Contact Dermatitis, First Edition. Edited by John McFadden, Pailin Puangpet, Korbkarn Pongpairoj, Supitchaya Thaiwat, and Lee Shan Xian.

© 2020 John Wiley & Sons Ltd. Published 2020 by John Wiley & Sons Ltd.

Companion website: www.wiley.com/go/mcfadden/common_contact_allergens

A patient demonstrated positive patch test reactions to ethanol and commercial cetyl and stearyl alcohols, but showed no reactions to chemically pure cetyl and stearyl alcohols. This indicated that the patient was allergic to the impurified components of cetyl and stearyl alcohols, rather than to the cetyl and stearyl alcohols themselves [8]. Of seven patients who were patch test positive to a commercial preparation of cetearyl alcohol, only one reacted to chemically pure cetyl alcohol on patch testing [9].

- Commercially available cetearyl alcohol appears to contain impurities which have a positive effect on its emulsifying properties [10].
- Stearyl alcohol can be contaminated with oleyl alcohol because oleyl alcohol is a residue of the hydrogenation step [3].

Frequency of sensitization

Contact allergy to cetearyl alcohol is uncommon [11, 12].

Europe

	(*n* = 1,664)	0.12%, (cetyl alcohol)	[13]
		0.24%. (stearyl alcohol)	
1986–1987	Finland (*n* = 1,374)	0.8%, (20% cetearyl alcohol)	[10]
	Belgium (*n* = 330)	11.2%, (30% cetyl alcohol)[a]	[14]
1986–1989	Italy (*n* = 737)	0.8% positive patch test reactions to 20% cetearyl alcohol in pet., but with clinical relevance only 0.4%	[15]
1992–1995	Italy (*n* = 146)	0% (purified cetyl alcohol 30% pet.) and 1.4% (purified stearyl alcohol 30% pet.)	[3]

[a] High numbers of leg ulcer patients, nevertheless, it is usually relevant when it is present and has major implications on the choice of topical treatments prescribed.

America

1975–76	North America (*n* = 172)	1.2% (stearyl alcohol)	[16]

Age

All ages can be affected.

Sex

The female:male ratio was approximately 2 : 1.

Clinical

Cetearyl alcohol is an important allergen amongst patients with stasis eczema and leg ulcers [3, 5, 10, 17]. A comparison study from Belgium demonstrated positive patch test reactions to cetyl alcohol in 21.6% and 7.4% of patients with and without leg ulcers, respectively [14].

The risk of developing cetearyl alcohol allergy seems to increase with polypharmacy. There were reports of patients showing positive patch test reactions to cetearyl alcohol together with reactions to multiple allergens, including fragrances, preservatives, vehicles, medicaments, and formaldehyde releasing agents [12, 18].

Clinical manifestations of cetearyl alcohol allergy, other than eczematous lesions, include:

- *Contact urticaria*: Patients with contact allergy to cetyl and/or stearyl alcohols can present with urticaria-like lesions [4].
- *Dermal reactions*: A 24-year-old female patient presented with erythematous and pruritic papules and plaques 3 months after using Metosyn cream intermittently for the treatment of psoriasis. Areas of edema were also noted. Patch testing showed ++ positive reactions to both stearyl alcohol and Metosyn cream (which contains cetearyl alcohol) [19].

Exposure

- As cetearyl alcohol acts as an emulsifier and stabilizer [7, 10, 11, 17, 19-21], it is found as an ingredient in many cosmetics, moisturizers, and topical medicaments such as steroid creams [19, 20, 22], 5-fluorouracil [6], topical gentamicin [15], ketoconazole cream [23], lanoconazole cream [24], sulconazole nitrate [8], silver sulfadiazine cream [8, 17], and Hirudoid cream [25].
- Importantly, there may be cetyl and/or stearyl alcohols in cosmetics even when they are not listed in the ingredient labeling. As cetearyl alcohol is usually considered part of the base, manufacturers may not include it in the product labeling [12]. In addition, small amounts of saturated and unsaturated fatty alcohols occur in natural vegetable and animal oils [3].

Patch testing

- The most appropriate concentration for the patch testing of cetyl alcohol is debatable. Concentrations of between 1% and 30% in petrolatum have been mentioned. Although cetyl and stearyl alcohols have the least irritating effects of all alcohols [8], irritant reactions and angry back syndrome are possible when high concentrations are used for patch testing [26].

- In the Federal Republic of Germany, there was a recommendation to add 20% cetearyl alcohol in petrolatum to the patch test series for lower leg dermatitis [27].

Co-sensitization/cross-reactivity

- Cetyl alcohol allergic patients generally have positive patch test reactions to stearyl alcohol. Stearyl alcohol may be present in concentrations of up to 30% in commercial cetyl alcohol [17].
- Patients who are sensitized to cetyl alcohol may co-react with wool alcohols [1, 17, 26].
- As previously mentioned, patients with cetearyl alcohol allergy may also show positive patch test reactions to multiple allergens, including fragrances, preservatives, vehicles, medicaments, and formaldehyde releasers [12, 18].

Case reports

- A 65-year-old man presented with severe dermatitis on the right hand 3 days after wearing a glove coated with a moisturizer only on his right hand whilst cleaning a shed. He was patch test positive to both the glove and cetyl alcohol. Cetyl alcohol was present in the moisturizer and steroid cream that he had used unsuccessfully to treat the inflammation. Chromatography and mass spectrometry identified cetyl alcohol in the glove extract. He had probably been sensitized to cetyl alcohol from a wound treatment 3 years ago [21].
- A 62-year-old woman, with an initial patch test demonstrating multiple sensitivities, presented with deteriorating chronic hand eczema despite allergen avoidance. Patch testing showed a +++ positive reaction to the Vanicream moisturizer that she had been applying regularly (which contained cetyl alcohol) and a ++ positive reaction to cetearyl alcohol [28].
- A 61-year-old woman developed dermatitis around her chronic leg ulcer after applying multiple topical products, including mupirocin ointment, doxepin cream, Benadryl Extra-Strength Itch Stopping Cream, and Vanicream moisturizer. Patch tests identified a ++ positive reaction to doxepin cream and + positive reactions to cetearyl alcohol and Benadryl Extra-Strength Itch Stopping Cream. Cetyl alcohol was an ingredient in the doxepin cream, Benadryl Extra-Strength Itch Stopping Cream, Vanicream moisturizer, and multiple other moisturizers that this patient had been using [28].
- A 24-year-old woman developed facial eczema after applying a cosmetic cream. Patch tests demonstrated ++ reactions to her face cream and cetyl alcohol [11].
- A 60-year-old man presented with localized eczema after using 1% lanoconazole cream to treat tinea pedis. The lesions developed after he had applied the cream for 1 year. Patch testing results showed positive reactions to lanoconazole cream ("as is") and three ingredients of lanoconazole cream, including lanoconazole (1% pet.), cetyl alcohol, and diethyl sebacate. The patient also had positive patch test reactions to several other antifungal creams which contained either cetyl alcohol or diethyl sebacate. The rash improved after changing the treatment to another antifungal drug which was negative on patch testing [24].
- A 60-year-old woman presented with dermatitis after using Mentholatum AD ointment. The patient had positive patch test reactions to both cetyl alcohol and crotamiton, which are both found in Mentholatum AD ointment. Patch testing with Mentholatum AD ointment ("as is") demonstrated ++ positive reactions at days 2, 3, and 4 with flare-up phenomena [7].

References

1 Marston, S. (1991). Contact dermatitis from cetearyl alcohol in hydrocortisone butyrate lipocream, and from lanolin. *Contact Dermatitis* 24 (5): 372.

2 Hong, L. and Altorfer, H. (2003). Radiolysis characterization of cetearyl alcohol by gas chromatography-mass spectrometry. *Journal of Pharmaceutical and Biomedical Analysis* 31 (4): 753–766.

3 Tosti, A., Vincenzi, C., Guerra, L., and Andrisano, E. (1996). Contact dermatitis from fatty alcohols. *Contact Dermatitis* 35 (5): 287–289.

4 Gaul, L.E. (1969). Dermatitis from cetyl and stearyl alcohols. *Archives of Dermatology* 99 (5): 593.

5 von der Werth, J.M., English, J.S., and Dalziel, K.L. (1998). Loss of patch test positivity to cetylstearyl alcohol. *Contact Dermatitis* 38 (2): 109–110.

6 de Berker, D., Marren, P., Powell, S.M., and Ryan, T.J. (1992). Contact sensitivity to the stearyl alcohol in Efudix cream (5-fluorouracil). *Contact Dermatitis* 26 (2): 138.

7 Oiso, N., Fukai, K., and Ishii, M. (2003). Concomitant allergic reaction to cetyl alcohol and crotamiton. *Contact Dermatitis* 49 (5): 261.

8 Ishiguro, N. and Kawashima, M. (1991). Contact dermatitis from impurities in alcohol. *Contact Dermatitis* 25 (4): 257.

9 Hannuksela, M. and Salo, H. (1986). The repeated open application test (ROAT). *Contact Dermatitis* 14 (4): 221–227.

10 Hannuksela, M. (1988). Skin contact allergy to emulsifiers. *International Journal of Cosmetic Science* 10 (1): 9–14.

11 Kieć-Świerczyńska, M., Krecisz, B., and Świerczyńska-Machura, D. (2005). Photoallergic and allergic reaction to 2-hydroxy-4-methoxybenzophenone (sunscreen) and allergy to cetyl alcohol in cosmetic cream. *Contact Dermatitis* 53 (3): 170–171.

12 Rademaker, M., Wood, B., and Greig, D. (1997). Contact dermatitis from cetearyl alcohol. *Australasian Journal of Dermatology* 38 (4): 220–221.

13 Hjorth, N. and Trolle-Lassen, C. (1963). Skin reactions to ointment bases. *Transactions of the St. John's Hospital Dermatological Society* 49: 127–140.

14 Blondeel, A., Oleffe, J., and Achten, G. (1978). Contact allergy in 330 dermatological patients. *Contact Dermatitis* 4 (5): 270–276.

15 Tosti, A., Guerra, L., Morelli, R., and Bardazzi, F. (1990). Prevalence and sources of sensitization to emulsifiers: a clinical study. *Contact Dermatitis* 23 (2): 68–72.
16 Rudner, E.J. (1977). North American Group results. *Contact Dermatitis* 3 (4): 208–209.
17 Degreef, H. and Dooms-Goossens, A. (1985). Patch testing with silver sulfadiazine cream. *Contact Dermatitis* 12 (1): 33–37.
18 Thormann, H., Kollander, M., and Andersen, K.E. (2009). Allergic contact dermatitis from dichlorobenzyl alcohol in a patient with multiple contact allergies. *Contact Dermatitis* 60 (5): 295–296.
19 Black, H. (1975). Contact dermatitis from stearyl alcohol in Metosyn (fluocinonide) cream. *Contact Dermatitis* 1 (2): 125.
20 Shore, R.N. and Shelley, W.B. (1974). Contact dermatitis from stearyl alcohol and propylene glycol in fluocinonide cream. *Archives of Dermatology* 109 (3): 397–399.
21 Vanden Broecke, K., Zimerson, E., Bruze, M., and Goossens, A. (2014). Severe allergic contact dermatitis caused by a rubber glove coated with a moisturizer. *Contact Dermatitis* 71 (2): 117–119.
22 Rademaker, M., Wood, B., and Greig, D.E. (1996). Multiple medicament allergies in two patients with chronic leg ulceration. *Australasian Journal of Dermatology* 37 (3): 151–152.
23 Garcia-Bravo, B., Mazuecos, J., Rodriguez-Pichardo, A. et al. (1989). Hypersensitivity to ketoconazole preparations: study of 4 cases. *Contact Dermatitis* 21 (5): 346–348.
24 Soga, F., Katoh, N., and Kishimoto, S. (2004). Contact dermatitis due to lanoconazole, cetyl alcohol and diethyl sebacate in lanoconazole cream. *Contact Dermatitis* 50 (1): 49–50.
25 Pecegueiro, M., Brandão, M., Pinto, J., and Conçalo, S. (1987). Contact dermatitis to Hirudoid cream. *Contact Dermatitis* 17 (5): 290–293.
26 van Ketel, W.G. (1984). Allergy to cetylalcohol. *Contact Dermatitis* 11 (2): 125–126.
27 Bandmann, H.J. and Keilig, W. (1980). Lanette-O – another test substance for lower leg series. *Contact Dermatitis* 6 (3): 227–228.
28 Aakhus, A.E. and Warshaw, E.M. (2011). Allergic contact dermatitis from cetyl alcohol. *Dermatitis: Contact, Atopic, Occupational, Drug* 22 (1): 56–57.

Exposure Color Code

- Clothing, jewelry, adornments
- Personal care products, cosmetics/cosmetic procedures
- Household products, domestic environment, including furniture and refurbishment
- Occupational dermatoses, work environment
- Medicines, surgical/dental procedures, herbal/alternative medicines
- Personal appliances/aids
- Leisure activities, sport, travel
- Other exposures (including dietary)
- Not relevant or multiple/general exposure

Index

Page locators underlined indicate derived from tables. Page locators in *italics* indicate derived from figures. Key index pages for subject are in **bold**. This index uses letter-by-letter alphabetization.

Common Contact Allergens: A Practical Guide to Detecting Contact Dermatitis, First Edition. Edited by John McFadden, Pailin Puangpet, Korbkarn Pongpairoj, Supitchaya Thaiwat, and Lee Shan Xian.

© 2020 John Wiley & Sons Ltd. Published 2020 by John Wiley & Sons Ltd.

Companion website: www.wiley.com/go/mcfadden/common_contact_allergens